CLINICAL RISK MANAGEMENT

Enhancing patient safety

Second edition

Edited by

CHARLES VINCENT

*Professor of Psychology, University College London,
London, UK*

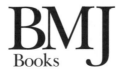

© BMJ Books 2001
BMJ Books is an imprint of the BMJ Publishing Group

First published in 1995
by the BMJ Publishing Group, BMA House, Tavistock Square,
London WC1H 9JR

www.bmjbooks.com

First edition 1995
Second edition 2001
Second impression 2001
Third impression 2003

British Library Cataloguing in Publication Data

A catalogue record for this book is available from the British Library

ISBN 0 7279 1392 1

Cover by Landmark Design, Croydon, Surrey
Typeset by J&L Composition Ltd, Filey, North Yorkshire
Printed and bound by MPG Books Ltd, Bodmin, Cornwall

Contents

Contributors

Alan Aitkenhead Professor of Anaesthesia, Department of Anaesthesia and Intensive Care, School of Medicine and Surgical Sciences, University of Nottingham, Nottingham, UK

Judith Allsop Professor in Health Policy, De Montfort University, Leicester, UK

Richard W Beard Professor of Obstetrics and Gynaecology, North West London Hospital's NHS Trust, Harrow, UK

Troyen A Brennan Professor of Medicine, Harvard Medical School and Harvard School of Public Health, Boston, USA

Henry Brown Solicitor, Penningtons, London, UK

Christopher Cassirer Associate Professor, Department of Healthcare, University of Minnesota, USA

E Jane Chapman General Manager, Risk & Legal Services, North West London Hospital's NHS Trust, Harrow, UK

Jan Davies Professor of Anaesthesia, Foothills Medical Centre, University of Calgary, Canada

Peter Dear Consultant in Neonatal Medicine, St James' University Hospital, Leeds, UK

Liam Donaldson Chief Medical Officer, Richmond House, London, UK

James Drife Professor of Obstetrics and Gynaecology, School of Medicine, University of Leeds, Leeds, UK

Peter Driscoll Consultant in Accident & Emergency Medicine, Hope Hospital, Manchester, UK

Martin Eccles Professor of Clinical Effectiveness, Centre for Health Services Research, University of Newcastle Upon Tyne, Newcastle upon Tyne, UK

Jenny Firth-Cozens Professor of Psychology, Centre for Clinical Psychology and Health Care Research, University of Northumbria at Newcastle, Newcastle upon Tyne, UK

Jane Fothergill Consultant in Accident & Emergency Medicine, St Mary's Hospital, London, UK

Robbie Foy MRC Training Fellow in Health Services Research, Department of Obstetrics and Gynaecology, University of Edinburgh, Edinburgh, UK

John Gosbee Director of the National Patient Safety Register, VHA National Center for Patient Safety, Michigan, USA

Jeremy Grimshaw Professor of Health Services Research, University of Aberdeen, Aberdeen, UK

David Hewett Assistant Medical Director, Winchester & Eastleigh Healthcare Trust, Winchester, UK

Gerald B Hickson Professor of Pediatrics, Vanderbilt University Medical Center, Nashville, USA

Laura Lin Human Factors Engineer, Logicon, Inc, Dayton, USA

Maurice Lipsedge Consultant Psychiatrist, South London and Maudsley NHS Trust, London, UK

Laura Morlock Professor of Health Policy and Management, Johns Hopkins University, Baltimore, USA

Fiona Moss Associate Dean, North Thames Department of Postgraduate Medical and Dental Education, University of London, London, UK

Linda Mulcahy Reader in Law, Birkbeck College, University of London, London, UK

Graham Neale Consultant Physician, Clinical Risk Unit, Department of Psychology, University College, London, UK

Anne O'Connor Risk Management Adviser, St Paul International Insurance Co Ltd, Redhill, UK

Elisabeth Paice Dean Director, North Thames Department of Postgraduate Medical and Dental Education, University of London, London, UK

James W Pichert Associate Professor of Education in Medicine, School of Medicine, Vanderbilt University, Nashville, USA

Peter Pronovost Assistant Professor of Anesthesiology and Critical Care Medicine, The Johns Hopkins Hospital, Baltimore, USA

James T Reason Professor of Psychology, University of Manchester, Manchester, UK

Gareth Rees Consultant in Clinical Oncology and Clinical Director, Bristol Haematology and Oncology Centre, Bristol Royal Infirmary, Bristol, UK

Stephen Rogers Senior Lecturer in Primary Care, Royal Free and University College Medical School, London, UK

Patricia Scott Risk Manager, Birth Unit, Hospital of St John and St Elizabeth, London, UK

Jonathan Secker-Walker Senior Lecturer, Department of Clinical Governance, University of Wales College of Medicine, Cardiff, UK

Arnold Simanowitz Chief Executive, Action for Victims of Medical Accidents, Croydon, UK

Lawrence Smith Shiftwork Research Group, School of Psychology, University of Leeds, Leeds, UK

Sally Taylor-Adams Senior Risk Management Consultant, Greenstreet Berman, Reading, UK

Eric J Thomas Assistant Professor of Medicine, Houston Medical School, University of Texas, Houston, USA

Martin Thomas Clinical Research Fellow, Accident and Emergency Department, Manchester Royal Infirmary, Manchester, UK

Robin Touquet Consultant in Accident and Emergency Medicine, St Mary's Hospital, London, UK

Charles Vincent Professor of Psychology, University College London, London, UK

Kieran Walshe Senior Research Fellow, Health Services Management Centre, University of Birmingham, Birmingham, UK

John Williams Consultant in Maxillofacial Surgery, St Richard's Hospital, Chichester, UK

To
Marjorie Howard

Acknowledgements

Many of the ideas underlying both the structure and contents of this book have been developed with colleagues at University College, particularly Pippa Bark, Graham Neale, Nicola Stanhope, Sally Taylor-Adams and Maria Woloshynowych. Clinicians and researchers in many fields and countries have also played a great part in shaping my approach and that of the book, but are too numerous to mention individually. I thank all the authors for the efforts they made and for their patience with the editing process. This book was a collaboration and any success it may have is due to everyone involved. At the BMJ Mary Banks stands out as an editor with a real interest in the books she commissions. Special thanks as before to Pam La Rose for help with all aspects of the book and to Angela for her (generally) calming influence on the editor.

Introduction

CHARLES VINCENT

Risk management was in the beginning primarily considered a means of controlling litigation, which has been a major worry for clinicians in the United States and Britain for a considerable time, and a growing problem in many countries. In the USA malpractice costs were over one billion dollars per annum by 1985 and were continuing to rise.[1] Early risk management strategies were dominated by attempts to reform the legal system and reduce the costs of compensation. Gradually the need to address the underlying clinical problems became apparent and the term risk management came to include strategies to reduce the incidence of harm and improve the quality of care. Crucially it began also to include positive efforts to care for injured patients and respond to their needs rather than simply treating them as potential litigants.

The introduction to the first edition of this book, published in 1995, distinguished two contrasting perspectives on risk management. In the narrow, defensive view, still regrettably to be found, the primary aim is to protect the hospital or other healthcare organisation from claims, with little regard for the origins of those claims or for the well being of the patients or staff concerned. The first edition, in contrast, endeavoured to promote a broader, more positive approach. In this broader view risk management is fundamentally a particular approach to improving the safety and quality of care, which places special emphasis on occasions in which patients are harmed or disturbed by their treatment, or where there is the potential for harm to result.

The last five years

Risk management in healthcare has developed and matured in the last five years in Britain, Europe and Australasia. Studies of medical error and adverse events in healthcare (see chapter 2) have brought a growing awareness of the scale of the problem of harm to patients. The financial costs of adverse events, in terms of additional treatment and extra days in hospital, are clearly vastly greater than the costs of litigation. The costs of lost working time, disability benefits and the wider economic consequences are greater still. There is also a much greater recognition of the human cost. Many patients suffer increased pain, disability and psychological trauma and may experience failures in their treatment as a terrible betrayal of trust. They may become depressed, angry and bitter, and a protracted adversarial legal process often compounds their problems. Staff may experience shame, guilt and depression after making a mistake, with litigation and complaints imposing an additional burden. A doctor or nurse whose confidence has been impaired will work less effectively and efficiently. At worst they may abandon medicine as a career.

Several important new initiatives in the last five years underline the increasing attention paid to patient safety. In the United States organisations such as the National Patient Safety Foundation are pioneering a much more sophisticated approach to patient safety, drawing on research and practice from a number of different industries. The recent report of the Institute of Medicine on *Building a Safer Healthcare System*[2] starkly set out the scale of harm to patients and an ambitious and radical agenda for change, which attracted presidential backing in the United States. In Australia the results of the Australian Quality in Healthcare Study[3] were initially marred by political interference, setting back the implementation programme that was to follow. However major initiatives are now underway at both a federal and national level. In Britain the Department of Health commissioned a major report on *Learning from Experience*, covering similar ground to the Institute of Medicine report, but in a British context. Again, ambitious and radical measures are proposed to tackle the major patient safety problems of the British National Health Service.

Risk management is also at the heart of the concept of clinical governance (see chapter 3), a wide ranging reform that, not before time, makes those in charge of NHS organisations accountable for the quality of care delivered, and not just the cost of it. The newly established Commission for Health Improvement will review organisations to establish that arrangements for clinical governance and risk management are effective, both in the hospital sector and in primary care and community settings. Further examples could be given of initiatives in Canada and several countries in Europe and Asia of an increasing interest in research on patient safety and practical approaches to the management of risk. Finally, the

British Medical Journal devoted an entire issue to the subject of medical error[4] in a determined effort to move the subject to the mainstream of academic and clinical enquiry.

Risk management is therefore evolving and expanding well beyond its roots in litigation, and beginning to benefit from contact with safety researchers and practitioners in other industries. The primary focus of risk management should now be patient safety and it should, of course, be closely integrated with approaches to improving other aspects of the quality of care – such as the appropriateness and acceptability of treatment. These other dimensions of quality are important in their own right, but safety is surely the foremost dimension of quality and the most important to patients and their families.[5]

Aims and structure of the book

As with the first edition, the book provides an overview of the major themes and principles underlying clinical risk management and acts as a handbook and source of reference for all those engaged in risk management. The second edition of the book is however very different from the first in a number of respects. With the field just emerging in Britain, the first edition had to be primarily straightforward and practical. In contrast chapters in the second edition, while retaining the ultimately practical aim of enhancing patient safety, have a stronger research emphasis and address a wider range of themes. All chapters have been updated, and many radically altered, in the light of new developments and new understanding of the nature of risk and safety in healthcare. There is also an entirely new section on the Conditions of Safe Practice, described below. As before a range of disciplines are represented, now including risk managers. There are many more American authors, reflecting the importance of developments in the United States.

Some chapters from the first edition are no longer included. The usual reason for this is the prescience of the authors of the original chapters. Roger Clements[6] for instance emphasised the central role of the medical director and Trust board in driving risk management. Fiona Moss[7] discussed the need to integrate risk management with other quality initiatives. Five years ago these things needed saying. However, in Britain at least, these ideas are now widely accepted and enshrined in the concept of clinical governance. Almost all the chapters that are no longer needed in this edition are still available in the special edition of *Quality in Healthcare* (June 1995) that was published in advance of the first edition.

Part I Principles of Risk Management

The book is divided into four parts. The first, Principles of Risk Management, provides essential background material for the more practical chapters that follow. The first chapter provides a theoretical framework for the understanding of accidents and adverse events. Many different studies and ideas are discussed, but one requires particular mention. Studies of accidents in other areas have led to a much broader understanding of accident causation, with less focus on the individual who makes an error and more on pre-existing organisational factors and conditions that provide the context in which errors occur. Conversely excellence arises partly through individual effort and partly because it is enabled by the wider organisation. This is a theme that runs throughout the book, and it provides the underlying rationale for the whole of Part III on the conditions of safe practice. The second chapter provides a comprehensive review of the nature and incidence of errors and adverse events in medicine, that should leave the reader in no doubt as to the scale and importance of the problem. The third chapter traces the development of risk management providing a critical history of its evolution, its successes and limitations. The fourth sets out the essentials of clinical governance, the context in which risk management operates in the British NHS and an essential support and structure for effective risk management.

Part II Reducing risk in clinical practice

In the second section experienced clinicians discuss the main sources of risk to patients in their particular speciality. Each chapter identifies high risk patient groups and procedures, discusses common causes of injury to patients and suggests how the various problems might be remedied. Adverse events of all kind are considered, not just those that lead to litigation. As many of the authors say, risk is inherent in the practice of medicine, and a single chapter can only highlight the most important areas in each speciality. Clinicians were also asked to discuss not only errors that are made, but also the circumstances that predispose to errors and accidents. These will include the characteristics of the patient and their condition, but may also involve such factors as the use of locums, communication and supervision problems, excessive workload, educational and training deficiencies and so on. Each chapter makes specific recommendations for the management of risk within that speciality.

Part III The conditions of safe practice

The view that harm to patients is simply a result of human error, in turn often associated with negligence, is giving way to a more sophisticated view of both error itself and the causes of sub-optimal care. Where care is sub-optimal, or harmful, the causes may lie less with the individual clinician and more in the conditions in which he or she works and the inherent uncertainty of clinical practice. Both success and failure are grounded in the overall system of healthcare and the multiple influences on clinical practice. Safety needs to be addressed on a number of different levels, including the individual staff, the tasks they undertake and the wider organisational structure.[8]

Clearly it is not possible to cover all conceivable factors that might impact on patient safety. These chapters are an attempt to identify some of the major themes and provide key targets for the reduction of risk and promotion of safety. These themes lie at different levels of a hierarchy of factors that are relevant to patient safety: the patient, the task, the individual member of staff, the team, the working environment and the wider organisational structure and context.[8] The first chapter addresses the crucial issue of communication with patients. The task dimension is illustrated by an examination of the role of guidelines and protocols, and by a discussion of the importance of the design of medical devices and medical systems. Individual and team factors are tackled in a chapter on training and supervision, and working conditions in the chapter that follows on stress, shift-work and fatigue. The next chapter in the section addresses the crucial role of teams in clinical practice, both in the delivery of care and in the management of change. The final chapter highlights the importance of the organisation of care and its impact on the outcome for patients. Where possible strategies for risk assessment and risk reduction are suggested, whether in the form of training, design of equipment or systems, team building, organisational change or other means.

Part IV The Implementation of Risk Management

The fourth section concerns the implementation of risk management, all chapters having a strong practical emphasis. The early chapters describe the systems and management structures that are needed for reporting, investigation and analysis of adverse events and the development of risk management protocols to reduce risk in clinical settings. Later chapters cover the response to adverse events. Here we should note that the term risk management has been extended to what would, in other contexts, be termed crisis management or disaster recovery. Clinical risk management is unusual in that the accident victims may be cared for in the same, or a similar, setting to that in which the accident occurred. The same professions, and perhaps the same people as those involved in the original injury will care for them. The continuing care of the injured patient must be considered as an integral part of risk management, especially as the original trauma is often made worse by insensitive handling after the event. The care of injured patients, the sensitive handling of complaints, the support of staff involved in serious incidents are all an integral part of clinical risk management. The last chapter considers the efficient and effective handling of claims. The decision to restrict the legal aspects to a single chapter on the management of claims is deliberate. Risk managers of course need to understand basic medical negligence law, but this is well covered elsewhere as indicated in the final chapter.

From risk management to a safety culture

Looking ahead there are, of course, many challenges for risk management and patient safety. In one particular area, however, there is still a long way to go and this may ultimately determine the long term impact of risk management. At the moment risk management is still the responsibility of a comparatively small number of people in each healthcare organisation. In contrast, in aviation, "safety is everyone's responsibility". Almost everyone working in healthcare cares about patient safety, in the sense of wanting to do their best for patients. However patient safety needs to become embedded in the culture of healthcare, not just in the sense of individual high standards, but of a widespread acceptance of a systemic understanding of risk and safety and the need for everyone to actively promote patient safety.

References

1   Dingwall R, Fenn P. Is risk management necessary? *Int J Risk Safety Med* 1991;2:91–106.
2   Corrigan J, Kohn L, Donaldson M, eds. *To err is human: building a safer healthcare system.* Committee on Quality of Healthcare in America, Institute of Medicine. National Academy Press 2000.
3   Wilson RM, Runciman WB, Gibberd RW, Harrison BT, Newby L, Hamilton JD. The Quality in Australian Health Care Study. *Med J Aust* 1995;**163**:458–71.
4   Leape L, Berwick D. Safe healthcare: are we up to it? *BMJ* 2000;**320**:725–6.
5   Vincent CA. Risk, safety and the dark side of quality. *BMJ* 1997;**3141**:1775–6.
6   Clements R. Essentials of clinical risk management. In Vincent CA ed, *Clinical risk management* (1st edition). BMJ Publications, 1995:335–49.
7   Moss F. Risk management and quality of care. In Vincent CA (ed), *Clinical risk management* (1st edition). BMJ Publications, 1995:88–102.
8   Vincent CA, Taylor-Adams S, Stanhope N. Framework for analysing risk and safety in clinical medicine. *BMJ* 1998;**316**:1154–7.

PART I: PRINCIPLES OF RISK MANAGEMENT

1 Understanding adverse events: the human factor

JAMES T REASON

A decade ago few specialists in human factors were involved in the study and prevention of medical accidents. Between the 1940s and 1980s the major concern of that community was to limit the human contribution to the conspicuously catastrophic breakdown of high hazard enterprises such as air, sea, and road transport; nuclear power generation; chemical process plants, and the like. Accidents in these systems cost many lives, create widespread environmental damage, and generate much public and political concern. By contrast, medical mishaps mostly affect single individuals in a wide variety of healthcare institutions. Only within the past few years has the likely extent of these accidental injuries become apparent (see chapter 2).

Since the mid-1980s several interdisciplinary research groups have begun to investigate the human and organisational factors affecting the safety of healthcare provision. Initially, these collaborations were focused around the work of anaesthetists and intensivists, partly because these professionals' activities shared much in common with those of more widely studied groups such as pilots and operators of nuclear power plants.[1] This commonality exists at two levels.

- At the "sharp end" (that is, at the immediate human–system or doctor–patient interface) common features include uncertain and dynamic environments, multiple sources of concurrent information, shifting and often ill-defined goals, reliance on indirect or inferred indications, actions having immediate and multiple consequences, moments of intense time stress interspersed with long periods of routine activity, advanced technologies with many redundancies, complex and often confusing human-machine interfaces, and multiple players with differing priorities and high stakes.[2]

• At the organisational level these activities are carried on within complex, tightly coupled institutional settings and entail multiple interactions between different professional groups. This is extremely important for understanding not only the character and aetiology of medical mishaps but also for devising more effective remedial measures.

In the last decade, the interest in the human factors of healthcare has spread to a wide range of medical specialties (for example, general practice, accident and emergency care, obstetrics and gynaecology, radiology, psychiatry, surgery, etc.). This burgeoning concern is reflected in an increasing number of texts and journal articles devoted to medical accidents.[3,4,5] One of the most significant consequences of the collaboration between specialists in medicine and in human factors is the widespread acceptance that models of causation of accidents, developed for domains such as aviation and nuclear power generation, can be applied to healthcare. The same is also true for many of the diagnostic and remedial measures that have been created within these non-medical areas.

I will first consider the different ways in which humans can contribute to the breakdown of complex, well-defended technologies. Then I will show how these various contributions may be combined within a generic model of accident causation and illustrate its practical application with a case. Finally, I will outline the practical implications of such models for improving risk management within the healthcare domain and consider the often neglected, positive contributions made by human factors.

Human contribution

A survey of published work on human factors estimated that the contribution of human error to accidents in hazardous technologies increased fourfold between the 1960s and 1990s, from minima of around 20% to maxima of beyond 90%.[6] The most likely explanation is that equipment has become more reliable and that accident investigators have become increasingly aware that safety critical errors are not restricted to the "sharp end". Figures of around 90% are hardly surprising considering that people design, build, operate, maintain, organise, and manage these systems. The large contribution of human error is more a matter of opportunity than the result of excessive carelessness, ignorance, or recklessness. Whatever the true figure, though, human behaviour – for good or ill – clearly dominates the risks to modern technological systems, medical or otherwise.

Not long ago, these human contributions would have been lumped together under the catch-all label of "human error". Now it is apparent that unsafe acts come in many forms – slips, lapses and mistakes, errors and violations – each having different psychological origins and requiring different countermeasures. Nor can we take account of only those human failures that were the proximal causes of an accident. Major accident inquiries (for example those for Three Mile Island nuclear reactor accident, *Challenger* [space shuttle] explosion, King's Cross underground fire, *Herald of Free Enterprise* capsizing, *Piper Alpha* explosion and fire, Clapham rail disaster, *Exxon Valdez* oil spill, Kegworth air crash, etc.) make it apparent that the human causes of major accidents are distributed very widely, both within an organisation as a whole and over several years before the actual event. In consequence, we also need to consider latent or delayed action failures that can exist for long periods before combining with local triggering events to penetrate a system's defences.

Human errors may be classified either by their consequences or by their presumed causes. Consequential classifications are already widely used in medicine. The error is described in terms of the proximal actions contributing to a mishap (for example, administration of a wrong drug or a wrong vessel unintentionally severed during surgery, etc.). Causal classifications, on the other hand, make assumptions about the psychological mechanisms implicated in generating the error. Since causal or psychological classifications are not widely used in medicine (though there are notable exceptions) a brief description of the main distinctions among types of errors and their underlying rationale is given below.[7,8]

Psychologists divide errors into two causally determined groups,[9] as summarised in Figure 1.1.

Slips and lapses versus mistakes: the first distinction

Error can be defined in many ways. For my present purpose an error is the failure of planned actions to achieve their desired goal. There are basically two ways in which this failure can occur, as follows.

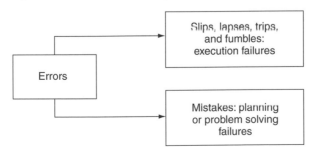

Figure 1.1 Distinguishing slips, lapses and mistakes.

- The plan is adequate, but the associated actions do not go as intended. These are failures of execution and are commonly termed slips and lapses. Slips relate to observable actions and are associated with attentional failures. Lapses are more internal events and relate to failures of memory.
- The actions may go entirely as planned, but the plan is inadequate to achieve its intended outcome. These are failures of intention, termed mistakes. Mistakes can be further subdivided into rule based mistakes and knowledge based mistakes (see below).

All errors involve some kind of deviation. In the case of slips, lapses, trips, and fumbles, actions deviate from the current intention. Here the failure occurs at the level of execution. For mistakes, the actions may go entirely as planned but the plan itself deviates from some adequate path towards its intended goal. Here the failure lies at a higher level: with the mental processes involved in planning, formulating intentions, judging, and problem solving.

Slips and lapses occur during the largely automatic performance of some routine task, usually in familiar surroundings. They are almost invariably associated with some form of attentional capture, either distraction from the immediate surroundings or preoccupation with something in mind. They are also provoked by change, either in the current plan of action or in the immediate surroundings. Figure 1.2 shows the further subdivisions of slips and lapses; these have been discussed in detail elsewhere.[9]

Mistakes can begin to occur once a problem has been detected. A problem is anything that requires a change or alteration of the current plan. Mistakes may be subdivided into two groups, as follows.

- Rule based mistakes, which relate to problems for which the person possesses some pre-packaged solution, acquired as the result of training, experience, or the availability of appropriate procedures. The associated errors may come in various forms: the misapplication of a good rule

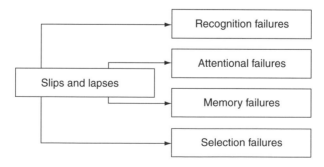

Figure 1.2 Varieties of slips and lapses.

12

(usually because of a failure to spot the contraindications), the application of a bad rule, or the non-application of a good rule.

- Knowledge based mistakes, which occur in novel situations where the solution to a problem has to be worked out on the spot without the help of pre-programmed solutions. This entails the use of slow, resource limited but computationally powerful conscious reasoning carried out in relation to what is often an inaccurate and incomplete "mental model" of the problem and its possible causes. Under these circumstances the human mind is subject to several powerful biases, of which the most universal is confirmation bias. This is particularly evident when trying to diagnose what has gone wrong with a malfunctioning system. We "pattern match" a possible cause to the available signs and symptoms and then seek out only that evidence that supports this particular hunch, ignoring or rationalising away contradictory facts. Other biases have been discussed elsewhere.[9]

Errors versus violations: the second distinction

Violations are deviations from safe operating practices, procedures, standards, or rules. Here, we are mostly interested in deliberate violations, in which the actions (though not the possible bad consequences) were intended. Violations fall into three main groups:

- Routine violations, which entail cutting corners whenever such opportunities present themselves
- Optimising violations, or actions taken to further personal rather than strictly task related goals (that is, violations for "kicks" or to alleviate boredom)
- Necessary or situational violations that seem to offer the only path available to getting the job done, and where the rules or procedures are seen to be inappropriate for the present situation.

Deliberate violations differ from errors in several important ways.

- Whereas errors arise primarily from informational problems (that is, forgetting, inattention, incomplete knowledge, etc.) violations are more generally associated with motivational problems (that is, low morale, poor supervisory example, perceived lack of concern, the failure to reward compliance and sanction non-compliance, etc.)
- Errors can be explained by what goes on in the mind of an individual, but violations occur in a regulated social context.

13

- Errors can be reduced by improving the quality and the delivery of necessary information within the workplace. Violations require motivational and organisational remedies.

Active versus latent human failures: the third distinction

In considering how people contribute to accidents a third and very important distinction is necessary – namely, that between active and latent failures. The difference concerns the length of time that passes before human failures are shown to have an adverse impact on safety. For active failures the negative outcome is almost immediate, but for latent failures dire consequences of human actions or decisions can take a long time to be disclosed, sometimes many years. The distinction between active and latent failures owes much to Mr Justice Sheen's observations on the capsizing of the *Herald of Free Enterprise*. In his inquiry report, he wrote:

> *At first sight the faults which led to this disaster were the . . . errors of omission on the part of the Master, the Chief Officer and the assistant bosun . . . But a full investigation into the circumstances of the disaster leads inexorably to the conclusion that the underlying or cardinal faults lay higher up in the Company . . . From top to bottom the body corporate was infected with the disease of sloppiness.*[10]

Here the distinction between active and latent failures is made very clear. The active failures – the immediate causes of the capsize – were various errors on the part of the ship's officers and crew. But, as the inquiry disclosed, the ship was a "sick" ship even before it sailed from Zeebrugge on 6 March 1987.

To summarise the differences between active and latent failures:

- Active failures are unsafe acts (errors and violations) committed by those at the "sharp end" of the system (surgeons, anaesthetists, nurses, physicians, etc.). It is the people at the human system interface whose actions can, and sometimes do, have immediate adverse consequences
- Latent failures are created as the result of decisions, taken at the higher echelons of an organisation. Their damaging consequences may lie dormant for a long time, only becoming evident when they combine with local triggering factors (for example, the spring tide, the loading difficulties at Zeebrugge harbour, etc.) to breach the system's defences.

Thus, the distinction between active and latent failures rests on two considerations: firstly, the length of time before the failures have a bad outcome and, secondly, where in an organisation the failures occur. Generally, medical active failures are committed by those people in direct contact with the patient, and latent failures occur within the higher echelons of the institution, in the organisational and management spheres. A brief account of a model showing how top level decisions create conditions that produce accidents in the workplace is given below.

Aetiology of "organisational" accidents

The technological advances of the past 20 years, particularly in regard to engineered safety features, have made many hazardous systems largely proof against single failures, either human or mechanical. Breaching the "defences in depth" now requires the unlikely confluence of several causal streams. Unfortunately, the increased automation afforded by cheap computing power also provides greater opportunities for the insidious accumulation of latent failures within the system as a whole. Medical systems and items of equipment have become more opaque to the people who work them and are thus especially prone to the rare, but often catastrophic, "organisational accident". Tackling these organisational failures represents a major challenge in medicine and elsewhere.

Figure 1.3 shows the anatomy of an organisational accident, the direction of causality being from left to right. The accident sequence begins with the negative consequences of organisational processes (that is, decisions concerned with planning, scheduling, forecasting, designing, policy making, communicating, regulating, maintaining, etc.). The latent failures so created are transmitted along various organisational and departmental pathways to the workplace (the operating theatre, the ward, etc.), where they create the local conditions that promote the commission of errors

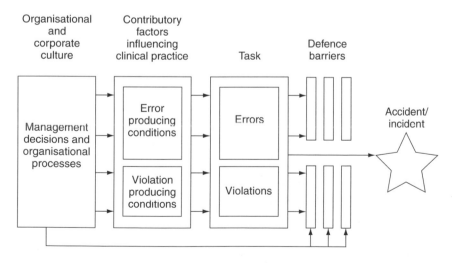

Figure 1.3 Stages of development of organisational accident.

and violations (for example, understaffing, high workload, poor human equipment interfaces, etc.). Many of these unsafe acts are likely to be committed, but only very few of them will penetrate the defences to produce damaging outcomes. The fact that engineered safety features, standards, controls, procedures, etc., can be deficient due to latent failures as well as active failures is shown in the figure by the arrow connecting organisational processes directly to defences.

The model presents the people at the sharp end as the inheritors rather than as the instigators of an accident sequence. This may seem as if the "blame" for accidents has been shifted from the sharp end to the system managers. But this is not the case for the following reasons.

- The attribution of blame, though often emotionally satisfying, hardly ever translates into effective countermeasures. Blame implies delinquency, and delinquency is normally dealt with by exhortations and sanctions. But these are wholly inappropriate if the individual people concerned did not choose to err in the first place, nor were not appreciably prone to error.
- High level management and organisational decisions are shaped by economic, political, and operational constraints. As with designs, decisions are nearly always a compromise. It is thus axiomatic that all strategic decisions will carry some negative safety consequences for some part of the system. This is not to say that all such decisions are flawed, though some of them will be. But even those decisions judged at the time as being good ones will carry a potential downside. The crux of the matter is that we cannot prevent the creation of latent failures; we can only make their adverse consequences visible before they combine with local triggers to breach the system's defences.

These organisational root causes are further complicated by the fact that the healthcare system as a whole involves many interdependent organisations: manufacturers, government agencies, professional and patient organisations, etc. The model shown in Figure 1.3 relates primarily to a given institution, but the reality is considerably more complex, with the behaviour of other organisations impinging on the accident sequence at many different points.

Applying the organisational accident model in medicine: a case study

A radiological case study is presented to give substance to this rather abstract theoretical framework and to emphasise some important points regarding the practice of high technology medicine. The case study below has all the causal hallmarks of an organisational accident but differs from most medical mishaps in having adverse outcomes for nearly 100 people. The accident is described in detail elsewhere.[11]

Omnitron 2000 accident at Indiana Regional Cancer Centre (1992)

An elderly patient with anal carcinoma was treated with high dose rate (HDR) brachytherapy. Five catheters were placed in die tumour. An iridium-192 source was intended to be located in various positions within each catheter, using a remotely controlled Omnitron 2000 afterloader. The treatment was the first of three treatments planned by the doctor, and the catheters were to remain in the patient for the subsequent treatments.

The iridium source wire was placed in four of the catheters without apparent difficulty, but after several unsuccessful attempts to insert the source wire into the fifth catheter, the treatment was terminated. In fact, a wire had broken, leaving an iridium source inside one of the first four catheters. Four days later the catheter containing the source came loose and eventually fell out of the patient. It was picked up and placed in a storage room by a member of staff of the nursing home, who did not realise it was radioactive. Five days later a truck picked up the waste bag containing the source. As part of the driver's normal routine the bag was then driven to the depot and remained there for a day (during Thanksgiving) before being delivered to a medical waste incinerator where the source was detected by fixed radiation monitors at the site. It was retrieved nearly three weeks after the original treatment. The patient had died five days after the treatment session, and in the ensuing weeks over 90 people had been irradiated in varying degrees by the iridium source.

The accident occurred as the result of a combination of procedural violations (resulting in breached or ignored defences) and latent failures.

Active failures

- The area radiation monitor alarm activated several times during the treatment but was ignored, partly because the doctor and technicians knew that it had a history of false alarms
- The console indicator showed "safe" and the attending staff mistakenly believed the source to be fully retracted into the lead shield
- The truck driver deviated from company procedures when he failed to check the nursing home waste with his personal radiation survey meter.

17

Latent failures

- The rapid expansion of high dose rate brachytherapy, from one to ten facilities in less than a year, had created serious weaknesses in the radiation safety programme
- Too much reliance was placed on unwritten or informal procedures and working practices
- There were serious inadequacies in the design and testing of the equipment
- There was a poor organisational safety culture. The technicians routinely ignored alarms and did not survey patients, the afterloader, or the treatment room after high dose rate procedures
- There was weak regulatory oversight. The Nuclear Regulatory Commission did not adequately address the problems and dangers associated with high dose rate procedures.

This case study illustrates how a combination of active failures and latent systemic weaknesses can conspire to penetrate the many layers of defences which are designed to protect both patients and staff. No one person was to blame; each person acted according to his or her appraisal of the situation, yet one person died and over 90 people were irradiated.

Principled risk management

In many organisations managing the human risks has concentrated on trying to prevent the recurrence of specific errors and violations that have been implicated in particular local mishaps. The common internal response to such events is to issue new procedures that proscribe the particular behaviour; to devise engineering "retro-fixes" that will prevent such actions having adverse outcomes; to sanction, exhort, and retrain key staff in an effort to make them more careful; and to introduce increased automation. This "anti-personnel" approach has several problems.

1 People do not intend to commit errors. It is therefore difficult for others to control what people cannot control themselves.
2 The psychological precursors of an error (that is, inattention, distraction, preoccupation, forgetting, fatigue, and stress) are probably the last and least manageable links in the chain of events leading to an error.
3 Accidents rarely occur as the result of single unsafe acts. They are the product of many factors: personal, task related, situational, and organisational. This has two implications. Firstly, the mere recurrence of some act involved in a previous accident will probably not have an adverse outcome in the absence of other causal factors. Secondly, so long as these underlying latent problems persist, other acts – not hitherto

regarded as unsafe – can also serve to complete an incipient accident sequence.

4 These countermeasures can create a false sense of security. Since modern systems are usually highly reliable some time is likely to pass between implementing these personnel related measures and the next mishap. During this time, those who have instituted the changes are inclined to believe that they have fixed the problem. But then a different kind of mishap occurs, and the cycle of local repairs begins all over again. Such accidents tend to be viewed in isolation, rather than being seen as symptomatic of some underlying systemic malaise.

5 Increased automation does not cure the human factor problem, it simply changes its nature. Systems become more opaque to their operators. Instead of causing harm by slips, lapses, trips, and fumbles, people are now more prone to make mistaken judgements about the state of the system.

The goal of effective risk management is not so much to minimise particular errors and violations as to enhance human performance at all levels of the system.[1] Perhaps paradoxically, most performance enhancement measures are not directly focused at what goes on inside the heads of single individuals. Rather, they are directed at task, team, situation, and organisational factors, as discussed below.

Task factors

Tasks vary widely in their liability to promote errors. Identifying and modifying tasks and task elements that are conspicuously prone to failure are essential steps in risk management.

The following simple example is representative of many maintenance tasks. Imagine a bolt with eight nuts on it. Each nut is coded and has to be located in a particular sequence. Disassembly is virtually error free. There is only one way in which the nuts can be removed from the bolt and all the necessary knowledge to perform this task is located in the world (that is, each step in the procedure is automatically cued by the preceding one). But the task of correct reassembly is immensely more difficult. There are over 40 000 ways in which this assemblage of nuts can be wrongly located on the bolt (factorial 8). In addition, the knowledge necessary to get the nuts back in the right order has to be either memorised or read from some written procedure, both of which are highly liable to error or neglect. Such an example may seem at first sight to be far removed from the practice of medicine, but medical equipment, like any other sophisticated hardware, requires careful maintenance – and maintenance errors (particularly omitting necessary reassembly steps) constitute one of the greatest sources of human factor problems in high technology industries.[9]

Effective incident monitoring is an invaluable tool in identifying tasks prone to error. On the basis of their body of nearly 4000 anaesthetic and intensive care incidents, Runciman *et al* at the Royal Adelaide Hospital[12] introduced many inexpensive equipment modifications guaranteed to enhance performance and to minimise recurrent errors. These include colour coded syringes and endotracheal tubes graduated to help non-intrusive identification of endobronchial intubation.[12]

Team factors

Multidisciplinary teams deliver a great deal of healthcare. Over a decade of experience in aviation (and, more recently, marine technology) has shown that measures designed to improve team management and the quality of the communication between team members can have an enormous impact on human performance. The aviation psychologist Robert Helmreich (one of the pioneers of crew resource management) and his colleagues at the University of Texas analysed 51 aircraft accidents and incidents, paying special attention to team related factors.[13] Their findings are summarised below.

These factors have a positive impact on survivability but, when absent, reduce safety. This list offers clear recommendations for the interactions of medical teams just as much as for aircraft crews. Recently, Helmreich and the anaesthetist Hans-Gerhard Schaefer studied team performance in the operating theatre of a Swiss teaching hospital.[14] They noted that "interpersonal and communications issues are responsible for many inefficiencies, errors, and frustrations in this psychologically and organisationally complex environment." They also observed that attempts to improve institutional performance largely entailed throwing money at the problem through the acquisition of new and ever more advanced equipment, whereas improvements to training and team performance could be achieved more effectively at a fraction of this cost. As has been clearly shown for aviation, formal training in team management and communication skills can produce substantial improvements in human performance as well as reducing safety-critical errors.

Situational factors

Each type of task has its own nominal error probability. For example, carrying out a totally novel task with no clear idea of the likely consequences (that is, knowledge based processing) has a basic error probability

Team factors in aviation

- Team concept and environment for open communications established
- Briefings are operationally thorough, interesting, and address crew co-ordination and planning for potential problems. Expectations are set for how possible deviations from normal operations are to be handled
- Cabin crew are included as part of the team in briefings, as appropriate, and guidelines are established for co-ordination between flight deck and cabin
- Group climate is appropriate to operational situation (for example, presence of social conversation). Crew ensures that non-operational factors such as social interaction do not interfere with necessary tasks
- Crew members ask questions regarding crew actions and decisions. Crew members speak up and state their information with appropriate persistence until there is some clear resolution or decision
- When conflicts arise the crew remains focused on the problem or situation at hand. Crew members listen actively to ideas and opinions and admit mistakes when wrong
- Captain co-ordinates flight deck activities to establish proper balance between command authority and crew member participation and acts decisively when the situation requires it
- Workload and task distribution are clearly communicated and acknowledged by crew members. Adequate time is provided for the completion of tasks
- Secondary tasks are prioritised to allow sufficient resources for dealing effectively with primary duties
- Crew members check with each other during times of high and low workload to maintain situational awareness and alertness
- Crew prepares for expected contingency situations
- Guidelines are established for the operation and disablement of automated systems. Duties and responsibilities with regard to automated systems are made clear. Crew periodically review and verify the status of automated systems. Crew verbalises and acknowledges entries and changes to automated systems. Crew allows sufficient time for programming automated systems before manoeuvres

From: Helmreich *et al*[13]

of 0·75. At the other extreme, a highly familiar, routine task performed by a well motivated and competent workforce has an error probability of 0·0005. But there are certain conditions both of the individual person and his or her immediate environment that are guaranteed to increase these nominal error probabilities (Table 1.1). Here the error producing conditions are ranked in the order of their known effects and the numbers in parentheses indicate the risk factor (that is, the amount by which the nominal error rates should be multiplied under the worst conditions). Notably, three of the best researched factors namely, sleep disturbance, hostile environment, and boredom carry the least penalties. Also, those error producing factors at the top of the list are those that lie squarely within the organisational sphere of influence. This is a central element in the present view of organisational accidents. Managers and administrators rarely, if ever, have the opportunity to jeopardise a system's safety directly. Their influence is more indirect: top level decisions create the conditions that promote unsafe acts.

For convenience, error producing conditions can be reduced to seven broad categories: high workload; inadequate knowledge, ability or experience, poor interface design; inadequate supervision or instruction; stressful environment; mental state (fatigue, boredom, etc.), and change. Departures from routine and changes in the circumstances in which actions are normally performed constitute a major factor in absentminded slips of action.[16]

Compared with error producing conditions, the factors that promote violations are less well understood. Broadly speaking, they concern lack of

Table 1.1 Summary of error producing conditions ranked in order of known effect (after Williams[15])

Condition	Risk factor
Unfamiliarity with the task	(× 17)
Time shortage	(× 11)
Poor signal:noise ratio	(× 10)
Poor human system interface	(× 8)
Designer user mismatch	(× 8)
Irreversibility of errors	(× 8)
Information overload	(× 6)
Negative transfer between tasks	(× 5)
Misperception of risk	(× 4)
Poor feedback from system	(× 4)
Inexperience – not lack of training	(× 3)
Poor instructions or procedures	(× 3)
Inadequate checking	(× 3)
Educational mismatch of person with task	(× 2)
Disturbed sleep patterns	(× 1.6)
Hostile environment	(× 1.2)
Monotony and boredom	(× 1.1)

safety culture, lack of concern, poor morale, norms condoning violation, "can do" attitudes, and apparently meaningless or ambiguous rules.

Organisational factors

Quality and safety, like health and happiness, have two aspects: a negative aspect disclosed by incidents and accidents and a positive aspect, which reflects the system's intrinsic resistance to human factor problems. Whereas incidents and accidents convert easily into numbers, trends, and targets, the positive aspect is much harder to identify and measure.

Accident and incident reporting procedures are a crucial part of any safety or quality information system. But, by themselves, they are insufficient to support effective quality and safety management. The information they provide is both too little and too late for this longer term purpose. To promote proactive accident prevention rather than reactive "local repairs" an organisation's "vital signs" should be monitored regularly.

When a doctor carries out a routine medical check he or she samples the state of several critical bodily systems: the cardiovascular, pulmonary, excretory, neurological systems, and so on. From individual measures of blood pressure, electrocardiographic activity, cholesterol concentration, urinary contents, reflexes, and so on the doctor makes a professional judgement about the individual's general state of health. There is no direct, definitive measure of a person's health. It is an emergent property inferred from a selection of physiological signs and lifestyle indicators. The same is also true of complex hazardous systems. Assessing an organisation's current state of "safety health", as in medicine, entails regular and judicious sampling of a small subset of a potentially large number of indices. But what are the dimensions along which to assess organisational "safety health"?

Several such diagnostic techniques are already being implemented in various industries.[17] The individual labels for the assessed dimensions vary from industry to industry (oil exploration and production, tankers, helicopters, railway operations, and aircraft engineering), but all of them have been guided by two principles. Firstly, they try to include those organisational "pathogens" that have featured most conspicuously in well documented accidents (that is, hardware defects, incompatible goals, poor operating procedures, understaffing, high workload, inadequate training, etc.). Secondly, they seek to encompass a representative sampling of those core processes common to all technological organisations (that is, design, build, operate, maintain, manage, communicate, etc.).

There is unlikely to be a single universal set of indicators for all types of hazardous operations. However, one example of a systematic approach to the measurement of such factors is Tripod-Delta, commissioned by Shell

International and currently implemented in several of its exploration and production operating companies, on Shell tankers, and on its contracted helicopters in the North Sea. Tripod-Delta assesses the quarterly or half-yearly state of 11 general failure types in specific workplaces: hardware, design, maintenance management, procedures, error enforcing conditions, housekeeping, incompatible goals, organisational structure, communication, training, and defences. A discussion of the rationale behind the selection and measurement of these failure types can be found elsewhere.[18]

The purpose of the measurements derived from Tripod-Delta is to identify the two or three factors most in need of remediation and to track changes over time. Maintaining adequate safety health is thus comparable with a long term fitness programme in which the focus of remedial efforts switches from dimension to dimension as previously salient factors improve and new ones come into prominence. Like life, effective safety management is "one thing after another". Striving for the best attainable level of intrinsic resistance to operational hazards is like fighting a guerrilla war. One can expect no absolute victories. There are no "Waterloos" in the safety war.

The positive face of the human factor

In a climate of growing concern about the adverse effects of medical errors, it is easy to lose sight of the far more important side of the human equation. Every medical practitioner has made errors – this is as much a part of being human as our dependence on oxygen. But very few of these errors have actually caused harm to a patient. The vast majority of potential adverse outcomes are detected and recovered long before any lasting damage is done. It is this remarkable ability to adjust and adapt, to make on-line corrections and compensations in a changing and uncertain world that raises people above even the cleverest of intelligent machines.

Unfortunately, it is in the nature of damaging mistakes to stand out from the normal run of medical practice, and it is just this singularity that gives error a public prominence that is out of all proportion to its consequences. We are far more likely to investigate the things that go wrong. This means that we know a good deal more about the bad days than the good days – but most days are good days, in the sense that the majority of patients gain some benefit from medical interventions. In this section, we will focus on the good days. The intention here is not to diminish the problem of human fallibility, only to place it in a much wider perspective than has hitherto been the case in this chapter.

One of the most important developments since the appearance of the first edition of this book has been a growing interest on the part of researchers in this more benign face of the human factor. As well as continuing to study how and why people fail, we have also been pursuing the – ultimately – more interesting question of how and why they succeed, often in the face of considerable adversity. An aviation case study will serve to echo the foregoing and introduce what follows. The incident has been termed the "Gimli glider" for reasons that will become evident.

Aviation case study: the Gimli glider

A Boeing 767 wide-bodied jet, en route from Ottawa to Edmonton, ran out of fuel about 60 miles from Winnipeg. The reasons for this occupied the greater part of the 100-plus page inquiry report (Lockwood). They included a diabolical conspiracy of all the usual suspects: human errors, faulty fuel gauges, systemic error traps and organisational failures.

Only three paragraphs were devoted to the most remarkable aspect of the incident: what happened immediately after the engines stopped. Each pilot possessed life-saving knowledge and skills. The co-pilot had trained with the military and remembered that he had flown in and out of a now deserted airstrip at Gimli, only a few miles away. The captain was, in his spare time, an enthusiastic glider pilot. Without engine power, the aircraft had no flaps or slats to control the rate of descent, and there was only a one-shot chance of landing.

After discussing the matter with his first officer, the captain decided to sideslip the aircraft on to the 7200ft runway at Gimli. Sideslipping is a manoeuvre used by gliders and small aircraft to get into small fields in a hurry. It puts the aircraft into an off-balance attitude with one wing advanced, and (with great skill) allows it to descend rapidly without gaining speed. Just before landing, the pilot must kick the aircraft straight using the rudder controls. This the captain did, touching down just past the runway threshold. All the passengers and crew disembarked safely and the aircraft was soon back in service after minor repairs.

It is likely that many doctors have witnessed – or even performed – similar heroic recoveries during the course of their training or practice. But this type of "grace under fire" is far more likely to be communicated by word of mouth than by the scientific literature. There are, however, two notable exceptions. The first body of publications relates to the study of high reliability organisations (HROs) – hazardous technologies that have fewer than their "fair share" of accidents.[19-23] The second set of papers is concerned with understanding the nature of excellence in athletics and surgery.[24] Although, in the former case, the focus was upon organisations, and, in the latter case, upon individuals, both research programmes have identified two very similar processes contributing to resilience or robustness. The first of these has to do with preparedness, the second with flexibility of action. They are summarised below.

- *Preparedness*: Perhaps the most important aspect of resilience, both in organisations and in individuals, is the knowledge that things can and will go wrong. They expect and prepare for nasty surprises. Thus, HROs know that their personnel will make errors and train them in recognising and recovering their slips, lapses and mistakes. HROs are continually reviewing the lessons of past failures and brainstorming new scenarios of system breakdown. They generalise rather than localise the lessons of past incidents or accidents. They have crisis management plans for dealing with a wide range of adverse events, both familiar and imagined. Similarly, excellence at the individual level is closely bound up with the mental rehearsal of possible eventualities and how to cope with them. Excellent surgeons, for example, spend a considerable amount of time before entering the operating theatre in visualising each stage of a procedure and working out ways of dealing with possible complications – of which their own errors are likely to form a major part. Both HROs and excellent performers understand that mental skills are just as important as technical skills. They also know that both types of skill need to be continuously practised and developed.
- *Flexibility*: Largely as a consequence of their mental readiness, both HROs and resilient individuals are able to reconfigure their plans, structures and actions to suit local circumstances. HROs, for example, adopt different organisational command structures in different circumstances. During high-tempo operations, control devolves to local experts and then reverts back to the normal hierarchical mode once routine activities have been resumed. Average performers at both the organisational and individual levels usually manage well enough when things go as planned, but often find themselves in severe difficulties in the face of unpleasant surprises. The ability to adapt and adjust places very heavy demands upon coping resources. These are limited. People are not usually at their best when required to think on their feet in an emergency. Successful compensations generally require some degree of pre-packaging, as well as the confidence to break out of routine modes of thinking and action that comes with mental preparedness.

Karl Weick, a social scientist at the University of Michigan, has made two very insightful observations about the adaptive processes discussed above. In the first place, he described reliability as a "dynamic non-event".[19,23] It is dynamic because it is achieved by the timely adjustments and compensations of a large number of people at the "sharp end". It is a non-event because safe outcomes attract little notice. He gives the following example from one of the high reliability organisations studied.

Air traffic controllers working in the Bay Area know that certain Asian pilots do not speak or comprehend English very well (the language of aviation). They also tend to arrive in the San Francisco airspace at fixed times of day. Just before they are due, the controllers start to stack aircraft with flight crew for whom English is the first language. This "cuts slack" in the system so that those pilots with less than fluent English have more time and space in which to make their approaches and landings. At the end of the day, everyone has landed safely and the passengers in the English-speaking carriers have been delayed by a barely noticeable few minutes. It is a non-event, but a very skilfully managed non-event.

Weick's second observation relates to the paradox of human variability.[23] The reduction of error has now become one of the primary objectives of those who manage hazardous technologies. Unsafe acts are viewed, not unreasonably, as arising from the unwanted deviations of human action. For most of these managers, reliability demands a prescribed consistency of action. They try to achieve this consistency by procedures, protocols, and, where possible, by increased automation. But, because it is a "dynamic non-event", they fail to appreciate that human variability – in the form of the moment-to-moment adjustments of the kind described above – is what preserves system safety in an uncertain and changing world. And therein lies the paradox. By striving to limit the variability of human action, they are also undermining the system's last and perhaps most important line of defence.

From their observations of HROs, Weick and his colleagues have distinguished two aspects of organisational functioning: cognition (what it thinks) and action (what it does). The cognitive element concerns the way the organisation views the hazards that beset its operations; the action element relates to how it carries out its activities. Traditional, "efficient" organisations strive hard to achieve invariant human performance, but they have variable mindsets – that is, they have different perceptions of risk before and after a bad accident. HROs, on the other hand, show the reverse pattern. They work very hard to achieve a consistent "collective mindfulness" of the ever-present dangers, while encouraging some variability of action. As Weick and his co-authors put it: "there is variation in activity, but there is stability in the cognitive processes that make sense of this activity".[23]

For a variety of practical, political and legal reasons, the medical profession is moving away from a culture in which individual practitioners were granted – and trained to exercise – a great deal of personal autonomy in how they diagnosed and treated their patients to one in which the practice of medicine is becoming increasingly governed by prescriptive protocols. Ironically, this is happening at a time when many tightly regulated and rule-driven industries (for example, railways, aviation, oil and gas exploration, etc.) are moving in the opposite direction – towards greater

27

self-determination, self-regulation and, in some cases, deregulation. Both medicine's move towards protocol-guided practice and the shift away by heavily proceduralised activities started from relatively extreme positions. Clearly, there is likely to be some optimal middle ground in which an appropriate balance is struck between procedures and protocols and individual discretion. In the case of medicine, however, it is important that the architects of the new protocols do not press their efforts to the point where the benign aspects of individual variability are overly restricted.

Summary and conclusions

1 Human rather than technical failures now represent the greatest threat to complex and potentially hazardous systems. This includes healthcare systems.
2 Managing the human risks will never be 100% effective. Human fallibility can be moderated, but it cannot be eliminated.
3 Different error types have different underlying mechanisms, occur in different parts of the organisation, and require different methods of risk management. The basic distinctions are between:

  • Slips, lapses, trips, and fumbles (execution failures) and mistakes (planning or problem solving failures). Mistakes are divided into rule based mistakes and knowledge based mistakes.
  • Errors (information-handling problems) and violations (motivational problems).
  • Active versus latent failures. Active failures are committed by those in direct contact with the patient, latent failures arise in organisational and managerial spheres and their adverse effects may take a long time to become evident.

4 Safety significant errors occur at all levels of the system, not just at the sharp end. Decisions made in the upper echelons of the organisation create the conditions in the workplace that subsequently promote individual errors and violations. Latent failures are present long before an accident and are hence prime candidates for principled risk management.
5 Measures that involve sanctions and exhortations (that is, moralistic measures directed to those at the sharp end) have only very limited effectiveness, especially so in the case of highly trained professionals.
6 Problems of human factors are a product of a chain of causes in which the individual psychological factors (that is, momentary inattention, forgetting, etc.) are the last and least manageable links. Attentional "capture" (preoccupation or distraction) is a necessary condition for the commission of slips and lapses. Yet its occurrence is almost impossible to predict or control effectively. The same is true of the factors

associated with forgetting. States of mind contributing to error are thus extremely difficult to manage; they can happen to the best of people at any time.

7 People do not act in isolation. Their behaviour is shaped by circumstances. The same is true for errors and violations. The likelihood of an unsafe act being committed is heavily influenced by the nature of the task and by the local workplace conditions. These, in turn, are the product of "upstream" organisational factors. Great gains in safety can be achieved through relatively small modifications of equipment and workplaces.

8 Automation and increasingly advanced equipment do not cure problems associated with human factors, they merely relocate them. In contrast, training people to work effectively in teams costs little, but has achieved significant enhancements of human performance in aviation.

9 Effective risk management depends critically on a confidential and preferably anonymous incident monitoring system that records the individual, task, situational, and organisational factors associated with incidents and near misses.

10 Effective risk management means, the simultaneous and targeted deployment of limited remedial resources at different levels of the system: the individual or team, the task, the situation, and the organisation as a whole.

11 While the greater part of this chapter has dealt with the problem of human error and its management, it is important to recognise that the human factor, especially in medicine, is also the last and most important defence against adverse events. It is hoped that the current salience of medical error in the minds of the managers of healthcare institutions and the general public does not blind them to the significance of the benign face of the human factor. The important challenge is not to eliminate fallibility, but to minimise its damaging consequences. Risk management should be focused upon the prevention of bad outcomes rather than the mere reduction of errors.

References

1 Cook RI, Woods DD. Operating at the sharp end: the complexity of human error. In: Bogner MS, ed. *Human errors in medicine*. Hillsdale, NJ: Erlbaum, 1994:255–310.
2 Gaba DM. Human error in dynamic medical domains. In: Bogner MS, ed. *Human errors in medicine*. Hillsdale, NJ: Erlbaum, 1994:197–224.
3 Vincent C, Ennis M, Audley RJ. *Medical accidents*. Oxford: OUP, 1993.
4 Bogner MS. *Human error in medicine*. Hillsdale, NJ: Erlbaum, 1994.
5 Vincent C. *Clinical risk management*. London: BMJ Publications, 1995.
6 Hollnagel E. *Reliability of cognition: foundations of human reliability analysis*. London: Academic Press, 1993.
7 Gaba DM. Human error in anaesthetic mishaps. *Int Anesth Clin* 1989;**27**:137–47.

8 Runciman W, Sellen A, Webb RK, *et al.* Errors, incidents and accidents in anaesthetic practice. *Anaesth Intensive Care* 1993;**21**:506–19.
9 Reason J. *Human error.* New York: Cambridge University Press, 1990.
10 Sheen J. *MV Herald of Free Enterprise. Report of court No 8074 formal investigation.* London: Department of Transport, 1987.
11 NUREG. *Loss of an iridium-192 source and therapy misadministration at Indiana Regional Cancer Centre, Indiana, Pennsylvania, on November 16, 1992.* Washington, DC: US Nuclear Regulatory Commission, 1993. (NUREG1480.)
12 Runciman WB. Anaesthesia incident monitoring study. In: *Incident monitoring and risk management in the healthcare sector.* Canberra: Commonwealth Department of Human Services and Health, 1994:13–15.
13 Helmreich RL, Butler RA, Taggart WIZ, Wilhem JA. *Behavioural markers in accidents and incidents: reference list.* Austin, Texas: University of Texas, 1994. (Technical report 94–3; NASA/University of Texas FAA Aerospace Crew Research Project.)
14 Helmreich RL, Schaefer H-G. Team performance in the operating room. In: Bogner MS, ed. *Human errors in medicine.* Hillsdale, NJ: Erlbaum, 1994.
15 Williams J. A data-based method for assessing and reducing human error to improve operational performance. In: Hagen W, ed. *1988 ILEEE Fourth Conference on Human Factors and Power Plants.* New York: Institute for Electrical and Electronic Engineers, 1988: 200–31.
16 Reason J, Mycielska K. *Absent-minded? The psychology of mental lapses and everyday errors.* Englewood Cliffs, NJ: Prentice-Hall, 1982.
17 Reason J. *Managing the risks of organisational accidents.* Aldershot: Ashgate, 1997.
18 Hudson P, Reason J, Wagenaar W, *et al.* Tripod Delta: proactive approach to enhanced safety. *J Petroleum Technology* 1994;**46**:58–62.
19 Weick KE. Organizational culture as a source of high reliability. *California Management Review* 1987;**29**:112–27.
20 LaPorte TR, Consolini PM. Working in practice but not in theory: Theoretical challenges of "high-reliability" organizations. *J Pub Admin Res Theory* 1991;**1**:19–47.
21 Rochlin G. High-reliability organizations and technological change: Some ethical problems and dilemmas. *IEEE Technology and Society Magazine.* September 1986:3–8.
22 Rijpma JA. Complexity, tight-coupling and reliability: Connecting normal accidents theory and high reliability theory. *J Contingencies Crisis Manage* 1997;**5**:15–23.
23 Weick KE, Sutcliffe KM, Obtsfeld D. Organizing for high reliability: processes of collective mindfulness. *Res Organiz Behav* 1999;**21**:23–81.
24 McDonald J, Orlick T, Letts M. Mental readiness in surgeons and its links to excellence in surgery. *J Paed Orthop* 1995;**15**:691–7.

2 Errors and adverse events in medicine: an overview

ERIC J THOMAS, TROYEN A BRENNAN

The body of scientific research on errors and adverse events in medicine is notable for both its diversity and its uniformity. Sociologists, psychologists, physicians, epidemiologists, lawyers, statisticians, nurses, and others have studied the topic. Errors and adverse events may occur in all types of patients, in all medical specialties, and throughout hospitals, nursing homes, and outpatient treatment areas. Thus it is not surprising to find that studies on this topic use a variety of methods and report a broad array of results. Nevertheless, there is one unifying theme of all these inquiries: errors and adverse events are common and a major problem in all healthcare settings that have been studied.

The goal of this chapter is to provide an overview of this diverse literature and an understanding of the importance of errors and adverse events. This is not a systematic review or meta-analysis and we do not attempt to mention every article or book written about this topic. Rather, we hope to convey the diversity of the methodological approaches to studying the epidemiology of this problem, and describe its impact and importance. Readers should look elsewhere in this book and in other publications for practical approaches to addressing errors and adverse events.[1]

This chapter is divided into three sections. First we provide an overview of definitions and methodological issues related to the study of errors and adverse events. Second, we review the methods and results of the four population-based studies of medical injury that have been conducted. And third, we overview the research on operative adverse events, adverse drug events, and adverse events in emergency rooms. These were chosen because the population-based studies either found that they were among the most frequent types of events or they were most often preventable.

Overview of definitions and methodological issues

Diverse investigative methods create difficulties for both the casual and professional reader of the literature on errors and adverse events in medicine. Almost every study uses different methods, terms, and definitions. It is therefore almost impossible to make direct comparisons among studies, even among studies that purport to use the same methods. This is an important limitation given the tendency to interpret rates of errors and adverse events as a measure of quality and then to compare one healthcare site to another. Ideally, we could directly compare among hospitals or clinics in order to focus quality improvement and risk management efforts. But determining whether or not one clinic has a problem compared to another depends upon what definition of injury was used, how data were collected, and upon the patient populations in each setting.

In general, the terms used to describe errors and adverse events can be grouped into two broad categories. In the medical literature, terms such as errors usually describe deviations in processes of care, which may or may not cause harm to patients. Terms such as adverse events refer to undesired patient outcomes that may or may not be the result of errors. In this chapter, we use both terms together when making general statements. Other examples of process-related terms like errors include mishaps and mistakes. Examples of other outcome-related terms like adverse events include negligent events, preventable adverse events, iatrogenic injuries, and complications.

Note that James Reason's definition of error as "occasions in which a planned sequence of mental or physical activities fails to achieve its intended outcome."[2] is perhaps the most inclusive, easily generalised, and well thought-out definition one could adopt, and was used by the US Institute of Medicine in their recent report on the subject.[3]

Although Reason and others have made fundamental insights into the causes of errors, most research in healthcare has focused on the consequences of errors the actual injury that occurred, often called an adverse event or complication. While this focus has allowed a better understanding of the costs, morbidity and mortality of errors and adverse events, prevention efforts will require an understanding of the errors that lead to adverse events. Another limitation of the current research is that investigators have used different definitions of adverse events and different methods to detect them.

For example, the Harvard Medical Practice Study[4] used the term adverse events and defined them as an injury that was caused by medical management (and not the disease process) that either prolonged the hospitalisation, produced a disability at the time of discharge, or both. After reviewing over 30 000 randomly selected medical records from the state of New York, they found that adverse events occurred in 3·7% of hospitalisations.

This is in contrast to studies by Steel[5] who found that 36% of 815 consecutive patients had an "iatrogenic illness". A more recent study by Andrews[6] found that 17·7% of patients admitted to a surgical service in a Chicago teaching hospital suffered at least one serious adverse event. "Serious" meant the patient suffered at least temporary physical disability.

Why is the rate of adverse events in the Harvard study 3·7% versus 17·7% in the Andrews' study? First, they defined adverse events differently; second, they used different methods to detect events; and third, they studied a different patient population. Regarding the definition of adverse event, although the Andrews' study states there was physical disability, they do not specify disability at the time of discharge, as in the Harvard study. This would result in a higher adverse event rate in the Andrews' study. Further, Andrews *et al* directly observed patient care so they were more likely to detect events compared to the Harvard study that relied completely upon medical records, thus increasing their rate relative to the Harvard study. Finally, Andrews studied surgical patients in a teaching hospital while the Harvard study reviewed a random sample of records from a random sample of hospitals. We know that more adverse events occur in surgical patients than non-surgical patients. This fact also makes the Andrews event rate higher.

Similar comparisons can be made for most studies of errors and adverse events. The take home message is: reader beware, especially when making comparisons of your own rates to those in published studies or from colleagues in other organizations.

Population based studies of iatrogenic injury

Four large population based studies of iatrogenic injury have been conducted, three in the United States and one in Australia. Although they have many methodological weaknesses, these studies reviewed thousands of randomly selected hospital records from large geographic regions and therefore provide the most easily generalized estimates available on the rate of injury in hospitals. These studies also reported which types of injuries occurred most often and therefore they can be used to focus additional research, quality improvement, and risk management activities.

The California Medical Insurance Feasibility Study

The California Medical Insurance Feasibility Study (CMIFS)[7] randomly sampled 20 864 hospitalisations from 23 hospitals in California in 1974. Of these, 4·65% of hospitalisations had a "potentially compensatable event" defined as an event due to medical management that resulted in disability which led to or prolonged a hospitalisation. Additional results will not be

33

described here because the data is 25 years old. However, this study is historically important because it developed the methodology used by the three more recent population-based studies described below.

The Harvard Medical Practice Study

The Harvard Medical Practice Study (HMPS)[4] reviewed patient records of 30 121 randomly chosen hospitalisations from 51 randomly chosen acute care, non-psychiatric hospitals in New York State in 1984. Their goal was to better understand the epidemiology of patient injury and to inform medical malpractice reform efforts. Because of this second goal they were trying to detect injuries that would potentially enter the tort system. Therefore they did not try to detect errors that did not harm patients nor did they count events that caused only minor physical discomfort. As noted above their definition was "an injury that was caused by medical management (and not the disease process) that either prolonged the hospitalisation, produced a disability at the time of discharge, or both".

Adverse events occurred in 3·7% of hospitalisations in New York in 1984 and 27·6% of these were due to negligence (defined as care that fell below the standard expected of physicians in their community). Of all adverse events, 47·7% were operative events (related to surgical care) and 17% of them were due to negligence. The most common non-operative adverse events were adverse drug events, followed by diagnostic mishaps, therapeutic mishaps, procedure related events, and others. Overall 37·2% of the non-operative events were negligent. As expected, the most common site for adverse events was the operating room followed by patients' rooms, the emergency room, labour and delivery room, and intensive care unit. Permanent disability resulted from 6·5% of adverse events and death from 13·6%.

The investigators subsequently reanalysed their data to determine preventability instead of negligence and found that 69·6% of adverse events were preventable.[8] Extrapolations of this data suggested that approximately 100 000 Americans died each year from preventable adverse events. They also identified the emergency room as the location with the highest percentage of preventable adverse events (93·3%), followed by labour and delivery (78·7%), intensive care units (70·3%) and operating rooms (71·4%).

The Quality in Australian Healthcare Study

The Quality in Australian Healthcare Study (QAHS) investigators based their study upon the HMPS methods.[9,10] Their goal was to inform quality improvement efforts, hence they measured preventability of adverse events instead of negligence. Negligent adverse events are those that fall below the standard of care in the community and are a subset of all preventable adverse events. By focusing on preventable events they identified a larger group of events to inform future quality improvement efforts.

They reviewed 14 179 randomly sampled records from hospitalisations in 8 randomly sampled hospitals in South Australia and 23 in New South Wales in 1992. Using the identical definition of an adverse event as the HMPS they found that 16·6% of hospitalisations were associated with an adverse event in 1992. When adjusted to count adverse events similar to the HMPS and thereby estimate the annual incidence, their rate was 13%, still four times higher than HMPS. Of all adverse events, 51% were judged preventable.

As in the HMPS most adverse events were related to surgical procedures (50·3%) followed by diagnostic errors (13·6%), therapeutic errors (12·0%) and adverse drug events (10·8%). Permanent disability resulted from 13·7% of adverse events and death from 4·9%. They also found that 34·6% of errors were related to technical performance, 15·8% to a failure to synthesise and/or act upon information, 11·8% failure to request or arrange an investigation, procedure, or consultation, and 10·9% due to lack of care and attention or failure to attend the patient.[9]

Utah and Colorado Medical Practice Study

The fourth population based study was the Utah and Colorado Medical Practice Study (UCMPS), conducted by some of the same investigators as the HMPS.[11] The primary goal of this study, like the HMPS was to inform malpractice reform efforts. They therefore used the same definition of an adverse event and judged negligence and preventability. They reviewed the records of 14 052 randomly selected hospitalisations from 28 hospitals in the American states of Utah and Colorado in 1992. Again using the HMPS definition they found that adverse events occurred in 2·9% of hospitalisations, that approximately 30% of all adverse events were due to negligence and that just over half were preventable. Permanent disability resulted from 8·4% of adverse events and death from 6·6%. Operative adverse events comprised 44·9% of all adverse events followed by adverse drug events (19·3%). Most adverse events occurred in operating rooms. Negligent adverse events were common in emergency rooms (and 94% of events attributed to emergency medicine physicians were judged negligent), intensive care units and patient rooms on general wards.

The investigators also estimated the total costs of adverse events (including direct healthcare costs and indirect costs such as lost household production and time off work). The cost in 1996 US dollars was $37·2 billion for all adverse events and $20·7 billion for preventable adverse events. The costs of adverse events were similar to the national costs of caring for persons with HIV/AIDS and totalled 4·8% of per capita healthcare expenditures in these states.[12]

In summary, these large population-based studies give us a view of the public health impact of errors and adverse events. For example, the most recent data from the Utah and Colorado study suggest that in 1997 approximately 44 000 persons died from preventable adverse events. If considered a disease, preventable adverse events would have been the eighth leading cause of death in the United States in 1997. Of course, many patients who died from preventable adverse events also had diseases that may have proved fatal, and it may not be appropriate to extrapolate data from two states to an entire country. Nevertheless, the incidence and cost data clearly demonstrate that errors and adverse events are a significant public health problem. These studies also consistently found that most adverse events occurred to patients undergoing surgical procedures. Adverse drug events were the most common non-operative event and preventable and negligent events were very likely in emergency rooms.

Research on specific types of adverse events

Operative complications

Although the above mentioned population-based studies identified operative complications as the most common type of adverse event, their very broad focus and reliance upon chart review provides limited information about the incidence of specific types of operative complications. The exception is the Utah Colorado Medical Practice Study that provided some additional data on operative events.[13]

These investigators found that the annual incidence rate of adverse events among hospitalised patients who received an operation was 3·0%. Among all surgical events, 54% were preventable. Eight operations were "high risk" based upon their preventable adverse event rate: lower extremity bypass graft (11·0%), abdominal aortic aneurysm repair (8·1%), colon resection (5·9%), coronary artery bypass graft/cardiac valve surgery (4·7%), transurethral resection of the prostate or of a bladder tumor (3·9%), cholecystectomy (3·0%), hysterectomy (2·8%), and appendectomy (1·5%). Among all surgical adverse events, 5·6% resulted in death, accounting for 12·2% of all hospital deaths in Utah and Colorado. Technique-related complications, wound infections, and postoperative bleeding produced nearly half of all surgical adverse events.

The National Veterans Affairs Surgical Risk Study has been collecting data on postoperative morbidity and mortality for most noncardiac surgical procedures in 44 Veterans Administration Medical Centers in the United States since 1 October 1991.[14] The study has contributed significantly to our understanding of postoperative adverse events, especially in advancing the field of risk adjustment to allow comparative assessments of quality among hospitals and in identifying patient[15,16] and organizational factors[17] that influence postoperative morbidity and mortality. In simple terms, risk adjustment is the process of accounting for the various patient characteristics such as age and other illnesses that contribute to outcomes. By measuring these factors and adjusting for them, the investigators were able to compare the postoperative outcomes among different sites. And since the same data collection methods and definitions were used at all 44 hospitals this allowed accurate comparisons of outcomes to be made despite differences in the types of patients at each institution. Any differences in postoperative complication rates after risk adjustment were attributed to differences in the process of care. A limitation of this study, especially for the focus of this chapter, is that it does not evaluate error or unexpected complications.

The overall 30-day mortality rate for patients in this study was 3·11%, ranging from 0·67% for urologic procedures to 5·91% for noncardiac thoracic surgery. The unadjusted mortality rate across all 44 hospitals varied from 1·2–5·4% and 93% of hospitals changed rank after risk adjustment. Overall 17·4% of patients experienced one or more postoperative morbidities with the most common being pneumonia (3·7%), superficial (2·6%) and deep (2·6%) wound infections, failure to wean from the ventilator after 48 hours (3·3%) and urinary tract infections (3·6%). The unadjusted postoperative morbidity rate by hospital varied from 7·4–28·4%.

Britain's Confidential Enquiry into Perioperative Deaths (CEPOD)[18,19,20] is a cooperative effort among surgeons and anaesthetists in the United Kingdom. It differs fundamentally from previously described studies in that it only focuses on deaths and relies upon provider reporting to gather data. The investigators identify all patients who die in hospital within 30 days of a surgical operation. Questionnaires are then sent to the consultant clinicians that cared for these patients and then an advisory group analyses the data. Examples of CEPOD recommendations include better supervision of trainees, assurance that hospitals have proper recovery rooms, and increase in the use of autopsy.

Such efforts to feedback data and improve quality of care have proven successful by studies such as the Northern New England Cardiovascular Disease Study Group.[21] This group implemented a process of continuous improvement focusing on systems and effected a 24% reduction in hospital mortality after cardiac surgery. The interventions included feedback of outcome data, training in continuous quality improvement techniques, and site visits to other medical centers.

While postoperative cardiac complications do not appear to be the most common complications they are definitely the best studied and therefore deserve mention. The literature in this field is vast and has been well summarised.[22,23] Many studies have been done that focus on preoperative screening to identify high risk patients[24] and recent data suggests that the combination of better screening and better treatment has lowered the incidence of postoperative cardiac complications.[25] This research provides an example that could be followed for focusing on other postoperative complications.

Other recent research on preventing operative adverse events has followed the lead of the airline industry by attempting to measure and improve teamwork in the operating room by surveying personnel about their attitudes toward teamwork and by using simulated surgical scenarios to improve performance.[26,27]

Adverse Drug Events

As noted above, the Harvard Medical Practice Study, the Quality in Australian Healthcare Study and the Utah and Colorado Medical Practice Study all found that adverse drug events were the most common type of nonoperative adverse events. Other, mostly single or two-institution studies confirm that adverse drug events are a significant problem. Bates *et al* found that adverse drug events (defined as an injury resulting from medical intervention related to a drug) occurred in 6·5% of hospitalisations.[28,29] Classen *et al* estimated the rate to be 2·5%.[30] The national direct costs of adverse drug events in the United States has been estimated to be $4–5 billion dollars per year.[30,31,32]

From 28% to 56% of adverse drug events are believed to be preventable,[28,29,30] but how can they be prevented? Obviously, one first has to identify and correct the errors that lead to these events. A comprehensive review of medication errors[33] cited 115 articles on the topic. This literature will not be re-reviewed here but examples of the basic types of medication errors include omission error, wrong-dose error, unordered-drug error, wrong-dosage-form error, wrong-time error, wrong-route errors, deteriorated-drug errors, wrong-rate-of-administration errors, wrong-administration-technique errors, wrong-dose-preparation errors and extra-dose errors.

The elucidation of the frequency and types of adverse drug events and the errors that lead to them has prompted many institutions to implement systems that track the occurrence of errors and adverse drug events. A recent survey of over 500 hospital pharmacies in the US found that the vast majority employ tracking systems for medication errors (98·4%), adverse drug reactions (98·0%), and pharmacist interventions (80·6%).[34] Some authors have called for national reporting systems for adverse drug events and errors similar to the anonymous reporting system used in the US airline industry.[35] Australians have developed an incident reporting system for anaesthesia[36,37] and there is also one being developed for transfusion medicine in the United States.[38]

Identifying the system errors that lead to adverse drug events has been a productive way of focusing interventions to decrease adverse drug events. For example, Leape and colleagues identified 16 major systems failures as the underlying causes of errors leading to adverse drug events.[39] The most common systems failure was the dissemination of drug knowledge, particularly to physicians, accounting for 29% of the errors. Inadequate availability of patient information, such as the results of laboratory tests, was associated with 18% of errors. Seven systems failures accounted for 78% of the errors and all could be improved by better information systems. This study also found that a single system fault could result in a variety of error types, so eradicating a single type of error is unlikely to have a major impact on the overall problem. Based upon this data, a computer order entry system was designed and it decreased the frequency of serious medication errors by 55%.[40] Other investigators have used computers to significantly improve the quality of antibiotic use in hospitals.[41]

Integrating pharmacists into clinical intensive care unit rounds also decreases errors and adverse drug events.[42]

The body of research and knowledge on adverse drug events and medication errors is extensive. Additional information on research into adverse drug events and its practical implications can be found in a new book published by the American Pharmaceutical Association,[43] and in the report on error in medicine by the US Institute of Medicine.[3]

Emergency rooms

As noted above, the Harvard Medical Practice Study found that the third most common site of adverse events in the hospital was the emergency room and 93·3% of these events were preventable.[44,8] The Utah and Colorado study found that 52% of adverse events in the emergency room were preventable and 94% of the adverse events attributed to emergency medicine physicians were preventable.[11] Given that trauma is a common problem in most countries (for example, over 500 000 Americans each year suffer some morbidity or mortality from trauma), the frequent occurrence of adverse events in emergency rooms and the very large proportion that were preventable is troubling.

Other studies confirm that errors are relatively common in emergency rooms. Between 2–9% of trauma patients die from preventable errors.[45,46,47,48,49,50] The majority (53%) of "significant" preventable errors that occur while caring for trauma patients occur during resuscitation (the initial care of the patient versus during the operative or postoperative period).[51]

In the same way as in the operating room investigators are focusing on measuring and improving teamwork during trauma resuscitation. Xiao *et al* analysed videotapes of trauma resuscitations and found a high level of complexity of work attribute termed tasks;[52] specifically, trauma resuscitation involved multiple and concurrent tasks, uncertainty (e.g. lack of complete medical history from an unconscious patient), changing plans, compressed work procedures, and high workloads. These factors seem likely to lead to preventable and even negligent errors. Because of this high level of task complexity, Xiao and colleagues suggested that trauma resuscitation teams should focus on improving communication and teamwork.

Several studies have in fact identified deficiencies in teamwork during trauma resuscitation. Analysis of videotapes of intubations during trauma resuscitation attributed 8 of 28 errors to poor teamwork.[53] Other reviews of videotaped trauma resuscitations identified interpersonal problems among team members,[54] deficiencies in leadership[55] (including poor communication with team members),[56] and lack of team member adherence to assigned responsibilities.[57,58] Finally, other emergency medicine researchers believe teamwork is important enough to develop high-fidelity simulation as a way to improve teamwork.[59]

Conclusions

The research findings reviewed in this chapter have several direct implications for risk managers and other individuals responsible for healthcare quality in hospitals. First, several large population-based studies reveal that errors and adverse events are a major public health problem in the United States and Australia. This also may be a problem for most western healthcare systems based upon preliminary results of similar studies in England and New Zealand. It is clear that more effort should go toward preventing errors and adverse events.

Second, the research tells us where prevention efforts should be directed. Errors and adverse events related to surgical procedures, drugs, and care in emergency rooms are especially common or preventable.

Finally, this chapter touched upon some examples of how errors and adverse events can be prevented. Other examples are detailed elsewhere in this book. In general terms, the approach to error reduction in healthcare has been best elucidated by Lucian Leape, who has argued that errors committed by healthcare professionals are often the result of systems failures rather than purely the fault of the individual who committed the error.[60] His reasoning arises in part from the experience of other industries which has shown that accidents are often the end result of a chain of events due to "latent" errors which exist within a system.[61,2] The exact nature of such latent system errors is in turn determined by overlying organizational features of the system, such as who owns the system and the regulatory environment within which it functions.[62]

Traditional efforts to control errors in medicine have focused on individual healthcare providers through the use of peer review and the medical malpractice system.[63] But humans will always make errors, and since some errors are due to characteristics of organizations and the processes they develop to deliver care, the way to prevent many errors and adverse events is to change the systems within which individuals work.

References

1 Vincent C, Taylor-Adams S, Stanhope N. Framework for analysing risk and safety in clinical medicine. *BMJ* 1998;**316**:1154–7.

2 Reason JT. *Human error*. New York: Cambridge University Press, 1990.

3 Kohn LT, Corrigan JM, Donaldson MS, eds. *To err is human*. Washington DC: National Academy Press, 1999.

4 Brennan TA, Leape LL, Laird NM, *et al.* Incidence of adverse events and negligence in hospitalized patients: results of the Harvard Medical Practice Study I. *N Engl J Med* 1991;**324**:370–6.

5 Steel K, Gertman PM, Crescenzi C, Anderson J. Iatrogenic illness on a general medical service at a university hospital. *N Engl J Med* 1981;**304**:638–42.

6 Andrews LB, Stocking C, Krizek T, *et al.* An alternative strategy for studying adverse events in medical care. *Lancet* 1997;**349**:309–13.

7 Mills DH, Boyden JS, Rubamen DS, eds. *Report on the Medical Insurance Study*. San Francisco: Sutter Publications, 1977.

8 Leape LL, Lawthers AG, Brennan TA, Johnson WG. Preventing medical injury. *Qual Rev Bull* 1993;**19**:144–9.

9 Wilson RM, Runciman WB, Gibberd RW, *et al.* The Quality in Australian Healthcare Study. *Med J Aust* 1995;**163**:458–71.

10 Wilson R McL, Harrision BT, Gibberd RW, Hamilton JD. An analysis of the causes of adverse events from the Quality in Australian Healthcare Study. *Med J Aust* 1999;**170**: 411–15.

11 Thomas EJ, Studdert DM, Burstin HR, *et al.* Incidence and types of adverse events and negligent care in Utah and Colorado in 1992. *Med Care* 2000 **38**:261–71.

12 Thomas EJ, Studdert D, Newhouse JP, *et al.* Costs of medical injuries in Colorado and Utah in 1992. *Inquiry* 1999;**36**:255–64.

13 Gawande AA, Thomas EJ, Zinner MJ, Brennan TA. The incidence and nature of surgical adverse events in Colorado and Utah in 1992. *Surgery* 1999;**126**:66–75.

14 Khuri SF, Daley J, Henderson W, *et al.* The National Veterans Administration Surgical Risk Study: risk adjustment for the comparative assessment of the quality of surgical care. *J Am Coll Surg* 1995;**180**:519–31.

15 Khuri SF, Daley J, Henderson W, *et al.* Risk adjustment of the postoperative mortality rate for the comparative assessment of the quality of surgical care: results of the National Veterans Affairs Surgical Risk Study. *J Am Coll Surg* 1997;**185**:315–27.

16 Khuri SF, Daley J, Henderson W, *et al.* Risk adjustment of the postoperative morbidity rate for the comparative assessment of the quality of surgical care: results of the National Veterans Affairs Surgical Risk Study. *J Am Coll Surg* 1997;**185**:328–40.

17 Young GJ, Charns MP, Desai K, *et al.* Patterns of coordination and clinical outcomes: a study of surgical services. *Health Services Res* 1998;**33**:1211–36.

18 Campling EA, Devlin HB, Hoile RW, Lunn JN. *Report of the National Confidential Enquiry into Perioperative Deaths, 1990*. London: National Confidential Enquiry into Perioperative Deaths, 1992.

19 Lunn JN. The National Confidential Inquiry into Perioperative Deaths. *J Clin Monit* 1994;**10**:426–28.

20 Lunn JN. The history and achievements of the National Confidential Enquiry into Perioperative Deaths. *J Qual Clin Pract* 1998;**18**:29–35.

21 O'Connor GT, Plume SK, Olmstead EM, *et al.* A regional intervention to improve the hospital mortality associated with coronary artery bypass graft surgery. *JAMA* 1996;**275**: 841–6.

22 Mangano DT, Goldman L. Preoperative assessment of patients with known or suspected coronary disease. *N Engl J Med* 1995;**333**:1750–6.

23 Mangano DT. Perioperative cardiac morbidity. *Anesthesiology* 1990;**72**:153–84.

24 Fleisher LA, Eagle KA. Screening for cardiac disease in patients having noncardiac surgery. *Ann Intern Med* 1996;**124**:767–72.

25 Lee TH, Marcantonio ER, Mangione CM, *et al.* Derivation and prospective validation of a simple index for prediction of cardiac risk of major noncardiac surgery. *Circulation* 1999;**100**:1043–9.

26 Helmreich RL, Davies JM. Human factors in the operating room: interpersonal determinants of safety, efficiency, and morale. *Baillière's Clinical Anaesthesiology* 1996;**10**:277–95.

27 Gaba DM, Howard SK, Flanagan B, Smith B E, Fish K J, Botney R. Assessment of clinical performance during simulated crises using both technical and behavioral ratings. *Anesthesiology* 1998;**89**:8–18.

28 Bates DW, Cullen DJ, Laird N, *et al.* Incidence of adverse drug events and potential adverse drug events. Implications for prevention. ADE Prevention Study Group. *JAMA* 1995;**274**:29–34.

29 Bates DW, Leape LL, Petrycki S. Incidence and preventability of adverse drug events in hospitalized adults. *J Gen Intern Med* 1993;**8**:289–94.

30 Classen DC, Pestotnik SL, Evans RS, Lloyd JF, Burke JP. Adverse drug events in hospitalized patients. Excess length of stay, extra costs, and attributable mortality. *JAMA* 1997;**277**:301–6.

31 Thomas EJ, Studdert DM, Newhouse JP, *et al.* Costs of medical injuries in Utah and Colorado. *Inquiry* 1999;**36**:255–64.

32 Bates DW, Spell N, Cullen DJ, *et al.* The costs of adverse drug events in hospitalized patients. Adverse Drug Events Study Group. *JAMA* 1997;**277**:307–11.

33 Allan EL, Barker KN. Fundamentals of medication error research. *Am J Hosp Pharm* 1990;**47**:555–71.

34 Ringold DJ, Santell JP, Schneider PJ, Arenberg S. ASHP National Survey of pharmacy practice in acute care settings: Prescribing and transcribing 1998. *Am J Health Syst Pharm* 1999;**56**:142–57.

35 Billings CE. Some hopes and concerns regarding medical event-reporting systems: Lessons from the NASA safety reporting system. *Arch Pathol Lab Med* 1998;**122**:214–15.

36 Runciman WB. Report from the Australian Patient Safety Foundation: Australasia Incident Monitoring Study. *Anaesth Intensive Care* 1989;**17**:1078.

37 Runciman WB, Holland RB. Symposium – The Australian Incident Monitoring Study. *Anaesth Intensive Care* 1993, **5**:502–694.

38 Battles JB, Kaplan HS, Van der Schaaf TW, Shea CE.The attributes of medical event-reporting systems: experience with a prototype medical event-reporting system for transfusion medicine. *Arch Pathol Lab Med* 1998;**122**:231–8.

39 Leape LL, Bates DW, Cullen DJ, *et al.* Systems analysis of adverse drug events. *JAMA* 1995;**274**:35–43.

40 Bates DW, Leape LL, Cullen DJ *et al.* Effect of computerized physician order entry and a team intervention on prevention of serious medication errors. *JAMA* 1998;**280**:1311–16.

41 Evans RS, Pestotnik SL, Classen DC *et al.* A computer-assisted management program for antibiotics and other anti-infective agents. *N Engl J Med* 1998;**338**:232–8.

42 Leape LL, Cullen DJ, Clapp MD *et al.* Pharmacist participation on physician rounds and adverse drug events in the intensive care unit. *JAMA* 1999;**282**:267–70.

43 Cohen MR (ed). *Medication errors.* American Pharmaceutical Association. 1999.

44 Leape LL, Brennan TA, Laird N, *et al.* The nature of adverse events in hospitalized patients. Results of the Harvard Medical Practice Study II. *N Engl J Med* 1991;**324**: 377–84.

45 Cales RH. Trauma mortality in Orange County: the effect of implementation of a regional trauma system. *Ann Emerg Med* 1984;**13**:1–10.

46 Cales RH, Trunkey DD. Preventable trauma deaths. A review of trauma care systems development. *JAMA* 1985;**254**:1059–63.

47 Lowe DK, Gately HL, Goss JR, *et al*. Patterns of death, complication and error in the management of motor vehicle accident victims: implications for a regional system of trauma care. *J Trauma* 1983;**23**:503–9.

48 Shackford SR, Hollingsworth-Fridlund P, Cooper GF, Eastman AB. The effect of regionalization upon the quality of trauma care as assessed by concurrent audit before and after institution of a trauma system; a preliminary report. *J Trauma* 1986;**26**:812–20.

49 Shackford SR, Hollingsworth-Fridlund P, McArdle M, Eastman AB. Assuring quality in a trauma system – the Medical Audit Committee: composition, cost, and results. *J Trauma* 1987;**27**:866–75.

50 West JG, Cales RH, Gazzaniga AB. Impact of regionalization. The Orange County experience. *Arch Surg* 1983;**118**:740–4.

51 Davis JW, Hoyt DB, McArdle MS, *et al*. An analysis of errors causing morbidity and mortality in a trauma system: a guide for quality improvement. *J Trauma* 1992;**32**:660–5.

52 Xiao Y, Hunter WA, Mackenzie CF, *et al*. Task complexity in emergency medical care and its implications for team coordination. LOTAS Group. Level One Trauma Anesthesia Simulation. *Hum Factors* 1996;**38**:636–45.

53 Mackenzie CF, Jefferies NJ, Hunter WA, *et al*. Comparison of self-reporting of deficiencies in airway management with video analyses of actual performance. LOTAS Group. Level One Trauma Anesthesia Simulation. *Hum Factors* 1996;**38**: 623–35.

54 Townsend RN, Clark R, Ramenofsky ML, Diamond DL. ATLS-based videotape trauma resuscitation review: education and outcome. *J Trauma* 1993;**34**:133–8.

55 Santora TA, Trooskin SZ, Blank CA, *et al*. Video assessment of trauma response: adherence to ATLS protocols. *Am J Emerg Med* 1996;**14**:564–9.

56 Sugrue M, Seger M, Kerridge R, *et al*. A prospective study of the performance of the trauma team leader. *J Trauma* 1995;**38**:79–82.

57 Hoyt DB, Shackford SR, Fridland PH, *et al*. Video recording trauma resuscitations: an effective teaching technique. *J Trauma* 1988;**28**:435–40.

58 Michaelson M, Levi L. Videotaping in the admitting area: a most useful tool for quality improvement of the trauma care. *Eur J Emerg Med* 1997;**4**:94–6.

59 Small SD, Wuerz RC, Simon R, *et al*. Demonstration of high-fidelity simulation team training for emergency medicine. *Acad Emerg Med* 1999;**6**: 312–23.

60 Leape LL. Error in medicine. *JAMA* 1994;**272**:1851–7.

61 Perrow C. *Normal accidents: living with high risk technologies*. New York: Basic Books, 1984.

62 Moray N. Error reduction as a systems problem. In: Bogner MS, ed. *Human error in medicine*. Hillsdale, NJ: Erlbaum, 1994.

63 Brennan TA, Berwick DM. *New rules: regulation, markets and the quality of American health care*. San Francisco, CA: Jossey-Bass Inc., Publishers, 1996.

Acknowledgments

Dr. Thomas is a Robert Wood Johnson Foundation Generalist Physician Faculty Scholar.

3 The development of clinical risk management

KIERAN WALSHE

Clinical risk management can be defined or described either in terms of its form or its function – through the processes involved or the outcomes it is intended to produce. For the former, the convention is to conceptualise risk management in three main processes or stages:

- identifying risk,
- analysing risk,
- controlling risk.

Risk is seen in broad terms as exposure to events which may threaten or damage the organisation and its interests, and risk management involves balancing the costs of risk (or the consequences of such exposure) against the costs of risk reduction. To do this, first the risks need to be identified – which can be done by analysing existing data on incidents or undertaking special surveys or assessments of services. Then the risks identified should be analysed, to understand their causes and consequences and establish a quantitative and qualitative assessment. That information is then used to make decisions about how to control the risk, by changing systems to prevent or reduce risk, acting to minimise the consequences, or preparing for the consequences through risk transfer.[1]

In this classical definition of risk management, used widely outside healthcare, the process can be characterised as financially driven and organisation-centred. It is financially driven, in that the costs of risk exposure and risk reduction predominate in decision making and other considerations or issues are therefore less important. It is organisation-centred, in that the process is focused on protecting the organisation and its interests against risk, and the interests or concerns of other stakeholders are not necessarily explicitly recognised. To the outside observer, this way of describing risk management makes it sound as if it has much in common with traditional insurance.

In healthcare, it may be more appropriate to define risk management in terms of its function rather than its form, and to make that function less oriented towards minimising the costs of risk and protecting the organisation itself, and more focused on improving quality and protecting patients.[2] For example, clinical risk management can be seen as one of a number of organisational systems or processes aimed at improving the quality of healthcare, but one which is primarily concerned with creating and maintaining safe systems of care. While the processes may be the same – identifying, analysing and controlling risk – the purpose is quite different. A definition of this form fits more comfortably with the culture and mission of healthcare organisations, especially those in the public sector, and is more likely to secure the support and involvement of clinical professionals because it better reflects their purpose and values. This form of definition makes risk management sound, to the observer, less concerned with insurance and more about improvement.

Clinical risk management has developed rapidly in the British National Health Service (NHS) during the 1990s. This chapter describes and reviews that development, in three main phases. Firstly, it considers why after many years with few if any formal risk management systems in place, it became necessary to develop arrangements for clinical risk management in the early 1990s. It then explores the early development of risk management, from the first national guidance to NHS organisations in 1993 to its establishment in most NHS organisations by 1997. Thirdly, the chapter reviews the quality reforms initiated in 1997, which represent a far reaching attempt to improve clinical performance in the NHS, and examines their impact on and implications for clinical risk management.

The need for clinical risk management

While in some countries such as the United States, systems for risk management in healthcare have been commonplace for two decades or longer,[3] it was not until the late 1980s that such arrangements began to develop in the NHS. Indeed, the last ten years have seen a growth of interest in clinical risk management internationally, with substantial developments in many countries in Europe and elsewhere.

The main impetus for the development of clinical risk management in the United Kingdom has come from the rising incidence and costs of litigation for clinical negligence against healthcare organisations. In 1975 there were about 500 claims a year across the NHS, but by 1992 this had risen to about around 6000 claims per annum.[4] In 1975, the total cost of claims to the NHS was around £1 million but by 1996, claims for clinical negligence cost the NHS about £200 million, and costs were predicted to reach £500 million per annum by 2001.[5] It has been estimated that during the 1980s, the frequency of claims rose fivefold, while the costs of each claim went up by 250%, and the rate of increase in clinical negligence costs for the NHS is expected to continue to be around 25% per annum.[6] Because there have been important changes in the way that the costs of such claims are accounted for, it is not straightforward to make comparisons over time[7] but it is undisputed that costs have climbed rapidly, and look likely to continue to rise for the foreseeable future.

These figures all represent settled or completed claims, and many claims take years to progress from initial claim to settlement. Therefore the future rate of increase in the costs of clinical negligence, over at least the next five years, is already largely determined by claims currently in hand. Estimating the costs of current claims in progress is difficult because of the assumptions that have to be made about whether they will be successful or not, what awards will be made if they are successful, and when that will be, but it has been suggested that these costs amount to between £1 billion and £2 billion. While these costs will be spread across a number of years, they still represent a substantial future commitment of NHS resources.

It is not straightforward to explain the rise in the numbers of claims for clinical negligence against the NHS. In part, it represents a wider trend towards litigiousness in British society (seen, for example, in the explosion of personal injury litigation, in rising settlements in other areas of civil law, and in the increasing use of the courts to challenge the decisions of public bodies and government). It may also result from changes in the civil litigation system, which made it easier for people to gain access to the law for redress, particularly for those who were entitled to legal aid. There may also have been a more subtle change in attitudes towards the NHS, in which people are less inclined to regard it with a special affection because of its history and public service status and so accept its failings, and are more likely to treat it as just another public or private service provider. The rise in the level of awards made in cases of clinical negligence may be easier to explain. It results in part from comparisons with award levels in other areas of civil law, from the courts being more willing to accept a wider definition of damages, but most of all from an increase in the number of large awards made primarily in obstetric cases.

It is very difficult to tell whether the rising level of clinical negligence litigation represents an increase in the level of risk within the NHS, or in the numbers of patients being injured by adverse events. It is recognised that the complexity of systems of care has increased, that the pace of care has been speeded up (with ever shorter lengths of stay and earlier discharges), and that therapeutic advance has created more complex technologies with greater risks as well as benefits. These trends might be expected to result

47

in an increase in the rate of adverse events. Moreover, the volume of care provided within the NHS (measured in terms of the numbers of inpatients and outpatients treated) has continued to rise, and this would result in a concomitant rise in the numbers of adverse events. However, research elsewhere has suggested that there is at best a tenuous link between litigation and adverse events, showing that very few adverse events actually result in litigation, and many instances of litigation are not based on actual adverse events.[8] For all these reasons, it seems unlikely that the rapid rise in claims for clinical negligence owes much to real changes in the underlying risk within the NHS.

However, even at their present levels the costs of clinical negligence litigation to the NHS do not, by themselves, explain the growing recognition of the need for clinical risk management. After all, these costs still only represent about 0·75% of total NHS spending each year, and clinical negligence litigation is focused mainly in a few clinical areas (such as obstetrics, accident and emergency, orthopaedics and gynaecology). In many areas of the NHS, negligence litigation is much rarer or even virtually unknown.

Some of the organisational and structural changes that have taken place in the NHS in recent years have indirectly promoted the development of risk management. For example, the creation of NHS trusts, healthcare providers which are public sector bodies but have a much greater degree of financial independence and freedom than in the past, meant that risks which in the past were shared and borne by the NHS as a whole now fall to individual NHS trusts. The ability of these smaller organisations to carry such risks themselves is much less, and so NHS trusts have needed to find ways to insure or share risk. NHS trusts have also now assumed the whole of the risk associated with clinical negligence – it used to be shared between healthcare providers and individual healthcare professionals who were required to buy their own professional indemnity insurance – and this too has increased their exposure to risk and hence their interest in risk management.

But, as the earlier definition of risk management in healthcare made clear, it should be seen in the healthcare context, and especially in the NHS, as being more about improvement than insurance. Over the last decade we have seen a dramatic growth in the structures and systems in the NHS for quality management and improvement[9] and a radical shift in attitudes towards clinical performance and quality issues. There has been a much greater recognition of the costs and consequences of adverse events, highlighted by this growing attention to the quality of healthcare, and this in itself has promoted the development of risk management. In addition, a series of high profile system failures in which major lapses in the quality of care have resulted in serious injuries to patients have done much to raise public awareness about the risks of healthcare and professionals' and managers' awareness of the need for risk management.[10] The rise of risk management should be seen as part of the wider move within the NHS towards modern and effective systems for quality improvement.

The rise of risk management in England in the 1990s

Until the late 1980s, no NHS organisations had a formal risk management function. Many had some of the components or apparatus of risk management in place – for example, most had some form of incident or accident reporting, many had health and safety committees and advisors, some had clinical pharmacists who collated data on medication errors and reactions, and most had people responsible for managing complaints and litigation. But these components were rarely connected, or made to work together, and there was little ownership at a corporate level of these processes or systems by senior managers and clinicians. The essentials of risk management – linked processes for identifying, analysing and then controlling risk – were definitely not in place.

Brighton Health Authority, on the south coast of England, was probably the first NHS organisation to establish a pilot risk management programme in 1989, and to begin to use more formal systems and approaches to manage risk. Through contacts with healthcare organisations in the USA, and their own experience in pioneering healthcare quality improvement in the UK,[11] senior executives and clinicians undertook a detailed risk assessment, and established a risk management group[12] with some local success. They went on, in partnership with a newly formed risk management consultancy, to share their experiences with a number of other NHS organisations.

In 1992, the Department of Health commissioned risk management consultants to develop a manual or training guide on risk management for the NHS, which was published in 1993, along with an Executive Letter which strongly encouraged NHS trusts to follow the manual's advice[13] and to establish their own arrangements for risk management. The manual provided a basic introduction to the ideas of risk management, and described a methodology for risk assessment, which had been used in two pilot projects in trusts in Essex and Leeds. It then set out a comprehensive analysis of the risks identified in those trusts (see Table 3.1).

The Department of Health's national endorsement of risk management certainly encouraged NHS trusts to take the issue more seriously and raised its profile nationally,[14] and by 1994 many trusts had undertaken initial risk assessments, either using the approach set out in the national risk management manual themselves or bringing in external risk management consultants to help them. But there were still no direct incentives for trusts to invest in risk management, and faced with cost constraints and controls on management costs, few had, for example, established and staffed a risk management function.

49

Table 3.1 Risk areas identified and described in pilot risk assessments in two NHS trusts

Area of risk	Description
Direct patient care risks	Standards of care Information, record keeping and confidentiality Consent to treatment and providing information to patients Working beyond one's competence Failures of communication within the NHS and between the organisation and patients or clients Delays in treatment
Indirect patient care risks	Personal safety, property and other security issues Fire Buildings, plant and equipment Waste collection, management and disposal Control of infection
Health and safety	Statutory obligations and legal implications Safe systems of work – lifting and handling, protective clothing, etc Control of substances hazardous to health Training and supervision of staff Safe work environment and risks to health
Organisational risk	Communication Provision of goods and services and liabilities Finance and insurance Information systems

However, in 1995, the establishment of the Clinical Negligence Scheme for Trusts and the introduction of national standards for risk management made it less a matter for individual trust discretion and more a national requirement that NHS trusts should have such systems in place.

After the introduction of Crown indemnity for clinical negligence in 1990, through which the NHS assumed all liability for clinical negligence in NHS trusts instead of requiring doctors to have their own professional liability insurance, it had been increasingly recognised that NHS trusts could not be expected simply to self-insure. It was clear that one or two major claims could have an enormous impact on a small trust's financial security. The Department of Health had ruled that NHS trusts should not seek commercial insurance for clinical negligence, as it was felt this would be expensive in the longer term. Instead, proposals were drawn up for a national risk-pooling arrangement, the Clinical Negligence Scheme for Trusts (CNST). This scheme would involve NHS trusts joining and paying a subscription based on their size and the clinical areas in which they worked. In return, most of the costs of claims for clinical negligence above a certain threshold (their "excess") would be met by the CNST. The subscriptions would be set each year at a level that covered the costs of claims met and administration for that year. Separate but similar arrangements were put in place to cover existing liabilities – claims that were already in existence before the inception of CNST in 1995.

The Department of Health set up the Clinical Negligence Scheme for Trusts, and then created a new special health authority – the NHS Litigation Authority (NHSLA) – to take charge of it and other matters related to clinical negligence. From the outset, CNST and NHSLA decided that NHS trusts wishing to join the scheme would be asked to meet a set of risk management standards, and those who met the standards would receive a discount on their subscription. Each trust would be assessed against the risk management standards by CNST assessors, and improved performance against higher level standards would be rewarded by increasing subscription discounts. Effectively, CNST and NHSLA had created a national set of risk management standards that NHS trusts were strongly encouraged to follow, and they had put in place financial incentives for good risk management.

Summary of the original CNST risk management standards[15]

- The Board has a written risk management strategy that makes their commitment to managing clinical risk explicit.
- An executive director of the Board is charged with responsibility for clinical risk management.
- The responsibility for management and co-ordination of clinical risk is clear.
- A clinical incident reporting system is operated in all medical specialties and clinical support departments.
- There is a policy for the rapid follow-up of major clinical incidents.
- An agreed system of managing complaints is in place.
- Appropriate information is provided to patients on the risks and benefits of the proposed treatment or investigation, and the alternatives, before a signature on a consent form is sought.
- A comprehensive system for the completion, use, storage and retrieval of medical records is in place; record-keeping standards are monitored through the clinical audit process.
- There is an induction/orientation programme for all new clinical staff.
- A clinical risk management system is in place.
- There is a clear documented system for management and communication throughout the key stages of maternity care.

The CNST's original risk management standards (see above) were relatively simple. For each main standard there was an accompanying series of statements and explanations in the standards manual. Each statement was categorised at either level 1 (the basic or minimum standard for risk management), level 2 (if it was rather more demanding or

Table 3.2 Standard 6 from the CNST standards – managing complaints

	Level 1	Level 2	Level 3
6.1.1 The method of dealing with complaints is clear and meets NHS guidelines	•	•	•
6.2.1 Examples of two changes that reduce risk as a consequence of complaints can be demonstrated		•	•
6.3.1 Examples of five changes that reduce risk as a consequence of complaints can be demonstrated			•

required more action) or level 3 (if it was more demanding still). An example, for standard 6 which concerned managing complaints is shown in Table 3.2.

The CNST risk management standards were not particularly demanding at level 1, but in the first two years of the Scheme only just over 50% of NHS trusts joining were able to comply with them.[15] Although all trusts joining the Scheme were required to undergo assessment, those who did not meet the standard still remained as members. They received no discount on their subscription, but there was no requirement for them to bring their arrangements for risk management in line with the standards in a certain period, or to undergo a further assessment, unless they wished to do so.[16]

Of course, the CNST standards only applied to NHS trusts – not to the primary care sector, in which medical care was provided by general practitioners working as independent contractors either by themselves or in small partnerships. Traditionally, the level of clinical negligence litigation against general medical practitioners had been low, and although costs had risen they had not reached levels which required a change to indemnity arrangements or the creation of a risk-pooling scheme. So while NHS trusts were being encouraged to develop systems for risk management, much less attention was given to primary care providers.

Risk management in NHS trusts: the emerging picture

Research undertaken in 1998[17] demonstrated that most NHS trusts had moved at least some way towards developing the systems for risk management envisaged in the CNST standards, and that some had made rapid progress in establishing risk management as part of their organisation. At that point in time, over 99% of the NHS trusts taking part in the research had a named member of the board who took responsibility for clinical risk management. Usually, this was either the medical director or nursing director, but less commonly the chief executive or another executive director (such as finance, operations or personnel). Nearly three in four trusts (74%) had explicitly mentioned their arrangements for clinical risk management in their current annual business plan, and 83% had discussed risk management at board meetings at least once in the last 12 months. The great majority of NHS trusts (96%) had some form of senior group or committee tasked with leading on clinical risk management across the trust, though the remit and makeup of these groups varied very widely. It seemed that there were relatively robust board level arrangements for clinical risk management in place in most NHS trusts, with clear responsibility assigned to individuals, and senior groups in place tasked with setting a strategic direction.

Risk management: whose job?

Most NHS trusts (85%) also had a nominated individual who took day to day responsibility for clinical risk management across the trust – a clinical risk manager. However, relatively few of the NHS trusts with a nominated individual responsible for clinical risk on a day to day basis (just 11%) had made it that person's sole or primary responsibility. In most trusts (89%) the clinical risk management role was combined with a range of other responsibilities. Frequently, this involved the clinical risk manager in areas like claims management, complaints, non-clinical risk management, or health and safety. Some clinical risk managers were also responsible for areas like quality and clinical audit. For most of them (81%) this was the first job in which they had taken responsibility for managing clinical risk, and most clinical risk managers had two years or less experience. There were, though, some clinical risk managers who had been in their current post for some time (managing, for example, complaints or litigation before they took on the remit for clinical risk). Clinical risk managers were drawn from a wide range of backgrounds. It was striking that most (72%) had some form of clinical qualification – usually, though not always in nursing – and many had backgrounds in managing claims or complaints. But almost 90% of clinical risk managers had no formal qualification related to managing clinical risk. Of course, such qualifications (either in risk management or more specifically in clinical risk management) had not been commonly available in the past.

Though at a trust level there were clearly structures for risk management in place, the embedding of these systems in clinical areas or directorates was less evident. Under half (44%) of NHS trusts had named individuals in each clinical directorate or service area with responsibility for clinical risk. A further 30% of trusts had such nominated leads established in at least some clinical directorates, but almost a quarter (24%) had no such arrangements in place. Only about one in eight NHS trusts (13%) reported that they had some kind of group taking responsibility for clinical risk in all clinical directorates (such as a directorate or departmental risk, audit or quality committee). Almost half (48%) said that such groups existed in at least some clinical directorates, but over a third (36%) had no such groups at all. These results reflected some confusion about what sort of structures or systems were needed at directorate level in trusts to manage clinical risk, and considerable diversity was found not just between but even within NHS trusts – with structures varying from directorate to directorate.

Incident reporting and risk assessment

NHS trusts had made use of two main tools for risk management – incident reporting, and risk assessment. The vast majority of trusts (96%) had some form of system for clinical incident reporting in place. Of those trusts, over three quarters (79%) indicated that their clinical incident reporting systems were being used across all clinical directorates or service areas, with the remainder using incident reporting in some areas only (such as those perceived to be at higher risk than others, like obstetrics or anaesthetics). Every trust involved in incident reporting had some kind of form that clinicians and others were expected to fill in when a clinical incident occurred, though some had different forms for different purposes – for example, for clinical incidents, equipment problems, fire and security incidents, staff accidents/injuries, and so on. Most trusts allowed clinicians to report incidents in other ways, as well as by completing an incident report form, such as by telephone, in person, through email, and via anonymous reports. There was, however, little consensus about what sort of clinical incidents should be reported. Perhaps for this reason, the numbers of incidents being reported varied very widely – the annual total ranged from 2 to 5000, with an average of 803. Most trusts (63%) reported that the numbers of clinical incidents being reported were rising – only 3% thought that numbers of incident reports were falling. But many attributed the rising rate of reports to an increased awareness among clinicians of the need to report clinical incidents, and a greater willingness to do so, rather than to any underlying change in the quality of care.

Trusts captured a substantial set of information about each clinical incident – including details of patients and staff involved, where and when it happened, what the incident was, and often what action had been taken following the incident. All trusts said that someone was responsible for reviewing every incident report – usually the clinical risk manager but sometimes also a manager in the area where the incident occurred. The great majority of trusts (91%) had a system for filtering out the few most serious and urgent incidents and subjecting them to some form of senior clinical and managerial review. Only half of trusts used some form of risk severity scoring to rate all clinical incidents to try to separate the important from the trivial and identify those which needed to be followed up. while only 16% of trusts always provided feedback to the person who reported an incident, on what had happened as a result. About 41% said they usually offered some feedback, and 38% did so sometimes.

In the great majority of trusts, it was the responsibility of the clinical risk manager to produce reports and analyses of clinical incidents. Only about 28% did so every month or more frequently. About 42% said that they produced reports each quarter, and the rest did so even less often than that. Usually, these reports were said to break down incidents either by the directorate in which they had occurred (82%), by the type of incident (82%) or by the frequency with which that sort of incident had happened (59%). About half of trusts (55%) said they produced regular reports on clinical incidents for all their clinical directorates or service areas, but 21% only did so for some directorates, and the rest did not do so at all. There were grounds to believe that more effort was being invested in collecting and managing incident data than in using it to reduce risk or improve quality, and that some trusts collecting large volumes of incident reporting data were making little use of most of it.

Clinical incident reporting is essentially reactive – when something happens, and is reported, then a risk may be identified and dealt with. But it may be unnecessary and undesirable to wait for risks to reveal themselves, and only to take action once some damage may have been done. Clinical risk assessment is a proactive process in which information is collected about an organisation or clinical service in order to identify what clinical risks may exist. Risk assessments may draw on data from clinical incident reporting, but are also likely to use other sources of information like surveys, interviews, and comparative data from elsewhere. In order to meet the more advanced CNST standards (level 2), NHS trusts were required to have carried out a trust-wide clinical risk assessment. The research found that just over half of NHS trusts (56%) had carried out some form of risk assessment in the last twelve months. Where trusts had focused on particular services, they had often been those perceived to be at highest risk of litigation – obstetrics, theatres, orthopaedics and accident and emergency in acute healthcare providers, and mental health services in non-acute NHS trusts. However, there were many other examples of risk assessments in less obvious areas, such as community nursing, learning disabilities, medical physics, sexual health, pharmacy and physiotherapy.

The impact of clinical risk management

Assessing the impact of clinical risk management in the NHS is difficult to do. The impacts that might be anticipated or expected, such as improved quality and safety, reduced levels of risk, the prevention of some adverse events, avoidance of potential litigation and so on, are very difficult to measure. The timescale for such changes may be long, and there may be many other influences or confounding factors. Moreover, because all NHS trusts have embarked on clinical risk management at around the same time, albeit with varying degrees of commitment and progress, it is very difficult to know how much of the change we see is due to systems for clinical risk management and how much might have happened anyway.

The research suggested that NHS trusts had seen some important changes as a result of the development of clinical risk management. Firstly, there had been some impact on the way that cases of clinical negligence are managed. Half of trusts reported that at least some claims had been first identified through their incident reporting arrangements, and they described advantages such as better documentation of events, faster settlement of claims, and damages minimisation which resulted from such advance warning of claims. Secondly, over half (54%) of trusts reported that some clinical audit had been initiated as a result of risk management activities (such as incident reporting and risk assessment). They offered a wide range of examples, concerning both clinical and organisational problems with the quality of care. But thirdly, and most importantly, almost three quarters of NHS trusts (74%) reported that their clinical risk management systems had brought about some changes in clinical practice. Those changes were very varied in nature, and some examples drawn from the research are described opposite.

Many of them concerned either the introduction of new policies, procedures, guidelines or protocols designed to define more clearly the way that care should be managed or delivered. Some also concerned changes to the way information was recorded, designed both to provide a more consistent and complete record and to improve interprofessional communication.

Risk management and the "new NHS" policy agenda

There can be no doubt that between 1995 and 1998, the NHS in England made great progress towards establishing a meaningful clinical risk management function, with both the corporate and organisational commitment and the operational systems needed to begin identifying, analysing and controlling clinical risk. It seems likely that much of that progress has been due to the work of CNST, and particularly to the national risk management standards developed by CNST and promoted for member NHS trusts. The process of external assessment by CNST assessors against these standards, and the existence of a financial incentive to comply with them, have certainly been important in providing both the motivation and the direction needed for the development of clinical risk management in NHS organisations. Throughout this period, the costs of clinical negligence have continued to rise as before, and this too has kept the issues of clinical negligence and clinical risk management on the agenda for NHS trusts.

In 1997, the new British government published a White Paper that set

Examples of changes in practice resulting from clinical risk management in NHS trusts

Use of bed rails and other measures to prevent falls.
Equipment and arrangements for manual handling changed.
Introduction of pre-operative clinics.
Consent practices changed.
Guidance issued on managing/using syringe drivers.
New prescription sheets introduced.
Management of suspected aortic aneurysms in A&E changed.
Training provided for use of tracheostomy tubes.
Move away from use of mercury thermometers.
Specimen labelling and transport tightened up.
Swab counting procedure in theatres improved.
Policy on use of heparin introduced.
X-rays taken in A&E now quickly reviewed by radiologist.
Procedure used for female sterilisation changed.
Syringes labelled when drugs drawn up but not used immediately.
CPR trolleys audited regularly.
Consultant responsible for labour ward identified.
All cardiac monitors changed due to fault.
Better policy for informed consent to treatment.
Development of patient information leaflets that cite risks as well as benefits.
Creation of a pump bank for all infusion pumps used to administer analgesia.
Theatre booking changed – more evenly spaced enabling better use.
Central referral point for "at risk children" with needs of child and *not* the client paramount.
Developed new policy for managing serious untoward events.
Children in A&E now seen by more experienced medical staff only.

out a new and challenging programme of quality reforms for the NHS[18] and marking a new chapter in the development of clinical risk management. Described in more detail in a subsequent consultation document in 1998,[19] these reforms included the establishment of new national mechanisms for setting standards of care, better local systems for delivering standards and improvement, and new arrangements for monitoring quality and performance and acting to deal with known problems or deficiencies. Chapter 4 provides a fuller account of these reforms which, taken together, represent the most radical attempt to date to establish comprehensive systems for quality improvement in the NHS.

The current quality reforms have introduced the concept of "clinical governance". This is defined officially as "a framework through which NHS organisations are accountable for continuously improving the quality of their services and safeguarding high standards of care by creating an environment in which excellence in clinical care will flourish". Clinical governance represents an explicit assertion that NHS organisations are responsible for the quality of clinical care they provide, and that those who lead them must ensure that systems for quality improvement are in place and being used and will be held accountable if they do not. Clinical governance is, in effect, an endorsement of the ideas of whole system quality improvement which have been increasingly influential in healthcare in the UK and elsewhere.[20] It is likely to bring greater investment in systems for quality improvement, including risk management, and to promote the integration of existing rather separate systems (such as risk management, clinical audit, complaints management, and so on) into a more coherent and corporately owned approach to quality improvement.

The reforms also involve major changes to the organisation of primary care – creating primary care groups and eventually primary care NHS trusts, which bring a number of general practices together into a single organisation. There is a striking imbalance between NHS trusts, where risk management is now well established, and primary care, where there is little activity at present. It seems likely that as a more managed form of primary care develops, primary care groups and NHS trusts will begin to develop their systems for risk management, though progress may be rather slower. Primary care NHS trusts will be eligible to join CNST if they wish to do so, and would then be subject to the CNST risk management standards like any other NHS trust.

Conclusions and future directions

From 1993 to 1998, clinical risk management in the NHS went through a period of rapid expansion and growth, as it was transformed from something of a sideline for a few interested clinicians and managers to a core function in most NHS trusts. That pace of development has not been without its costs, as clinicians and managers with limited experience of risk management have been required to put systems in place before they necessarily knew best what was needed or what would work. Nevertheless, it is an impressive achievement. It seems that now we are moving on from that initial phase of rapid expansion, into a more mature period of consolidation and integration.

In consolidating the progress that has been made, more consideration should be given to the effectiveness of the systems of risk management that have been put in place.[14] A great deal of time and resources have been invested in ensuring that NHS trusts comply with the CNST risk management standards, and that those standards have widespread acceptance and high face validity. However, there is little empirical evidence that compliance will result in reduced risk, few clinical negligence claims, improved quality, and so on. More research is needed to evaluate approaches to clinical risk management and systems like incident reporting, so that our future decisions about what risk management arrangements to put in place can be better informed.

There is no doubt that clinical risk management has become established in the NHS largely because of the pressures of litigation for clinical negligence, and few people would argue that such rapid progress would have been made without the stimulus of a litigation crisis. As a result, risk management activities can sometimes seem to be overly concerned with litigation and its consequences for the organisation, and not as focused on quality improvement and patient safety as they might be. Perhaps the real test of maturity in clinical risk management systems and processes is whether they succeed in escaping their origins in negligence and litigation and become real contributors to quality improvement. In the future, our ideas of risk in healthcare might be less immediately concerned with individual instances of suboptimal clinical practice, and more directed at larger and more significant risk issues, such as the safety and reliability of processes of care and the risks associated with routine clinical practice.[21] In other words, risk management might move its attention from the outliers of clinical practice which are often rare, unusual or idiosyncratic cases from which little can be learnt, to the mainstream of clinical practice where even small changes might make a substantial difference to the quality of care for many patients.

As the definition with which this chapter commenced made clear, clinical risk management is just one facet of quality improvement. In the future, the connections between clinical risk management and other systems for quality improvement need to be made more explicit and meaningful. The rather separate development of clinical risk management to date has probably been helpful in allowing the rapid progress referred to above. However, isolated systems of clinical risk management may be rather ineffective, because the information that is collected about clinical risks does not get used properly in quality improvement activities to change clinical practice. The concept of clinical governance is predicated on this idea of greater integration, in which current rather disparate and stand-alone systems of quality improvement are brought together to create a coherent whole which is more than the sum of its parts. By linking existing data and information systems, and joining up quality improvement staff and other resources, a more robust and effective approach to quality improvement incorporating clinical risk issues can be created. In the future, this may mean that the risk management function in NHS organisations becomes less separately identifiable than it has been up to now, but more effective in achieving quality improvements.

References

1 Dickson G. Principles of risk management. *Qual Healthcare* 1995;4:75–9.
2 Vincent C. Risk, safety, and the dark side of quality. *BMJ* 1997;314:1775–6.
3 Mills DH, von Bolschwing GE. Clinical risk management: experiences from the United States. In: Vincent C, ed. *Clinical risk management* (1st edition). London: BMJ Publishing Group, 1995.
4 Dingwall R, Fenn P. Risk management: financial implications. In: Vincent C, ed. *Clinical risk management* (1st edition). London: BMJ Publishing Group, 1995.
5 NHS Executive. FDL(96)39. *Clinical negligence costs*. London: NHS Executive, 1996.
6 Evans D. Where next for the hospital clinical claims manager? *Clin Risk* 1998;4:66–8.
7 Towse A, Danzon P. Medical negligence and the NHS: an economic analysis. *Health Econ* 1999;8:93–101.
8 Harvard Medical Practice Study. *Patients, doctors and lawyers: medical injury, malpractice litigation and patient compensation in New York*. Harvard College, 1990.
9 Taylor D. Quality and professionalism in health care: a review of current initiatives in the NHS. *BMJ* 1996;312:626–9.
10 Smith R. All changed, changed utterly. British medicine will be transformed by the Bristol case [editorial]. *BMJ* 1998;316(7149):1917–18.
11 Walshe K, Lyons C, Coles J, Bennett J. Quality assurance in practice: research in Brighton Health Authority. *Intern J Health Care Qual Assur* 1991;4(2):27–35.
12 Bowden D. Risk management in the health service. *Health Serv Manage* 1993;89(5): 10–12.
13 EL(93)111. *Risk management in the NHS*. London: Department of Health, 1993.
14 Mant J, Gatherer A. Managing clinical risk: makes sense but does it work? *BMJ* 1994;308:1522–3.
15 NHS Litigation Authority. *CNST risk management standards and procedures: manual of guidance*. Bristol: NHSLA, 1997.
16 Sanderson IM. The CNST: a review of its present function. *Clin Risk* 1998;4:35–43.
17 Walshe K, Dineen M. *Clinical risk management: making a difference?* Birmingham: NHS Confederation, 1998.
18 Department of Health. *The new NHS: modern, dependable*. London: HMSO, 1997.
19 Department of Health. *A first class service: quality in the new NHS*. London: Department of Health, 1998.
20 Berwick D. A primer on leading the improvement of systems. *BMJ* 1996;312:619–22.
21 Walshe K, Sheldon TA. Dealing with clinical risk: implications of the rise of evidence-based healthcare. *Public Money and Management* 1998;18(4):15–20.

4 Clinical governance: the context of risk management

JONATHAN SECKER-WALKER, LIAM DONALDSON

For most of the 51 years of the existence of the National Health Service (NHS) in Britain, the quest for improved quality has been a fragmented affair. In the early days it rested on the notion of improving health facilities, supplying well trained staff and enabling them to deliver a service which was presumed to be inherently of a generally high standard. In the 1960s and 1970s, quality improvement initiatives, such as medical audit, were largely uniprofessional activities and, even then, were by no means comprehensive. There were few examples of where they contributed to corporate quality strategies within individual health organisations.

The late 1980s and early 1990s saw a major change of emphasis. Medical and later clinical audit became a requirement[1] for hospital doctors working in the NHS. Hospitals and community health services became managed organisations bringing clearer accountability for results, and hence a more critical focus on the performance of services.[2] The concept of clinical effectiveness[3] gained widespread acceptance within the health professions, and stimulated activity in producing guidelines and protocols to improve clinical decision-making.[4] The repeated observation that the benefits of research were slow to become part of routine practice[5] yielded to an evidence-based medicine movement,[6] with its origins in North America. It rapidly became international in its application.

Despite these developments, which strengthened the attention which the NHS gave to the quality of the services it provided, by the mid-1990s, there was still no unifying concept or system to drive progress comprehensively. It was not until 1998, with the new Labour Government's White Paper on the NHS, that this development came.[7] The 1999 Health Act introduced, for the first time, a statutory duty on NHS trusts and primary care trusts to assure and improve the quality of healthcare that they deliver. In practice, this duty will be met by the implementation of clinical governance.

In this chapter, we describe the concept of clinical governance, discuss how it can be implemented and developed within a health organisation, and describe how it sets the context for clinical risk management.

Clinical governance: a unifying quality concept

Clinical governance aims to produce within every health organisation a structure and systems to assure and improve the quality of clinical services. Clear accountability is placed on the Chief Executive of the health organisation, underpinned by a statutory duty of quality on provider organisations.

Clinical governance is defined as:

"A framework through which NHS organisations are accountable for continuously improving the quality of their services and safeguarding high standards of care by creating an environment in which excellence in clinical care will flourish."[8]

The prevention of service failure

The introduction of clinical governance came at a time of increasing publicity and public concern about serious service failures. Such occurrences had attracted extensive media coverage in the past. For example, in the 1980s, concern about the Birmingham bone tumour service led to an inquiry that demonstrated service failings. This in turn led to the misdiagnosis of cancer and, in some cases, to patients having radical surgery unnecessarily.[9] However, during the 1990s, instances of patients suffering harm as a result of the poor performance of services or of individual practitioners led to heightened public concern. A specific instance of this were the serious questions raised over standards of care in the Bristol Children's Heart Surgery Service,[10] events which undoubtedly represent a watershed in public and professional attitudes to such matters in Britain.

The prevention of service failure is only one of the products of successful clinical governance. Indeed, it might be argued that, because they are relatively uncommon, service failures should not receive undue emphasis. However, such events can have a major impact on the lives of individual patients and their families, sometimes a catastrophic impact, as illustrated by some of the very large medical negligence settlements that have occurred. Moreover, well-publicised service failure has the potential to damage public confidence in services: for example, failings in women's cancer screening programmes[11] are bound to be of concern to women considering whether to take up such services.

There has been little systematic study of the reasons why health services fail, aside from the work of investigations and inquiries into specific incidents. This is in contrast to other sectors where "disasters and crises" is an established field of research.[12]

Experience suggests that a cycle of prevention in the NHS (Figure 4.1) would be weak at most points.

- Problems are often formally recognised only when there is a major incident but may have been known on informal networks for years.[13]
- Methodologies for organisational analysis are not well developed.[14]
- Short-term corrective action is usually put in place but may not be sustained.
- There are problems in dealing with the aftermath of service failure which often compound the sense of grievance of the victims and their families.

Most importantly, the recognition that service failures are most often due to systems malfunctioning, as well as individuals under-performing,[15] is the underpinning philosophy for risk management.

Much more needs to be done to build up the evidence base to understand what makes health organisations fail, as well as how to recognise and correct

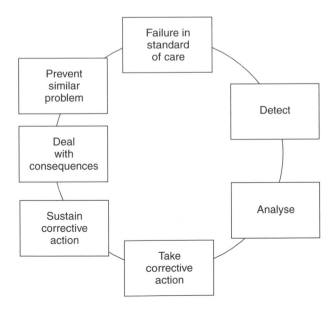

Figure 4.1 Cycle of prevention.

a failure prone environment. Similarly, much more needs to be learned from the approach to understanding errors in medicine in the most technical and high risk areas of healthcare (for example, cardiothoracic surgery).[16]

Learning from good practice

Clinical governance also seeks to create health organisations that are able to routinely adopt good practice. It is fundamentally inequitable that in a national health service, demonstrable benefit to patients gained from innovation in a service in one part of the country, can be denied to patients in other parts of the country simply because mechanisms for systematic learning do not exist.

A learning network was launched in the NHS in 1999[17] aimed at promoting the spread of good practice in service delivery and management. It aims to make more information available on services that have achieved practical improvements in the care of patients, so that other staff and services can learn from such experience. Amongst the elements of this system are Specialist Learning Centres, which have demonstrated major innovation and excellence in particular aspects of healthcare quality improvement and which can be visited by other services. In addition, nearly 300 sites in the NHS were identified as Beacon Services in 1999 for demonstrating excellence in particular aspects of care (for example, mental health, reduction of waiting times, cancer services). Further, a Learning Zone has been created on the NHS Web that contains a database of service delivery practice and benchmarking data.

The emphases of these learning activities are around whole services or organisations. Better clinical decision-making is also a key element of the process of improving the quality of healthcare. Action here tends to be focused more on the individual and clinical team and be derived from the philosophy of evidence based medicine.[6] Part of good clinical governance, therefore, is to ensure that health organisations develop the information systems, the infrastructure and the training to enable access and use of research evidence to become part of routine clinical practice.

Transforming health organisations

The organisational transformation required to achieve successful clinical governance is a major one, with an emphasis on establishing clear accountability and leadership at all levels, a positive culture in which education and research are valued, an emphasis on teamwork, and much greater involvement of patients and users in the process of quality improvement than has been the case in the past.

In 1999, every health organisation in the NHS[18] was required to:

- establish leadership, accountability and working arrangements for clinical governance
- carry out a baseline assessment of capacity and capability
- formulate and agree a development plan in the light of this assessment
- clarify arrangements for reporting progress and future plans, both internally and publicly, in the organisation's annual report.

National structures

The new duty of quality, which finds its expression through local clinical governance, is supported and reinforced by the other key components of a wider government strategy for NHS quality improvement. The new National Institute for Clinical Excellence (NICE) and National Service Frameworks (NSFs) provide mechanisms for setting clear and authoritative quality standards. Modern professional self-regulation and lifelong learning will underpin clinical governance locally. The Commission for Health Improvement (CHI) and a new NHS Performance Assessment Framework have been developed as effective, quality-focused monitoring mechanisms. The Commission will look explicitly at local performance in implementing clinical governance as a key component of its rolling review programme, and failure to abide by the standards likely to be required by the CHI will prove a significant risk for board members and managers of trusts. Health authorities, primary care groups and trusts commissioning for care are likely to take the Commission's findings into account. Progress in implementing clinical governance has been established as a prerequisite for primary care groups to progress to primary care trust status.

Accountability

The legislation underpinning clinical governance places on the boards of NHS provider organisations a duty[18] of ensuring that the quality of care is regularly monitored with the same rigour as the health organisation's financial regime. To be able to fulfil this statutory role the chief executive will need to be assured that he or she is provided with regular information relating to the complex clinical environment. In an NHS trust, this organisational accountability for the quality of care, cascades down the organisation from the chief executive, through the medical director and director of nursing, to clinical directors and directorate managers. There is thus a clear and fairly simple chain of delegated autonomy downwards, and an equally straightforward path of responsibility upwards. The links between organisational accountabilities for quality and professional accountabilities through the regulatory bodies are also being clarified, for example with the publication for consultation of new proposals for dealing with issues of poor clinical performance.[19]

The absence of clear accountability for safety was a feature of disasters in other sectors in the United Kingdom (for example, the *Herald of Free Enterprise* sinking). The significance of this is that it will no longer be advisable, as a clinical director, to know that something is wrong without attempting to rectify it or, if the directorate cannot resolve the problem, to alert the next management level up.

Organisational structures

The health organisation board and chief executive need to be confident that clinical quality is monitored and that they are provided with regular reports to warn of problems or deficiencies, in much the same way that monthly financial reports are scrutinised.

It is difficult to monitor quality without a standard against which to measure. Many NHS trusts have no formal mechanism for agreeing and setting trust-wide clinical policy. Individual directorates may work to guidelines – for instance, the agreed treatment of asthma in young adults. Often these guidelines fail to cross directorate boundaries to reach, for example, such as orthopaedic or mental health patients who happen to suffer from asthma. New primary care organisations face particular challenges given both their formative state and the added complexities of independent contractor status.

NHS trusts and primary care trusts will be assessed by the CHI on their adherence to guidelines to be produced by NICE and to standards set in National Service Frameworks. Furthermore, unjustifiable departure from some national guidelines may lead to difficulties in mounting a legal defence[20] in allegations of clinical negligence. Guidelines will, therefore, need to be formally accepted (or rejected if there are particular reasons), adopted and then widely publicised by organisations to form local protocols. Key elements of clinical governance therefore will be clinical policy setting and clinical policy monitoring.[21]

Clinical governance leads and the clinical governance committee

All NHS bodies need to have in place mechanisms to enable these functions of clinical policy setting and clinical policy monitoring to be delivered. The reasons for clear lines of accountability have already been discussed. NHS organisations must have in place a lead clinician who is responsible to the chief executive for the implementation of clinical governance. This individual can be from any clinical discipline, but the most important factors are that he or she should command the respect of clinicians at all levels within the organisation and have the support and backing of the chief executive and the board. In particular, clinical governance is not solely a medical activity; it is for all health professions with nursing in particular having a key leadership role.

Within a NHS Trust, the process of clinical governance implementation must be supported by a dedicated committee of the board. This committee will provide a focus for the component parts of clinical governance within an organisation. It is responsible for gathering data, which may come from existing committees, such as risk management, complaints, claims and other information sources or from other mechanisms established in the trust. Models will vary from organisation to organisation, but the principle should be that the committee should have access to, and act on, all relevant information impacting on the clinical services of the NHS body. It needs to monitor both the vertical implementation of clinical quality through the directorates and the horizontal issues exposed by its supporting mechanisms reflecting activity across the Trust (e.g. diagnostic testing).

The clinical governance committee should co-ordinate the work of a wide range of groups within the organisation, including clinical governance teams, drug and therapeutic committees, and complaints data. It may be chaired by the trust's lead clinician for clinical governance, or by another executive or non-executive board member. Many NHS trusts have already subdivided the task. An example of this is reflected in the structure illustrated in Figure 4.2.

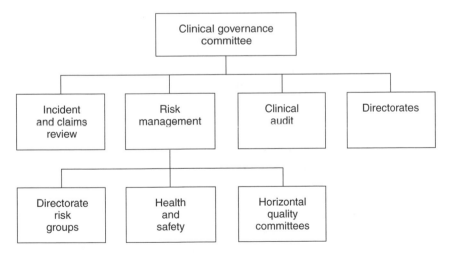

Figure 4.2 Clinical governance committee.

Such a structure will suit some organisations, but others will need to think carefully about the most appropriate structure for them. What ever that structure turns out to be, it must bring together the component parts into a sensible whole that enables the board through its committee to undertake its duty of quality.

The clinical governance committee can provide a mechanism for drawing together information from a wide range of sources to form a broad-based picture of service quality across the whole organisation. For example, Royal College reports on junior staff training, reports of Health and Safety Executive inspections, post-graduate deans' visits and accreditation visits to pathology laboratories would all yield valuable external feedback on the quality of services.

It should also act as a forum for clinical policy setting, bringing together work from parts of the organisation to learn from and disseminate good practice. It will need to ensure that national standards set through NICE and NSFs are being effectively implemented within the organisation and that there is coherence in the ways in which clinical treatment is provided to patients. It will need to work across many of the organisation's functions to ensure that clinical governance is properly implemented. For example, it will need to understand the organisation's approach to information technology, to training and education and to other key functions such as research and development. The committee must therefore aid its board in the setting of its strategic agenda – its policy for clinical services, as well as monitoring effective service delivery.

Clinical information and information technology

Clinical governance makes effective clinical systems a major priority and provides a specific focus for their development. Most NHS information has, up until now, been used in the contracting process and, in many organisations, the emphasis has not been on the use of clinical information for clinical care – indeed many clinicians are unaware of the data that is available on their work. Current systems in secondary care can only judge outcomes in terms of discharge or death (and that only if it occurs in hospital). Rates of medication error or post-operative infection may or may not be entered onto the dataset, depending on the quality of the written notes and the time that the coding staff have to enter codes that are not compulsory. Primary care information systems have tended to focus principally on prescribing activity. Outside specific national audit projects, attempts to benchmark between organisations have been severely limited by the quality of available information. A comprehensive information strategy was launched in the NHS in 1998, which has at its heart an electronic patient record.[22]

Role of the individual doctor

In 1998, the General Medical Council published its new guidelines[23] on Good Medical Practice and Maintaining Good Medical Practice, and sent a copy to each registered doctor. These documents are more comprehensive than previous advice and lay explicit individual responsibilities on medical staff, strongly supporting the philosophy of clinical governance. Clinicians individually are responsible and accountable for their clinical practice; to this end they must ensure that they have the appropriate skills to deliver care safely and therefore ensure that their continuous professional development programme is aimed at the maintenance or acquisition of new skills if these are required.

Over time, appraisal for all staff will be the cornerstone of good clinical governance and professional self-regulation. Whilst nurses and junior doctors are familiar with regular appraisal, older doctors will find this a strange new world, and the culture change required should not be underestimated, but the potential benefits for individuals in both primary and secondary care and the organisations themselves are enormous.

Risk management

Risk reduction programmes and critical incident reporting make up some of the main components of clinical governance described in the consultation document *A First Class Service*.[8]

Several studies suggest that, whilst the rate of negligent accidents appears to affect around 1% of inpatients, the overall rate of injuries or adverse outcomes as a result of medical or clinical management – and therefore the extra cost – is considerably greater (see Chapter 2). A pilot investigation similar to the New York State and Australian studies of adverse events (see Chapter 2) has been carried out in England. This pilot study found that 10% of patients admitted to hospital had sustained an adverse event. Each adverse event led to an average of seven extra days in hospital.[24]

Clear evidence that risk management in healthcare institutions improves quality and reduces the number of accidents to patients is hard to come by. However hospitals in Maryland that had implemented programmes relating to physician and nurse responsibilities in quality assurance and risk management, have been shown by Morlock[25] to reduce both the number of claims and the quantum awarded. Workplace risks to staff and the public are covered by health and safety legislation. Meeting the standards required by the Central Negligence Scheme for Trusts in England or the Welsh Risk Pool which are intended to improve patient safety, has the advantage of reducing premiums.

Staff working at the front-line in hospital or in primary care are a valuable and informed source of knowledge about risks in their area, and the collection of information about such perceived risks through an incident reporting system is impossible without the assistance of all staff. Monitoring of incidents depends on staff reporting organisational process failures as well as their own errors. It provides essential data for directorate managers and for clinical governance leads. However, comprehensive systems of incident reports do not exist in the present NHS. If they are to be developed there are fundamental issues to be resolved such as how to create a reporting culture and practical matters such as how to standardise definitions, how to synthesise and disseminate findings and how to implement change (see Chapter 22). In order to capture environmental and organisational issues the definition of an adverse event will need to become broader than that used by Leape and Brennan.[26]

Clinicians who have been involved in an accident involving a patient will recognise that it was seldom a single isolated event but a constellation of numerous factors, many outside the clinician's control, that ultimately led to the error. Reason[27] quotes Mr Justice Sheen's report[28] into the capsizing of the *Herald of Free Enterprise* in 1987. This highlights the distinction between active human failures – the sailor who did not shut the bow doors – and latent human failures – the inadequate organisational policies or inappropriate decisions that sculpted the environment in which active failures were more likely to thrive. These latent human failures can be likened to resident pathogens just biding their time for appropriate conditions in which to strike (see Chapter 1).

Making the link between risk management and human factors research into industrial, transport or medical accidents, appears to persuade sceptical clinicians to support concepts and methods of managing risk. For many years, aviation has learnt detailed lessons after investigation of its disasters and near-misses to make flying safer; healthcare could use incident analysis to achieve the same end. In fact, this could be considered to be its most important facet, for it enables the organisation as well as the individual to learn from events to enhance safety and the quality of care in the future.

Clinical audit

Since its inception in 1989, clinical audit has not achieved all that was expected of it and it is an essential component of clinical governance and a requirement for clinical practice set by the General Medical Council.[23] Nevertheless it is likely that the nature of audit will alter from being "clinician-led", for example, projects suggested by the directorate and often needed by junior staff to satisfy their training requirements, to a "service-led" method by which the organisation satisfies itself that appropriate areas are being targeted and that particular policies or guidelines are being followed. For instance, a trust might wish to ensure that night-time operating was on appropriate patients and being undertaken by staff of sufficient seniority.

Claims and complaints review

The positive management of clinical incidents, complaints and actual civil legal actions brought against a Trust is an integral part of the risk management process. Management of such events serves four purposes.

- It saves considerable sums of money by assembling material evidence and witness statements as close in time to the incident as possible.
- It can obtain swift resolution of complaints or early settlement with claimants where clinical care is considered to be below standard, preferably before both sides' lawyers get involved.
- Where necessary, by getting early expert opinion, it empowers lawyers acting for the trust to fight unwarranted claims forcefully, thereby reducing the frequency of going to court.
- It reduces the trauma to patients and staff of the litigation process.

Some trusts have developed a mechanism to take an early view of the standard of care delivered after a patient accident, claim or complaint and then make a decision about a satisfactory resolution of the problem. Because swift resolution of appropriate cases depends on early warning from incident reporting by staff that an error has occurred, it is very important that the risk manager and the complaints and litigation officers work closely together.

The effective management of complaints is of prime importance in an organisation committed to improvement in the quality of care. The manner in which a complaint is received, and the speed and integrity with which issues are addressed contribute to the perception of the organisation by users of its services, members of staff and the wider community. Key areas for attention in any complaints system will include:

- Ease of access and ease of use for complainants.
- Ensuring particular groups are not disadvantaged.
- Improved training for complaints managers.
- Local resolution to be the aim.
- Consistency of approach.
- Clear process for dealing with multi-agency complaints.
- Better feedback for complainants and staff.
- Educating the public and their advocates.
- Good practice should be disseminated.

Clinical governance requires that the health organisation can be assured that complaints' management is satisfactory and that the organisation has a mechanism of learning lessons from complaints.[29]

Conclusion

Clinical governance is a cornerstone of the modernisation agenda of the NHS. It aligns professional and organisational responsibilities and priorities, and provides a means of translating the national drive for improved clinical quality into better services for patients. The components that make up the means to deliver clinical governance are already available and in use in many NHS organisations, and a large part of the task is to co-ordinate and develop them. This chapter has not sought to discuss regular appraisal for all clinical staff, continuing development plans or revalidation since these relate to staff training and development. Yet they will be crucial in underpinning the delivery of clinical governance locally.

References

1 Department of Health. *Medical audit in the hospital and community services*. Health Circular 91(2). London: HMSO, 1991.
2 Griffiths R. *NHS Management enquiry*. London: DHSS, 1983.
3 Department of Health. *Improving clinical effectiveness*. London: DoH, 1993. (Executive Letter: EL(93)115.)
4 Grimshaw JM, Russell IT. Effect of clinical guidelines on medical practice: a systematic review of rigorous evaluations. *Lancet* 1993;**342**:1317–22.
5 Eddy DM. Clinical policies and the quality of clinical practice. *N Engl J Med* 1982;**307**: 343–7.
6 Evidence-based Medicine Working Group. Evidence-based medicine: a new approach to teaching the practice of medicine. *JAMA* 1992;**268**:2420–5.
7 Department of Health. *The new NHS: modern, dependable*. London: HMSO, 1997.
8 Department of Health. *A First Class Service: quality in the new NHS*. London: DoH, 1998 (Health Service Circular: HSC(98)113.)
9 Malcolm AJ. *Enquiry into the bone tumour service based at the Royal Orthopaedic Hospital*. Birmingham: Birmingham Health Authority, 1995.
10 Smith R. Regulation of doctors and the Bristol inquiry. Both need to be credible to both the public and doctors. *BMJ* 1998;**317**:1539–40.
11 NHS Executive (South Thames). *Review of cervical cancer screening services at Kent and Canterbury hospitals*. London: NHS Executive, 1997.
12 Toft B, Reynolds S. *Learning from disasters: a management approach* (2nd edition), Leicester, Perpetuity Press, 1997.
13 Donaldson LJ. Doctors with problems in an NHS workforce. *BMJ* 1994;**308**:127–82.
14 Donaldson LJ, Gray JAM. Clinical governance: a quality duty for health organisations. *Qual Health Care* 1988;7(suppl 1):S37–S44.
15 Donaldson LJ. Medical mishaps: a managerial perspective. In: Rosenthal MM, Mulcahy L, Lloyd-Bostock S, eds. *Medical mishaps: pieces of the puzzle*. Buckingham, Open University Press, 1999.
16 De Leval, MR, François K, Bull C, *et al*. Analysis of a cluster of surgical failures. *J Thoracic Cardiovasc Surg* 1994;**107**:914–24.

17 NHS Executive. *NHS Magazine* 1999, Issue No 17. Leeds: Atlas Public Relations Ltd.
18 Department of Health. *Clinical governance: quality in the new NHS.* London: DoH, 1999 (Health Service Circular: HSC(99)065.)
19 Department of Health. *Supporting doctors, protecting patients.* London: DoH, 1999.
20 Bolitho v City and Hackney Health Authority [1998] 9 Med LR 29.
21 Lugon M, Secker-Walker J. Organisational framework for clinical governance In: Lugon M and Secker-Walker J, ed. *Clinical governance; making it happen.* London: RSM Press, 1999.
22 NHS Executive. *Information for health.* Leeds: NHS Executive, 1998.
23 *Good medical practice.* London: GMC, 1998.
24 *An organisation with memory: learning from adverse events in the NHS.* London: The Stationery Office, 2000.
25 Morlock LL, Malitz FE. Do hospital risk management programs make a difference?: relationships between risk management programme activities and hospital malpractice claims experience. *Law Contemp Problems* 1991;**54**:1–22
26 Leape LL, Brennan TA, Laird N *et al.* The nature of adverse events in hospitalised patients. Results of the Harvard Practice Study II. *N Engl J Med* 1991;**324**:377–84.
27 Reason JT. Understanding adverse events: human factors. In: Vincent CA, ed. *Clinical risk management.* London: BMJ Publications, 1995.
28 Sheen J. *MV Herald of Free Enterprise.* Report of court No 8074 formal investigation. London: Department of Transport, 1987
29 Hobbs S. Learning from complaints. In: Lugon M, Secker-Walker J, ed. *Clinical governance; making it happen.* London: RSM Press, 1999.

PART II: REDUCING RISK IN CLINICAL PRACTICE

5 Reducing risk in obstetrics

JAMES DRIFE

Obstetrics is an unusual specialty. Its core business is a physiological process which usually ends successfully without medical intervention. When it does not, however, the consequences can be disastrous – medically, emotionally and financially. The risks involved in pregnancy and childbirth have changed over the years and are continually being reassessed. The important question of how these risks are perceived by professionals, consumers and policymakers remains poorly researched. Within the NHS, obstetricians are mainly concerned with complicated pregnancies, while midwives deal mainly with normal pregnancy and childbirth: it is almost inevitable that these two groups of professionals will have different perceptions of risk. Consumers' perceptions are affected by many factors including personal or family experience and information given in the media and at childbirth preparation classes. The same probably applies to policymakers' perceptions, which are the least researched of all.

Partly because of these differences, the relationship between obstetricians and midwives has not always been easy. The post-feminist era renewed some of the old antagonisms but by the end of the 1990s there was again a spirit of co-operation. In 1999, for the first time, the Royal College of Midwives and the Royal College of Obstetricians and Gynaecologists (RCOG) produced a joint document on risk reduction in childbirth. *Towards Safer Childbirth* is a landmark statement about the management of labour in UK hospitals.[1]

General practitioners take part in antenatal and postnatal care but only a few want to be involved in labour and delivery. This may limit the options available to some women. In 1994 a government expert report, *Changing*

Childbirth, recommended that women should have more choice in maternity care.[2] The number choosing home delivery remains low but some health authorities are planning a return to "midwife led" units which may be distant from obstetric units. This is viewed with apprehension by many obstetricians. On the other hand, during the 1990s hospital delivery was associated with a sharp rise in caesarean section rates and this is viewed with equal apprehension by consumer groups, who suggest that it is due to flawed perceptions of risk.

Reducing risk in obstetrics therefore raises complex questions about how risks are measured and perceived. On a practical level, however, there is ample evidence that errors occur in obstetric units. Risk reduction requires identification and analysis of the patterns of such errors, followed by improvements in clinical practice focused on the problem areas.[3] In obstetrics this process has been under way for some time.

Consumers' expectations

In developed countries like the UK the risks of childbirth are very different from those faced by most of the world's women. In Britain almost all mothers now survive pregnancy, as do 99% of babies. Safety is a recent phenomenon, however, in historical terms. Between 1935 and 1985 the UK maternal mortality rate fell from 1 in 200 pregnancies to 1 in 10 000, and the perinatal mortality rate from 60 per thousand to under 10 per thousand. These dramatic improvements have led to a change in people's expectations. Women and their partners now want childbirth to be an emotionally rewarding experience. Safety is still a top priority but is almost taken for granted.

Women also know that caesarean section is no longer an operation fraught with risk, and for some women "choice" means freedom to request a caesarean delivery. A Scottish survey in 1994 suggested that 7·7% of caesarean sections were done because of maternal request.[4] Consumer groups have blamed obstetricians for the rise in Britain's caesarean section rate, which is now above 20% in some hospitals, but it is becoming clearer that the reasons for this rise are complex and that the threshold for caesarean section has fallen for both women and obstetricians.[5] Most pregnant women are unwilling to tolerate small risks that seem acceptable to obstetricians[6] and the same applies to their partners.

Litigation

Increasing public expectations lead to increasing litigation when these expectations are not met. In the 1980s obstetrical and gynaecological claims accounted for nearly 20% of the workload of the Medical Protection

Society and 23·7% of total settled claims to the Medical Defence Union.[7] These proportions have probably altered little and may even have increased since Crown Indemnity was introduced in 1990, but Health Authorities and NHS Trusts have yet to build up significant experience of these patterns.

Obstetric cases may involve very large settlements. A child who requires constant nursing may be awarded over a million pounds in damages, and the resultant publicity may encourage other people towards litigation. Such large awards give the impression of serious clinical incompetence but a case may in fact be settled because of a minor lapse in care.

The current pattern of care

Pregnancy care can be divided into three parts – antenatal, intrapartum and postnatal. Until very recently obstetric involvement in these areas has not reflected a policy of risk reduction. The reverse was the case, with consultant involvement being concentrated on antenatal care.

Antenatal care

Antenatal care is usually shared between hospital, general practitioner and community midwife. Clinic visits are monthly in the first two-thirds of pregnancy and more frequent thereafter, so a healthy woman may make more than a dozen visits to the clinic. This naturally raises her expectations that conscientious attendance will be rewarded by a trouble-free labour, but this is by no means always the case. The traditional number of antenatal visits can safely be reduced,[8] though this may cause women some anxiety.

At each visit the woman is checked for complications such as diabetes and hypertension. Fetal growth is assessed by palpation of the abdomen, though this misses about 25% of cases of growth retardation. The fetal condition can be more accurately checked by cardiotocography, ultrasound measurements and blood flow assessment. These require the mother to spend time in the ultrasound or fetal assessment unit and they are used only for high-risk cases.

Care in labour

Almost all British babies are born in NHS hospitals, and around 70% are delivered by midwives. Home delivery accounts for less than 1% and private obstetric practice for very few. Intrapartum care is crucially important to risk reduction but is often provided by staff under stress because of limited resources and minimal consultant support.

Fetal monitoring during labour

The fetal condition in labour is assessed through the fetal heart rate, auscultated by the midwife every fifteen minutes. She also observes the colour of the amniotic fluid, which is normally clear but turns green if the fetus releases meconium (bowel contents) – a possible sign of lack of oxygen. This is one of the reasons for artificial rupture of the membranes early in labour, though some women refuse this as they feel it makes labour unnatural. Abnormalities of the fetal heart rate or amniotic fluid are the traditional signs of "fetal distress" – a term which lacks a precise definition.

Electronic fetal monitoring (EFM) has been in widespread use for nearly 30 years and involves continuous recording of the fetal heart rate. Signs of fetal distress are reduced heart-rate variability, a rate that is too fast or too slow, or decelerations that are not synchronous with uterine contractions.[9]

These abnormalities, however, are not diagnostic of fetal distress, and there is a high level of inter-observer variation among obstetricians.[9,10] Even with the most sinister abnormalities there is only a 50% chance that the fetus is suffering oxygen deprivation. Thus if EFM is the sole guide to fetal condition, unnecessary caesarean sections or instrumental deliveries will be done. EFM was intended as a screening test to decide which babies should be assessed by fetal blood sampling (FBS), which allows more direct estimation of the amount of oxygen in the blood. Even when lack of oxygen is accurately diagnosed by FBS, however, only a small minority of affected babies will develop long-term problems.[11]

FBS is more difficult than EFM: it involves inserting a tubular instrument through the cervix, collecting a blood sample and analysing it in a machine that must be carefully maintained. Not every unit that uses EFM has access to FBS and in those that do, it is not always used. In a Plymouth study of 30 caesarean sections for fetal distress, 17 were not preceded by FBS: in 10 cases this was for sound reasons but in the other seven there was "overhasty intervention".[12]

EFM is important in high-risk labour but there has been controversy about its use in low-risk cases. Nevertheless, nowadays a low-risk woman is often checked with a short interval of EFM on admission to the labour ward. Intermittent EFM is as safe as continuous EFM in low risk labours.[13] Computerised analysis of EFM may reduce but not eliminate false positive and false negative cases.[14]

Instrumental delivery and caesarean section

Rates of caesarean section and instrumental delivery vary widely between hospitals.[15–17] Different hospitals serve different populations, some with a high proportion from ethnic minority groups, but this is unlikely to explain such wide variations in clinical practice. Rates of forceps delivery fell sharply in the late 1970s in British hospitals, and have recently fallen again as rates of vacuum extraction have increased.[15] Vacuum extraction has been recommended in preference to forceps when the obstetrician feels there is a choice but long term effects of forceps and vacuum are similar.[18] Rates of caesarean section have risen steadily over the last half-century but the rise accelerated in the 1990s. As mentioned above, this seems partly to be due to women's wishes.[19] Among women who request caesarean section, fear of perineal damage is a major reason for doing so.[20]

Postnatal care

The lying-in period has greatly reduced over the years. The community midwife has a statutory duty to give care, as required, for up to 28 days after delivery but postnatal care is the Cinderella of the service: much of the morbidity of pregnancy occurs after delivery but little of it is recognised by professionals.[21]

Standardisation of practice

Obstetric management varies between consultants and between hospitals. Case notes also vary, though there are moves to standardise maternity notes throughout England. Many British hospitals have labour ward guidelines but there is no national protocol. *Towards Safer Childbrith*[1] sets out general principles for managing labour wards, not detailed protocols for managing labour. Some midwives dislike protocols, feeling that they limit individual judgement, and some doctors fear that national guidelines would make it easier for plaintiffs to sue hospitals.

Effective Care in Pregnancy and Childbirth

This book, first published in 1989 and now in its third edition, applied science to the debates about different styles of practice. It attempted to review all published and indeed unpublished trials of obstetric management.[22] It has a continuously updated database in electronic form, and includes lists of interventions that are of proven effectiveness, those that are unproven and those that are definitely ineffective.

This evidence-based approach is important and is attractive to midwives and obstetricians but its limitations are now becoming more apparent. For example, randomised trials conducted in Britain in the 1980s, when most intrapartum care was given by doctors in training, may not be applicable to the practice of fully trained specialists.[23] Some important clinical questions may now be impossible to answer by randomised trials, because fully-informed women are unwilling to submit themselves to a study in which treatment (for example, caesarean section or vaginal breech delivery) is randomly allocated.[24] Finally, "we should recognise that [evidence-based] reviews may be as much subject to bias and wrong conclusions as individual studies".[25] Too often they are not subject to the usual scientific checks and balances.[23,25]

Staffing

Midwives

Community midwives are usually attached to one or more groups of GPs. Midwives conduct virtually all deliveries in "general practitioner" units and the great majority in obstetric units.[26] Hospital midwives work shifts and most women are delivered by a midwife whom the woman has never met before. Flexible schemes have been introduced, such as the "domino" scheme, in which the community midwife accompanies the woman to hospital and supervises the delivery and her return home a few hours later. Birth centres staffed only by midwives are associated with less medical intervention,[27,28] and overall satisfaction with care is higher in some but not all midwife-led units.[29,30] Criteria for booking vary widely.[31] Midwife-led units are viewed with mistrust by obstetricians[32] and research conducted by midwives has raised concerns that although risks are low, proof is still lacking that they are as safe as obstetric units.[27,28]

Hospital doctors

Hospital medical staffing is hierarchical and the most junior doctor is first on call. He or she will have been qualified for at least a year but may have only a few months' obstetric experience.

Larger obstetric units also have a resident middle-grade doctor – usually a registrar with several years' obstetric experience. There is a limit on the number of registrar posts in the UK, and because planned consultant expansion in the 1990s[33] did not occur there is currently an "excess" of trainees. The number of training posts is therefore being reduced and in future many obstetric units may have little or no middle-grade cover. This will throw an increased burden on consultants, who, like all doctors, are subject to European legislation on their working hours. Possible solutions to the obstetric staffing crisis include consultant expansion (albeit belated), the appointment of non-consultant specialists, or a reduction in elective gynaecological work.

At night consultants are on call from home and at present their involvement in the labour ward during the day is variable. *Towards Safer Childbirth* recommends that all labour wards except the very smallest should have a consultant present for 40 hours a week, and the RCOG will require this to be implemented by the spring of 2001.

Relationships between professionals

Midwives are independent practitioners but in the past were bound by the Midwives' Rules to call a doctor when they judged this necessary.

Often this meant an experienced midwife in hospital calling an inexperienced doctor. In 1998 the Midwives' Rules were changed to allow her to call an appropriately experienced midwife colleague,[1,34] removing one potential source of friction between the professions.

Towards Safer Childbirth recommends that the main organisational drive for the labour ward should come from a Labour Ward Forum, including as a minimum the lead obstetrician, the clinical midwife manager, an obstetric anaesthetist, a neonatal paediatrician, a risk manager, representatives from the junior medical and midwifery staff, and a consumer representative from the Maternity Services Liaison Committee.

Audit in obstetrics

For many years obstetricians led the way in audit. Confidential enquiries into maternal deaths have been systematically carried out for 50 years to identify and correct avoidable factors.[35] More recently a review of stillbirths and deaths in infancy has been instituted on a national and regional basis.[36] Most maternity hospitals hold regular meetings at which doctors and midwives review cases of stillbirth and neonatal death, again with the aim of improving practice. As obstetric care improved, however, "mortality" meetings became less useful, and systems for identifying "near misses" have been developed,[37] though they are being used locally rather than nationally.[38] As part of clinical governance hospitals are holding meetings to discuss "incidents" and guidelines on the types of incidents to be discussed have been published.[39] A "process clinical audit tool" has been developed which allows routine identification of management which falls outside agreed guidelines.[40]

Sources of risk to babies

Stillbirth or handicap may arise from congenital abnormality, complications before labour, premature delivery or lack of oxygen in labour. At present premature delivery is almost impossible to predict and prevent, but to some extent the other causes are theoretically preventable.

Congenital abnormalities

These could be reduced by pre-pregnancy counselling (e.g. to improve diabetic control or give vitamin supplements to prevent spina bifida) or by prenatal diagnosis followed by termination of pregnancy. Prenatal diagnosis is now offered routinely in antenatal clinics in the form of an ultrasound scan – usually at 19 weeks' gestation – to detect fetal anomalies. The range of anomalies that can be detected is steadily increasing but district hospitals may not match the standards of tertiary referral centres. Screening for Down syndrome involves offering a blood test, either to all women or to those above a certain age. A woman who gives birth to an abnormal baby may blame the hospital for not offering her the appropriate test or not referring her to a tertiary centre.

Antepartum causes of stillbirth

Death in utero before labour sometimes has a specific cause such as maternal diabetes or infection. When a stillbirth occurs, maternity hospitals have a protocol of tests on the baby and mother but nevertheless a cause may not be identified. Growth retardation may be recognised after delivery but as mentioned above it can be hard to diagnose before delivery.[41]

Intrapartum stillbirth

In 1995 the Confidential Enquiry into Stillbirths and Deaths in Infancy (CESDI) estimated that the loss of a normally formed, non-premature baby due to problems in labour occurs in 1 in 1561 deliveries. Of 873 cases reviewed by expert panels convened by CESDI, no fewer than 78% were criticised for suboptimal care and in over 50% of the 873 cases better care "would reasonably have been expected" to have made a difference – in other words, to save the baby's life. Often there has been a failure to recognise a fetal heart rate abnormality that seems glaringly obvious in retrospect. Nevertheless, it is difficult to predict some obstetric disasters, such as shoulder dystocia,[42] and in a survey of babies who developed encephalopathy, over 50% had suffered events that were outside the control of the obstetrician.[43]

Handicap

Avoidable handicap is first and foremost a tragedy for the affected individual but it is also a major concern for the NHS because the ensuing litigation is often extremely expensive. A large proportion of mental handicap cases (often misleadingly called "brain damage") are not avoidable in our present state of knowledge because they are due to genetic causes, i.e. the problem lies in abnormal development of the brain and not in outside influences. Prenatal diagnosis has a limited role, with tests for chromosomal abnormalities such as Down syndrome, but other types of mental handicap cannot be detected by ultrasound or other tests during pregnancy.

Birth injury due to forceps can cause mental handicap if intracranial bleeding occurs, but direct injury is unlikely to be a cause without such bleeding.[44] Intrapartum hypoxia is often blamed for causing mental handicap or cerebral palsy but in fact less than 10% of cases of cerebral palsy are due to asphyxia.[9,45] Nevertheless, whatever the cause of the child's disability there may be a coincident abnormality on the cardiotocograph trace, and if it was not acted upon a court may link it with the child's subsequent condition and award damages to the child.

"Brain damage"

In such legal cases the condition of the child in the days after birth may be crucial. The newborn is routinely assessed by the Apgar score, which notes the baby's colour, tone, breathing, heart rate and response to stimulation but has little prognostic value. Taking a sample of blood from the umbilical cord and measuring its oxygen tension and pH gives a more accurate assessment but is not routine practice.

A better guide to prognosis is the baby's condition in the first days after delivery. Abnormal neurological signs may amount to hypoxic–ischaemic encephalopathy, a condition caused by brain cell death.[46] Ultrasound scans may show signs of bleeding within the brain, and later cavitation due to lack of oxygen. It can be hard to tell whether such deprivation of oxygen occurred during or before labour. Freeman and Nelson[47] suggested that if "brain damage" is due to asphyxia four questions should be answered positively.

1 Is there evidence of marked and prolonged intrapartum asphyxia?
2 Did the infant show signs of moderate or severe hypoxic–ischaemic encephalopathy during the newborn period, with evidence also of asphyxial injury to other organ systems?
3 Is the child's neurologic condition one that intrapartum asphyxia could explain?
4 Has the work-up been sufficient to rule out other conditions?

The incidence of cerebral palsy due to encephalopathy is thought to be between 1 in 2000 and 1 in 4000 births.[48] Therefore, in a medium sized maternity hospital there will be one case every year which could result in the award of over £1 million in damages.

Deficiencies in care

The systematic investigation of adverse and potentially adverse outcomes in medicine is relatively new in Britain.[49] Procedures are being introduced into individual hospitals as part of risk management but the analysis of the causes of "incidents" remains relatively unsophisticated, compared with such analysis in some areas of industry. Nevertheless some research has been done.

Over ten years ago, Ennis and Vincent[50] reviewed 64 cases that came to litigation over stillbirth, perinatal or neonatal death or other problems. They identified three main concerns – inadequate fetal heart monitoring, mismanagement of forceps and inadequate supervision by senior staff. In addition, women reported that sometimes staff were unsympathetic and gave too little information.[51] Five years later, little had changed. Over half of a group of women who had experienced stillbirth or neonatal death had poor or confused knowledge of what had happened, and only 29% were satisfied with the information they had received.[52]

Murphy *et al*[53] carried out a study in which the intrapartum cardiotocograph records of severely asphyxiated babies were compared with those of healthy infants. Investigators unaware of the clinical outcome agreed that abnormalities were present in the traces of 87% of the asphyxiated infants and 29% of the controls. They diagnosed severe abnormalities in 61% of the asphyxiated infants and 9% of the controls. Fetal blood sampling was indicated in 58% of cases in the asphyxia group but was actually carried out in only 16%. The response of staff to the abnormalities was slow and the authors of this study concluded that "the interpretation of cardiotocograph records during labour continues to pose major problems for practising clinicians."

In a study of the training of obstetric senior house officers in teaching hospitals and district general hospitals, Ennis[54] found that most of these doctors received only one or two hours' teaching a week and some received even less. Half of the doctors had had no formal training in interpreting or recognising abnormal or equivocal cardiotocograms. When they were questioned at the end of their jobs about training in the use of forceps, 23% of the senior house officers said they had had no training, and 35% of the remainder thought their training had been less than adequate. In a study of GP trainees' views on hospital obstetric training, Smith[55] found that less than 40% believed at the end of their six months that they were competent to perform a simple forceps delivery. Most of those questioned believed that more than six months' hospital training was necessary for a general practitioner who wished to provide care in labour.

Reducing risk

"The real answer to the question 'How to avoid medico-legal problems in obstetrics and gynaecology' is good practice and good communication."[56] Good practice is the best form of defence, and several improvements are necessary.

Focusing care

Resources need to be directed to where they are needed most. This applies, for example, to the senior medical staff. Much of their time and attention has been devoted to antenatal care, on the basis that many problems during labour are predictable and preventable. This approach led to "cattle-market" antenatal clinics, and has detracted from intrapartum and postnatal care. It raised expectations but has not abolished medico-legal problems. Most litigation arises from events in labour, and most dissatisfaction arises from postnatal care. Strategies for risk reduction should focus on both these areas, but particularly on care in labour.

Focusing care

- Most litigation arises from events in labour
- Most unhappiness arises from postnatal care.

Equipment

Fetal monitoring equipment is often used long after it has become obsolete. The danger is that staff learn to mistrust unreliable equipment, making them slow to react to genuine abnormalities. An inventory of monitoring equipment should be maintained and there should be planned programmes of replacement.

Fetal blood sampling equipment should be available in all units that use electronic fetal monitoring. Fetal blood sampling equipment is prone to technical problems and requires careful maintenance on a daily basis.

Consultant involvement

The RCOG will shortly require all accredited hospitals to have a consultant present without other commitments for 40 hours a week on the delivery suite. The Department of Health is reducing the long hours worked by junior doctors in "hard-pressed" specialties and trainee numbers are being reduced. However, insufficient consultant posts are being created to maintain service provision. There will be considerable difficulties in the short term but in the long term the move towards a specialist-provided service will continue. This has led to anxieties among some consultants, who feel they have become deskilled. Updating courses will be needed. The RCOG already has a programme of continuing medical education for consultants[57] and publishes the names of those who complete it.

Training of junior doctors

The need for better training of senior house officers is becoming glaringly apparent. As NHS managers become more aware of the importance of risk management, pressure to improve training will increase. There has been excessive complacency in British hospital practice that learning by osmosis is adequate for junior doctors: the studies reviewed above have revealed how far training is falling short of what is needed.

A distinction needs to be made between "teaching" (often directed towards future practice or examinations) and "training" to do the job in hand. As far as risk management is concerned, the immediate need is to ensure that senior house officers are trained in the interpretation of cardiotocographs and in the procedures they are expected to undertake unsupervised.

Resources for teaching are now being identified more clearly and should in future be better directed as postgraduate deans control budgets. It has been suggested that attitudes towards general practitioner training should change and that only those vocational trainees who wish to contribute to intrapartum care should be specially trained to do this.[58]

A significant minority of trainees did not have access to computers or sufficient IT training to run basic tutorial programmes or access the Internet.[59]

Specific requirements

- Training of new senior house officers should include an introductory session to orientate them to the organisation of the hospital, and its clinical guidelines. Most hospitals already hold such sessions.
- At present, teaching sessions for junior staff are often poorly attended due to pressure of clinical work. Arrangements should be in place to ensure that such sessions are not interfered with by other commitments.
- Some emergencies – such as major haemorrhage or eclampsia – occur so infrequently in most hospitals that staff do not get regular experience in dealing with them. Hospitals should have protocols to guide staff dealing with obstetric emergencies and it may be helpful to hold irregular "fire drill" exercises to test how well these protocols work. Courses on managing emergencies, using models and reality-based scenarios are now available.[61]
- There should be formal mechanisms for reviewing the effectiveness of training.[60] District tutors of the RCOG should liaise with postgraduate deans and hospital managers to ensure that weaknesses in training are identified and remedied.

Doctors' work

Guidelines

As mentioned above, most hospitals have guidelines to the management of routine cases and emergencies. These should be regularly reviewed and updated.

Handovers

With the new restrictions on junior doctors' working hours, hospitals are introducing partial shifts and split weekends. This has increased the need for formal handovers between medical teams at the start of each shift. Traditionally such handovers have been part of nursing and midwifery practice: they should now be part of routine medical practice on the delivery suite.

Support

A problem that has received little attention is that a doctor managing a case for a prolonged period of time may sometimes not notice signs that later seem obvious and important. This problem may be reduced by shorter shifts, as a new team will review problems with fresh eyes. It could also be tackled by the junior reporting regularly to a senior doctor (perhaps by phone) and by ensuring that the midwifery staff can speak direct to the duty consultant if they have any concerns.

Midwives' work

Antenatal care

Schemes are being introduced to standardise antenatal care while allowing it to be shared appropriately between midwife, hospital clinic and general practitioner. These should include clear guidelines, agreed between midwives and doctors, about when medical referral is required.

Care in labour

In the delivery suite, the use of electronic fetal monitoring seems likely to continue even if midwives gain more autonomy and run sections of the delivery suite without doctors in attendance. Many midwives do not feel comfortable with the interpretation of cardiotocograph traces and better training is required to teach them which types of pattern require further investigation. Such training should not be provided as a "one-off" session but should include regular revision and updating.

Some hospitals are relying increasingly on staff from a "bank" or a nursing agency. The dangers of this trend should be obvious from this article. It is impossible to be sure that temporary staff are adequately trained in the hospital's procedures. Reliance on them should be kept to an absolute minimum.

89

Relationships between professions

Ideally labour should be supervised by an experienced midwife who has immediate support from an experienced doctor.[62] The place of the inexperienced doctor on the labour ward will become more and more that of a trainee, learning from senior doctors and midwives.[59]

In general, consultants and midwives have good working relationships, particularly in the private sector. To provide this level of cover in the NHS will require increased resources from Health Authorities, who will need to be educated that increased investment in experienced staff will save money in claims as well as providing a better service for women.

Specific measures

As mentioned above, the senior midwife on duty should have direct access to the consultant on call.

The relationship between midwives and junior doctors can be made less difficult by guidelines defining as clearly as possible their roles and responsibilities in each particular hospital. These guidelines should of course be drawn up by the consultants and midwives together.

Regular meetings should be held to review the work of the delivery suite. The atmosphere in perinatal mortality meetings and "near miss" meetings can be tense and it is better to hold regular meetings to discuss interesting cases and matters of current concern as well as cases which have a poor outcome.

"Team building" is necessary in the delivery suite as in any other organisation where staff need to interact under pressure. Social occasions have an important part to play in this process. They occur infrequently, however, because doctors socialise with doctors and midwives with midwives. This problem needs to be recognised and addressed.

Communication with patients

The importance of a good rapport with the woman and her partner is now recognised and communication is being given a higher priority by doctors as well as midwives. "The best protection for the doctor remains the one of talking to the patient and recording an outline of what is said."[56] Good communication is essential once a problem has arisen, but good rapport with women throughout pregnancy and labour will create a sound basis for full explanations if anything goes wrong.

Good communication as a routine

Midwives and doctors often feel offended if it is suggested that they are poor communicators. They protest that such skill is fundamental to their job. Nevertheless, they receive little feedback on these skills and often do not realise how they are perceived by women and their partners. Over half of a

Checklist for risk reduction

Equipment	No obsolete monitors Fetal blood gas equipment available
Staffing levels	Minimal use of agency and "bank" staff Workload includes time to talk to patients
Consultants' role	Dedicated sessions in delivery suite Sessions dedicated to training
Juniors' training	Introductory training at start of post Regular *protected* teaching sessions Occasional "fire drill" exercises Regular formal feedback on training quality
Juniors' work	Guidelines on routine and emergency practice Formal handovers between shifts Support from seniors and midwives
Midwives' work	Regular training sessions on fetal monitoring Clear definition of role *vis-à-vis* SHOs Senior midwife has access to duty consultant
Staff communication	Regular delivery suite meetings Team-building social occasions
Communication with patients	Regular feedback from patients' advocates Consultant promptly notified of problems Explanations are consultant's responsibility

group of women who had had a caesarean section reported that they had not had a discussion about the reasons before being discharged from hospital.[63]

The delivery suite has the dual function of dealing with life-threatening emergencies and creating a relaxed atmosphere for normal childbirth. These functions do not easily mix. Efficiency may be perceived as abruptness, and communication problems are likely to be worse if staff are under pressure. Communication takes time, and therefore adequate numbers of staff must be on duty.

There is a need for sessions providing feedback to staff from patients' advocates, who can tactfully identify any shortcomings in attitudes to women and their partners. This is particularly important in units dealing with a high proportion of patients from ethnic minorities.

Communication in problem cases

If a problem does arise, whether or not it is thought likely to lead to litigation, it should be notified as soon as possible to the consultant – ideally to the woman's own consultant but if not, to the consultant on duty. Whenever possible, explanations to the woman and her relatives should be given by the consultant, in conjunction with other staff as necessary. This is not to say that consultants are always the best communicators, but litigation sometimes arises because the woman feels the problem has not been taken seriously at a senior level.

A single explanation may not be enough, and it may be necessary for the same doctor to see the couple again to answer further questions. More often, however, the couple will ask the same questions of different members of staff. It is helpful if a note is made of what the patient has been told, so that unnecessary confusion can be avoided.

Conclusion

Risks in obstetrics are already low and reducing them still further is a challenging task. A major problem is that both professionals and the public have forgotten how much has already been achieved. Obstetricians sometimes have a poor image and indeed a poor self-image. Constant criticism from consumer groups and an increasing burden of litigation has left many obstetricians demoralised. The image of the specialty may be improved by the imminent change in its gender balance (over 50% of trainees are women) and by the extension of fetomaternal medicine as a subspecialty. Perhaps the best hope for the future, however, lies in the implementation of the principles of risk management. These will not only make childbirth even safer for women but should also make obstetrics enjoyable again for its beleaguered practitioners.

References

1   Royal College of Obstetricians and Gynaecologists and Royal College of Midwives. *Towards Safer Childbirth: minimum standards for the organisation of labour wards.* London: RCOG, 1999.
2   Department of Health. *Changing Childbirth.* London: HMSO, 1993.
3   Capstick B. Risk management in obstetrics. In: Clements RV, ed. *Safe practice in obstetrics and gynaecology: a medico-legal handbook.* Edinburgh: Churchill Livingstone, 1994, 405–16.
4   Wilkinson C, McIlwaine G, Boulton-Jones C, Cole S. Is a rising caesarean section rate inevitable? *Br J Obstet Gynaecol* 1998;**105**:45–52.
5   Leitch CR, Walker JJ. The rise in caesarean section rate: the same indications but a lower threshold. *Br J Obstet Gynaecol* 1998;**105**:621–6.
6   Thornton J. Measuring patients' values in reproductive medicine. *Contemp Rev Obstet Gynaecol* 1988;**1**:5–12.
7   B-Lynch C, Coker A, Dua JA. A clinical analysis of 500 medico-legal claims evaluating

the causes and assessing the potential benefit of alternative dispute resolution. *Br J Obstet Gynaecol* 1996;**103**:1236–42.

8 Clement S, Candy B, Sikorski J, *et al*. Does reducing the frequency of routine antenatal visits have long term effects? Follow up of participants in a randomised controlled trial. *Br J Obstet Gynaecol* 1999;**106**:367–70.

9 Spencer JAD, Badawi N, Burton P, *et al*. The intrapartum CTG prior to neonatal encephalopathy at term – a case-control study. *Br J Obstet Gynaecol* 1997;**104**:25–8.

10 Umstad MP, Permezel M, Pepperell RJ. Litigation and the intrapartum cardiotocograph. *Br J Obstet Gynaecol* 1995;**102**:89–91.

11 Ingemarsson I, Herbst A, Throngren-Jerneck K. Long term outcome after umbilical artery acidaemia at term birth: influence of gender and duration of fetal heart rate abnormalities. *Br J Obstet Gynaecol* 1997;**104**:1123–7.

12 Westgate J, Greene K. How well is fetal blood sampling used in clinical practice? *Br J Obstet Gynaecol* 1994;**101**:250–1.

13 Herbst A, Ingemarsson I. Intermittent versus continuous electronic monitoring in labour: a randomised study. *Br J Obstet Gynaecol* 1994;**101**:663–8.

14 Chung TKH, Mohajer MP, Yang ZJ, *et al*. The prediction of fetal acidosis at birth by computerised analysis of intrapartum cardiotocography. *Br J Obstet Gynaecol* 1995;**102**:454–60.

15 Drife JO. Choice and instrumental delivery. *Br J Obstet Gynaecol* 1996;**103**:608–11.

16 Hemminki E, Gissler M. Variation in obstetric care within and between hospital levels in Finland. *Br J Obstet Gynaecol* 1994;**101**:851–7.

17 Middle C, MacFarlane A. Labour and delivery of "normal" primiparous women: analysis of routinely collected data. *Br J Obstet Gynaecol* 1995;**102**:970–7.

18 Johanson RB, Heycock E, Carter J, *et al*. Maternal and child health after assisted vaginal delivery: five-year follow up of a randomised controlled study comparing forceps and ventouse. *Br J Obstet Gynaecol* 1999;**106**:544–9.

19 Mould TAJ, Chong S, Spencer JAD, Gallivan S. Women's involvement with the decision preceding their caesarean section and their degree of satisfaction. *Br J Obstet Gynaecol* 1996;**103**:1074–7.

20 Sultan A, Stanton S. Preserving the pelvic floor and perineum during childbirth – elective caesarean section? *Br J Obstet Gynaecol* 1996;**103**:731–4.

21 Glazener CMA, Abdalla M, Stroud P, *et al*. Postnatal maternal morbidity: extent, causes, prevention and treatment. *Br J Obstet Gynaecol* 1995;**102**: 282–7.

22 Chalmers I, Enkin M, Keirse MJNC. *Effective care in pregnancy and childbirth.* Oxford: OUP 1989.

23 Grant JM. The whole duty of obstetricians. *Br J Obstet Gynaecol* 1997;**104**:387–92.

24 Penn ZJ, Steer PJ, Grant A. A multicentre randomised controlled trial comparing elective and selective caesarean section for the delivery of the preterm breech infant. *Br J Obstet Gynaecol* 1996;**103**:684–9.

25 Gardosi J. Systematic reviews: insufficient evidence on which to base medicine. *Br J Obstet Gynaecol* 1998;**105**:1–5.

26 Graham W. Midwife-led care. *Br J Obstet Gynaecol* 1997;**104**:396–8.

27 Waldenstrom U, Nilsson CA, Winbladh B. The Stockholm Birth Centre Trial: maternal and infant outcome. *Br J Obstet Gynaecol* 1997;**104**:410–18.

28 Waldenstrom U, Turnbull D. A systematic review comparing continuity of midwifery care with standard maternity services. *Br J Obstet Gynaecol* 1998;**105**:1160–70.

29 Brown S, Lumley J. Changing childbirth: lessons from an Australian survey of 1336 women. *Br J Obstet Gynaecol* 1998;**105**:143–55.

30 Hundley VA, Milne JM, Glazener CMA, Mollison J. Satisfaction and the three C's: continuity, choice and control. Women's views from a randomised controlled trial of midwife-led care. *Br J Obstet Gynaecol* 1997;**104**:1273–80.

31 Campbell R. Review and assessment of selection criteria used when booking pregnant women at different places of birth. *Br J Obstet Gynaecol* 1999;**106**:550–6.

32 Cheyne H, Turnbull D, Lunan CB, *et al*. Working alongside a midwife-led care unit: what do obstetricians think? *Br J Obstet Gynaecol* 1995;**103**:485–7.

33 Calman K. Hospital doctors: training for the future. *Br J Obstet Gynaecol* 1995;**102**:355–6.

34 United Kingdom Central Council for Nursing, Midwifery and Health Visiting. *Midwives Rules and Code of Practice.* London: UKCC, 1998.

35 Department of Health. *Report on Confidential Enquiries into Maternal Deaths in the United Kingdom 1994–96.* London: HMSO, 1998.

36 *Confidential Enquiry into Stillbirths and Deaths in Infancy. Fourth Annual Report, 1 January – 31 December 1995.* London: Maternal and Child Health Consortium, 1997.

37 Mantel GD, Buchmann E, Rees H, Pattinson RC. Severe acute morbidity: a pilot study of a definition for a near miss. *Br J Obstet Gynaecol* 1998;**105**:985–90.

38 Drife JO. Maternal "near miss" reports? *BMJ* 1993;**307**:1087.

39 Royal College of Obstetricians and Gynaecologists. *Maintaining Good Medical Practice in Obstetrics and Gynaecology: the role of the RCOG.* London: RCOG, 1999.

40 Halligan AWF, Taylor DJ, Naftalin NJ, *et al.* Achieving best practice in maternity care. *Br J Obstet Gynaecol* 1997;**104**:873–5.

41 Gardosi J, Mui T, Mongelli M, Fagan D. Analysis of birthweight and gestational age in antepartum stillbirths. *Br J Obstet Gynaecol* 1998;**105**:524–30.

42 Hope P, Breslin S, Lamont L, *et al.* Fatal shoulder dystocia: a review of 56 cases reported to the Confidential Enquiry into Stillbirths and Deaths in Infancy. *Br J Obstet Gynaecol* 1998;**105**:1256–61.

43 Westgate JA, Gunn AJ, Gunn TR. Antecedents of neonatal encephalopathy with fetal acidaemia at term. *Br J Obstet Gynaecol* 1999;**106**:774–82.

44 Drife JO. Intracranial haemorrhage in the newborn: obstetric aspects. *Clin Risk* 1998;**4**: 71–4.

45 Pharaoh POD. Cerebral palsy and perinatal care. *Br J Obstet Gynaecol* 1995;**102**:356–8.

46 Longo L, Packianathan S. Hypoxia–ischaemia and the developing brain: hypotheses regarding the pathophysiology of fetal–neonatal brain damage. *Br J Obstet Gynaecol* 1997;**104**:652–62.

47 Freeman J, Nelson K. Intrapartum asphyxia and cerebral palsy. *Pediatrics* 1988;**82**: 240–9.

48 Hall DMB. Intrapartum events and cerebral palsy. *Br J Obstet Gynaecol* 1994; **101**:745–7.

49 Stanhope N, Vincent C, Taylor-Adams SE, *et al.* Applying human factors methods to clinical risk management in obstetrics. *Br J Obstet Gynaecol* 1997;**104**: 1225–32.

50 Ennis M, Vincent CA. Obstetric accidents: a review of 64 cases. *BMJ* 1990;**300**:1365–7.

51 Vincent CA, Martin T, Ennis M. Obstetric accidents: the patient's perspective. *Br J Obstet Gynaecol* 1991;**98**:390–5.

52 Crowther ME. Communication following a stillbirth or neonatal death: room for improvement. *Br J Obstet Gynaecol* 1995;**102**:952–6.

53 Murphy KW, Johnson P, Moorcraft J, *et al.* Birth asphyxia and the intrapartum cardiotocograph. *Br J Obstet Gynaecol* 1990;**97**:470–9.

54 Ennis M. Training and supervision of obstetric senior house officers. *BMJ* 1991;**303**: 1442–3.

55 Smith LFP. GP trainees' views on hospital obstetric vocational training. *BMJ* 1991;**303**: 1447–50.

56 Clements RV. Litigation in obstetrics and gynaecology. *Br J Obstet Gynaecol* 1991;**98**: 423–6.

57 Burr R, Johanson R. Continuing medical education: an opportunity for bringing about change in clinical practice. *Br J Obstet Gynaecol* 1998;**105**:940–5.

58 Pogmore, JR. Role of the senior house officer in the labour ward. *Br J Obstet Gynaecol* 1992;**99**:180–1.

59 Draycott T, Cook J, Fox R, Jenkins J. Information technology for postgraduate education: survey of facilities and skills in the South West Deanery. *Br J Obstet Gynaecol* 1999;**106**: 731–5.

60 Konje JC, Taylor DJ. Formative assessment within structured training in obstetrics and gynaecology. *Br J Obstet Gynaecol* 1998;**105**:139–41.

61 Johanson R, Cox C, O'Donnell E, *et al.* Managing obstetrics emergencies and trauma (MOET): Structured skills training using models and reality-based scenarios. *Obstetr Gynaecol* 1999;**1**:46–52.

62 Drife JO. My grandchild's birth. *BMJ* 1988;**297**:1208.

63 Graham WJ, Hundley V, McCheyne AL, *et al.* An investigation of women's involvement in the decision to deliver by caesarean section. *Br J Obstet Gynaecol* 1999;**106**:213–20.

6 Reducing risk in paediatrics and neonatal intensive care

PETER DEAR

No area of medical practice is free from the risk of causing harm to patients but in paediatric medicine the chances and consequences of doing so are generally greater than in many other specialities. This is particularly true in the case of very young children where every aspect of investigation and treatment is difficult and where the consequences of any harm done may have to be borne for a full lifetime. The most extreme example is neonatal intensive care.

From the medico-legal point of view paediatricians are in double jeopardy. Firstly, a doctor or health authority can be sued for medical negligence up until the time that the child reaches 21 years of age, or indeed at any age if the child is so disabled that a state of independence is never reached. Secondly, eligibility for legal aid is based on the child's earnings and therefore easily obtained if there seems to be a prima facie case.

The need for paediatricians to be risk conscious in the interests both of their patients and themselves is obvious. Although the stakes are high, paediatricians are clearly not expected to perform at a higher level than other doctors. They, like others, are expected to take all reasonable precautions to avoid inflicting preventable and foreseeable harm on their patients and to communicate effectively when there has been a misadventure. Recognising the main areas of risk is an essential pre-requisite for their prevention and this chapter is devoted to just that in relation to paediatric practice. The first section of the chapter addresses general areas of risk, common to almost all of paediatric practice, while the second section addresses a selection of risks related to neonatal medicine.

95

Areas of risk in general paediatric practice

Children have in common the facts that they are small, generally unco-operative, difficult to evaluate medically and mostly have parents who watch over them and guard their best interests. These features alone create potential problems for the doctor attempting to provide a high quality of care and to stay out of court. Some barriers to these endeavours as well as some possible solutions will be discussed.

Benefits of specialisation

Paediatricians are often heard to say that "children are not simply small adults". Although now a cliché, this vitally important message is by no means redundant in the current state of organisation of medical services for children in this country.

The first and most important step in reducing clinical risk in paediatric practice is to ensure that medical care for children is provided by clinical staff with appropriate training and experience in purpose-designed accommodation. A good illustration of the risks associated with not doing so was provided by the 1989 National Confidential Enquiry into Peri-Operative Deaths (NCEPOD), in relation to paediatric anaesthesia and surgery. One of the main recommendations of that report was that "surgeons and anaesthetists should not undertake occasional paediatric practice". Reassuringly, the 1999 NCEPOD discovered considerable improvements – for example, the proportion of anaesthetists not undertaking the care of infants of less than six months had increased from 16% to 58% since the earlier report. No similar investigation has yet been conducted into other areas of hospital care for children but it is likely that similar findings would be obtained, for example, in intensive care, A & E attendances and so on. This is a matter of healthcare planning and organisation and it is the responsibility of all those engaged in this activity to ensure that these initial conditions for risk reduction in paediatric practice are met. To persist with the surgical example – when every young child who needs an operation sets out from a children's surgical ward in the company of its parents and a children's nurse to be anaesthetised by a paediatric anaesthetist and operated on by a surgeon trained in the management of small children in a designated paediatric operating theatre we will have got it right. Another good example of the benefits of a centralised and specialised unit for children is the Paediatric Sedation Unit in which appropriate and safe sedation and analgesia can be provided for distressing procedures.[1]

An extension of the above line of argument to sub-specialisation within paediatric medicine is also appropriate to a consideration of risk reduction. Paediatrics has been slower than adult medicine in recognising the place of the specialist. The general paediatrician is certainly able to deal effectively with most problems but as the scientific knowledge on which paediatric practice is based continues to expand, and in the face of increasing public awareness and expectation, the doctor who does not know when to refer is increasingly vulnerable. A possible solution to this might be to form closer links between central and peripheral units so that the care of children with less common problems can be shared rather than devolved. In that way the best interests of the child can be combined with professional interest.

Communication with parents

One of the peculiar features of paediatric practice is the tripartite relationship between the doctor, the child and the parents. Although most experienced paediatricians regard this as one of the more interesting and challenging aspects of the speciality, less experienced doctors often find the situation daunting and may perform poorly as a result. To an extent this reflects the insecurity of the doctor in dealing with non-dependent adults who often seem to want to know an awful lot about what is going on. In terms of risk management, it is essential for parents to be thoroughly well informed on every point including an understanding of the risks as well and the benefits associated with the investigation or treatment to be undertaken, especially in emergency or intensive care settings. Parents embarking on legal action do so for a variety of motives but a recurring theme is a feeling that they have not received adequate explanation and that they are victims of a "cover-up". We cannot prevent parents from suing us because the public provision for handicapped children is lamentably inadequate but we can prevent them from suing us because we did not talk to them.

Another very important area of communication is telling parents that their child has a serious, chronic condition such as cystic fibrosis or cerebral palsy. If done badly this can lead to long-lasting resentment. The task should not be left to juniors, although they should be present in order to learn. Repeated interviews with both parents and the provision of written information is valuable.[2]

Handover and continuity of care

Young children cannot explain that they have already had their evening medication or that they are supposed to be fasting prior to surgery. As a result they are so much more vulnerable to the risks of mishap through failures of communication. Nurses are generally good at handover[3] but doctors are generally less so and the changes in training and working patterns that are developing are bound to make matters worse. Handover rounds between junior staff are a crucial component of any risk reduction strategy and it is incumbent on senior staff to insist that they be done and to demand the resources required to enable them.[4]

Communication with the general practitioner on discharge is immensely important. Discharge summaries should be short, delivered quickly and concentrated on discharge information.[5]

Cross-infection

Too many children admitted to hospital acquire infection from others as the result of inadequate isolation facilities or poor prevention measures such as handwashing. It is a serious deficiency in the service when a baby admitted for a minor operation contracts a major respiratory illness such as bronchiolitis[6] or when a child with cystic fibrosis acquires a problematic organism like *Burkholderia cepacia* for the first time in hospital.[7,8] The current recommendation is for 50% of all children's beds to be in cubicles but this is probably an underprovision. The problem with more cubicles is that more nurses are generally required to look after them but the costs of unnecessary morbidity generated by cross-infection may outweigh this.

Prescribing for children

Medication errors in paediatric practice are relatively common, especially in children under 2 years of age and in emergency or intensive care settings.[9,10,11,12,13,14] The majority of errors are in prescribing, predominantly incorrect dosage. Such errors often relate to careless transcribing (such as a misplaced decimal point), computational mistakes[15,16] or an incorrect body weight being recorded. Prescribing errors occur with increased frequency when junior doctors first move into paediatrics and when trainee paediatricians rotate through subspecialties.[13]

Fortunately, the vigilance of nursing and pharmacy staff prevent most medication errors from harming patients but more needs to be done. Suggested approaches to reducing medication errors in paediatrics include encouraging their voluntary reporting as part of a Continuous Quality Improvement System;[13,17] formal training of junior medical staff on the pitfalls of prescribing; improving the quality of handover information, especially when children move from one unit to another; greater use of computerised prescribing.[18]

Unfortunately, knowledge of paediatric pharmacology, particularly in the younger age groups, lags well behind knowledge of adult pharmacology, partly because of the ethical and technical difficulties involved in studying children but partly because it is a commercially less attractive area. As a result many drugs are not licensed by the controlling authorities for the way they are currently prescribed or dispensed. This unsatisfactory situation has been much improved by the Royal College of Paediatrics and Child Health publication *Medicines for Children*.[19]

Record keeping

There are a couple of particular points to be made about record keeping in paediatrics. The first is the importance of recording normal findings and it relates particularly to the screening examinations that are part of normal child health surveillance. There is a natural tendency when writing notes to concentrate on the abnormal findings but failure to record the fact that an infant's hips examined normally at one week of age can create a serious problem if dislocation is diagnosed later on.

The other is the fact that all children under five years of age now have a personal health record held by their parents. This contains (or would if it was completed properly by the professionals) important information that, in some circumstances, it might be deemed negligent not to have discovered. A note about drug allergy for example!

Follow-up

The need to organise appropriate follow-up is common to all branches of medicine. The need to take steps to ensure that it takes place is peculiar to specialities like paediatrics in which the patients cannot be expected to take responsibility for their own actions. If a child fails to attend for a hearing test following meningitis or is discharged on heavy medication for asthma and does not attend for review it is the responsibility of the medical staff concerned to do something. Sometimes just informing the general practitioner will be enough but on other occasions it will be necessary to pursue the family with the aid of the health visitor or social services.

Following up the results of tests is another aspect of this. It is especially important in paediatrics where a battery of tests may be requested at once in order to avoid repeated venepuncture. The results of every test performed must be seen and signed by somebody and not just filed in the notes. An abnormal test result that was not pursued is difficult to explain.

Child protection

Most children are fortunate enough to have parents who try to meet their needs and guard their interests. An extremely unfortunate minority inherit parents who have no interest in them or in some way abuse them. This distortion of the expected parent–child relationship is difficult for health professionals to come to terms with but when it goes undetected children are put at great risk.

99

Child abuse, in any one of its varied forms, is much more likely to be suspected by clinical staff specialising in the care of children than by those not doing so. Some doctors and nurses outside paediatric practice do not seem to be able to accept that so many apparently normal parents do such terrible things to their offspring. Until we achieve the ideal of having all children cared for by children's nurses, hospitals should at least ensure that there is good liaison between departments such as the orthopaedic wards and the A&E department and the paediatricians. Each district has a Designated Doctor for Child Protection who will be a useful source of advice. There should be a low threshold for consulting the Child Protection Register whenever suspicions are aroused. The register is held by Social Services and a child's name can be added or removed only as a result of a decision reached by a case conference. The child's name remains on the register as long as there is a current child protection plan in operation. As well as the names of children who have been officially placed on the register the registry keeps a log of the names of children about whom there have been enquiries.

Particularly difficult to recognise are cases of emotional deprivation and cases of what has become known as Münchhausen syndrome by proxy.[20] Children may be murdered, repeatedly poisoned, suffocated or subjected to innumerable, unnecessary investigations in the pursuit of an organic disease. The parent responsible is often highly inventive and plausible and the only way that the risks associated with this and other forms of child abuse can be minimised is for clinical staff caring for children to be fully aware of such possibilities and to become suspicious when there are features of the case that do not feel right. These are difficult cases that may demand considerable expertise to unravel but there are plenty of sources of expert advice and by far the most common reason for children to remain at risk from their own parents is that the problem remains unsuspected.[21] Continuing medical and nursing education has a vital role to play here as in so many other areas of risk reduction.

The possibility that children might be at risk of deliberate harm perpetrated by healthcare professionals was thrown into sharp focus by the Beverley Allitt affair. The recommendations of the Clothier Committee should reduce the risk of a recurrence of this tragedy. The main recommendations are:

- more stringent assessment of the physical and mental health of nurses caring for children
- better access to paediatric pathology services
- improved reporting of untoward incidents and better collating of reports
- better implementation of the recommendations of the DoH report *Welfare of Children and Young People in Hospital.*

Neonatal medicine

Neonatal medicine is unquestionably one of the most venturesome areas of medical practice, for patients and doctors alike. It is also one of the few specialities in which a mistaken diagnosis can have serious legal implications for doctors in another speciality. I refer here to the consequences for obstetricians of a false diagnosis of birth asphyxia. This section begins by addressing that particular issue and then goes on to consider some of the commoner hazards associated with intensive care of the newborn.

Birth asphyxia

The diagnostic label "birth asphyxia" (or "birth trauma") should be used with great care. A significant proportion of litigation against obstetricians is started on the basis of a mistaken diagnosis of birth asphyxia. In these cases it is usually the paediatric staff who have used the term inappropriately and usually without realising the potential repercussions.

The term "birth asphyxia" is likely to be used as a diagnostic term when babies present with one or more of the following features:

- Obstetric evidence of "fetal distress", usually in the form of fetal heart rate abnormalities on the cardiotocograph[22]
- Poor condition at birth, usually described by low Apgar scores and the need for resuscitation
- A metabolic acidosis in umbilical cord blood or blood taken soon after birth
- A neurological illness during the first few days of life, characterised by irritability, seizures, and abnormalities of conscious level, posture and muscle tone. When such an illness is genuinely the result of acute asphyxial brain injury it is properly termed a "post-asphyxial" or "hypoxic / ischaemic" encephalopathy. When the cause is less certain the implication-free term "neonatal-encephalopathy" is more appropriate.

Although these features are indeed the hallmark of intrapartum asphyxia, it is also true that any one of them, and some combinations of them, may have quite a different aetiology. It is only when all of the evidence is taken together and alternative explanations have been excluded by appropriate investigation that the diagnosis of birth asphyxia can be made with reasonable confidence. Even when that situation is reached, however, it does not necessarily follow that any subsequent disabilities are the result of birth asphyxia. The fetus with a serious intrinsic abnormality of the nervous system or one who has sustained antepartum central nervous system damage may not be able to cope with the stresses imposed by birth and may present many of the features of an asphyxiated baby without necessarily having been damaged further in the process. Such babies may, for

101

example, appear very floppy and unresponsive at birth, to the extent of requiring ventilatory support, and may then go on to exhibit abnormal neurological features.

In most cases of cerebral palsy associated with problems at birth and in the neonatal period, appropriate investigation, including brain imaging and a search for metabolic disorders, usually allows the formation of a reasonably clear view on the likelihood of the cerebral palsy being due to intrapartum asphyxia.[23] Too often, though, the necessary analytical thinking and investigation is performed as part of the medical litigation process and by the time it is concluded that a child's disabilities are probably due to something other than intrapartum asphyxia a good deal of stress has been imposed on all those involved and a good deal of public money has been wasted. It is the responsibility of all paediatricians to avoid the false attribution of the term "birth asphyxia" and to hold such discussions with parents as are necessary, sometimes in conjunction with colleagues in obstetrics, to convey as clear a picture as possible of the likely causation of the child's problems.

It seems likely that less than 20% of cerebral palsy is due to asphyxial brain injury acquired intrapartum (which is a helpful perspective) but it is unlikely that we will ever be able to prevent all of these cases from occurring.[24,25] The public at large is not as acutely aware as are obstetricians and neonatologists of the hazards associated with birth. It is sometimes necessary to confess that a baby has been damaged by intrapartum asphyxia that could not have been prevented, other than by a prior caesarean section for which there was no indication.

Resuscitation

It is possible to predict the majority of instances when resuscitation of the newborn might be required but it is not, and never will be, possible to predict them all. At present about 7% of babies needing resuscitation are born normally at term. This means that every birth must be attended by someone capable of assessing an asphyxiated baby, establishing a clear airway and administering effective bag-and-mask ventilation. This is the key to neonatal resuscitation and the vast majority of asphyxiated babies need no more than lung inflation and improved arterial oxygenation in order to recover fully.[26] For the benefit of non-paediatric readers it should perhaps be pointed out that drugs are rarely needed during resuscitation of the newborn and the trappings of the adult resuscitation scene such as cardiac monitors and defibrillators are redundant. When the birth occurs in hospital it is reasonable to expect that someone with the ability to intubate and provide advanced resuscitation if necessary will be available within five minutes. For births taking place outside a hospital with resident paediatric cover this will not usually be possible and this constitutes an area of small, but finite, risk. Women choosing to give birth under such circumstances should be fully informed about what will and will not be available in the event that an unexpectedly asphyxiated baby is born. They should not be encouraged to believe that giving birth at home is as safe as doing so in hospital; it can never be so.[27]

Accurate documentation of resuscitation is important both in demonstrating that it was performed properly and in assessing the likely severity of asphyxia present at birth. A specially designed pro-forma for recording details of resuscitation is useful.[28]

Neonatal intensive care

Despite the associated high mortality and morbidity neonatal intensive care is relatively rarely the subject of litigation. This may be chiefly because the hazardous nature of the undertaking is explicit, and quite different from an event like childbirth which is perceived to be a normal process which should have a normal outcome. Yet, paediatricians can take some of the credit for effectively communicating with parents and involving them in decision making and aspects of care. We must not become complacent, though, as the climate may change and there is invariably room for improvement. This section deals with aspects of some of the commonest avoidable mishaps.

Hypoglycaemia

All newborn infants are liable to become hypoglycaemic if they do not receive adequate nutrition. Some infants are particularly predisposed to do so because of reduced endogenous nutrient stores, increased glucose utilisation, disordered metabolism or endocrine imbalance. Most important among these are the small-for-gestational-age infant and the infant of a diabetic mother. Hypoglycaemia of sufficient severity and duration can cause irreversible brain injury, through mechanisms believed to be similar to those occurring during hypoxia, leading to mental retardation and cerebral palsy. It is thought that only symptomatic hypoglycaemia is likely to damage the brain. The symptoms of hypoglycaemia are too subtle and varied, however, especially in the immature or sick infant, to be relied upon and adherence to biochemical limits is a safer approach. A particularly difficult situation is hypoglycaemia following birth asphyxia when it is impossible to disentangle the contributions from the two possible causes of abnormal neurological signs.

Recent research suggests that to be on the safe side the blood glucose concentration should be maintained above 2·7 mmol/L.[29,30] Babies known to be at increased risk of hypoglycaemia should receive regular monitoring of blood glucose concentration, as ever with documentation of the results! If the blood glucose concentration falls below 2·7 mmol/L, other than transiently, steps must be taken to bring it to a safer level by whatever means necessary. Too often there is procrastination. In circumstances of significant clinical risk an intravenous infusion should be set up and the concentration of glucose should be increased until normoglycaemia is achieved. If that means a central venous catheter and 20% dextrose so be it! Untreated, sustained hypoglycaemia in the newborn is generally indefensible.

Neonatal sepsis[31]

Newborn infants, particularly those born prematurely, have poor defences against infection and yet are exposed to a wide variety of potentially pathogenic micro-organisms during early postnatal life. The rapidity with which an infected infant can deteriorate and the non-specific nature of the presenting signs make sepsis a very serious threat. Among the most notorious pathogens are group B streptococci, *Staphylococcus aureus*, *Listeria monocytogenes*, *Haemophilus influenzae* and *Escherichia coli*. All are capable of causing the death of a previously well infant within a matter of 24 hours. Delays in the diagnosis and treatment of neonatal sepsis are all too common and it is incumbent on all maternity units to ensure that their staff are well trained in recognising the early signs of neonatal infection. Loss of signs of well-being in any young infant should raise the suspicion of sepsis and always merits a careful clinical appraisal. Among presenting features demanding urgent evaluation are grunting or moaning respiration, lack of interest in feeding, pallor, mottling of the skin and loss of muscle tone. By no means are all babies presenting with such signs suffering from infection but the penalties for delayed diagnosis and treatment are so severe as to demand a screening approach that emphasises sensitivity over specificity. That is, it is preferable to make false-positive diagnoses of sepsis than to make false-negative ones. An unnecessary septic screen and a 48-hour course of antibiotics is the price that some babies have to pay for the safety of others.

Vascular access procedures

Securing and maintaining safe vascular access is a challenging task in all young children but nowhere more so than in neonatal intensive care. No type of vascular access is totally free of risk and a complete list of possible adverse events is too frightening to contemplate. It would certainly include the loss of limbs and sudden death from perforation of the myocardium. However, vascular access is often essential and all that can be asked is that appropriate measures are taken to minimise the risk of serious complications.

Arterial lines

Gaining and maintaining arterial access is an essential component of neonatal intensive care. In any objective appraisal of risks and benefits, catheterisation of the umbilical artery (UAC) using a catheter bearing a continuous-reading oxygen-electrode has to be best value. Locating the tip of the catheter in the lower thorax possibly has less complications than placing it at the bifurcation of the aorta but both approaches have their advocates. Placing the catheter tip anywhere between these locations is taboo. A well recognised hazard of umbilical artery catheterisation in very immature babies is burning of the skin by the fluid used to clean the peri-umbilical area. This is especially likely to occur if excess cleaning fluid soaks into the bedding and remains in contact with the skin of the back and buttocks. As a precaution the minimum amount of fluid should be used and the baby's bedding should be replaced after the procedure. Regular checks must be made of the circulation to the buttocks and lower limbs and these should be documented. Any non-transient compromise of the circulation should trigger the immediate removal of the catheter under virtually all circumstances. UACs will often continue to function for many weeks but should be removed once the baby's condition is sufficiently improved for the benefits to become outweighed by the risks. There are no hard and fast rules.

Next in order of preference is the radial artery cannula. This does not have the benefits of continuous oxygen monitoring but does allow continuous arterial blood pressure monitoring and frequent arterial sampling. Before catheterising the radial artery it is mandatory to ensure that the corresponding ulnar artery is able to maintain a satisfactory circulation to the hand by using what has become knows as Allen's test. This is too widely known to paediatricians to require description here. In common with the UAC, and every other form of arterial line, if there is more than a transient compromise of the circulation the line should be removed. There may occasionally be circumstances in which the benefits of maintaining arterial access are thought to outweigh a significant risk of ischaemic injury to the tissues but these are few and far between and in such circumstances it would be wise to share a discussion of the risks and benefits with the parents.

All other sites of arterial access are less desirable than the two outlined above although ulnar arteries, brachial arteries, femoral arteries, posterior tibial arteries and superficial temporal arteries are all acceptable sites when necessary as long as careful monitoring for complications is undertaken and documented.

Whichever artery is cannulated it is absolutely vital to ensure that vasoactive drugs such as adrenaline and dopamine are never infused through an arterial line. The consequences can be disastrous.

105

Venous access

Venous access is generally far less problematic than arterial access but by no means free from potentially serious complications. The main risks associated with peripheral venous access are those related to leakage of the infusion fluid into the tissues, which may cause serious scarring even in very immature babies who normally heal well.[32] Large extravasated volumes of any fluid are capable of causing ischaemic tissue injury but quite small volumes of some fluids are notorious for causing tissue necrosis. Among the worst offenders are solutions containing calcium, some antibiotics and concentrated glucose solutions. All infusion devices should have pressure alarms and infusion sites should be inspected at least hourly and some form of simple documentation of this process must be undertaken.[33] Once again, no documentation may be interpreted as a lack of observation.

Retinopathy of prematurity (ROP)

The development and growth of the blood vessels of the retina is normally an antenatal event but following preterm birth it occurs postnatally, particularly in the peripheral retina which is the last part to be reached by the advancing tide of capillaries. In babies born at less than 32 weeks of gestation this vascularisation can progress abnormally leading to disruption of the retina and blindness. The chief, but not the only, factor predisposing to ROP is an excessively high oxygen tension (commonly designated "pO_2") in arterial blood. Meticulous control of arterial pO_2 below 10 kilopascals until retinal vascularisation is complete will prevent the development of significant ROP in the vast majority of susceptible infants. In order to achieve this aim, arterial pO_2 must be monitored carefully in all babies of less than 32 weeks' gestation receiving supplemental oxygen, especially during their period of intensive care. By far the best way to do this is to use an umbilical artery catheter with a continuous reading pO_2 electrode but regular intermittent sampling of arterial blood, supported by some form of continuous non-invasive monitoring, is an acceptable alternative. It is not sufficient to rely on pulse oximetry, transcutaneous pO_2 monitoring or capillary blood gas sampling alone and a claim of medical negligence would be difficult to defend if significant ROP occurred in the absence of attempts to secure some form of direct arterial pO_2 monitoring. It is of course not always possible to achieve arterial access but it is always possible to make a determined effort to do so and to record these efforts in the notes.

As babies improve and move out of intensive care their vulnerability to ROP generally declines and less intensive monitoring of pO_2 is appropriate even if oxygen therapy is continued on account of chronic lung disease. This is just as well as arterial access may be difficult to maintain for prolonged periods. The emphasis at that stage is on the prevention of hypoxia and pulse oximetry is now the best technique for this.

Screening

From about 1992 onwards it has been essential to ensure that babies at risk of ROP are screened by an ophthalmologist so that those few babies who develop progressive ROP despite primary prevention measures (almost all below 28 weeks' gestation[34]) can benefit from retinal treatment with cryosurgery or, preferably, laser photocoagulation.[35] Current recommendations are that all babies born at less than 1500 g birthweight or 31 weeks' gestation should be screened from 6 to 7 weeks postnatal age.[36] If abnormalities are noted, repeated examinations are required to check for progression to severe disease and to determine when therapy is indicated. Such screening and treatment can substantially reduce the expected rate of severe visual impairment and scrupulous efforts at primary prevention coupled with an effective screening programme make blindness from ROP a rare event.[37] Unfortunately, screening for ROP requires considerable ophthalmological skill, patience and experience and it may be difficult to offer an effective screening programme to every at risk infant. It is unlikely that failure to screen could be successfully defended if potentially treatable visual impairment developed. This still represents a significant area of risk for many hospitals in the UK at the present time.

Conclusions

There are probably more specific risks in paediatric practice than there are words in this chapter and so I have been highly selective. The more general issues are as usual the most important ones and the following check list reiterates a few key points.

- Children should be cared for in designated children's wards, outpatient clinics, A & E departments, operating theatres etc. They should not share accommodation with adult patients. Apart from permitting a "child-orientated" physical environment, including suitable cross-infection measures, the segregation of children's services helps to ensure that child- and family-centred care can be developed and sustained. This usually means good communication, a holistic approach to the child's needs and the early detection of disturbed family relationships.
- Children should be cared for and treated by healthcare professionals specialising in paediatrics. This includes medical, nursing and paramedical staff. In this way the risk of children coming to harm out of ignorance is minimised.

107

- The recommendations of key advisory documents such as the report of the Clothier Committee and the "Welfare of Children and Young People in Hospital" should be implemented. There is a great measure of risk reduction implicit in many of the recommendations contained in these reports.
- Effective child protection procedures should be in place and arrangements for educating staff and publicising networks of communication should be established and kept up to date.
- Adequate medical and nursing notes should be maintained as a permanent record of the high quality of care provided and as a means of ensuring effective transfer of information between professionals. The Parent Held Record is a part of this.
- As well as providing good quality care, communicating with parents is vital. Not the transatlantic approach of detailing every conceivable potential hazard but rather showing a willingness to explain and, when appropriate, share decision-making. Parents generally have a right to know exactly what is going on and are probably less likely to embark on legal action if they feel they are partners with the staff in the care of their child than if they are treated in a high-handed and paternalistic manner.

References

1 Lowrie L, Weiss AH, Lacombe C. The Pediatric Sedation Unit: A mechanism for pediatric sedation. *Pediatrics* 1998;**102**:e30.
2 Jedlicka-Kohler I, Gotz M, Eichler I. Parents' recollection of the initial communication of the diagnosis of cystic fibrosis. *Pediatrics* 1996;**97**:204–9.
3 Lally S. An investigation into the functions of nurses' communication at the inter-shift handover. *J Nurs Manag* 1999;**7**:29–36.
4 Roughton VJ, Severs MP. The junior doctor handover: current practices and future expectations. *J R Coll Physicians, Lond* 1996;**30**:213–14.
5 Van Walraven C, Rokosh E. What is necessary for high-quality discharge summaries? *Am J Med Qual* 1999;**14**:160–9.
6 Sims DG, Downham MA, Webb JK, *et al.* Hospital cross-infection with respiratory syncytial virus and the role of adult carriage. *Acta Paediatr Scand* 1975;**64**: 541–3.
7 Whiteford ML, Wilkinson JD, McColl JH, *et al.* Outcome of *Burkholderia (Pseudomonas) cepacia* colonisation in children with cystic fibrosis following a hospital outbreak. *Thorax* 1995;**50**:1194–8.
8 Ledson MJ, Gallagher MJ, Corkill JE, *et al.* Cross infection between cystic fibrosis patients colonised with *Burkholderia cepacia*. *Thorax* 1998;**53**:432–6.
9 American Society of Hospital Pharmacists ASHP guidelines on preventing medication errors in hospital. *Am J Hosp Pharm* 1993;**50**:305–14.
10 Raju TNK, Kecskes S, Thornton JP, *et al.* Medication errors in neonatal and paediatric intensive care units. *Lancet* 1989;**2**:374–6.
11 Williamson JA, Mackay P. Incident reporting. *Med J Aust* 1991;**155**:340–4.
12 Folli HL, Poole RL, Benitz WE. Medication error prevention by clinical pharmacists in two children's hospitals. *Pediatrics* 1987;**79**:718–22.
13 Wilson DG, McArtney RG, Newcombe RG, *et al.* Medication errors in paediatric prac-

tice: insights from a continuous quality improvement approach. *Eur J Pediatr* 1998;**157**: 769–74.

14 Selbst SM, Fein JA, Osterhoudt K, Ho W. Medication errors in a paediatric emergency department. *Pediatr Em Care* 1999;**15**:1–4.

15 Koren G, Barzilay Z, Greenwald M. Tenfold errors in administration of drug doses. A neglected iatrogenic disease in paediatrics. *Pediatrics* 1986;**77**:848–9.

16 Perlstein PH, Callison C, White M. Errors in drug computations during newborn intensive care. *Am J Dis Child* 1979;**133**:376–9.

17 Gitlow HS, Melby MJ. Framework for continuous quality improvement in the provision of pharmaceutical care. *Am J Hosp Pharm* 1991;**48**:1917–25.

18 Leape LL, Bates DW, Cullen DJ, *et al.* Systems analysis of adverse drug events. *JAMA* 1995;**274**:35–43.

19 *Medicines for Children.* London: RCPCH Publications Ltd, 1999.

20 Meadow R. Münchhausen syndrome by proxy. *Arch Dis Child* 1982; **57**:92–8.

21 Meadow R. Unnatural sudden infant death. *Arch Dis Child* 1999;**80**:7–14.

22 Rommal C. Documentation issues in electronic fetal monitoring. *J Healthc Risk Manag* 1997;**17**:27–34.

23 Freeman JM, Nelson KB. Intrapartum asphyxia and cerebral palsy. *Pediatrics* 1988;**82**: 240–9.

24 Blair E, Stanley FJ. Intrapartum asphyxia: a rare cause of cerebral palsy. *J Pediat* 1988;**112**:515–19.

25 Stanley FJ. The aetiology of cerebral palsy. *Early Human Develop* 1994;**36**:81–8.

26 Royal College of Paediatrics and Child Health. *Resuscitation of babies at birth.* London: BMJ Publishing Group, 1997.

27 Bastian H, Keirse MJNC, Lancaster PAL. Perinatal death associated with planned home birth in Australia: population based study. *BMJ* 1998;**317**:384–8.

28 Rommal C. Risk management issues in the perinatal setting. *J Perinat Neonat Nursing* 1996;**10**:1–31.

29 Lucas A, Morley R, Cole T. Adverse neurodevelopmental outcome of moderate neonatal hypoglycaemia. *BMJ* 1988;**297**:1304–8.

30 Koh TH, Eyre JA, Aynsley-Green A. Neural dysfunction during hypoglycaemia. *Arch Dis Child* 1988;**63**:1386–8.

31 Dear PRF. Infection in the newborn. In *Textbook of neonatology*, Rennie J, Robertson NRC eds. 3rd edition. Edinburgh: Churchill Livingstone, 1999:1127–1132.

32 Morrison WA, Hurley JV, Ahmad TS, Webster HR. Scar formation after skin injury to the human fetus in-utero or the premature neonate. *Br J Plast Surg* 1999;**52**:6–11.

33 Wynsma LA. Negative outcomes of intravascular therapy in infants and children. *AACN Clin Issues* 1998;**9**:49–63.

34 Hussain N, Clive J, Bhandra V. Current incidence of retinopathy of prematurity, 1989–1997. *Pediatrics* 1999;**104**:e26.

35 Paysse EA, Lindsey JL, Coats DK, *et al.* Therapeutic outcomes of cryotherapy versus transpupillary diode laser photocoagulation for threshold retinopathy of prematurity. *J AAPOS* 1999;**3**:234–40.

36 Fielder AR, Levene MI. Screening for retinopathy of prematurity. *Arch Dis Child* 1992;**67**: 860–7.

37 Connolly BP, McNamara JA, Regillo CD, *et al.* Visual outcomes after laser photocoagulation for threshold retinopathy of prematurity. *Ophthalmology* 1999;**106**: 1734–7.

Further reading

Reports advising on aspects of healthcare for children

Children First. A Study of Hospital Services. Audit Commission 1993.
Children's Surgical Services. Royal College of Paediatrics and Child Health 1996.
Management Models in Established Combined or Integrated Child Health Services. BPA 1992.
Outcome Measurements for Child Health. BPA 1992.
Parent Held and Professional Records Used in Child Health Surveillance. BPA 1993.

Purchasing Health Services for Children and Young People. BPA 1994.
The Report of the National Confidential Enquiry into Perioperative Deaths. HMSO 1989.
The Report of the National Confidential Enquiry into Perioperative Deaths. 1999.
Welfare of Children and Young People in Hospital. HMSO 1991.
Working Together. Under the Children Act 1989. HMSO 1991.

7 Clinical risk management in anaesthesia

JAN DAVIES, ALAN AITKENHEAD

The state of anaesthesia may be considered to be intrinsically unsafe. The anaesthetised patient is at risk of complications from many contributory factors, including the actions or inaction of the anaesthetist and other associated healthcare workers, and from the absence, malfunction or failure of anaesthetic equipment. Patients are given drugs that have side effects, particularly on the cardiovascular and respiratory systems. Unconsciousness carries with it risks of airway obstruction, soiling of the lungs and inability to detect peripheral injury. Pharmacological muscle paralysis necessitates the use of artificial ventilation, making the patient dependent on the anaesthetist and anaesthetic equipment for the fundamental functions of oxygenation and excretion of carbon dioxide. The anaesthetist may also deliberately alter physiological functions, for example, by inducing hypotension or ventilating only one lung.

Human error in anaesthetic practice

An anaesthetist obtains information about the physiological state of the patient and the progress of the anaesthetic from observing the patient, the monitors, and the anaesthetic machine. All of this information is collated and used to make decisions about the anaesthetic. Any required change will necessitate an action, such as adjusting a control, which must be correctly executed to achieve the desired end. Consequently, human errors may occur during the observation (input of information), decision making (processing of information), or action (output of responses) stages.

Input errors can be minimised by good equipment design. Advances in the design of monitors have eliminated many subjective errors and introduced a range of important measurements not previously available. New generations of anaesthetic monitors using computer technology can integrate and display physiological information and raise alarms when predetermined limits are transgressed. The overall aim is to provide information that is clear and easily assimilated, thus reducing the risk of mental overload.

Traditionally, constant vigilance is expected of the anaesthetist, yet it is clear that continuously maintaining total alertness and vigilance is not possible, as confirmed by critical incident studies. Well-designed equipment and physiological monitors trigger a return to total vigilance at appropriate times.

When making decisions the anaesthetist has to decide not only whether or not something is wrong but also why. The monitors indicate which vital signs are abnormal, but the anaesthetist must piece the various items of information together and choose a hypothesis that will lead to the correct action. Often the anaesthetist will follow some, perhaps unconscious, mental rule and select the most common explanation that matches the situation. When confronted with a novel problem, an anaesthetist is required to use abstract reasoning. This knowledge-based behaviour is slower and requires more effort.

Anaesthetists need to be taught to question their decisions because clinging to false hypotheses or an inappropriate rule is a well-known cause of accidents. In one instance, a patient was left in a persistent vegetative state after a hypoxic cardiac arrest caused by disconnection from the ventilator. The hypoxaemia initially caused increases in heart rate and blood pressure, which the anaesthetist interpreted as indicating inadequate anaesthesia. He increased the inspired concentration of anaesthetic agent, and administered an intravenous β-blocker. He attributed the subsequent progressive decreases in heart rate and blood pressure, and the cardiac arrest, to administration of the β-blocker. The possibility that profound hypoxaemia was the cause of all of these physiological changes escaped him.

What are the risks associated with anaesthesia?

Numerous publications describe anaesthetic-related risks. Traditionally these publications have described the results of mortality, morbidity, and litigation reviews. In addition, critical incident studies provide some estimate of anaesthetic-related risks. Each of these types of publications has advantages and disadvantages (see Table 7.1).

Estimates of mortality

Mortality is a vital estimate of risk associated with anaesthesia, the most important reason being that the definition is clear, in contrast to the

112

Table 7.1 Advantages and disadvantages of methods of evaluating anaesthetic-related risk

Type of study	Advantage	Disadvantage
Mortality	Well-defined	Infrequent
Morbidity	Greater frequency than mortality	Ill-defined
Litigation	Severe outcomes or patterns	Biased
Critical incident	What can go wrong	Anecdotal

more debatable definitions of morbidity. However, mortality or "flower-bedecked failure"1 is a somewhat crude estimate of risk, because of the relative rarity of this complication.

During the three decades up to 1980, a number of investigators in various countries attempted to estimate the frequency with which death was associated with anaesthesia.[2-15] There was a general trend towards reduced mortality attributable primarily to anaesthesia (from about 1:2500 to about 1:5000). However, the studies continued to identify the same principal causes of death, such as inadequate supervision of trainees and lack of postoperative care.

One of the problems that renders comparison among these studies difficult is that different criteria were used to define "anaesthetic death". A spectrum of time limits has been used, starting with all deaths occurring before the time of transfer of the patient from the operating theatre or from the recovery room. A limit of deaths occurring within 24–48 hours after anaesthesia has reflected coronial requirements in many jurisdictions, with a period of 7–10 days used in other studies. However, some patients who suffer anaesthetic-related complications may not die for weeks, months or even years after the anaesthetic. These deaths would not be captured in studies using such limits. In addition, some studies of anaesthetic mortality have included patients who suffered hypoxic cerebral damage, with resultant persistent coma.

In 1982, the Association of Anaesthetists of Great Britain and Ireland (AAGBI) published the results of a major study of mortality in the United Kingdom. An anonymous and confidential system was established to report deaths that occurred within six days of surgery. During the study, an estimated 1 147 362 operations took place,[16] with an overall perioperative mortality of 0·53%. Anaesthesia was considered totally responsible for death in less than 1:10 000 operations, but might have contributed to death in 1:1700 operations.

Many of the conclusions are still relevant today. The overwhelming message was that the process of anaesthesia is remarkably safe. However, many patients suffer from intercurrent disease and the implications for the anaesthetist are often ignored. While mistakes occur in the hands of all grades of anaesthetist, trainee anaesthetists are often unsupervised and abandoned by their assistants. There also appears to be insufficient consultation between surgeon and anaesthetist. Anaesthesia may contribute to deaths that occur more than 24 hours after its administration and autopsy reports alone are of limited value in explaining deaths associated with anaesthesia.[16]

Because of the importance of these findings, and because of the difficulty in separating anaesthetic and surgical factors when reports came only from anaesthetists, the AAGBI initiated the first Confidential Enquiry into Perioperative Deaths (CEPOD) in conjunction with the Association of Surgeons of Great Britain and Ireland. Over a 12-month period, the overall perioperative mortality was 0·7% (2928 deaths after 555 258 anaesthetics).[17] Of the 410 deaths associated with anaesthesia, expert assessors considered that only three deaths resulted solely from anaesthesia, an incidence of 1 in 185 086 anaesthetics.

Studies from other countries have suggested higher rates of death related to anaesthesia than that reported in the CEPOD study. From 1978 to 1982, the French Health Ministry conducted a prospective nationwide survey of major complications during anaesthesia. A representative sample of 198 103 anaesthetics (~ 8% of the total estimated number of anaesthetics in France) was analysed from 460 randomly selected institutions.[18] The incidence of death and persistent coma (after 24 hours) attributable totally to anaesthesia was 1:7924; death due solely to anaesthesia occurred with an incidence of 1:13 207.

In New South Wales, Australia, a system for the confidential investigation of deaths within 24 hours of, or as a result of, anaesthesia, has been in place since 1960. The Special Committee Investigating Deaths Under Anaesthesia (SCIDUA) classifies deaths as anaesthetic, surgical, inevitable, fortuitous or unassessable. Between 1960 and 1985, the incidence of death attributable to anaesthesia decreased from 1:5500 to 1:26 000.[19] The proportion of deaths attributable to anaesthesia in which no error in management could be found increased from 2·8% between 1960 and 1969 to 10% between 1983 and 1985. Over the same period, the proportion of specialist anaesthetists involved in deaths attributable to anaesthesia increased from 27% to 62%.

Between 1984 and 1990, SCIDUA assessed 1503 deaths, attributing 11·4% to factors under anaesthetists' control. About 10% of these deaths occurred in patients undergoing urgent non-emergency operations, of which 31·3% were attributed to anaesthetic factors.[20,21] The calculated rate of death attributable to anaesthesia was 1 in 20 000 operations.

Also from Australia are triennial reports collated from each of the state-based, government-supported committees that collect data about anaesthetic-related deaths. The fourth and latest report, for 1994–1996,[22] concluded that anaesthetic-related deaths occurred with a frequency of no more than 1:63 000 operative or diagnostic procedures. The death rate attributable to anaesthesia alone was considered to be about 1 in over 150 000 procedures.

In the Netherlands, a retrospective study of faults, accidents, near accidents and complications associated with anaesthesia in one institution was conducted between 1978 and 1987.[23] During that period, 97 496 anaesthetics were administered for non-cardiac procedures. Cardiac arrest occurred with an incidence of 1:3362 anaesthetics, and mortality from cardiac arrest in these patients occurred with an incidence of 1:5417 anaesthetics. Anaesthesia was considered to have contributed to cardiac arrest in 1:7500 anaesthetics, with a fatal outcome in 1:16 250 anaesthetics.

In Canada, the risk factors associated with death within seven days of anaesthesia were analysed in a study involving 100 000 surgical procedures.[24] There were 71 deaths per 10 000 patients, and differences in anaesthetic practice were much less important in contributing to death than were patient variables (age >80 years, concurrent severe disease) and surgical variables (major versus minor, emergency versus elective).

In a prospective study conducted in Denmark,[25] mortality attributable to anaesthesia occurred with a frequency of 1:2500 (0·04%). The overall perioperative mortality rate was 1·2%, and 0·05% of patients died during anaesthesia. Patients who developed postoperative cardiovascular complications had a mortality rate of 20%.

In the USA, an incidence of 1·7 cardiac arrests per 10 000 anaesthetics was reported in 1985,[26] although not all were fatal. The study involved 163 240 anaesthetics administered over a 15-year period. Of 449 cardiac arrests, 27 were judged to be attributable solely to anaesthesia, and mortality was 0·9 per 10 000 anaesthetics. Three-quarters of these cardiac arrests were considered to be preventable. In 1991, the same authors published results relating to 241 934 anaesthetics given between 1969 and 1988. Cardiac arrest related to anaesthetic causes decreased from 2·1 per 10 000 anaesthetics in the first decade to 1·0 per 10 000 in the second decade, when pulse oximetry and capnography were introduced.[27] Most of the difference was due to a decrease in cardiac arrests from preventable respiratory causes.

In 1998, there were five deaths in the United Kingdom associated with dental anaesthesia in which a specific inhalational agent, halothane, was employed. It is likely that, in most cases, the precipitating factor was a ventricular arrhythmia. A recent study[28] identified that the frequency of cardiac arrhythmias during dental surgery in children anaesthetised with halothane was six times higher than when another agent (sevoflurane) was used (48% vs. 8%). The Committee on Safety of Medicines has now recommended that halothane should not be used for dental anaesthesia outside hospitals.

115

Estimates of morbidity

Reference has been made above to some studies that have estimated the frequency of serious morbidity as well as mortality. Pedersen[25] reported a very high incidence (9%) of intra-operative cardiopulmonary complications associated with anaesthesia or surgery, and requiring intervention during the procedure. One-third of all complications were considered preventable.

Cooper et al [29] studied patients admitted to an intensive care unit as a result of serious complications of anaesthesia. Over the decade of the study, 2% of ICU admissions were related to complications of anaesthesia (1 in 1543 anaesthetics). The majority of complications (62%) occurred in the recovery period and most involved the heart or lungs. One quarter of the complications were judged to have been avoidable, and 17% of the patients died.

The Multicenter Study in the United States[30-32] was conducted in an attempt to analyse predictors of severe perioperative adverse outcome related to general anaesthesia using four specific anaesthetic agents. A total of 17 201 patients were followed up for seven days for the occurrence of certain specified outcomes, such as changes in blood pressure, heart rate and rhythm, myocardial infarction, and respiratory failure. The major risk factors for severe outcome included type of surgery (such as cardiovascular surgery) and patient history (such as heart failure). The study was too small to detect any important differences (if they existed) among the four anaesthetic agents.

In Canada, data relating to complications from anaesthesia were collected over two decades, between 1975 and 1983.[33] Follow-up of 112 961 patients showed that nearly 10% of patients were either inconvenienced or suffered some morbidity as a result of the anaesthetic, while 0·45% suffered significant morbidity. The most common complications were nausea, vomiting and sore throat.

The Canadian Four-Centre Study reported on follow-up of 27 184 patients who underwent anaesthesia and surgery between 1987 and 1989.[34,35] A panel of experts defined 115 major events, and classified them into anaesthesia-related, surgery-related or disease-related categories. There was an anaesthetic involvement in 10·3% of major events but no anaesthetic deaths.

Recently, Myles and colleagues[36] developed a 40-item questionnaire, which covered various aspects of recovery: physical comfort, pain, physical independence, emotional state and psychological support. In an accompanying paper,[37] the authors compared the occurrence of specific outcomes, such as nausea, vomiting, pain and other complications, with patient satisfaction. The level of satisfaction was high (96·8%) and the level of dissatisfaction low (0·9%). There was a strong correlation between dissatisfaction and the occurrence of intraoperative awareness, severe nausea and vomiting, or moderate or severe postoperative pain.

These reports of morbidity show that the risk of non-lethal complications is greater than the risk of death related to anaesthesia. However, one of the problems with these studies is that there is a great range of what constitutes morbidity. Indeed, the study by Myles and colleagues illustrates the trend toward considering patients' psychological well being, as well as their physical outcome, and the importance of the link between the two.

Data from litigation

Because of the high rate of litigation against anaesthetists in some countries, analysis of claims for compensation has been used to examine the pattern of injury which patients may suffer, or believe that they have suffered, as a result of the actions of anaesthetists. There is a risk of bias in analysing claims for compensation, in that the complaints relate predominantly to events that the patient does not expect. For example, a patient may not expect to suffer blindness after undergoing a lumbar laminectomy and might well institute medico-legal proceedings. In contrast, totally inept treatment of postoperative pain is very unlikely (at present) to result in a claim for compensation, because the patient expects to experience postoperative pain. While patients are prepared to accept that surgery may not be entirely successful, or may be associated with a small incidence of complications, they are often unwilling to acknowledge that any consequence which they attribute to anaesthesia, or the anaesthetist, is acceptable. In one extreme example, a patient attempted to sue her anaesthetist for failing to diagnose breast cancer at the pre-operative visit when she underwent cystoscopy; the tumour was diagnosed six months later. In addition, the pattern of claims is influenced by the personality of the patient, and, in some countries, by the availability of free legal advice.

Analysis of cases reported to the Medical Defence Union between 1970 and 1982 showed that anaesthetic-related death or cerebral damage was most often related to error rather than to misadventure. Faulty technique (43%) and failure of postoperative care (9%) were the most common errors.[38] Recently, death attributable to negligence by anaesthetists has resulted in convictions for manslaughter[39] as well as civil litigation. In addition, an anaesthetist was jailed in Canada for criminal negligence in the case of a young man left permanently brain-damaged.[40]

Patients may also suffer less serious physical injury or distress, which may be followed by claims for compensation. Damage to teeth is by far the single most common complaint, accounting for 52% of reports to the Medical Defence Union[38] and 14% of closed claims from the Canadian Medical Protective Association for 1987–90.[41]

In the 1980s in the USA, the Committee of Professional Liability of the American Society of Anesthesiologists began a structured evaluation of adverse anaesthetic outcomes to improve safety by devising strategies to prevent anaesthetic mishaps. Data was extracted from "closed claims" files of 17 insurance organisations that indemnify doctors. The first report[42] reviewed 14 cases of unexpected cardiac arrest in healthy patients who had received spinal anaesthesia. In a number of cases, it was postulated that respiratory insufficiency had occurred in relation to administration of sedatives. In others, death was related to cardiovascular insufficiency that had been treated inappropriately. The second report[43] assessed the potential role of monitoring devices in the prevention of anaesthetic mishaps. Reviewers considered that 31·5% of negative outcomes in 1097 claims could have been prevented by the use of additional monitors, particularly pulse oximetry and capnography. Outcomes considered preventable by this mechanism were more severe in terms of injury and cost of settlement, for both regional and general anaesthesia.

The third closed claim report[44] concerned adverse respiratory events, which constituted the single largest category of injury – 34% of 1541 files examined. (Dental damage was excluded from the studies.) Death or brain damage occurred in 85% of cases with adverse respiratory events compared with 30% for non-respiratory events. The percentage of claims in which anaesthetic management was considered to have been substandard was much higher for respiratory than for non-respiratory events.

Subsequent reports have focused on less frequent respiratory events,[45] obstetric anaesthetic practice,[46] paediatric anaesthetic practice[47] and burns during anaesthesia.[48]

Critical incident reporting

Critical incident studies in medicine were pioneered in anaesthesia. Depending on how the study is structured, the results may provide a picture of what could go wrong, rather than what did (e.g. morbidity or mortality). Studies of potential problems ("near hits") have the dual advantages of greater frequency of occurrence and a lack of guilt on the part of the reporter. Critical incident studies that also collect "hits" provide essentially anecdotal data, in that the numerator and denominator are often unknown, particularly when reports are collected on a voluntary and anonymous basis. (This is in contrast to critical incident studies in aviation, which may be mandatory and confidential, thus providing a more accurate assessment of frequency.)

The first application of the critical incident analysis technique from aviation to anaesthesia was made by Blum in 1971,[49] when he described ambiguity of the oxygen pressure gauge design. He also noted the importance of the layout of the anaesthetist's work place. He recognised the concepts of "vigilance" and "negative transfer". He even criticised equipment manufacturers for continuing to produce their own (different) designs without consideration for ergonomics and the needs of the users of the equipment.

Cooper *et al*[50] applied a version of the critical incident technique to anaesthetic practice to examine errors and equipment failures. Their definition of a critical incident was:

an occurrence that could have led (if not corrected and discovered in time) or did lead to an undesirable outcome ranging from increased length of hospital stay to death. It must also involve error by a member of the anaesthetic team or a failure of the anaesthetists' equipment to function; occur while the patient is under anaesthetic care; be described in clear detail by an observer or member of the anaesthetic team; and be clearly preventable.

This definition was a mixture of what could and did happen. In addition, incidents could lead to a change in Process of care, as in increased length of hospitalisation, or to Outcome, such as permanent disability or death.

In their first study,[50] Cooper *et al* employed an interview technique. Both consultant and trainee anaesthetists were asked to describe preventable happenings which they had observed involving either equipment failure or human error. Three of the most frequent events involved breathing system disconnections, problems with gas supply, and errors with syringes. One important finding was that more reported incidents occurred during the day (79%) than at night (21%), although the day/night case distribution was 85/15. One interpretation is that more daytime incidents were reported – a potential problem with voluntary reporting.

In subsequent studies,[51,52] the same group collected data prospectively, using anonymised reporting. They evaluated the effect of a relief anaesthetist and produced a more specific analysis of mishaps with substantive negative outcomes. These were defined as death, cardiac arrest, cancelled operation, extended stay in the recovery room, intensive care unit or hospital. (Some of these "outcomes" in fact represented Process, such as cancelled operation.) Those critical incidents that did not progress to an actual complication had on average 2·5 associated factors, whereas those that were associated with a complication had on average 3·4 associated factors. There was also a higher frequency (71%) of adverse outcomes of errors versus critical incidents only (41%) in moderately or severely ill patients, reflecting the smaller margin for safety in less healthy patients.

Critical incident reporting has been adopted widely over the last decade. Many anaesthetic departments collect data internally,[53] using the data to identify and correct faults with specific items of equipment, to modify protocols, guidelines and training, and to provide feedback at departmental meetings.

One of the largest studies is the Australian Incident Monitoring Study,[54] which, in 1993, reported in detail the findings from analysis of the first 2000 incident reports. Minor physiological changes occurred in association with 30% of incidents, major physiological changes but no injury followed 18%, physical morbidity occurred in 6%, and awareness in 1%. Death was associated with 1·5% of incidents.[55]

Examples of the most commonly quoted critical incidents	Examples of the commonest human factors associated with critical incidents
Problems with the anaesthetic breathing system <ul><li>disconnections</li><li>misconnections</li><li>leaks</li></ul> Problems in the administration of drugs <ul><li>overdosage</li><li>underdosage</li><li>wrong drug</li></ul> Problems with intubation and control of the airway <ul><li>failed intubation</li><li>oesophageal intubation</li><li>endobronchial intubation</li><li>accidental or premature extubation</li><li>aspiration</li></ul> Failure of equipment <ul><li>laryngoscopes</li><li>intravenous infusion devices</li><li>breathing system valves</li><li>monitoring devices</li></ul>	Inexperience Lack of <ul><li>skilled assistance</li><li>supervision</li></ul> Failure of planning Equipment <ul><li>lack of familiarity</li><li>failure to check</li></ul> Poor communication Restricted visual field or access Haste Fatigue and decreased vigilance Distraction Inattention/carelessness

The commonest incidents reported in critical incident studies and the most commonly quoted associated human factors are shown above. There is a close similarity with the factors that contributed to death in the CEPOD study,[17] in particular, inexperience and fatigue. However, it should be noted that in many of these studies, particularly those from litigation, the focus of the analysis has been the behaviour of the anaesthetist and his or her failings. In others, the actions of the surgeon and a contribution by the patient are also included. Very few studies take a truly systems-oriented view of anaesthetic risk by encompassing such latent system factors as the organisation (management attitudes, policies and procedures, budgetary restrictions) and the regulatory agencies (licensing and disciplinary bodies).

Managing risk

A risk management programme in anaesthesia should aim to identify areas of risk before a patient is harmed. There should also be continuous review, and where necessary, improvement of all aspects of anaesthesia delivery. Because human error is inevitable, risk management programmes should endeavour to manage error. In any system there are three levels at which human error can be managed. The first level seeks to decrease the probability of errors occurring, through shaping the behaviour of the individuals involved: careful selection, appropriate training, continuing medical education, and good working conditions. (These factors are to be found in the Structure of any system.) The second level encourages the detection of errors. (These activities are based in Process and represent event-shaping factors.) The third level reduces the consequences of errors. (The severity of an Outcome may be diminished, unchanged or magnified by factors subsequent to the error.)[56] Of these three levels, the first – efforts to reduce the probability of errors occurring – is the most important.

Decreasing the probability of errors occurring

Selection of anaesthetists

Anaesthetists are recruited from medical graduates, and their selection is therefore influenced by the methods of selection of medical students. The qualities which have been suggested as ideal in those seeking to embark on a career in anaesthesia are aptitude as a physician, academic ability, enthusiasm and energy, humanity, team membership concept, health, mental stability, sense of humour and conscientiousness.[57]

Attitudes are an important component of ability. Psychologists studying judgement in aviators have identified five attitude types as being particularly hazardous, and they have developed specific antidote thoughts for each hazardous attitude.[58] These are shown below.

Examples of hazardous attitudes and their antidote*

Hazardous attitude	*Antidote*
Anti-authority: "Don't tell me what to do. The policies are for someone else."	"Follow the rules. They are usually right."
Impulsivity: "Do something quickly – anything."	"Not so fast. Think first."
Invulnerability: "It won't happen to me. It's just a routine case."	"It could happen to me. Even routine cases develop serious problems."
Macho: "I'll show you I can do it. I can intubate anybody."	"Taking chances is foolish. Plan for the future."
Resignation: "What's the use? It's out of my hands. It's up to the surgeon."	"I'm not helpless. I can make a difference. There is always something else to try that might help."

*Adapted from *Aeronautical Decision Making* [58]

The invulnerability and macho attitudes are particularly dangerous in anaesthetists. These may be compounded by pressure from surgeons, heads of department or hospital managers to do more cases in less time, with less opportunity for pre-operative evaluation and with fewer cancellations. The belief that accidents only happen to other people, and that skill and knowledge will enable the individual to retrieve every situation successfully, can lead to cavalier behaviour and poor planning. In addition, just as pilots assess their ability to fly each day, anaesthetists should assess their ability to provide anaesthetic care. A simple list of questions that will aid in this self-assessment is shown below.

The I'M SAFE self-evaluation*

I   **Illness** – am I suffering from an illness that might interfere with my ability to provide safe anaesthetic care?

M   **Medication**–have I taken any prescription, over-the-counter or recreational drugs?

S   **Stress** – am I under any psychological pressure from my job, my family, my income or my own health?

A   **Alcohol** – have I had anything to drink in the last 24 hours and am I hung-over?

F   **Fatigue** – how much sleep have I had since I last worked during the day or was on-call? Did I sleep well last night and am I adequately rested?

E   **Eating** – have I eaten enough of the proper foods to keep me adequately nourished during the entire case and will I be able to obtain something to eat and drink if I get a break between cases?

*Adapted from *Human Factors for Aviation*[58]

Training and education

Syllabus   In some countries, there is a tendency to train anaesthetists in accordance with an examination syllabus. In some ways, this is inappropriate. The syllabus may rapidly become outdated. The existence of the syllabus may discourage the active search for knowledge beyond that specified by the syllabus, and so diminish interest in clinical learning. An important part of any training programme should be the development of appropriate attitudes towards learning and towards patient care. The trainee should want to learn, should want to acquire practical skills, and should want to become a safe anaesthetist.

Examinations The principal benefits of examinations are that they have a positive influence on motivation and study, and that, within certain limitations, they provide an objective and uniform standard for assessment of knowledge. However, they have a number of disadvantages. Written papers are useful tests of factual knowledge but are poor at assessing clinical skills. Oral examinations test factual knowledge, and can assess judgement, problem-solving ability and attitudes. Clinical skills are more difficult to assess formally.

Training devices and anaesthesia simulators Many life-threatening emergencies occur during anaesthesia with a frequency of one in 10 000 or less. An anaesthetist can complete his or her training without being exposed to these situations. Some emergencies are so rare that an anaesthetist may encounter only one during a working lifetime.

Training devices and simulators can be used to learn practical skills or rehearse clinical actions without risk. Training devices or part-task trainers permit individuals to acquire both knowledge and skills, although the emphasis usually focuses on specific skills, for example, intubation manikins and devices for practising central venous cannulation. A true simulator mimics the environment and phenomena as they appear in the real world, providing a learning experience that has the look and feel of a real operating theatre and real patient.[59] Simulators are valuable for training and expert practice but are not necessarily good for systematic learning of new skills and knowledge. Advantages of simulators are listed below. It should be noted that this list starts with an absence of risk to patients and ends with an absence of risk to the anaesthetist and other team members.

Advantages of simulators in anaesthesia

For the patients
- No risk from errors

For the trainee
- Scenarios involving uncommon but serious problems can be presented
- Recording, replay and critique of performance are facilitated

For the educator
- Same scenario can be presented to many trainees
- Scenarios can be repeated
- Simulation can be stopped for teaching, and restarted
- Errors can be allowed without any risk to the anaesthetist and other team members

---

Continuing medical education For many specialist anaesthetists, the scope of practice narrows. Specialists may lack expertise in new fields, and may fail to keep up-to-date within their own field. This is perhaps more likely in anaesthesia than in many other medical specialties because anaesthetists often work alone, and outdated practices may not be apparent either to the individual or to other members of the department.

Human factors

Two of the most important human factors in anaesthetic practice are fatigue and performance degradation because of drugs or illness.

Fatigue It is widely accepted that 24–36 hours of continuous duty is an absolute limit for anaesthetists. It is already common in many anaesthetic departments to limit duty to a maximum of 24 hours, followed by a full day off for recuperation. However, this practice is not followed uniformly. Significant acute and chronic fatigue may still develop even with the day off duty, because sleep will probably be disturbed during the recuperation period and many individuals will not take full advantage of the time to sleep because of other demands of their life.

Illness and drug abuse The specialty of anaesthesia has recognised the risks associated with impairment of function as a result of illness or drug abuse, and has implemented mechanisms of dealing with those in whom problems are detected. Menk *et al*[60] conducted a survey of teaching hospitals, and found that 113 trainees in whom drug abuse had been detected were re-admitted to the training programmes. The success rate associated with re-admission was 34% for opioid abusers and 70% for those who had abused other groups of drugs. Fourteen of the trainees committed suicide or died as a result of a self-administered drug overdose. In 13 of 79 opioid abusers re-admitted to training programmes, death was the first sign of relapse. The authors concluded that drug rehabilitation followed by redirection into an alternative specialty was the most prudent course of action for trainee anaesthetists in whom opioid abuse was recognised. Although the main risk appears to be to the individual's own safety, concerns about patient safety can never be eliminated.

A number of studies suggest that many senior doctors suffer high levels of stress, both anxiety and depression (see Chapter 17). Other studies have found similar problems in junior doctors. Psychological ill health often leads to excessive alcohol use or drug dependency. These are conditions that are dangerous for the patients of any doctor but can be quickly lethal for patients of an anaesthetist. In addition, the ageing anaesthetist may not recognise limitations imposed by failing eyesight, hearing, motor skills or cognition. All departments should have a plan for dealing with individuals who can no longer function at an appropriate level. This plan might include medical and/or psychological assessment, a change in work assignments, retraining, relief from night call, and phased or active retirement.

Team organisation

Staffing The numbers and grades of staff employed within an anaesthetic department must be commensurate with its clinical, professional and contractual obligations. These obligations include service provision, training, continuing education, research, audit and management. Allowance must be made for annual leave, study leave and external professional commitments. Failure by a department to make appropriate staffing arrangements may result in a mismatch between the capability of the anaesthetist and the nature of the work expected of him or her. For example, a relatively inexperienced trainee may be required to undertake anaesthesia for a patient with complex needs because inadequate provision has been made to cover the absence of a consultant.

Orientation All anaesthetic staff should take part in a formal induction programme before starting their clinical duties. An example of such a programme is shown on page 126.

Failure to implement an appropriate programme may result in anaesthetists using equipment with which they are unfamiliar, being unaware of the location of emergency equipment in the operating theatre, or being unaware of the location of a ward or department to which they may be called in an emergency.

Supervision Only consultants work independently. Other grades of staff, including trainees, work under direct or indirect supervision. All of these staff should know the identity and whereabouts of the responsible consultant, and should be taught to communicate any potential problems and to seek help or advice as appropriate. They should be firmly discouraged from undertaking any activity which is not comfortably within their competence and experience in the absence of such help, except in a life-threatening emergency.

Consultant emergency cover As anaesthesia becomes more highly specialised, there is a risk that consultant anaesthetists may be required to undertake procedures in an emergency which are outside their recent knowledge and experience. This is a risk particularly in departments in which consultants' elective clinical practice is fixed. Steps should be taken either to ensure that there are subspecialist on-call rotas (easier in large hospitals than in small ones), or to increase the flexibility of elective work so that consultants do not become de-skilled.

Sample orientation procedure for staff

This is an example of information which is required by new members of staff. The specific information that needs to be made available in each department of anaesthesia will vary, and this example should not be interpreted as a standard.

The Clinical Director is responsible for ensuring that, before working unsupervised, all new members of the department of anaesthesia (including locum appointments) are:

1 familiarised with the layout of the operating theatres, accident and emergency department and hospital wards, to ensure that they know where to attend if called to assist in an emergency

2 shown how to gain access to the hospital at night, and how to gain access to pertinent areas of the hospital protected by security locks

3 familiarised with the anaesthetic and monitoring equipment used in all locations in which the new member of staff may be expected to work

4 familiarised with the procedures for recovery from anaesthesia and for discharge to surgical wards

5 shown the locations of emergency equipment (e.g. defibrillator, difficult intubation kit) and emergency drugs (e.g. dantrolene)

6 told about the expectations of the department with regard to preoperative assessment, postoperative follow-up and reporting of complications

7 told about the system in force for checking anaesthetic and monitoring equipment before use

8 shown the anaesthetic record, and told the expectations of the department regarding its completion

9 told about the procedures for ordering urgent investigations and for obtaining blood or blood products in an emergency

10 informed about local protocols for clinical management, e.g. protocols used in the obstetric unit, criteria for notifying a more senior anaesthetist including the on-call consultant

11 informed about local protocols for specific emergency situations, e.g. malignant hyperthermia, difficult intubation, or anaphylaxis

12 told about the role of the department of anaesthesia in the hospital's major incident plan, and how to initiate the department's involvement in a major incident

13 informed about local educational and audit activities, including critical incident reporting.

It may be appropriate for items 6–13 to be presented in written form as an "Information Pack", together with a list of useful paging system and telephone numbers.

Reproduced with the permission of the Association of Anaesthetists of Great Britain and Ireland.[61]

Evaluating risks associated with new techniques   Anaesthesia has to adapt to changing surgical requirements, and hazards that may be peculiar to a new operation or anaesthetic technique need to be considered. In the early days of laparoscopy, patients were occasionally anaesthetised solely with a mask and spontaneous ventilation, with inevitably serious consequences. Laparoscopic cholecystectomy under general anaesthesia has cardiovascular effects on older patients that might not have been expected and laser surgery to the lower respiratory tract to relieve the dyspnoea of bronchial tumour is a procedure potentially fraught with hazard. Such procedures need consideration and evaluation by senior anaesthetists, as well as discussion with consultant surgeons, before a protocol is developed and junior staff left unsupervised.

Preoperative assessment

The anaesthetic management of any patient due to undergo surgery begins with the preoperative visit. Usually, the decision to operate has already been taken, but the anaesthetist has a vital contributory role, particularly in respect of preparation of the patient and the timing of surgery. The perceived benefit of surgery must be balanced against any risks inherent to the perioperative period. The anaesthetist's duty is to ensure that the patient is offered the best care, with anaesthesia and surgery taking place under conditions of maximum safety. The overall aims of assessment include:

- anticipation of difficulties
- making advanced preparation regarding facilities, equipment, and expertise
- enhancing patient safety and minimising the chance of errors
- assessing the risks of anaesthesia and surgery, and, where appropriate, discussing these with the patient
- allaying any relevant fears or anxieties perceived by the patient.

Unless there are overriding circumstances, patients should be assessed by their anaesthetist before transfer to the operating theatre suite; assessment in the anaesthetic (induction) room can result in pressure being applied on the anaesthetist to proceed when the patient is in suboptimal condition, or has been inadequately prepared or investigated. In recent years, there has been financial pressure to admit patients very close to the time of surgery. Departments of anaesthesia must ensure that hospital admission policies take account of the need for thorough assessment and preparation by an anaesthetist.

Information and consent

Although these subjects do not influence the risk of an error occurring, they may affect the risk of litigation. Recently the Association of

Anaesthetists of Great Britain and Ireland recommended[62] that patients should be told what they will experience in the perioperative period.

If a local or regional anaesthetic technique is to be used, then patients should be informed of the nature of the technique, and that numbness and/or weakness may be experienced in the first few postoperative hours. The patient should be told also that alternative techniques, including the use of general anaesthesia, may be required if the block is unsuccessful. If local or regional anaesthesia is to be used alone, then this should be explained to the patient. Some patients do not wish to remain conscious during an operation, and they may reject these techniques. In those who consent, it should be explained that they may experience some sensations during surgery, including possibly a degree of pain, even if a sedative drug is to be administered concurrently. Furthermore, if a technique of a sensitive nature, such as the insertion of an analgesic suppository, is to be employed during anaesthesia, then the patient should be informed.

Anaesthetists should normally warn patients of common complications, such as sore throat after laryngoscopy, muscle pains following administration of suxamethonium, and postural headache after spinal anaesthesia. The patient should normally be told that there is a small risk of more serious complications associated with any anaesthetic, and the anaesthetist should provide details if asked to elaborate, for example about awareness, nerve damage, cerebral damage, death. In addition, patients who are at increased risk from anaesthesia and surgery should be told the nature and magnitude of the increased risk.

If a patient is expected to go to a high dependency or intensive care unit postoperatively, then appropriate information should be given, including information relating to any invasive monitoring techniques which are planned. Day-stay patients in hospitals or dental surgeries must be supplied with clear and comprehensive pre- and postoperative instructions, and told that, when they leave the premises, they must be accompanied by a responsible adult.

All patients should be given the opportunity to ask questions, and honest answers should be provided. The anaesthetist should then make a record of the anaesthetic techniques (e.g. general anaesthesia, regional anaesthesia, local anaesthesia, or a combination) which have been discussed with and agreed by the patient. There is some disagreement as to listing the risks that have been explained, related to the fact that not all possible complications can be so listed.

Communication with colleagues

There must be good communications between anaesthetists and surgeons, physicians and operating theatre staff. The aim is to ensure that the extent of the proposed operation is understood by the anaesthetist, that non-urgent surgery is conducted only when the patient is in optimal condition and that the appropriate equipment and assistance are available in the operating theatre when the patient arrives. Where, exceptionally, the preoperative assessment and the anaesthetic are carried out by different anaesthetists, it is essential that there is good communication between them.

Identification of patient and operation

Appropriate policies must be in place to ensure that the correct patient arrives in the appropriate operating theatre, and that the correct operation is performed on (where ambiguity exists) the appropriate side of the body. It is the responsibility of the surgical team to mark the operative side or site before the patient comes to the operating theatre. An identity bracelet should be attached to the patient at the time of admission to hospital, and a system of checks put in place to ensure that the patient who is brought to the anaesthetic room corresponds to the patient described on the operating list. Alterations to the operating list should be discouraged, and hospitals should develop guidelines to ensure that all relevant staff are made aware of changes if they become necessary.

It may be necessary to remove an identity bracelet to allow access for arterial or venous cannulation. This creates a risk if accurate identification of the patient is required during the procedure, e.g. when blood is checked before transfusion. If an identity bracelet is removed, then the patient's identity and hospital number should be written on the skin with an indelible marker.

Operating theatre environment

Personnel   The anaesthetist should have the appropriate training and experience to deal with the proposed procedure and the condition of the patient. In complex or prolonged procedures, more than one anaesthetist should be present.

The anaesthetist must have skilled, dedicated assistance throughout the procedure. In the United Kingdom, this assistance may be provided by a suitably qualified anaesthetic nurse, an operating department assistant or an operating department practitioner. There should be sufficient operating theatre staff to provide all services necessary in the operating theatre without depriving the anaesthetist of his or her dedicated assistant.

Equipment   Faulty equipment rarely causes serious accidents or critical incidents, but the low frequency of this type of problem can lead to a risk of complacency. A system should be in place to ensure that all staff are aware of current hazard warnings and safety action bulletins, and of relevant information relating to the Control of Substances Hazardous to Health. In a survey conducted in south-west England only 66% of consultant anaesthetists and 33% of junior anaesthetists were moderately confident that they had seen relevant notices.[63]

129

The commonest cause of "equipment failure" is a failure to detect a fault in assembling the equipment before anaesthesia begins. Several studies have indicated that, in up to 33% of cases in which death or misadventure occurred in association with anaesthesia, no preoperative check of the anaesthetic machine had been undertaken. Protocols and checklists for anaesthetic and monitoring equipment have been published by a number of individuals and professional bodies.[64] A survey found that between 30% and 41% of anaesthetists perform no checks and, of those who do, few follow the guidelines of the Association of Anaesthetists.[65]

Some checklists are very time-consuming. However, in one study of a checklist procedure published by the AAGBI,[66] faults were detected in 60% of the machines checked, and of these, 18% were deemed to be serious. Thus, the checklist appears to justify the expenditure of time. To ensure compliance, a logbook should be kept for each anaesthetic machine, and signed each day when the machine is checked. The anaesthetist is solely responsible for ensuring that the anaesthetic equipment functions correctly at the start of every operating session, and for rechecking the equipment if any alteration is made to its configuration during an operating session.

Each department of anaesthesia should have an agreed-upon equipment standard for anaesthetic and monitoring equipment. This standard should take into account any regional or national standards or guidelines. The equipment should be adequate to cope safely with the diversity of the department's workload. All anaesthetic staff and their assistants should be trained in the safe use of the equipment supplied, and instruction manuals should be available and easily accessible. One survey[65] disclosed that 48% of anaesthetists use new equipment without reading the instruction manual. All equipment should be subject to regular maintenance and servicing.

Syringe labels should be available, and their use encouraged, to minimise the risk of drug administration errors. Pre-printed adhesive labels can also be used to minimise the risk of errors in prescribing postoperative analgesic and anti-emetic drugs.

Monitors   In addition to the clinical skills of the anaesthetist in diagnosis and management of abnormalities, monitoring equipment is valuable in detecting changes from normal with sufficient speed to allow detection, absorption or recovery from errors before injury occurs.

Most national professional bodies have recommended minimal monitoring standards in anaesthesia. In some states in the USA, the use of these standards has become mandatory by law and enforced by state inspectors.[67] The adoption of improved monitoring has led to reduced premiums for malpractice insurance in the United States. It has been assumed that the reductions in premiums have been the result of improved safety. However, better monitoring, in conjunction with good record keeping, makes claims for compensation defensible in situations in which there was no fault. In such cases, the absence of adequate monitoring and records might have made it impossible to demonstrate that anaesthesia or the anaesthetist was not responsible. For example, in 1974, anaesthesia was responsible for between 3% and 5% of malpractice claims handled by one American insurer,[68] and for 11% of the total sum of money paid in compensation. By 1989, the number of claims remained at 3·5%, but the total cost had dropped to 3·6% of the total. It is therefore important to examine closely the evidence that relates improvements in monitoring to improvements in safety rather than reductions in insurance premiums.

Eichhorn et al[69] compared two groups of patients anaesthetised at the Harvard group of hospitals. From 1976 until 1985, 757 000 patients were studied; there were 10 serious accidents and 5 deaths. In 1985, when minimal monitoring standards were introduced, there was one accident and no deaths among 244 000 patients. However, this difference is not statistically significant, there was no control group, and over the period studied there had been many changes in technique and training other than the introduction of (predominantly) pulse oximetry and capnography.

Keenan and Boyan[26] also compared two periods of anaesthetic practice before and after the introduction of monitoring standards. Between 1969 and 1983, in 163 240 cases, there were 27 cardiac arrests during anaesthesia, from which 14 patients died. After adoption of monitoring standards, there were no cardiac arrests in a study of 25 000 cases. However,[27] the incidence of cardiac arrests was decreasing before the standard of monitoring was improved.

Cullen et al[70] reported a decrease in the number of patients admitted unexpectedly to the intensive care unit following the introduction of pulse oximetry during anaesthesia. However, this finding was not replicated by Moller et al,[71,72] who conducted a randomised, controlled investigation of the impact of pulse oximetry in the peri-operative period in over 20 000 patients in five Danish hospitals. There were no differences between the groups in respect of death, non-lethal postoperative complications or duration of hospital stay; 10% of patients in the oximetry group developed one or more postoperative complications compared with 9·4% in the non-oximetry group. The only benefit was to the anaesthetists, 80% feeling "more secure" when oximetry was available.

In a study carried out before use of oximetry was routine, McKay and Noble[73] determined that the use of pulse oximetry shortened the time to detection of an increased risk of a complication in 4% of cases. The authors calculated the cost of pulse oximetry to be about $2·40 per case, in contrast to the cost of more than $1 million (CAD 1988) for a patient with hypoxic brain damage.

The AIMS study found that 52% of critical incidents were detected first by a monitor; the pulse oximeter and capnograph detected the first changes in more than half of these cases, and ECG, blood pressure monitor or low pressure breathing system alarm in a further 39%.[74] A theoretical analysis predicted that a pulse oximeter, on its own, would have detected 82% of applicable incidents (nearly 60% before any potential for organ damage), and that a combination of pulse oximetry, capnography and blood pressure monitoring would have detected 93% of applicable incidents.

However, in view of the range of injuries which patients suffer at the hands of anaesthetists, it is foolish to assume that improved monitoring can abolish risk. Some errors, for example, the administration of an inappropriate drug, are likely to cause damage irrespective of the standard of monitoring. In other cases, although monitors are connected, they are not always heeded. Every treatment in medicine carries its own risks and anaesthetic monitoring is no exception. Anaesthetists may rely entirely on numbers generated by monitoring devices, even if they are incompatible with the clinical condition of the patient. Anaesthetists may treat "abnormal" numbers generated by monitoring devices, even when the degree of abnormality is so small that no injury can result. However, the treatment itself results in injury.

If monitors are to achieve their full potential in improving safety, then they must be used appropriately, alarms must be set at appropriate levels, and the information provided by the monitors must be scanned regularly and interpreted in conjunction with the results of clinical monitoring. Monitors must not be used as an alternative to vigilance by the anaesthetist, but as an adjunct.

Checklists, guidelines and protocols   Anaesthetists are required to rely heavily on memory for essential facts when carrying out routine and emergency procedures. Many anaesthetists eschew clinical practice guidelines and protocols as contrary to "clinical freedom". Anaesthetists have also expressed concerns that lawyers might interpret any deviation from a published guideline as representing an inadequate standard of care. In most countries, protocols and guidelines are developed within a department to inform trainees about standard methods of dealing with specific clinical problems (for example, routine practices in the obstetric department) and to establish the limits of unsupervised practice (for example, the minimum age of children who can be treated without reference to a consultant). The scope and content of such departmentally-based documents will vary widely from centre to centre. Standardised protocols for management of rare emergencies (for example, severe anaphylaxis or malignant hyperthermia) are valuable, as anaesthetists of all grades are likely to benefit from a checklist. Although such protocols are available, their distribution is often patchy, even within an institution.

Medical records   Not only do good anaesthetic records provide vital information for anaesthetists who treat the patient subsequently, but they also reduce the risk of litigation. The development of modern complete monitoring systems allows continuous printouts of information monitored, with the ability for the anaesthetist to mark drugs and events on the same chart. These printouts provide valuable evidence of exactly what took place at what time, but it is important to note artefacts and to add any necessary explanation.

Postoperative care

The postoperative period is potentially hazardous, and many legal claims relating to surgical patients allege inadequate postoperative care. Recovery rooms should be available to receive all postoperative patients 24 hours a day.[17] The precipitate return to a surgical ward places sick postoperative patients at risk of complications going unrecognised,[75] because of an inadequate degree of supervision of patients, as a result of inadequate staffing or staff training in the interests of economy. High dependency units or post-anaesthetic care units (PACUs) have much to commend them. The anticipated level of postoperative care should be determined before anaesthesia begins, and non-urgent procedures postponed if the required level is unavailable. Support for recovery rooms came from the French mortality study, which showed that postoperative respiratory depression was responsible in half of all the patients who died or suffered coma. A high proportion of patients who died were returned directly to the ward after anaesthesia because of the infrequent use of recovery rooms.[18]

Reducing the consequences of errors

An integral part of any risk management programme is the reporting of adverse processes and outcomes. Although completely computerised hospital reporting systems are still fairly uncommon in the United Kingdom, anaesthetic audit systems have been recording critical incidents and complications in many hospitals for some years. To be of use, serious or repeated problems must be investigated and recommendations made to reduce the likelihood of recurrence. Most importantly, should a patient suffer a complication, then those involved should apologise for the occurrence of the complication while not admitting blame or liability. While this simple act will not increase patient safety, it may reduce the risk of litigation and all its attendant consequences.

Conclusions

Recognition of the risks associated with anaesthesia is the first step to improving safety. This is not a new concept. In 1949, Professor (later Sir)

Robert Macintosh drew attention to the dangers of suppressing information about fatal accidents in anaesthetic practice. The result of such suppression was that similar accidents occurred elsewhere, which could have been avoided if the causes of earlier problems had been identified.[76] However, this lesson was learnt only slowly.

The second step is to recognise the contribution of human error in all parts of the anaesthetic and healthcare system. The third step to improving safety is to recognise the positive contribution to safety of a well-staffed, well-equipped and well-organised department, with thoughtful development and implementation of guidelines, policies and procedures.

References

1 Owens WD, Spitznagel EL. Anesthetic side effects and complications: an overview. *Int Anesth Clinics* 1980;**18**:1–9.
2 Beecher HK, Todd DP. *A study of the deaths associated with anesthesia and surgery.* Springfield, Illinois: Charles C Thomas, 1954.
3 Dornette WHL, Orth OS. Death in the operating room. *Anesth Analg* 1956;**35**:545–51.
4 Schapira M, Kepes ER, Hurwitt ES. An analysis of deaths in the operating room and within 24 hours of surgery. *Anesth Analg* 1960;**39**:149–52.
5 Phillips OC, Frazier TM, Graff TD, DeKornfeld TJ. The Baltimore Anesthesia Study Committee. A review of 1024 postoperative deaths. *JAMA* 1960;**174**:2015–20.
6 Dripps RD, Lamont A, Eckenhoff JE. The role of anesthesia in surgical mortality. *JAMA* 1961;**178**:261–6.
7 Clifton BS, Hotten WIT. Deaths associated with anaesthesia. *Br J Anaesth* 1963;**35**:250–9.
8 Memery HN. Anesthesia mortality in private practice. *JAMA* 1965;**194**:1185–8.
9 Gebbie D. Anaesthesia and death. *Can Anaesth Soc J* 1966;**13**:390–6.
10 Minuck M. Death in the operating room. *Can Anaesth Soc J* 1967;**14**:197–204.
11 Harrison GG. Anaesthetic contributory death – its incidence and causes. *S Afr Med J* 1968; **42**:514–18, 544–9.
12 Marx GF, Matteo CV, Otkin LR. Computer analysis of post anesthetic deaths. *Anesthesiology* 1973;**39**:54–8.
13 Bodlander FMS. Deaths associated with anaesthesia. *Br J Anaesth* 1975;**47**:36–40.
14 Harrison GG. Death attributable to anaesthesia: a 10 year survey (1967–1976). *Br J Anaesth* 1978;**50**:1041–6.
15 Hovi-Viander M. Death associated with anaesthesia in Finland. *Br J Anaesth* 1980;**52**:483–9.
16 Lunn JN, Mushin WW. *Mortality associated with anaesthesia.* London: Nuffield Provincial Hospitals Trust, 1982.
17 Buck N, Devlin HB, Lunn JN. *Report on the confidential enquiry into perioperative deaths.* London: Nuffield Provincial Hospitals Trust, The Kings Fund Publishing House, 1987.
18 Tiret L, Desmonts JM, Hatton F, Vourc'h G. Complications associated with anaesthesia – a prospective survey in France. *Can Anaesth Soc J* 1986;**33**:336–44.
19 Holland R. Anaesthetic mortality in New South Wales. *Br J Anaesth* 1987;**59**:834–41.
20 Horan BF, Warden JC, Dwyer B. Urgent non-emergency surgery and death attributable to anaesthetic factors. *Anaesth Intensive Care* 1996;**24**:694–8.
21 Warden JC, Horan BF. Deaths attributed to anaesthesia in New South Wales, 1984–1990. *Anaesth Intensive Care* 1996;**24**:66–73.
22 Davis NJ ed. *Anaesthesia related mortality in Australia.* 1994–1996. Aust N Z Coll Anaesth. Melbourne, 1999.
23 Chopra V, Bovill JG, Spierdijk J. Accidents, near accidents and complications during anaesthesia: a retrospective analysis of a 10-year period in a teaching hospital. *Anaesthesia* 1990;**45**:3–6.

24 Cohen MM, Duncan PG, Tate RB. Does anesthesia contribute to operative mortality? *JAMA* 1988;**260**:2859–63.
25 Pedersen T. Complications and death following anaesthesia. A prospective study with special reference to the influence of patient-, anaesthesia-, and surgery-related risk factors. *Dan Med Bull* 1994;**41**:319–31.
26 Keenan RL, Boyan CP. Cardiac arrest due to anesthesia: a study of incidence and causes. *JAMA* 1985;**253**:2373–7.
27 Keenan RL, Boyan CP. Decreasing frequency of anesthetic cardiac arrests. *J Clin Anesth* 1991;**3**:354–7.
28 Blayney MR, Malins AF, Cooper GM. Cardiac arrhythmias in children during outpatient general anaesthesia for dentistry: a prospective randomised trial. *Lancet* 1999;**354**: 1864–6.
29 Cooper AL, Leigh JM, Tring IC. Admissions to the intensive care unit after complications of anaesthetic techniques over 10 years. *Anaesthesia* 1989;**44**:953–8.
30 Forrest JB, Rehder K, Goldsmith CH, *et al.* Multicenter study of general anesthesia. I. Design and patient demography. *Anesthesiology* 1990;**72**:252–61.
31 Forrest JB, Cahalan MK, Rehder K, *et al.* Multicenter study of general anesthesia. II. Results. *Anesthesiology* 1990;**72**:262–8.
32 Forrest JB, Rehder K, Cahalan MK, Goldsmith CH. Multicenter study of general anesthesia. III. Predictors of severe perioperative adverse outcomes. *Anesthesiology* 1992;**76**:3–15.
33 Cohen MM, Duncan PG, Pope WDP, Wolkenstein C. A survey of 112 000 anaesthetics at one teaching hospital (1975–83). *Can Anaesth Soc J* 1986;**33**:22–31.
34 Cohen MM, Duncan PG, Tweed AW, *et al.* The Canadian four-centre study of anaesthetic outcomes. I. Description of methods and populations. *Can J Anaesth* 1992;**9**:420–9.
35 Cohen MM, Duncan PG, Pope WDB, *et al.* The Canadian four-centre study of anaesthetic outcomes. II. Can outcomes be used to assess the quality of anaesthesia care? *Can J Anaesth* 1992;**39**:430–9.
36 Myles PS, Weitkamp B, Jones K, *et al.* Validity and reliability of a postoperative quality of recovery score: the QoR-40. *Br J Anaesth* 2000;**84**:11–15.
37 Myles PS, Williams DL, Hendrata M, *et al.* Patient satisfaction after anaesthesia and surgery: results of a prospective survey of 10 811 patients. *Br J Anaesth* 2000;**84**:6–10.
38 Utting JE. Pitfalls in anaesthetic practice. *Br J Anaesth* 1987;**59**:877–90.
39 Brahams D. Medicine and the law. Two anaesthetists convicted of manslaughter. *Lancet* 1990;**336**:430–1.
40 Williams LS. Anaesthetist receives jail sentence after patient left in vegetative state. *Can Med Assoc J* 1995;**153**:619–20.
41 Davies JM, Robson R. The view from North America and some comments on "Down Under". *Br J Anaesth* 1994;**73**:105–17.
42 Caplan RA, Ward RJ, Posner K, Cheney FW. Unexpected cardiac arrest during spinal anesthesia. A closed claims analysis of predisposing factors. *Anesthesiology* 1988;**68**:5–11.
43 Tinker JH, Dull DL, Caplan RA, *et al.* Role of monitoring devices in prevention of anesthetic mishaps: a closed claims analysis. *Anesthesiology* 1989;**71**:541–6.
44 Caplan RA, Posner KL, Ward RJ *et al.* Adverse respiratory events in anesthesia: a closed claims analysis. *Anesthesiology* 1990;**72**:828–33.
45 Cheney FW, Posner KL, Caplan RA. Adverse respiratory events infrequently leading to malpractice suits, a closed claims analysis. *Anesthesiology* 1991;**75**:932–9.
46 Chadwick HS, Posner K, Caplan RA, *et al.* A comparison of obstetric and nonobstetric anesthesia malpractice claims. *Anesthesiology* 1991;**74**:242–9.
47 Morray JP, Geiduschek JM, Caplan RA, Posner K, Gild WM, Cheney FW. A comparison of pediatric and adult anesthesia closed malpractice claims. *Anesthesiology* 1993;**78**:461–7.
48 Cheney FW, Posner KL, Caplan RA, Gild WM. Burns from warming devices in anesthesia: a closed claims analysis. *Anesthesiology* 1994;**80**:806–10.
49 Blum LL. Equipment design and "human" limitations. *Anesthesiology* 1971;**35**:101–2.
50 Cooper JB, Newbower RS, Long CD, McPeek B. Preventable anesthesia mishaps: a study of human factors. *Anesthesiology* 1978;**49**:399–406.
51 Cooper JB, Long CD, Newbower RS, Philip JH. Critical incidents associated with intraoperative exchanges of anesthesia personnel. *Anesthesiology* 1982;**56**:456–61.

52 Cooper JB, Newbower RS, Kitz RJ. An analysis of major errors and equipment failures in anesthesia management: considerations for prevention and detection. *Anesthesiology* 1984;**60**:34–42.

53 Kumar V, Barcellos WA, Mehta MP, Carter JG. An analysis of critical incidents in a teaching department for quality assurance. *Anaesthesia* 1988;**43**:879–83.

54 Holland R. Symposium – The Australian Incident Monitoring Study. *Anaesth Intensive Care* 1993;**21**:501.

55 Webb RK, Currie M, Morgan CA, *et al* The Australian Incident Monitoring Study: an analysis of 2000 incident reports, *Anaesth Intensive Care* 1993,**21**:520–8.

56 Davies JM. Application of the Winnipeg model to obstetric and neonatal audit. *Topics Health Information Manage* 2000;**20**:12–22.

57 Adams AP. Safety in anaesthetic practice. In: Atkinson RS, Adams AP eds. *Recent advances in anaesthesia and analgesia.* 17. Edinburgh: Churchill Livingstone 1992;1–24.

58 *Aeronautical Decision Making. Advisory Circular Number 60–22.* Washington, DC: Federal Aviation Administration, 1991.

59 Helmreich RL, Davies JM. Human factors in the operating room: interpersonal determinants of safety, efficiency and morale. In: Aitkenhead AR ed. *Quality Assurance and Risk Management in Anaesthesia.* Baillière's Clinical Anaesthesiology International Practice and Research. London Baillière Tindall 1996;**10**:277–95.

60 Menk EJ, Baumgarten RK, Kingsley CP, *et al.* Success of re-entry into Anesthesiology training programs by residents with a history of substance abuse. *JAMA* 1990;**263**:3060–2.

61 *Risk management.* London: Association of Anaesthetists of Great Britain and Ireland, 1998.

62 *Information and Consent for Anaesthesia.* London: Association of Anaesthetists of Great Britain and Ireland, 1999.

63 Weir PM, Wilson ME. Are you getting the message? A look at the communication between the Department of Health, manufacturers and anaesthetists. *Anaesthesia* 1991;**46**:845–8.

64 *Checklist for Anaesthetic Apparatus 2.* London: Association of Anaesthetists of Great Britain and Ireland, 1997.

65 Mayor AH, Eaton JM. Anaesthetic machine checking practices: a survey. *Anaesthesia* 1992;**47**:866–8.

66 Barthram C, McClymont W. The use of a checklist for anaesthetic machines. *Anaesthesia* 1992;**47**:1066–9.

67 Moss E. New Jersey enacts anesthesia standards. *American Patient Safety Foundation Newsletter* 1989;**4**(2):13–18.

68 Pierce EC. Anesthesia: standards of care and liability. *JAMA* 1989;**262**:773.

69 Eichhorn JH, Cooper JB, Cullen DJ, *et al.* Standards of patient monitoring during anesthesia at Harvard Medical School. *JAMA* 1986;**256**: 1017–20.

70 Cullen DJ, Nemaskal JR, Cooper JB, *et al.* Effect of pulse oximetry, age, and ASA physical status on the frequency of patients admitted unexpectedly to a post-operative intensive care unit. *Anesth Analg* 1992;**74**:181–8.

71 Moller JT, Pedersen T, Rasmussen LS, *et al.* Randomized evaluation of pulse oximetry in 20 802 patients. I. Design, demography, pulse oximetry failure rate, and overall complication rate. *Anesthesiology* 1993;**78**:436–44.

72 Moller JT, Johannessen NW, Espersen K, *et al.* Randomized evaluation of pulse oximetry in 20 802 patients. II. Perioperative events and postoperative complications. *Anesthesiology* 1993;**78**:444–53.

73 McKay WP, Noble WH. Critical incidents detected by pulse oximetry during anaesthesia. *Can J Anaesth* 1988;**35**:265–9.

74 Webb RK, Van der Walt JH, Runciman WB, *et al.* Which monitor? An analysis of 2000 incident reports. *Anaesth Intensive Care* 1993;**21**:529–42.

75 Leeson-Payne CG, Aitkenhead AR. A prospective study to assess the demand for a high dependency unit. *Anaesthesia* 1995;**50**:383–7.

76 Macintosh RR. Deaths under anaesthetics. *Br J Anaesth* 1949;**21**:107–36.

8 Risk management in surgery

JOHN WILLIAMS

Surgical interventions by their very nature are accompanied by a degree of risk. All specialties in surgery have their own particular risks, which are well known and identified. The object of this chapter is not to discuss these specific risks but to look at the generality of surgery to assess how risks can be reduced. However, potentially catastrophic surgical events are fortunately rare and when encountered, are usually dealt with promptly and efficiently, resulting in a satisfactory outcome. It is much more frequently the small cumulative events which individually might pass unnoticed, that are likely to lead to a hazardous situation. It is the identification and management of these risks that enable surgery to be practised safely.

An operation is only a single point in a pathway of care and it is by looking at the total process that the various aspects of risk can be identified and actions taken to minimise the chance of harm occurring. It is important that risks should be identified and analysed to eliminate them where possible. If they cannot be eliminated, the effects must be reduced to a minimum and as a result, the chance of harm occurring also minimised. Clinical skills are all important in determining the ultimate quality of surgical care received by patients, but so too is professional judgement. This applies not only to surgeons but to all members of the surgical team. However, no matter how finely tuned are these skills, organisational and managerial aspects of care are equally important in the safe conduct of surgical practice. Surgery is particularly affected by nationally determined priorities of care which, if not managed carefully, have a detrimental effect at local level and can adversely affect clinical priorities. It is particularly noticeable where priorities may be subject to sudden change in funding and pressures of work have to be changed in the face of unforeseen

137

emergencies. The waiting time targets for planned surgery are unduly influenced as a result of the sheer weight of emergency admissions, shortage of available staff and hence beds during the winter months. The increased pressures placed upon surgeons to satisfy political targets may well be at the expense of clinical priorities for other groups.

What are the risks?

Operations on fit healthy adults carry significantly lower risks than those on patients at the extremes of age or with significant comorbidities.[1] The surgeon has, therefore, to decide in these groups whether it is:

- appropriate to operate on the patient
- whether he or she is the right person to do the procedure.

The answer to the first question must be determined not only by the surgeon but also by the anaesthetist and where appropriate, by the physician responsible for the more general care of the patient. Where comorbidities do exist, the opportunity for the physician to minimise the influence of these on the surgical procedure preoperatively is important in terms of the postoperative outcome.[2]

Avoidable risks

There are certain obvious and avoidable risks. Obesity is a problem from both the anaesthetic and surgical point of view. Not only do obese patients carry a significantly higher anaesthetic risk, particularly since their metabolism becomes increasingly less predictable, the physical bulk of the patient carrying a large volume of fat makes the technical surgical aspects increasingly difficult. There are clear risks in handling a patient of this type, since moving them from beds to trolleys and to theatre tables all mean an increased potential hazard, not only to the patient themselves but particularly to the staff responsible for that exercise. With such patients, it becomes increasingly difficult to position them in the most advantageous way on the operating table. The greater the level of obesity, the greater becomes the problem of access and surgical management.

A further avoidable hazard is that of smoking. People who are long term smokers not only have significant change in their respiratory function, they are also more likely to produce problems postoperatively as a result of their decreased respiratory function, increased secretions and persistent coughing. Not only does persistent coughing produce increased discomfort at the operation site, it is likely to increase the venous pressure and hence may well cause the development of large haematomas. The risk of postoperative respiratory infection is greatly enhanced and with this, the likelihood of an increased hospital stay. Excessive alcohol consumption and the habitual abuse of drugs are well-recognised complications of anaesthesia and surgery. It is an interesting observation that these are frequently found together in people whose social circumstances are less than ideal. The consequence of this summation tends to result in a patient who is poorly nourished, inadequately mobile, with little physical resilience to withstand the surgical insult.

Unavoidable risks

Unavoidable risks which must be overcome include the comorbidities associated with medication for these other medical conditions, such as the need for antibiotic cover, modification of insulin regimes or adjustment to anticoagulant or steroid medication. For all concerned however, there is a far greater hazard from patients who may be carrying potentially lethal infectious diseases without their own knowledge. The surgical team are particularly exposed to this hazard since the risk from those carrying transmittable disease is greater among the patients who are carrying them unknowingly than amongst those who openly admit to having a problem. Surgery does not carry risks to the patient alone, a needle and sharp instrument injury to the surgeons or their assistants is a source of potentially lethal transmittable disease. Similarly, aerosol spray of infected material may occur from rotatory surgical drills. Precautions against such injuries are well established and protocols must be followed.[3]

Where a surgeon decides to operate outside his sphere of expertise, risk to the patient is significantly increased and this applies particularly to the care of children. In the patient's best interest the decision to refer a patient to a colleague should be taken at an early stage. With increasing sub-specialisation in surgery, the need for cross referral between consultants is increased.[4–6]

The greatest number of claims laid against surgeons are for operations carried out on either the wrong patient, the wrong side, the wrong digit, or the wrong organ, all potentially avoidable factors.

A detailed working knowledge of the anatomical proximity of structures is part of a surgeon's basic skills. However, there is no doubt that disease tends significantly to distort normal anatomy and it is this distortion that is more likely to produce accidental damage to adjacent organs than simply failure to recognise the structures being dealt with. The more experienced the surgeon, the less likelihood there is that he will not recognise distorted anatomy. However, experience only comes with time and it is inevitable, therefore, that the more junior the surgeon, the greater becomes this potential risk. The greatest risks to adjacent structures affect particularly nerves and blood vessels and failure to recognise a structure may lead to permanent disability. Where blood vessels are concerned, damage to their integrity may result in a persistent slow leak of blood and a haematoma developing sometimes insidiously and in large volume. Not only does a haematoma increase the risk that healing will be delayed, it also significantly increases the risk of subsequent secondary infection providing an ideal medium in which bacteria can grow. Intra-abdominally, unrecognised damage to the intestine or adjacent viscera can produce serious postoperative complications necessitating additional surgery. In all these cases, the risks are enhanced by either the disease process, trauma, or the inexperience of the operator.

Postoperative complications

In addition to these obvious intra-operative complications, even with the best of care, postoperative complications may still occur. The most notable amongst these in the immediate postoperative period is the development of infections, either of the wound site, the chest or the urinary tract. The fitter the patient, the less likely are the chances of this occurring but unfortunately the presence of hospital resistant infections is increasingly affecting even the fitter patients.

The potential hazard of the development of deep vein thromboses and subsequent pulmonary embolism has been recognised for many years. It is known that the chances are increased from the tenth postoperative day. All the factors that produce a reduction in mobility of the patient are likely to increase the risk of this unfortunate occurrence. However, prevention of deep vein thrombosis by prophylaxis still lacks robust scientific evaluation. Even when all precautions are observed, cases are recorded of deep vein thrombosis occurring in fit healthy adults for no apparent reason.[7] With older patients, those who are less mobile, the potential for developing pressure sores or even cerebrovascular accidents in the postoperative period are well recognised complications. Although steps could be taken to avoid these untoward incidents, they are potential hazards that may occur despite prophylactic precautions.

Emergency surgery

The risks so far identified in relationship to elective surgery are enhanced in emergency situations. Although the risks mentioned for elective inpatient admissions remain, the situation in emergency admissions carries additional risks that need to be recognised and appropriate actions taken. This was demonstrated clearly in the NCEPOD 1997 – *Report On*

Who Operates When.[2] One of the greatest risks associated with out of hours admissions is that those on duty are inevitably the most inexperienced team members, staffing numbers are reduced and supporting services and facilities less available. Not only is this a time when communication between the various levels of staff is critical, but also it is essential that the seniority of the clinicians involved, of all disciplines, matches the severity of the patient's condition. The collective impact of all these factors increases the potential for errors.

Out of hours operating is accompanied by increased risk. Not only may surgery be carried out inappropriately by clinicians with inadequate experience, but also the optimum conditions for operating are not in place. There is a need, therefore, for consultant surgeons, anaesthetists and hospital managers to plan together the administration and management of emergency admissions and procedures in order to eliminate these elements of risk.

In the young and the very old where particular problems of comorbidity may make immediate resuscitation essential, these additional risk factors demand even greater attention. It is important under these circumstances that a multidisciplinary team is involved both pre- and postoperatively if the patient is to achieve the best chance of a successful outcome.

To avoid queuing for theatre space it may be necessary to nominate an arbitrator in theatres who would decide the relative priority of cases. This practice is successfully used in many hospitals and could be more widely practised. Consultant trauma lists are now commonly practised on weekdays but problems still arise out of hours, both in the evenings and more particularly at weekends. These areas are a potential for increased risk and need to be addressed in planning emergency services. Cancellation of patients either because of a failure to complete preoperative investigations, a lack of preoperative care, or shortage of time are accompanied by a reduction in the quality of care received by a patient already in a compromised state. This is not conducive to a good outcome. A further hazard to patients under emergency circumstances is that the surgeon is unfamiliar with the patient and consequently, unless a thorough preoperative evaluation is undertaken, the surgeon is disadvantaged when operating. NCEPOD 1999[8] demonstrated again that elderly patients in particular, benefit significantly from adequate resuscitation before being taken to theatre. They suggest the need for a period of intensive multidisciplinary care, which will increase the likelihood of a successful outcome. This in itself poses additional problems because of lack of continuity of care, since the juniors admitting the patient are unlikely to be those who are able to take the patient to theatre on the following day. Thus, although the consultant may be available to carry out the work, the continuity of care provided by junior medical staff is likely to be missing. The lack or unavailability of particular medical equipment, high dependency or intensive care facilities provides additional risk.

141

The immediate resuscitation of patients is a major concern in emergency admissions. In the elderly this problem becomes more hazardous for the reasons already outlined. It is necessary, therefore, to evaluate such patients thoroughly on a multidisciplinary basis if the patient is going to be presented with an optimum chance of avoiding postoperative complications. Fluid balance is particularly difficult in the elderly and evidence suggests that it is frequently inadequately managed.[8] Failure adequately to address these important considerations preoperatively results in an increased likelihood of postoperative complications which may keep the patient bed bound. This is likely to be associated with further complications, notably chest infection, deep vein thrombosis, pressure sores and reduced mobility. As a simple rule, doubling the time in bed doubles the stay in hospital. Postoperative care may involve a critical care period in a high dependency or intensive care area. At such times communication between all members of the clinical team is of greatest importance. Detailed written clinical notes following agreed protocols are the surest way of avoiding misunderstandings and mistakes. Similarly, the discharge of the patient from hospital must be accompanied by careful communication with the primary care team.

Transfer of patients admitted as emergencies to the receiving hospital tends to be hazardous but, nevertheless, it is an essential element of emergency work. This means that before transfer the airway must be secured and circulating fluid volume stabilised. Appropriately trained staff must accompany all patients with life threatening conditions during transfer between and within hospitals.

With increasing subspecialisation, fewer surgeons and anaesthetists are prepared to operate on young children. This is a healthy state of affairs but it means that children who are seriously ill will have to be transferred to a paediatric centre. In these circumstances, the risks are significantly reduced if a specialist recovery team from the paediatric centre is able to retrieve the patient from the initial receiving hospital.

Where common emergency conditions are concerned, particularly head injuries, ruptured aortic aneurysms and gastrointestinal bleeding it is appropriate that in addition to any clinical guidelines that may exist, integrated care pathways and protocols should be established in order to minimise risk.[1]

The reasons things go wrong

Risks start from the point at which patients are referred by general practitioners. It is easy for the general practitioner, when sitting on the opposite side of the table to a patient, to confuse right and left and this simple error can be perpetuated in a chain unless corrected early on. The clinician initially seeing the patient on referral may simply copy down the complaint from the referral letter as the first item on the hospital clinical notes. Similarly, the use of signs L or R for left and right are causes of confusion, particularly when written in a hurry. Many general practitioner referral letters are still hand written and the legibility of handwriting, particularly of clinicians in a hurry, is notoriously bad. This can lead to simple errors in assessment of urgency by the consultant when ascribing a priority to a given case, which in turn can mean that a patient with a serious condition is erroneously given a non-urgent priority which might prejudice the ultimate outcome of treatment. The onus is on the referring clinician to assess the degree of urgency with which the patient is being referred. To categorise a patient as urgent when they are not can be just as hazardous to overall care as can failure to identify the true seriousness of a given complaint.

Further delays may be introduced by referring the patient to the wrong type of surgeon or the wrong hospital. Outpatient clinics are excessively busy and the levels of referral far exceed the values set by various surgical associations in conjunction with the Royal College of Surgeons, as recommended norms for outpatient activity. With these pressures, more patients are being referred to outpatient consultations year by year and unless patients are channelled in the right direction and with the right priorities, the risks of inappropriate action being taken are increased.[9]

There is a plethora of people with whom patients may come into contact during the course of their process through a hospital: clinical staff at all levels, secretarial, managerial, nursing staff, and staff in professions ancillary to medicine. By reducing the number of visits to a minimum, the chances of risk are in turn reduced. National CEPOD in its 1990 recommendations[10] came to the conclusion that decisions for or against operations should be made by surgeons of consultant status. This ensures that no matter how many people have been involved, the final arbiter is the person who carries the ultimate responsibility.

Once the decision to operate has been taken, therefore, patients placed on the waiting list should be in a position to give their informed consent as a result of that consultation. This decision may be helped by the provision of information leaflets written in simple English or, where appropriate, alternative languages, which are carefully constructed for the lay reader. These significantly reduce the ever present difficulty of communication between the profession and their patients, thereby reducing the risk of misunderstanding. If a booked admission is organised, the number of occasions on which patients return to the hospital should be minimised. This ideal arrangement cannot always be achieved, but where possible it reduces the potential for errors later on. If the process is kept strictly to given protocols, chances of error creeping in are reduced significantly. This means that the surgeon is in a position not only to inform the patient, but

143

also the general practitioner, of what decisions have been taken and what the patient has been told, including the options and potential hazards and a realistic estimate of the time when the operation is likely to take place. Such a streamlined process is in everyone's best interests, but in the face of intense pressures for increased throughput of elective surgical cases to meet tight contractual obligations, it is all too frequently unachievable. Without significant attention, attempting to meet such obligations may place the most vulnerable party, the patient, at greatest risk.

For patients undergoing elective surgery the process of admission to hospital and preoperative assessment will bring them into contact with a variety of clinical and non-clinical staff of all grades. Unless a clear understanding exists of the responsibilities of each individual in that team, the possibility for confusion to arise, errors to creep in and hence for risks to be increased, has to be acknowledged. This can be reduced or minimised by the adoption of pre-assessment clinics some 2–4 weeks before admission. At that time, in addition to a thorough medical history, including medication and any known allergies, the patient is seen again by the surgeon who took the original decision to operate (this should be the consultant) for a final review. It is a further opportunity for informed consent to be taken as well as patients being provided with information leaflets.

Once the patient is admitted to hospital, they are likely to come across junior doctors who may not have met them before and indeed because of the shorter training times and reduced hours of duty may have little experience in the specialty. It is important, therefore, that when the patients are seen and clerked at that stage, the process should not increase risks but indeed eliminate them. The consent having been obtained in the outpatient department, at a time when the patient is more receptive to the issues in question, is one way of ensuring this aspect of risk is eliminated. Equally, the difficulty of patients being admitted without x ray films or even without their notes is, hopefully, eliminated. These processes collapse when patients cancel an admission or are unable to be admitted at the last minute and short notice replacements are admitted instead. These replacement patients may not have been through the same pre-admissions process and hence the risk to them is significantly greater, demanding a heightened awareness amongst all staff at a time of increased pressure.

In an analysis of some 1200 completed claim cases by Health Care Risk Resources International,[11] the following areas were identified of particular risk:

- theatre   32%
- ward areas   28%
- A/E departments   22%
- outpatients   18%
- others   0·2%

Therefore, the greatest area of hazard to the patient occurs either in the ward area, which includes the physical transfer of a patient to the operating table and careful positioning, as well as during the operative procedure itself. In the same series, they identified that during surgery, unintentional damage was the greatest risk at 28% followed by a diagnostic error at 27%. The responsibility, therefore, for ensuring minimisation of risk rests singularly with those directly responsible for the patient immediately before, during and after surgery. The advent of a significant reduction in junior doctors' hours has resulted in a lack of continuity of care by a single person, an area identified by the Royal College of Surgeons and the Royal College of Nursing as being of particular concern in the overall quality of care for surgical patients.

The responsibilities of the operating surgeon, as well as junior members of the team, to ensure that the correct limb and digit are marked in a site that will remain visible even after drapes have been applied in the operating theatre, is recognised as one of the most significant sources of error. It is essential that the correct marks are made and that this is reconfirmed against the notes, the consent form and with the patient. The use of integrated care pathways and also the insistence of daily entries in the medical records are important steps to be taken to avoid the possibility of risks.

Managing and reducing risks

Staffing and supervision

Trainees

Reference should be made to the need to supervise trainees. If risks are to be minimised, it is important that the level of expertise of the operating surgeon matches the severity of the condition with which he/she is dealing. With a reduction both in junior doctors' hours and the duration of training, it is important that time be set aside for surgeons to supervise trainees, particularly when dealing with emergency surgery. However desirable it may seem to be, the fact has to be recognised that there are an inadequate number of consultants to mount cover 24 hours a day for all procedures. Rationalisation of activities to ensure that consultants are available to cover trainees during the times when they are operating, is not only good practice from a training standpoint, but also safe practice if risk management is to be practised in the most effective manner. It has been difficult to attribute a direct relationship between the volume of procedures carried out by a surgeon and the outcome; there is a strong feeling that unless an operation is done sufficiently frequently, the surgeon will not demonstrate consistently good outcomes. However, risks to

145

patients, the doctors in training, and the hospital, are all reduced by appropriate supervision from people with experience.

Non-trainee staff

It is a statutory responsibility of consultants to supervise all staff of non-consultant grade, which includes the non-consultant career grades within a hospital. Most particularly, the need for supervision of locums is of greatest importance. NCEPOD 1997[2] commented on the fact that lack of supervision of untrained staff was particularly noticeable when, for whatever reason, weekday operations were postponed until out of hours periods, despite their previous comments on this potentially hazardous practice.[5,7]

Work pressures

This aspect of risk management has gained increasing importance in recent years. However, the problem has not necessarily been adequately matched by changing clinical practice within trusts simply because of increasing pressures of clinical work being recorded on a year on year basis. Unless adequate clinical staff are available to provide this degree of supervision, it is inevitable that risks to patients will increase. The staffing of trusts does need to take into account the relative skills and competencies of those involved and their job plans do need to be realistic in terms of their ability to carry out the work expected of them. Failure in this area, in the same way as any lack of facilities, is likely to result in a reduction of the standards of care to patients. It is essential that people are not placed in a situation where they are working beyond their level of competence or without the necessary support and facilities to achieve an optimum outcome.

Clinical guidelines

Nationally agreed clinical guidelines do not exist for many procedures. Where they do exist, however, there can be little doubt that the risk to patients' care is significantly reduced by adherence to these valuable pieces of advice. It is reasonable to assume that unless a surgeon has a good reason for not following clinical guidelines, they should be regarded as the gold standard of care at any given time. In future these will be issued under the banner of the National Institute for Clinical Excellence (NICE). In the same way, documents issued by that body through their Appraisals Panel, such as that covering the removal of wisdom teeth and a choice of hip prostheses must be regarded as the best available advice.

Many hospital protocols exist covering management of individual conditions. These are there for the advice and guidance of all members of the surgical team and in many instances are embodied within clinical care

146

pathways, adherence to which will ensure the best possible care within that team.

Resuscitation and prioritisation of emergencies

As has already been mentioned, NCEPOD have recommended repeatedly the need for adequate resuscitation of emergency patients before conducting emergency surgery. Attention to the needs of patients in this area is even more vital for those in the extremes of age. It is particularly important if risks are to be avoided that resuscitation is carried out promptly and expertly and that the patient, once resuscitated, receives their definitive surgery without further delay. All too frequently, elderly patients in particular, having suffered orthopaedic injuries, have their definitive surgery delayed due to lack of operating time. These patients do badly under such circumstances and once resuscitated should receive the definitive surgery without further delay.

Management of this is always difficult. In hospitals where a facilitator has been appointed to expedite the treatment of emergency patients, where surgeons are available when on call to carry out the surgery, and where dedicated theatres have been set aside to cope with this additional load, the outcome of surgery is improved. Attention to all these areas, therefore, reduces the surgical risk and needs to be encouraged.

Out of hours surgery

In the past it has been the practice to carry out surgery throughout the night. Under these circumstances, not only is the surgeon likely to be fatigued, the person on duty and performing the surgery is unlikely to be a consultant. It is important that the severity of the patient's condition is matched by the skill of the operator. It is equally important that the patient is adequately resuscitated. As shown by NCEPOD, only in dire emergencies should a patient be taken straight to theatre and whilst this may still apply, the number of cases where it is necessary to take a patient to theatre without adequate resuscitation are very few. Better practice is to ensure that the patient is adequately resuscitated and to have the facilities for dealing with that case during daylight hours at the next available opportunity.

Pre-assessment clinics and booked admissions

In order to ensure a smooth passage for patients, the ideal situation is that every patient should know exactly when they are coming into hospital by having a booked admission date for their operation. Although this has been seen as impossible due to the current pressures of work, many hospitals have now demonstrated that it can be achieved and, furthermore, it

147

has become a political priority. The inexorable rise in emergency admissions has meant that many hospitals find themselves inadequately staffed to cope with the anticipated demand for elective procedures. Reference to Healthcare Needs Assessment Tables demonstrates the anticipated surgical needs of any demographic group in the country. It is, therefore, theoretically possible to ring fence this facility for elective surgery. In practical terms this cannot be achieved because of the competing demands within the acute hospital for beds.

However, careful planning and management, particularly facilitated by modern technology have been demonstrated to improve the throughput of patients by the introduction of booked admission dates along with pre-assessment clinics. Whilst this process is relatively straightforward for day case admissions, it is achievable for inpatient elective surgery in well-run systems. Not only does such a system decrease the risk to patients, it has also been demonstrated to decrease the non-attendance rate and hence improve efficiency all around. Improvements of efficiency of this type also reduce the chance of risk.

Postoperative complications

Management of infection

The risk of infection is ever present in surgical procedures. Risks are reduced significantly when adequate control of infection procedures are in place. It is important that these protocols are followed and that consultation with consultant microbiologists is conducted whenever postoperative infection rates show signs of exceeding acceptable limits. Equally, when unusual organisms are encountered, it is imperative that junior staff, in particular, do not take their own decisions on choice of antibiotics but follow recommendations of more senior microbiologists. Increasingly in surgery, implantable devices are being used. These carry with them an enhanced risk of infection requiring the utmost care in their perioperative management if the potential hazards are to be reduced.

Management of deep vein thrombosis

The second commonest problem in association with surgery is the risk of a deep vein thrombosis and the possible lethal sequelae of the development of pulmonary emboli. It is normally recognised that the risk of developing a deep vein thrombosis is increased in patients with decreased mobility. This applies particularly after intra-abdominal operations and orthopaedic operations involving the lower limbs. However, the problem is not as simple as this and deep vein thrombosis may develop both early and in seemingly fit people. In the apparently fit patient where the risk of deep vein thrombosis is low, the use of simple techniques such as full-length compression stockings and elevation of the foot of the bed may prove adequate. However, in those who are already on anticoagulant therapy or have a significantly increased risk of developing a deep vein thrombosis, perioperative cover by the use of heparin or alternatively modification of their anticoagulant regime is to be recommended. Prophylaxis against deep vein thrombosis is an area which does need much greater attention and research.[7] There is no foolproof protocol to be followed.

Investigation/results

It is important that surgeons pay attention to the outcome of both pathology and imaging results. Failure to take note of the outcome of laboratory investigations of this type may mean that potentially hazardous situations are able to pass unrecognised. Although this may seem an obvious point, medical records are frequently given inadequate attention, which increases the risks to patients.

Summary

The issues described in this chapter emphasise the need for strict attention to the processing of patients through their hospital stay. Risks are only reduced when attention to detail is strictly observed, the number of people involved in handling a patient reduced to a minimum, and the optimum conditions for surgery are ensured.

References

1 *The Report of the National Confidential Enquiry into Perioperative Deaths 1993/94*. London, 1996:11.
2 Campling EA, Devlin HB, Hoile RW, *et al*. Who operates when? *A report by the National Confidential Enquiry into Perioperative Deaths*. London, 1997:9.
3 Royal College of Surgeons Symposium. *Risks to surgeons – A Practical Guide to Risk Management in Surgery*. London: Royal College of Surgeons, 1999.
4 Gallimore SC, Hoile RW, Ingram GS, Sherry KM. *The Report of the National Confidential Enquiry into Perioperative Deaths 1994/95*. London, 1997:9.
5 Campling EA, Devlin HB, Hoile RW, Lunn JN. *The Report of the National Confidential Enquiry into Perioperative Deaths 1992/93*. London, 1995:17.
6 Campling EA, Devlin HB, Lunn JN. *The Report of the National Confidential Enquiry into Perioperative Deaths 1989*. London, 1990:15.
7 Campling EA, Devlin HB, Hoile RW, Lunn JN. *The Report of the National Confidential Enquiry into Perioperative Deaths 1991/92*. London, 1993:10.
8 *Extremes of Age: The 1999 Report of the National Confidential Enquiry into Perioperative Deaths*. London, 1999:xix.
9 *Out patient referrals – quarterly statistics*. London: DoH, 2000.
10 Campling EA, Devlin HB, Hoile RW, Lunn JN. *The report of the National Confidential Enquiry into Perioperative Deaths 1990*. London, 1992:11.
11 Wilson, J. *A practical guide to risk management in surgery: Developing and planning*. Health Care Risk Resources International – Royal College of Surgeons Symposium, 1999.

149

Further reading

All National Confidential Enquiry into Perioperative Deaths reports, both annual and specific issues reports, available from: National CEPOD, 35–43 Lincolns Inn Fields, London, WC2A 3PN.

9 Risk management in accident and emergency medicine

PETER DRISCOLL, MARTIN THOMAS,
ROBIN TOUQUET, JANE FOTHERGILL

Accident and emergency medicine is a relatively new speciality, with the first 30 consultants being appointed in 1974. Though the number of these senior doctors has increased to about 280, accident and emergency departments remain largely staffed by inexperienced senior house officers, working in shifts and changing jobs every six months.[1]

As the speciality has matured, expectations of what it can provide have increased. The pressures on overstretched accident and emergency staff can be very great because, of all the hospital specialties, they see and treat the greatest number of patients. Indeed the amount is larger than the total number seen in the outpatient department.[2,3] New patient attendances are increasing at a rate of 2% per annum, and departments often have to cope with rising numbers of acute medical admissions.[4] As some of these patients have to remain in accident and emergency if no inpatient beds are available, accident and emergency nurses have to spend more time performing ward duties rather than their accident and emergency-based roles. The open-door access, 24 hours per day, further exacerbates the situation by producing a vast range of presenting conditions. Accident and emergency medicine is a specialty where patients of any age can present at any time with any condition!

Although accident and emergency departments vary considerably in shape and size, all will have, as a minimum, the following three key clinical sectors for both adults and children:

- A resuscitation room for seriously ill or injured patients
- Cubicles or rooms for patients who need to lie down on a trolley
- Cubicles or rooms for patients who can walk.

151

Around 60% of patients attending accident and emergency departments in the UK fall into this latter category. They generally have soft tissue conditions or skeletal problems and once treated, over 90% will be able to go home. In contrast, patients in the first two categories have a higher chance of requiring admission. Furthermore, they take longer to sort out and utilise a greater amount of both human and technical resources.

Nature and frequency of errors

When these pressures of accident and emergency medicine are combined with the heterogeneous patient population, it is not really surprising that mistakes occur. As with any department there are many more "near miss" episodes than adverse outcomes. Nevertheless accident and emergency medicine has a high incidence of complaints and medical negligence cases.[5-8] Figures from the North West Regional Health Authority, place accident and emergency third in the league table of incidence of claims made against specialties. The commonest claims are listed in Table 9.1 but nationally over half involve radiology, usually pertaining to a missed fracture or dislocation.

Misdiagnosis in other clinical situations occurs less frequently but can have much more serious consequences. The most worrying of these are the patients who are inappropriately discharged because their underlying life threatening condition has been missed (Table 9.2).

Table 9.1 Reasons for common claims in accident and emergency in the North West Regional Health Authority

Nature	Frequency
Missed fracture	42%
Misdiagnosis	9%
Poor fracture management	7%
Nerve, tendon or ligamental injury	6%
Poor wound healing and missed foreign body	5%
Missed dislocation	3%

Table 9.2 Common misdiagnosis of life threatening conditions

Life threatening condition	Misdiagnosis
Subarachnoid haemorrhage	Non specific headache; migraine
Myocardial infarction	Indigestion; angina
Pulmonary embolus	Indigestion; angina
Ectopic pregnancy	Period pain; salpingitis
Abdominal aortic aneurysm	Renal colic; pancreatitis
Gastro-intestinal perforation	Gastro-enteritis

Human factors affecting clinical performance in accident and emergency

Mistakes made in accident and emergency rarely result from a single error. Usually there is an interplay between human, environmental and equipment factors which increases the chances of an error happening (see Chapter 1). In the following sections we review some of the more important factors affecting clinical performance.

Experience and Training

A particular skill required by accident and emergency personnel is the ability to correctly prioritise, or triage, patients so that the sickest can be treated first. For the individual patient the most dangerous condition always takes priority. When these skills are lacking, serious errors can occur and whole groups of patients may be allowed to deteriorate before it becomes apparent that they require urgent attention.

Another essential skill is the ability to manage critically ill patients, where the chance of errors occurring increases if inexperienced staff are left unsupervised.[9,10] Indeed, studies have shown that many junior doctors lack even the most rudimentary knowledge and skills needed to manage such patients.[11] Trauma patients have a significantly better outcome when they have been treated by a consultant rather than by junior staff.[12] It is therefore worrying that there are still accident and emergency departments where junior doctors work without adequate experienced cover.[4] While staff ratios are undoubtedly improving, there is still a long way to go before ideal consultant and middle grade levels are reached.

Lack of supervision not only allows mistakes to occur but also limits education and training. Accident and emergency staff, like all adults, learn best by acquiring knowledge and skills and then applying them in a safe and supportive environment. In this way the effect of their actions can be assessed. However, lack of feedback allows inappropriate actions to develop into bad habits, which may be handed on from one member of staff to another.

Shift patterns and fatigue

Working in accident and emergency departments can be physically tiring. Personnel need to remain on their feet for many hours as they move around the department assessing and treating the constant stream of patients. Therefore, without proper organisation, personnel may become exhausted, especially by the end of a shift in a busy, large department.

Emergency physicians in the United States commonly work 12-hour shifts. In the United Kingdom, however, shifts vary between 8 to 24 hours.

There is therefore a tendency to fatigue and this becomes more marked the longer the shifts are. For example, fatigue and reduced alertness are likely in the last few hours of a 12-hour shift, especially if the person is on a new night rotation. Interestingly, at the beginning of shifts certain tasks are also carried out less effectively, especially by inexperienced staff. For example, radiological interpretation by junior staff is more likely to be faulty at the beginning and end of the shift compared with that carried out in the middle.

Adjustments to shift working is most difficult when the rotation lasts less than 3 weeks.[13] A further insult occurs if the shift rotation occurs in a counter-clockwise rotation, because the biological clock is totally disrupted. Changes in shifts are another significant cause of variation in the functional ability of accident and emergency staff. In the United States they are cited as a major cause of stress and dissatisfaction in emergency medicine and the principal reason for the annual 12% attrition rate in the speciality.[14]

The shift system also means that some patients will not have been completely managed by the time the doctor or nurse has to leave. Consequently the departing staff need to hand over the patient's continuing care to other personnel. This process is susceptible to errors. For example, a clinician may fail to reassess a patient handed onto him/her by a colleague. In doing so s/he is in danger of perpetuating an error made by the departing doctor.

Vigilance and alertness

The detection of subtle abnormalities is particularly difficult if they occur rarely compared to the number of normalities. For example, a common presenting complaint to accident and emergency is the painful, swollen ankle following an inversion injury. The vast majority of these patients will be suffering from ligamental sprain, with only the minority having a fracture. Nevertheless, most of these patients will require a radiograph so that skeletal damage can be excluded.[15] Doctors can become less vigilant after inspecting many normal radiographs – that is, their mind may already be made up before looking at the film. It follows that unless they maintain a disciplined systematic approach to examining these patients and their radiographs, mistakes will occur.

Kadzombe and Coals have also shown that complaints are at their highest when SHOs are in their last month in the department.[5] Another small study found that, while actual numbers of incidents relating to SHO performance were similar between the first and the sixth month of an attachment, the causes of these incidents were different, showing a shift towards errors related to failures of verification and execution of procedures.[16] Though further work is needed to confirm this finding, it may reflect both misplaced confidence and a fall in alertness during the final month of the doctor's attachment.

Stress

Accident and emergency medicine has stresses beyond those found in other branches of clinical medicine. Accident and emergency doctors deal with excessive patient loads and treat people, with incomplete information, for conditions which vary from the trivial to the immediately life threatening. They often work under time pressure and continually have to negotiate with admitting teams. Dealing with patients attending accident and emergency departments is sometimes difficult for inexperienced staff. Many patients are anxious and agitated by delays. When drunkenness or drug abuse is added to this, verbal and sometimes physical aggression towards staff can result. The high incidence of drug use by emergency residents in the United States is probably a reflection of the levels of stress facing these doctors.[17,18]

In addition, accident and emergency doctors routinely have to manage several patients at once. These patients may have a wide variety of conditions of varying severity, but the doctor still needs to move smoothly from one patient to the other. Needless to say, with an increase in patient numbers, or clinical severity, there is a greater risk of mistakes being made. These usually take the form of omissions, for example incomplete documentation, inadequate investigations or lack of reassessment. There is also potential for serious confusion if patients' histories are written in the wrong notes and inappropriate treatment prescribed.

Doctors and nurses working in the accident and emergency department experience emotional upheavals both within and outside the work place. Though all healthcare professionals learn to detach themselves from these issues, occasionally this is not possible. Bereavement, illness in a loved one or the ending of a close relationship are obvious examples. Compared to married non-clinicians, doctors who are married have a higher incidence of divorce, troubled relationships and drug and alcohol abuse.[19] However, marriages that endure are protective in that married doctors experience fewer symptoms of stress and depression than their unmarried counterparts.[20] Nevertheless, during bereavement or when long-term relationships are ending, there may be a lengthy period of emotional turmoil which may affect performance at work.

The British Association of Accident and Emergency Medicine recommends that all departments should have a scheme to deal with problems and provide support for colleagues.[21] Doctors should be made aware of whom they can turn to in times of need, both within the department and outside. All doctors should be encouraged to register with a general practitioner and to make use of them. Self-diagnosis and self-treatment should be strongly discouraged. Other agencies, for those concerned about their own health or that of a colleague, exist, and their contact numbers should be available to anyone who may need them. These include the National Counselling Service for Sick Doctors (Tel. 0870 241 0535) and the BMA Stress Counselling Service for Doctors (Tel. 0645 200169).

Environment and equipment

Accident and emergency departments are often noisy, with poor acoustics and frequent disturbances from bleeps and intercoms. Lighting is often inadequate, space is at a premium and there can be a variety of unpleasant smells. All these factors may affect clinical performance. If the adverse environmental features are only present in a particular area of the department, then personnel will try to avoid working there and delay returning to review a patient. Faulty, inadequate or absent equipment also leads to a poor clinical performance and so increases the risks of mistakes being made. For example, lack of standard equipment, such as auroscopes, ophthalmoscopes and page-writing 12-lead ECG machines, leads to staff taking short cuts and not undertaking a sufficiently detailed examination.

Managing risk in accident and emergency

In the remainder of the chapter we consider the conditions of safe practice and the implementation of practical methods of reducing risk to patients. A major aspect in attempting to achieve this is to establish an appropriate number of trained staff, in departments that are well laid out, organised, and fully supported by other specialities and services.[3]

Staffing, training and supervision

Appropriate number and type of staff

The British Association for Accident and Emergency Medicine has provided recommendations on staffing levels.[2] Full details are available from the Association and only an outline is given here. It is strongly advised that there is one SHO for each 3500 patients attending annually, with a minimum complement of 6 to maintain 24-hour cover by shiftwork. Minimum consultant cover varies from three (30 000 patients per annum) to six for departments seeing over 100 000 patients per annum. In 1996, The Audit Commission found that only 25% of accident and emergency departments had the number of consultants recommended by the British Association for Accident and Emergency Medicine at that time.[4]

Staffing levels below those recommended will lead to a deterioration in service due to lack of supervision, teaching, audit, and time available to spend with each patient. In addition, there is prolongation of the waiting times, which aggravates the situation further. Therefore for overall patient care, it is essential that accident and emergency departments have adequate senior cover. Unfortunately this is not cheap and hospital trusts may express concern as to the costs. The counter argument is that the cost is considerably less than the financial penalty resulting from a medical negligence claim.[22]

By a combination of identifying potential mistakes as well as being a source of information and advice, the immediate availability of experienced staff helps prevent errors occurring. Though this is particularly noticeable in cases of critically ill patients, it also extends to the less severely injured.[23] For example, apparently innocent lacerations to the hand or wrist could overlie significant damage which, if missed, can result in marked morbidity.[22,24,25]

Training

This should take place at a formal and informal level. A formal, or planned teaching programme for the medical staff is essential. Minimum requirements are departmental induction, departmental medical guidance notes, an induction course and regular teaching. New senior house officers (SHOs) should not be expected to see patients as soon as they arrive on their first day. Time must be spent teaching them the departmental organisation, local management protocols, and essential practical skills. The SHOs must also be told clearly the tasks and roles expected of them. Not only are these essential factors in ensuring work satisfaction, but they also enhance team work and reduce stress.[18] This teaching is helped greatly if the doctors are given copies of the department's medical guidance notes. Several units achieve this by giving all new members of staff a filofax with the departmental policies and protocols printed inside.

Experience has shown that trying to cram too much teaching into the first day is counter-productive. Instead it should be considered part of an ongoing training programme which will last the entire duration of the doctors' stay in the department. Nevertheless, those conditions which are most serious and/or most common must be covered sooner rather than later. Examples of these core topics include all types of resuscitation, myocardial infarction and unstable angina, asthma, musculoskeletal problems, tendon injuries, wounds, bleeding in pregnancy, head injury with alcohol intoxication, and investigations, especially radiology. The ease with which certain serious conditions, such as those shown in Table 9.2, are misdiagnosed should be stressed.

An integral part of the SHO teaching is the induction course. All new SHOs working in the department must attend this within the first month of their attachment. Usually they are run at a regional level and aim to cover the common presenting clinical problems, national protocols and training in resuscitation skills. How this formal training programme is put into effect will depend upon staffing numbers and local expertise.

Teaching sessions following the first day should be held at least weekly and the time protected – that is, the doctors should not be clinically on duty. A way forward is to dedicate 2 to 4 hours per week as paid "Protected Education Time". As an accident and emergency department cannot close for "staff training", adequate clinical cover is essential. Attendance at the formal teaching sessions must be compulsory and part of the doctors' contracted hours of work.

Informal teaching takes place at several levels. Situational, or shop floor teaching enables junior doctors to be taught about clinical problems as they occur. During these sessions, advice on communication, prioritisation, documentation, and how to avoid distractions can be given along with basic clinical training, including history taking and examination.[24] This teaching is the responsibility of both the consultants and other middle grade staff. Only by having a sufficient number of staff can this service be provided throughout the day and evening.

It is important to ensure that the educational aims are being met. This can come from constructive feedback during informal teaching sessions or audit. Allocating each doctor a senior accident and emergency doctor to act as their mentor also helps. A further way is to give staff logbooks to fill in. This enables the doctors and their mentor to see how they are progressing and which areas still require attention.

Staff organisation and shift patterns

When a department has the correct number of adequately trained SHOs they can be built into a team, with two SHOs rotated each month to cover for those who are away. SHOs appreciate their rotas being organised by the consultant personally. This brings home to junior doctors how important it is to turn up for work on time and breeds self respect and a strong team spirit for that particular group. Members of a happy team will be more responsive to patients' needs (reducing the likelihood of complaints) and also more likely to help each other, minimising the chance of mistakes. The incidence of sickness also usually falls, reducing the costs of locums, and allowing reasonable staffing levels.

Having departments of sufficient size so that a doctor is never working on his/her own reduces tiredness, stress, and enables peer stimulation and security. Tiredness can also be minimised by carefully planned shift patterns and by good departmental organisation.[18] For example, it is strongly recommended that the optimum shift rotation is in a clockwise direction with at least a one month period between rotations to allow for circadian stabilisation.[14] Furthermore, it is important to match peaks in patient arrivals with appropriate numbers of both medical and nursing staff.

Senior personnel must be on the look-out for mistakes, particularly at the beginning and end of shifts where the chances of their occurring are highest. Furthermore, all medical personnel should be made aware of how their performance will vary during the day so that they can be extra vigilant. Shifts must be arranged so that there is an hour's overlap period between the doctor who is leaving and the one who is starting work so that the handover of patients is not hurried. The doctor or nurse on a new shift should assess all the patients in their area of responsibility who still require investigation or treatment. In this way errors of judgement made by the outgoing team are not perpetuated. Furthermore, any deterioration in the patient's condition can be detected at an early stage.

Personal workload organisation

Doctors working in accident and emergency need to be taught to organise their workload into manageable tasks. They should concentrate on what they are doing and aim to complete as much as possible before taking on another problem. On those occasions when the task is interrupted by an emergency, the doctor is strongly advised to review the situation from the beginning once s/he returns to the patient.

Breaks are essential for both physical and mental recuperation. Therefore senior staff must ensure that personnel take time for meals as well as time to come away from the intensity of the department. Rotating personnel to different parts of the department is also a good idea because it prevents staff becoming stale due to seeing the same types of conditions for long periods.

The doctor or nurse on a new shift should assess personally all the patients in their area of responsibility who still require investigation or treatment. In this way errors of judgement made by the outgoing team are not perpetuated. Furthermore, any deterioration in the patient's condition can be detected at an early stage.

Errors resulting from mixing up patients are best prevented by training doctors to complete any documentation during the patient consultation or immediately afterwards. A personal self-inking name stamp for each accident and emergency doctor facilitates clarity and responsibility because signatures are often difficult to read and accident and emergency SHOs change jobs every six months. Having the nursing staff aware of each patient in their area of responsibility also helps because it reduces the chances of inappropriate treatment being given.

Performance and stress

During the course of a single shift, accident and emergency personnel may be exposed to a whole spectrum of emotions and be expected to provide the appropriate response in each case. However, this continuous adaptation can lead to emotional fatigue that will be manifested as irritability, anxiety, depression, or a blunted affect. Critical incident debriefing can go some way to reducing emotional stress. It is important that seniors are sensitive and supportive to the emotional thresholds of

159

personnel in the department. Taking time to listen is an important first step. Without this, the staff will go on to develop low levels of alertness, physical fatigue and eventually absenteeism from work.

Communication

There are many examples where poor communication significantly increases the risk of mistakes. Not listening to patients, or not understanding them, means that diagnosis is almost completely dependent upon the physical examination. This incomplete assessment greatly increases the chance of incorrect diagnosis and incorrect management decisions. Failures of communication also occur between medical and nursing staff, and between the accident and emergency department and other departments, especially when discussions are carried out by telephone. Not only does this allow mistakes to be perpetuated, it also introduces "conceptual" errors because medical staff differ in what they consider terms such as "exhaustion", "cyanosis", "pallor" and "sickness" to mean.

Communication with patients

In the drive to perfect clinical and diagnostic skills, the human side of practising medicine must not be forgotten. Studies have shown that failures in communication are usually an important aspect of all types of complaints, including those primarily dealing with missed diagnosis and dissatisfaction with treatment.[5-7,26] Communication skills can be taught, particularly by using videoed consultations or role play with actors. This training is now widespread in general practice but is not yet an accepted part of medical or nursing training in accident and emergency medicine, although some departments are running pilot training schemes for staff.

Key points on communication with patients*

- Listen and ensure that you understand what the patient is saying.
- Ensure that patients and/or relatives understand what you are saying.
- Prior to any procedure, explain carefully why and what you are doing.
- Do not speak down to patients either figuratively or literally.
- Control your own emotions.
- Avoid unintended communication such as disparaging asides.
- Do not criticise previous advice or treatment unless you have all the facts.

*Adapted from Hill[26]

The initial impression given to the patient is vital. Not only will this affect the consultation but it will also encourage the patient to complain if they are dissatisfied with the treatment. Furthermore, when giving advice, the clinician must ensure that the patient understands the instructions and can carry them out. It is important that the patient is fully informed before they are asked to consent to a particular procedure. If this is not done, the doctor could be considered negligent if the patient went on to develop a complication following the treatment. The number of possible misadventures following most medical procedures is large, but the chance of most of them occurring is very remote. It is however considered essential that the patient is told about complications with a greater than 10% chance of occurring. Other possibilities should be discussed if the patient asks or the doctor feels it appropriate in that particular case.[27]

There are several reasons for patients leaving against medical advice, but the most common are misunderstanding, anger, fear, and loss of control.[28] As these patients are potentially putting their own health at risk, as well as that of others, it is important that they are persuaded to stay. Often, timely explanation, reassurance, and involvement of friends and relatives can help prevent the patient leaving. However, it is the patient's right to refuse treatment, provided they are able to understand fully the risks they are facing. In these situations it is important that the clinician documents his/her advice and has this witnessed by a senior member of staff (see below).[28]

Crucial documentation when a patient leaves against medical advice

- reasons why the patient was thought to be competent
- the patient's reason for leaving
- what management has been recommended and its risks and benefits
- the reasonable alternative approaches to care which have been discussed
- the risks associated with leaving which have been discussed
- confirmation that the patient can return following a change of mind.

In cases where the patient is incapable of comprehending the risks, s/he can be restrained and retained in the department pending a Section 2 by an approved psychiatrist and social worker or relative. An NHS Trust, as an employer, has a duty to protect their staff and therefore must provide the necessary security staff. This is especially so now that a greatly increased number of psychiatric patients are managed in the community and attend accident and emergency departments out of hours.

Communication with hospital medical staff

As discussed previously, there is great potential for mistakes occurring when patients are handed on to other healthcare professionals. To try and prevent such errors, Hill suggests that certain key facts must be born in mind (see below).[26]

Key points on communication with healthcare professionals

- Write legible and comprehensible notes.
- Pass on in person any clinically vital pieces of information.
- Provide sufficient clinical details when requesting investigations.
- Only accept second opinions if the patient has been seen.
- Verbal instructions on further management must be supplemented by written notes.

Adapted from Hill[26]

Obviously care must be taken that the notes are both legible and comprehensible. This can be helped greatly by having structured accident and emergency cards, which prompt the doctor to elicit certain pieces of information. This concept has been used for many years in the documentation of trauma resuscitations. More recently, documentation sheets for other conditions, such as head injuries, have also been developed.[29] Nevertheless, irrespective of which type of documentation sheet used, it is also advisable to hand over directly any vital clinical details. Consequently the clinician is not dependent upon the receiving doctor reading the notes.

Communication between doctors is also helped if the one initiating the exchange is clear about what s/he wants from their colleagues. It is also important that only unambiguous terms and phrases are used. For example, following a head injury the individual components of the Glasgow coma score should be given rather than their sum total. This gives a clearer assessment of the patient and reduces the chances of misinterpretation. Similarly, the accident and emergency doctor must provide clear and appropriate clinical information when requesting any investigation. This enables the investigating team to contribute much more in excluding or diagnosing specific conditions.[30] Occasionally patients can be so ill or injured that they have to be transferred rapidly through the department with only a limited assessment and investigation carried out. Examples of this include the tender abdominal aortic aneurysm or the multiply-injured patient who is haemodynamically unstable. In these circumstances it is important that the accident and emergency staff document what has and has not been carried out and that the receiving team are fully aware of this.

Telephone communication between accident and emergency personnel and patients is becoming more common in the UK.[31] These advice lines provide patients with a fast and convenient source of medical help. For the accident and emergency department it represents a method of reducing patient attendance. However, as the doctor or nurse cannot see the patient there is always a risk that errors of judgement may occur. To help reduce the chances of this happening it is essential that certain safeguards are in place (see below).

Safeguards for accident and emergency telephone advice lines

- Only experienced clinical A&E personnel should be involved.
- The time and date of the call must be recorded.
- The patient's name, telephone number and complaint must be recorded.
- The A&E personnel involved and the advice given must be recorded.
- All advice should comply with the standard treatment of care.
- All telephone records must be regularly assessed.

The recent introduction of NHS Direct advice lines may reduce the numbers of calls to departments, though its impact and performance have yet to be fully evaluated.

Communication with the community

Good communication must also extend out into the community. For example, the patient's general practitioner must be informed if s/he is not ill enough to be admitted, but doubt remains as to the cause of the condition. Several departments have computerised systems which enable letters to be generated automatically. Though these can be given to the patient to hand to the general practitioner, only about 60% will arrive.[32] It is therefore preferable to post the letter and, in appropriate cases, to phone the general practitioner and discuss the management with them.

Environment and working conditions

The layout of the department should be optimised so that staff do not feel uncomfortable or cramped whilst working. Equipment must be adequate, checked regularly, and positioned so that it is close to the patients. The accident and emergency consultant must also ensure that distracting and intrusive environmental conditions are kept to a minimum. Occasionally this is unavoidable, such as during structural alterations. Other sources, for example the volume of departmental intercoms, should be adjusted so they get the message over but allow people to carry on working.

Lighting has to be adequate and non-flickering. It has been found that exposure to bright light (for instance, 10 000 lux) shifts the temperature curve, affects the subjective assessment of alertness, and improves cognitive performance.[14] However, the actual level required varies with the activity. High levels are required for patient assessment, surgical procedures and radiological interpretation.

Departmental organisation

Triage

This process enables patients to be sorted into categories of increasing urgency. In this way personnel and equipment can be used most effectively. Furthermore, the awareness of staff will be heightened before seeing the urgent cases because of the prior warning made by the person triaging the patient.

Once triage is introduced, accident and emergency personnel soon find it an essential element in the department's overall organisation. However, incorrect triage, when the patient is sent to the wrong part of the department to be seen by the wrong person, greatly increases the chances of mismanagement. To overcome this three rules need to be obeyed:

• Triage MUST be carried out by experienced staff
• Triage MUST be repeated
• Triage MUST be audited

The risk of incorrect triage will be reduced by having only experienced accident and emergency personnel carrying it out. As a patient's condition may alter rapidly it is also essential that triage is carried out several times during his/her stay in the department. This also helps to minimise the effect of any initially incorrect triage decisions. Auditing triage enables the sensitivity and specificity to be assessed and appropriate training or adjustments to be made. The Manchester Triage System has been introduced into many accident and emergency departments in an attempt to provide an objective, robust, and consistent triage tool.[33] A study has found it to be sensitive in the identification of critically ill patients, though the investigators stressed the need for triage to be dynamic, so that deterioration after initial assessment can be detected.[34]

Departmental protocols

The aim of these is to stipulate a course of action that is considered to be the most appropriate by the senior members of the department, hospital, or indeed specialty. Protocols cover aspects of patient management, data interpretation and radiological assessment and minimise risks of mistakes being made. The "10 commandments of Accident and Emergency Radiology" is one such system of good practice: [35]

The "10 commandments of accident and emergency radiology"

1 Treat the patient, not the x ray film.
2 Take a history and examine the patient before requesting an x ray film.
3 Request an x ray film only when necessary.
4 Never look at an x ray film without seeing the patient; never see the patient without looking at the x ray film.
5 Look at every x-ray film, the whole x ray film and the x ray film as a whole.
6 Re-examine the patient when there is an incongruity between the x ray film and the expected findings.
7 The rule of twos: two views, two joints, two sides.
8 Take x ray films before and after procedures.
9 If an x ray film does not look quite right, ask and listen: there is probably something wrong.
10 Ensure you are protected by fail-safe mechanisms.

Another example of good practice is not discharging patients until the social situation has been determined. This ensures that patients with missed fractures can get back to hospital if their condition does not improve. All the people working in the department should be aware of these policies and, ideally, have a personal copy. Compliance with these protocols, and their effectiveness can be audited.

Referral procedures

An accident and emergency department cannot work in isolation from the rest of the hospital. Key support staff must be on site 24 hours per day to provide experienced medical and surgical back up, as well as all the appropriate investigations.[3] This process is helped greatly by the accident and emergency consultant developing with these specialities an inpatient referral system of particular patient groups. This must include generally accepted recommendations for groups such as patients with head injuries, asthmatics, suspected myocardial infarction, sexual assault, and injuries to children.

The accident and emergency consultant must establish a robust system of outpatient referral to ensure patient follow-up of appropriate cases. In this way the initial treatment can be assessed and continuing management provided. A common example is the referral of fractures and dislocations to the hospital's orthopaedic clinic. However, links with other specialties, including general practice, is also desirable. Feedback from these specialists is an important element in the training of accident and emergency doctors.

Children and the elderly

Children and the elderly represent two groups of patients well recognised for presenting accident and emergency personnel with both puzzling and potentially dangerous diagnostic dilemmas.[36, 37] To help prevent mistakes being made, a systematic assessment needs to be carried out by experienced personnel with early recourse to investigative tools such as plain radiography and ultrasonography.[36] Other diagnostic aids need to be available to accident and emergency staff because they have a role in certain situations, such as the assessment of abdominal pain and ECG interpretation.[38]

Around 20% of attendees at accident and emergency departments are children under the age of 16 years, with a disproportionately high number of patients who are under 5 years old. SHOs may have little postgraduate experience in paediatrics, and yet they must be able to distinguish those few children with early, possibly extremely subtle, signs of serious illness from the majority who will have only minor complaints. It is therefore vital not only that SHOs receive formal teaching in paediatrics, but also that a second opinion is readily available from middle-grade and consultant accident and emergency staff as well as from paediatric registrars and above.

A joint statement produced in 1988 by the British Paediatric Association, the British Association of Paediatric Surgeons and the Casualty Surgeons Association (now the British Association for Accident and Emergency Medicine) laid down the minimum requirements for the management of children in accident and emergency departments.[39] These requirements include a consultant paediatrician who has responsibility for liaison with the consultant in accident and emergency medicine as well as a liaison health visitor to facilitate communication between the accident and emergency department and the community. The accident and emergency consultant must ensure that there is good liaison between his/her department, the paediatricians and the community.

All patients either under 16 years or over 65 years who have been discharged from the department must be followed up by a health visitor liaison officer. As both groups are particularly sensitive to poor social situations, it is important to determine if they and their relatives are coping, if any new symptoms have developed, and that their general practitioners know of their plight. When funding for a liaison health visitor post is not provided by the community, there is a risk of serious consequences to the care of children attending accident and emergency departments. This is because an isolated problem may not assume its correct significance when viewed without all other information relating to the child's social circumstances and previous health record.

Transfer of patients

To facilitate a smooth transfer, it is important to ensure the receiving facility and personnel have been contacted. If an intra-hospital transfer is envisaged, the clinicians must also decide on the most suitable method of transportation and how the patient should be stabilised and prepared for the journey.[40]

All aspects of the patient's airway, breathing, and circulation must be reassessed before the patient leaves and appropriate adjustments made. For example, the patient who tolerates an oropharyngeal airway should be intubated and ventilated so that the airway can be protected and hypoxia and hypercarbia prevented. All cannula, catheters, tubes, and drains must be secured.

Monitoring during the transfer period must be continued to ensure that ventilation and tissue perfusion are adequate. During transit, the patient needs to be accompanied by appropriately trained and equipped staff to enable them to monitor and intervene with any ventilatory or perfusion problems. All the medical and nursing notes, radiographs, blood tests, identifying labels, and, if necessary, consent forms must also be taken with the patient. Upon arrival the transfer team must hand over to the personnel who will be in charge of the patient's definitive care. In this way, important events during transfer as well as a summary of the initial resuscitation can be provided.

Quality control

No matter how good an accident and emergency department is, errors will occur. It is therefore important that a quality control system is in place, which can identify errors quickly so that patients can be recalled and any harm minimised. As there are several aspects of accident and emergency work that must be routinely checked, adequate staffing levels are essential (see below).

Accident and emergency activities subjected to routine quality control

- Radiology
- ECG
- Telephone advice records
- Laboratory records
- Children and the elderly
- Discharge summaries.

Most missed diagnoses in the accident and emergency department result from misinterpretation of radiographs. Error rates of 2·8–35% have been found, but this number can be reduced when a system is set-up whereby all radiographs are reported by radiologists.[41-46] It is important that all x rays carried out on accident and emergency patients are reviewed by an experienced radiologist within three working days. In carrying this out, s/he must have an adequately completed request card (see before) and the accident and emergency doctor's radiological opinion. Should an abnormality be missed, the radiologist will immediately inform the accident and emergency department so that that the patient can be recalled.

A similar quality control system for all the ECGs carried out in the department is also essential.[22,47] As with radiographs, this is particularly important when the investigation was carried out on patients who were subsequently discharged from accident and emergency. A system also needs to be in place for assessing the telephone advice records, discharge summaries and all laboratory results returned to accident and emergency.[48] The latter must be checked, and acted upon, prior to filing. Unfortunately, there is usually a considerable gap between the time the patient was in the department and when the discharge letter is written by the in-house team. Nevertheless, analysis of these reports by senior accident and emergency personnel provides important feedback as well as pointers for quality control.

Near misses

Near misses are unfortunately difficult to detect and are therefore rarely recorded. However, they represent an invaluable source of information on errors occurring in the department. A system which has been used to some effect in clinical practice, with particular success in the field of anaesthetics and ICU medicine, is the anonymous documentation of clinical incidents.[49] Furthermore, certain specialties have enhanced this system by employing a "risk management" officer to specifically assess near misses so that lessons can be learnt before a patient suffers. It would be interesting to see whether the introduction of such a system into Emergency Medicine would have a beneficial effect. In the meantime, departments will have to continue to rely on other time honoured ways of detecting near misses, such as return visits, review clinics and card review.

Return visits

Special attention must be given to patients who return with the same condition because it is no better or has got worse. Studies have shown that 9–20% of these patients have conditions missed on their first visit and initial care had been inappropriate in 5–23% of cases.[50-52] These people must be completely reassessed and any investigation reviewed, to make sure that a mistake has not occurred. Ideally such patients should be seen by a doctor, more senior than an SHO, whilst they are in the department or, if this is not possible, referred to the next accident and emergency review clinic.

Review clinics

Most accident and emergency departments run review clinics to which SHOs refer patients for follow-up of specific conditions (for example, burns) or for review by a senior doctor for confirmation of their diagnosis. However, at the present time few departments have enough staff to provide 24-hour senior cover. Consequently these clinics tend to be used to provide a second opinion. When used in this way they provide a safety net for the patient (and junior staff), as well as giving the seniors a chance to informally assess medical management and record keeping by the referring staff.

Card review

A further method of identifying near misses and assessing the performance of accident and emergency personnel, utilised by some departments, is daily review of accident and emergency cards by senior accident and emergency staff. In this way, the seniors can ensure that patients are being treated and referred appropriately. Both near misses and actual incidents can be identified and patients recalled or their general practitioner informed if necessary. Card reviewing is considered to be time-consuming, though its exponents find that with experience the time required lessens considerably. However, it may not be feasible in all departments, particularly where there are low numbers of senior doctors available.

Complaints

An essential aspect of quality control is analysis of the complaints against the department. They have a frequency of approximately 0·2–0·4 per 1000 new patients seen and cover a wider range of quality issues including communication, diagnostic and therapeutic matters.[5,6,53] Addressing these issues will lead to improvements in the quality of care as well reducing the risk of mistakes. Once a mistake is identified by the quality control system, it should be studied so that the reasons for it can be determined. The lessons learnt from this can then be fed back into the appropriate part of the departmental system to reduce the chances of this error occurring again.

Audit

The UK Trauma Audit and Research Network (UKTARN) represents a national based audit system.[54] However, highly effective audit can also be carried out at a local level.[46,55,56] The number and depth of clinical topics covered is dependent upon the administrative resources available but all

169

should be quantifiable, repeatable and relevant to accident and emergency.[57] The choice of clinical topics audited depends upon the incidence of the particular condition in accident and emergency patients, its morbidity and mortality. Examples include resuscitation attempts, the "door to needle time" for administration of streptokinase and the management of adults or children with asthma. Triage decisions and record-keeping must also be audited frequently, as inaccurate initial patient assessment can have such serious consequences.

Departmental and hospital medical guidance notes, along with clinical protocols, should be used as a basis for clinical audit. Where audit highlights difficulties in the provision of clinical care or outmoded protocols, it may be appropriate to update them. In this way doctors and nurses throughout the hospital can develop a feeling of ownership for clinical protocols, which as a result are more likely to be adhered to.

Integrated Care Pathways (ICPs) are a relatively new natural progression from clinical audit. ICPs are protocols for the management of patients with particular conditions (for instance, asthma) which are available at the patients' bedside to inform and guide them, the doctors, nurses, and all other heath care professionals on the likely plan for their care during a hospital admission. Overall patient care involves management, resources, and a multidisciplinary team. Scrutiny of ICPs for areas where a patient's care does not follow the anticipated route is a helpful form of audit, which may highlight areas of risk in an accident and emergency department. Most accident and emergency departments now regularly audit the clinical record-keeping of their nursing and medical staff. This is most valuable if a structured audit form is used so that individual feedback can be given on areas of good and poor practice.

It is very important that all recommendations made are documented so that follow up audits can ascertain whether these policies have been carried out and whether their execution has had the effect of improving the service to patients.

Incident analysis in accident and emergency

Recent attempts have been made to introduce risk management procedures from the industrial field into accident and emergency medicine. The first of these was called PRISMA (Prevention and Recovery Information System for Monitoring and Analysis), which was originally developed for use in chemical engineering,[58] and later adapted for use in medicine.[59,60] Further modifications were made by van Vuuren *et al*,[61] to make the system more easily applicable in the medical domain. This latest system was named MECCA (Medical Errors and Complications Causal Analysis), and describes a process in which critical incidents are identified and analysed for human, environmental and organisational root causes.

Thus far, studies using PRISMA and MECCA have been of small scale, but a larger scale study using MECCA as a tool for comparing root causes between four different accident and emergency departments is currently under way. It remains to be seen whether or not these tools will have a practical application in the day-to-day quality control and risk management procedures in other departments.

Summary and conclusion

1 Mistakes occurring in the accident and emergency department rarely result from one catastrophic error.
2 Invariably the chances of a mistake being made are already high because a catalogue of human, environmental, and equipment problems coexist.
3 People responsible for running accident and emergency departments must reduce the chances of human mistake by adequate training, staffing, and optimal shift patterns.
4 Accident and emergency personnel should be provided with an environment and equipment that facilitate effective and efficient work.
5 By appropriate departmental organisation, people responsible for running accident and emergency departments must ensure that human, environmental, and equipment problems do not occur in combination.
6 Finally it is important that a good quality control system is present to minimise the effect of any mistake as well as to investigate why it occurred.

References

1 Information supplied by British Association for Accident and Emergency Medicine.
2 British Association for Accident and Emergency Medicine. *The Way Ahead 1998*. October 1998.
3 National Audit Office. *NHS Accident & emergency departments in England*. Report by the Controller and Auditor General. HMSO, 1992.
4 Audit Commission National Report. *By accident or design: Improving A & E services for England and Wales*. HMSO, 1996.
5 Kadzombe E, Coals J. Complaints against doctors in an accident and emergency department: A 10 year analysis. *Arch Em Med* 1992;9:134.
6 Hunt T, Glucksman M. A review of 7 years of complaints in an inner-city department. *Arch Em Med* 1991;8:17.
7 Reichl M, Sleet R. Complaints against an accident and emergency department: Current trends. *Arch Em Med* 1990;7:246.
8 Gwynne A, Barber P, Tavener F. A review of 105 negligence claims against departments. *J Accid Em Med* 1997;14(4):243–5.
9 *Report of the working party on the management of major trauma*. Royal College of Surgeons of England, 1988.
10 Cooke MW, Kelly C, Khattab A, *et al*. 24-hour senior cover – a necessity or a luxury? *J Accid Em Med* 1998;15:181–4.
11 Morris F, Tordoff S, Wallis D, Skinner D. Cardiopulmonary resuscitation skills of pre-registration house officers: Five years on. *BMJ* 1991;302:626.

12 Wyatt JP, Henry J, Beard D. The association between seniority of doctor and outcome following trauma. *Injury* 1999;**30**:165–8.
13 Coleman R. *Wide awake at 3:00 am.* New York: Freeman and Co, 1986.
14 Whitehead D. Using circadian principles in emergency medicine scheduling. In: Andrew A, Pollack M, eds. *Wellness for emergency physicians.* Dallas: American College of Emergency Physicians, 1995.
15 Stiell I, Greenberg G, McKnight B, *et al.* Decision rules for the use of radiographs in ankle injury: Refinement and prospective validation. *JAMA* 1993;**269**:1127.
16 Mackway-Jones, K. Personal communication.
17 McNamara R, Margulies J. Chemical dependency in emergency medical residency programs: Perspective of the program disorder. *Ann Em Med* 1994;**23**:1072.
18 Heyworth J, Whitley T, Allison E, Revicki D. Predictors of work satisfaction among SHOs during medicine training. *Arch Em Med* 1993;**10**:279.
19 LeWinter J. The medical family. In: Andrew A, Pollack M, eds. *Wellness for emergency physicians.* Dallas: American College of Emergency Physicians, 1995.
20 Kelner M, Rosenthal C. Postgraduate medical training, stress and marriage. *Can J Psychol* 1986;**31**:22.
21 British Association for Accident and Emergency Medicine. *Stress in medicine.* December 1998.
22 Touquet R, Fothergill J, Harris N. Accident and emergency department; the speciality of medicine. In: Powers M, Harris N, eds. *Medical negligence.* London: Butterworths, 1994.
23 Driscoll P, Vincent C. Variation in trauma resuscitation and its effect on outcome. *Injury* 1992;**23**:111.
24 Guly H. Missed tendon injuries. *Arch Em Med* 1991;**8**:87.
25 Guly H. Medico-legal problems in departments. *J Med Defence Union* 1993;**2**:36.
26 Hill G. *A & E risk management.* London: The Medical Defence Union, 1991.
27 Sidaway v. Board of Governors of the Bethlem Royal and the Maudsley Hospital. 2 WLR 480, 1985.
28 Rice M. Emergency department patients leaving against medical advice. *Foresight* 1994;**29**:1.
29 Wallace S, Gullan R, Byrne P, Bennett J, Perez-Avila C. Use of proforma for head injuries in departments – the way forward. *J Accid Emerg Med* 1994;**11**:33.
30 Rickett A, Finlay D, Jagger C. The importance of clinical details when reporting radiographs. *Injury* 1992;**23**:458.
31 Egleston C, Kelly H, Cope A. Use of telephone advice lines in an accident and emergency department. *BMJ* 1994;**308**:31.
32 Sherry M, Edmunds S, Touquet R. The reliability of patients in delivering the letter from the hospital department to their general practitioner. *Arch Em Med* 1985;**2**:165.
33 Manchester Triage Group. *Emergency triage.* BMJ Publications, 1997.
34 Cooke MW, Jinks S. Does the Manchester triage system detect the critically ill? *J Accid Em Med* 1999;**16**(3):179–81.
35 Touquet R, Driscoll P, Nicholson D. Teaching in Medicine – 10 commandments of radiology. *BMJ* 1995;**310**:642.
36 Advanced Life Support Group. *Advanced paediatric life support: A practical approach.* London: BMJ, 1997.
37 Caesar R. Dangerous complaints: The acute geriatric abdomen. *Em Med Repts* 1994;**15**:190.
38 Stonebridge P, Freeland P, Rainey J, Macleod D. Audit of computer aided diagnosis of abdominal pain in departments. *Arch Em Med* 1992;**9**:271.
39 Morton R, Phillips B. *Accidents and emergencies in children.* Oxford: Oxford University Press, 1992.
40 Intensive Care Society. *Safe transfer of the criticially ill.* Intensive Care Society, 1999.
41 DeLacey G, Barker A, Harper J, Wignall B. An assessment of the clinical effects of reporting radiographs. *Br J Radiol* 1980;**53**:304.
42 Mucci B. The selective reporting of x ray films from departments. *Injury* 1983;**14**:343.
43 Wardrope J, Chennels P. Should casualty radiographs be reviewed? *BMJ* 1985;**290**:1638.
44 Gleadhill D, Thomson J, Simmons P. Can more efficient use be made of x ray examinations in the department? *BMJ* 1987;**294**:943.

45 Vincent C, Driscoll P, Audley R, Grant D. Accuracy of detection of radiographic abnormalities by junior doctors. *Arch Emerg Med* 1988;**5**:101.
46 Thomas H, Mason A, Smith R, Fergusson C. Value of radiographic audit in an accident service department. *Injury* 1992;**23**:47.
47 McCallion W, Templeton P, McKinney L, Higginson J. Missed myocardial ischaemia in the department: ECG a need for audit? *Arch Em Med* 1991;**8**:102.
48 Verdile V. The telephone in emergency practice. *Foresight* 1993;**27**:1.
49 Webb RK, Currie M, Williamson JA, *et al*. The Australian Incident Monitoring Study: An analysis of 2000 incident reports. *Anaesth Intens Care* 1993;**21**(5):520–8.
50 Wilkins P, Beckett M. Audit of unexpected return visits to an accident and emergency department. *Arch Em Med* 1992;**9**:352.
51 O'Dwyer F, Bodiwala G. Unscheduled return visits by patients to the department. *Arch Em Med* 1991;**8**:196.
52 Pierce J, Kellerman A, Oster C. "Bounces": An analysis of short-term return visits to a public hospital emergency department. *Ann Em Med* 1990;**19**:752.
53 Richmond P, Evans R. Complaints and litigation – three years experience at a busy department 1983–85. *Health Trends* 1989;**21**:42.
54 Yates D, Woodford M, Hollis S. Preliminary analysis of the care of injured patients in British hospitals: First report of the United Kingdom major trauma outcome study. *BMJ* 1992;**305**:737.
55 Yates D, Bancewicz J, Woodford M, *et al*. Trauma audit – closing the loop. *Injury* 1994;**25**:511.
56 Tulloh B. Diagnostic accuracy in head injured patients: An emergency department audit. *Injury* 1994;**25**:231.
57 Driscoll P. Audit in A&E departments. *Med Audit News* 1991;**1**:8.
58 van der Schaaf TW. PRISMA: *A risk management tool based on incident analysis*. The Netherlands: Paper for the Safety Management Group at Eindhoven University of Technology, 1995.
59 van der Hoeff B, van der Schaaf TW. *Risk management in hospitals: predicting versus reporting risks in a surgical department*. The Netherlands: Paper for the Safety Management Group at Eindhoven University of Technology, 1995.
60 Shea CS. *The organization of work in a complex and dynamic environment: the department*. PhD Thesis, University of Manchester, 1996.
61 van Vuuren W, Shea CS, van der Schaaf TW. *The development of an incident analysis tool for the medical field*. Report EUT/BDK/85. The Netherlands: Eindhoven University of Technology, Faculty of Technology Management, 1997.

10 Reducing risks in the practice of hospital general medicine

GRAHAM NEALE

"Medicine used to be simple, ineffective and relatively safe. Now it is complex, effective and potentially dangerous."[1]

Risks are inevitable in any human endeavour. Yet clinical audit was not introduced into the NHS until 1989[2] and risk management not until 1994.[3] For some well-defined clinical activities such as maternal deaths,[4] stillbirths and deaths in infancy[5] and perioperative deaths[6] confidential studies have been undertaken since the 1930s and such studies have had significant effects in improving practice. But clinicians have been slow to grasp the much more difficult problem of determining the incidence and nature of adverse events in general medicine.

This chapter is devoted to specific problems predisposing to adverse events in general (internal) medicine; how to identify risks in practice and how these risks may be minimised.

The practice of medicine in hospitals – the changing scene

The provision of care in general medical wards has changed dramatically over the past 30–40 years. In the fifties and sixties individual house staff had overall responsibility for patients admitted to designated beds in one or two wards. Overall responsibility meant providing care from admission to discharge – writing all the notes; charting the history of the disease process; planning clinical care under supervision and explaining the nature of the disease to patient and relatives. The house doctor was guided by registrars and one or two consultants and worked closely with senior ward nursing staff. Special investigations were few. Dramatic happenings were rare. There were no means of cardiac resuscitation; no pacemakers; no ward artificial ventilators; no intensive care units. There was minimal use of intravenous fluids (through rubber tubing and glass drip chambers). The pharmacopoeia was limited – the first antibiotics and psychotropic drugs had recently been added

The house staff lived in the hospital 24 hours a day, 7 days a week. They were "on call" for their patients throughout, except perhaps for half a day a week and one weekend in three, but the emphasis was on caring rather than dramatic intervention. Patients were docile and accepting. They virtually never complained and medico-legal actions were extremely rare. It was generally accepted that hospital staff were doing their best to provide a uniformly high standard of care.

Over the past 30–40 years the rapid advances in medical technology and medical treatment have had a double-edged effect. The general population became caught up in the excitement of the next "medical breakthrough" yet at the same time increasingly dissatisfied with the Victorian hospital buildings and the wartime "pre-fabs" in which they were nursed. As the health of the population improved (and people lived longer) far from a lessening demand for hospital services the pressure mounted. Patients expected prompt relief of their ills and prolonged high-tech care for chronic disease. The problem of providing that care has been compounded by government intervention – the repeated re-structuring of hospital services; the introduction of the techniques of management not always suited to the provision of healthcare; the emasculation of consultant staff councils; the reduction in working hours; changes in nurse training, and changes in the organisation of service provision.

Ward doctors became increasingly unhappy as they were subjected to the strain of increasing numbers of patients, shorter hospital stays, a perpetual shortage of beds and coping with clinical crises. The highly experienced and supportive ward sisters disappeared to be replaced by young managers who rarely worked directly with patients (and then often for no more than three years as they climbed the career ladder); the links between the nursing and medical professions were rapidly eroded and patients were cared for wherever a bed could be found. A consultant with a nominal cohort of 20 beds may find himself advising on up to 40 or so patients, depending on a cycle of admissions which are outside his direct control. These patients may be spread over 7–10 wards; under the care of individual named nurses who are often not on duty during ward rounds; and clerked by four or five house staff not all of whom may be present on ward rounds because of the introduction of shift work.

Ninety per cent of patients in general medicine are admitted with emergency problems. They are allocated to the firm "on take" and will normally be under the care of a succession of students/junior doctors before being reviewed by a consultant. Most patients do not understand the hierarchy of care. In worst case scenarios consultants go to the ward twice a week with a retinue of doctors who do their best to up-date everyone on the progress of individual patients. There may be minimal consultation with patients or nurses before decisions are made. Arrangements for the discharge of a patient from hospital care are usually left to the houseman and nursing staff. Fragmentation of professional care combined with interventional medical practice has inevitably increased the risk of adverse events.

Adverse events in medical practice – critical points in the process of care

The causes of adverse events in hospital practice are analysed in depth elsewhere in this book (see Chapter 2). In the practice of general (internal) medicine causation is usually complex. Most patients are elderly and often have underlying chronic pathology (especially conditions leading to cardiovascular and respiratory insufficiency) as well as that of their presenting disease. Thus diagnosis may not be straightforward and the results of treatment may be difficult to predict. Management becomes problematical. After patients have recovered from the condition that brought them into hospital they are often left less able to look after themselves. The perpetual pressure on beds; the lack of nurses to provide high dependency care when needed; and the inadequate facilities for rehabilitation place high demands on overworked hospital doctors. These are factors that predispose to adverse events.

It is in adapting to modern medical practice that we have to consider the causes of adverse events and to determine ways of limiting risks. Training in medicine in the UK and Ireland produces dedicated and conscientious doctors of a remarkably uniform high standard. But it is difficult to devise a system that will protect acutely sick patients against every eventuality over every hour of every day. It is against this background that I shall attempt to define critical points in the care of patients admitted to a NHS hospital with general medical problems (see below).

Critical points in hospital medicine

- Providing care in the emergency room
- Making a diagnosis
- Ordering investigations and interpreting the results
- Undertaking invasive procedures
- Drug treatment
- Ward management

Care in the emergency room

There is no uniform approach to the care of medical emergencies. However, in many hospitals there have been few organisational changes over the past 40 years. The medical house officer or senior house officer on call sees the patient; initiates investigations; informs a clinician of intermediate grade; and together they make a decision. If that decision is incorrect the patient may suffer a serious adverse event before a fully trained specialist becomes involved.

Example 1

> *A 58-year-old man had pain in his chest when moving a heavy cupboard. He thought that he had strained a muscle. The following day the discomfort returned and he became cold and sweaty for a short period. His wife took him to the local hospital emergency department where he was detained for three hours. The attending staff (non-consultant) read the ECG and chest radiograph as showing no abnormalities. Circulating cardiac enzymes were at the upper limit of normal. The patient was discharged with a diagnosis "chest pain – ?muscular". Later that day he collapsed and died. Review of the ECG showed early but clear-cut ischaemic changes.*

Inadequate supervision of insufficiently experienced staff in the care of patients presenting as emergencies is a common cause of serious errors.[7]

Making a diagnosis

Making the correct diagnosis is the key to effective management. In clinical practice diagnosis is often straightforward and only one reasonable diagnosis is tenable (for example, as with an exacerbation of bronchial asthma) but it is easy to follow the wrong line of reasoning (for example, all who wheeze do not have bronchial asthma). The acute condition has to be set in context. Retrospective analysis of case records show that adverse events are far more likely to occur in patients who have an acute illness superimposed on pre-existing pathology such as that associated with hypertension and diabetes mellitus.[8]

Example 2

> *At a general practitioner screening examination a 65-year-old man with a somewhat raised blood pressure reported lower chest pain. The GP thought that the pain might be angina although there were atypical features and the pain was not related to exercise. He referred the patient to a cardiologist who noted tenderness in the right hypochondrium and arranged for a barium meal in addition to electrocardiography (ECG) and a stress test. The barium study showed what was thought to be a bulbar duodenal diverticulum and the stress test was stopped because of ST segment depression although the patient was asymptomatic. The patient was treated for angina but a few days later had a massive bleed from a duodenal ulcer as a result of which he died.*

The specialist allowed his special interest in heart disease to dominate in the assessment of this patient's condition. Abdominal tenderness and an

178

abnormal duodenal bulb should have led to endoscopic examination of the duodenum (and the correct diagnosis of a deep duodenal ulcer).

Interpreting investigations

Most diagnoses in general medicine are apparent from a carefully taken history[9] but medical practice has become dominated by investigation. It is true that investigation is needed to confirm the suspected diagnosis; maybe to exclude other diagnoses; and to plan the most appropriate treatment. But investigations must be carefully performed and accurately interpreted.

Example 3

A 74-year-old man had had repeated attacks of altered consciousness and confusion sometimes associated with sweating, often precipitated by exercise and always in the morning. He was treated unsuccessfully with anti-epileptic drugs. A neurologist suspected recurrent hypoglycaemic attacks and admitted the patient to hospital to test the effects of prolonged fasting. A ward doctor conducted the test poorly and misinterpreted the result. The patient had attacks for a further six years before he was correctly diagnosed as having an insulinoma.

This patient had a "benign" tumour producing insulin. As a result his blood sugar fell to dangerous levels especially before breakfast. The condition is rare but the clinical story is so striking that the diagnosis should never be long delayed.

Undertaking invasive procedures

It is now possible to intervene in the function of all bodily organs without open operation. This has brought enormous benefits such as balloon angioplasty for coronary artery disease; the insertion of cardiac pacemakers; the endoscopic removal of gastro-intestinal tumours; the placement of stents across narrowed ducts; and the drainage of abscess cavities in the chest and abdomen. Inevitably such procedures carry risks. These need to be clearly defined for each specialty.

Example 4

A 73-year-old woman presented with episodic diarrhoea. Examination by barium enema showed no abnormality and her symptoms settled only to recur a year later. The diarrhoea settled promptly on treatment with loperamide or codeine phosphate. The clinicians then decided to look for evidence of organic pathology that could cause diarrhoea. They arranged for examination by sigmoidoscopy, barium follow-through, upper intestinal endoscopy with biopsy, ultrasound examination of the gall bladder and pancreas. No abnormality was found. The consultant decided that chronic pancreatic disease had not been completely excluded and arranged for examination of the pancreas by ERCP, a procedure known to carry a risk of serious complications of about 5%. During the examination the ampulla of Vater was biopsied and the patient went home. A day later, she was re-admitted very seriously ill (with a probable retroperitoneal bleed). She was in intensive care for five days and

179

in hospital for a further three weeks. During this period she required drainage of the stomach via a nasogastric tube. This led to severe inflammation and stricturing of the oesophagus. The patient was left with severe dysphagia and her oesophagus needed dilatation every few weeks By now her presenting symptoms had long since been forgotten.

In this case no clinician took a detailed history of the patient's illness and no one examined the patient's stools. Chronic pancreatic insufficiency was a very unlikely diagnosis and one that could have been excluded by examining the patient's stools and testing the response to treatment with pancreatic supplements. The likely diagnosis was an irritable bowel.

Drug treatment

In the US it is estimated that 1–2% patients admitted to hospital are harmed by drugs.[10] Errors are of two main types: prescribing errors and administration errors (including failure to monitor drug levels and the side-effects of treatment).

Example 5

A 20-year-old woman developed inflammatory bowel disease. After treatment for a year she was found to have a mild anaemia and iron was prescribed. After several months the haemoglobin remained low (Hb 9·6 g/100 ml with a normal mean corpuscular volume that pointed against a diagnosis of iron deficiency) yet more iron was prescribed. The patient's wellbeing deteriorated although there was little evidence of active inflammation in the bowel. The Hb fell to 7·6 (normal value 12·5–14·0). The patient was admitted to hospital for "a whole body iron infusion". At this stage she was found to have proteinuria and a serum creatinine of 455 μmol/l indicating severe renal damage which was the cause of the anaemia. The patient had interstitial nephritis caused by mesalazine.

In this case the clinician was probably unaware of mesalazine-induced nephritis. In fact at that time there were only nine reported cases. But mesalazine carries a long list of possible side-effects including anaemia. This patient's blood count warranted investigation rather than further treatment with iron.

Ward management

The problem of maintaining high quality care in general medical wards has become increasingly difficult with the reduction of junior doctors' working hours and the changes in nursing practice. The consultant can no longer rely on obtaining accurate information from a good house officer and an effective senior nurse. Weekend cover for the care of patients is often dangerously inadequate. A house officer may be "on call" for more than 100 patients with medical problems. Instructions will have been left at the nursing station for tasks that need doing such as checking the level of anti-coagulation for a patient with pulmonary embolism or the circulating electrolytes of a patient who has had a major disorder of fluid balance. The nurses will contact the house staff for advice about analgesia or sedation. If the patient "collapses" the nurses will usually call the "crash" team and the house officer will attend to provide background data. These tasks may seem to be more than enough responsibility for a doctor who has not been qualified for a year and is not on the medical register. But general medical cover has also to be provided. Nursing staff have to be able to recognise when a patient is not progressing as well as expected; then the house doctor has to be competent to assess the problem; and finally he or she has to take appropriate action. The "on call" doctor has access to the expertise of the doctors on duty for new emergency admissions and he or she may be able to contact a member of staff of the team caring for the patient. But the risks are obvious. The problem may develop insidiously; the "on call" doctor is always relatively inexperienced; and usually there is a natural reluctance to call for help if the patient does not seem seriously ill. And for some ward doctors there will be the thought that the end of the shift is only an hour away.

Many conscientious consultants try to keep in touch with the wards over weekends and holiday periods. They will ensure that patients with unstable disorders are reviewed either by themselves or by an experienced registrar. But practice in this respect is very variable.

Example 6

> Late one evening a 58-year-old man presented to a large city hospital after passing three melena stools. His pulse rate was 88/minute; blood pressure 110/60 and haemoglobin 9·8 g/100 ml. He was admitted to a medical ward. He was not given fluid (blood) intravenously, blood was not cross-matched, he was not assessed by a surgeon and his condition was not monitored closely. Six hours after admission he had a large haematemesis and died.

The case notes do not disclose why the care of this patient was so poor. The doctors who admitted the patient may have violated a well-defined protocol but the summary letter sent to the GP suggested that the organisation for the care of patients with gastrointestinal bleeding was seriously deficient. Correct management would have included blood transfusion and emergency endoscopy. If the bleeding could not have been controlled by endoscopic injection then surgical intervention was indicated.

Discharge from hospital

It is common practice to leave arrangements for the discharge of patients from hospital care to house doctors. The majority of patients discharged from medical wards are elderly. Most have more than one disease process and are being treated with several drugs. Common defects in discharging a patient include failure to ensure that an acute-on-chronic condition (such as congestive heart failure) has been stabilised; failure to provide patients and their GPs with coherent plans for conditions that often lead to recurrent hospital admission (such as epilepsy, asthma and chronic lung disease); and failure to provide a multidisciplinary care plan for chronically disabled patients, especially for those living alone.

Example 7

> *A 60-year-old Asian man who was a smoker and who had type 2 diabetes mellitus had a chest radiograph that showed a shadow in the left upper zone. His GP referred him to a chest clinic where sputum was examined (negative for TB) but no further tests done. He was treated for suspected tuberculosis with full doses of rifampicin and pyrazinamide. Over the next month he lost his appetite (possibly because of the drugs) and was admitted to hospital with hypoglycaemic attacks. He was found to be anaemic (Hb 9·5); had a raised blood urea and biochemical signs of osteomalacia. After three days he was discharged home without further investigation. A month later he was re-admitted for five days with fever and chest pain. Radiograph of the chest showed no abnormality. He was treated with antibiotics. Within three weeks he was re-admitted for three days with recurrent fever and diarrhoea. No cause was found and he was sent home. A week later he was brought to the emergency department "short of breath" and sent home only to be admitted 24 hours later moribund. Chest radiography showed an opaque left lung. He was given antibiotics and died. Autopsy showed pulmonary oedema and bronchopneumonia.*

This patient had four admissions under four different consultants. He was not reviewed by the chest physician. On each admission he was treated symptomatically and sent home without a full assessment. There were no discharge summaries. This tragic set of circumstances occurred during the economy drive of the early 1990s ("efficiency savings") and would have made a good statistical impression – four medical admissions with an average length of stay of three days!

Identifying risks in the practice of general medicine

It is much more difficult to identify risks in the practice of general medicine than in areas which have well-defined hazards at specific times such as anaesthesia, obstetrics, intensive care and the surgical specialties. In these fields specially designed retrospective studies[4-6] and critical incident reporting[11,12] have been shown to be of considerable value in modifying practice to reduce risks. In general medical practice the periods of risk are often prolonged and not infrequently errors go unrecognised. Several method have been used to assess risk:

- Audit – analysing processes and assessing the end-results
- Critical incident reporting – analysing adverse events in hospital

- Analysis of autopsy reports
- Assessing reports of "closed" complaints and claims
- External retrospective analysis of case records
- Prospective reporting studies
- Prospective observational studies.

Audit

Ten years ago, following publication of the Department of Health document *Working for Patients*,[13] audit was introduced into hospital medical practice. It was generally believed that by analysing the care of patients with common conditions, weaknesses in management would be identified and corrected (preferably by using written protocols or guidelines). Doctors in the Department of Health, aided and abetted by prime movers in the Royal Colleges and the BMA, accepted the idea of audit with enthusiasm. The medical profession would be seen to be capable of self-regulation. Appropriate instructions were delivered to Regional Health Authorities and within four years £220m were spent in setting up an appropriate bureaucracy.[14] In essence the plan was simple. Heads of units were to identify key processes; the care of patients who had been through the chosen process would be examined in detail; the end-results would be determined; and ideas formulated to improve care. The proposed changes would then have to be implemented and the process repeated to determine their efficacy.

It was soon shown that audit was not very effective in general medicine. Initially this was believed to be due both to a lack of understanding by clinicians and to methodological deficiencies.[15,16] Since then, despite repeated efforts to improve the process, it has been found that effective audit is hard to achieve, time-consuming and relatively complex.[17] In fact much of so-called audit has not been audit at all – simply a consideration of local practice followed by a commentary from the heads of units.[18] It has been estimated that less than 5% of audits have led to changes that were then re-audited. Analyses of the value of audit suggest that improvements in the care of defined problems such as haematemesis or a severe attack of bronchial asthma have been established by enthusiastic consultants who then used audit to back up their proposals, i.e. the cart preceded the horse.[14]

In the practice of general medicine audit may be useful in defining a process of care, for example, the rate and timing of thrombolytic therapy for acute myocardial infarction, but it has proved unsatisfactory as a means of defining risks in clinical practice.[17] Moreover it is probably not cost-effective. In addition to the central funding through regions it was estimated that the practice of audit in each NHS Trust took away time from clinical care equivalent to £500 000 to £1 000 000 per annum.[14] With

183

changes in the structure of the NHS the central funding for audit disappeared and the issue has been left to negotiation between purchasers and providers. We now await the results of the deliberations of the Commission for Health Improvement to determine the future role of clinical audit.

Critical incident reporting

Clinicians are reluctant to face up to errors;[19,20] important errors are often not recognised especially when they occur outside normal working hours; and objective analysis is difficult to achieve. Nevertheless critical incident reporting in the practice of general medicine should be encouraged. Hospital doctors should be able to face the issues honestly and without feeling threatened. In fact only those involved directly with the incident truly know what happened and even then they may find it difficult to recall events accurately. To what extent such an ethos of openness can be extended throughout the NHS remains to be defined.

Analysis of autopsy data

Until the 1960s autopsy was regarded as an important tool for teaching hospital medicine. Consultants, their junior staff, and students attended the demonstrations by pathologists (usually at lunchtime) and there was considerable interest in knowing whether or not the clinician had "got it right". Over the last three decades in the UK autopsy rates have declined from more than 50% to around 20% of deaths[21] and clinical interest has fallen despite repeated pleas to reverse the change.[22] Trends are similar in the USA where "low-tech" autopsies in the era of "high-tech" medicine are regarded as having a continuing value for quality assurance and patient safety.[23] In a recent study of 108 autopsies in a district general hospital (patients' mean age – 78 years; range 54–94) 61 clinical diagnoses were inconsistent with the pathological findings. The most common causes of death, not suspected clinically, were pulmonary embolism (23%), bronchopneumonia (25%), ischaemic heart disease (13%) and malignancy (10%). The clinical sensitivity of ante-mortem diagnosis was particularly low for peritonitis (25%) and pulmonary embolism (24%).[24] It may be argued that the elderly should be "allowed to die in peace" but data from autopsies allows the clinician to identify weaknesses in clinical diagnosis that it may be possible to correct. Overall it is estimated that there are 550 000 deaths a year in the UK. 135 000 cases go to autopsy of which 125 000 are at the request of the coroner (many occurring outside hospital practice). However few coroners in England and Wales are prepared to explore the cause of an adverse event in medical practice unless the death is the result of a glaring error.

Assessing records of "closed" complaints and claims

In the previous edition of this book I demonstrated how a database of key issues arising from complaints and claims could be analysed to reveal the nature of errors.[25] This database has now been extended to cover 350 separate cases of adverse events in hospital medical practice. It has become large enough to allow organisational errors in distinct segments of medical practice to be defined such as the care of medical emergencies,[7] and the practice of gastroenterology (including endoscopy).[26] There seems to be a place for further studies.[27]

External retrospective analysis of case records

Case record analysis provides interesting comparative data (see Chapter 2) but is of limited value for risk management in individual hospitals. In a pilot retrospective analysis of hospital case records in the NHS it has been shown possible to build on American and Australian experience by redesigning and adding to the questionnaire in order to define organisational causes of preventable adverse events (Table 10.1).[8] Such data would be invaluable in determining the cost-benefit of specific interventions designed to reduce adverse events.

Prospective reporting studies

With some clearly defined parts of medical practice it is possible to identify risks by getting doctors to complete questionnaires at the time of undertaking procedures and analysing collected data. This may be useful in comparing practices between units and individuals within units.[28]

Table 10.1 Organisational problems identified by retrospective analysis of case records[8]

Organisational error	Possible means of reducing error
Failure to find details of previous problems in poorly organised case records	Frontispiece record of ongoing problems Develop SMART cards for healthcare
Diagnostic/operative errors by trainees	Improve supervision and training
Drugs leading to adverse events	Pharmacists to monitor prescribing and administration Computerise
Poor teamwork leading to adverse events	Integrate work profiles and record-keeping of clinicians and other carers
Adverse events occurring after discharge	Integrate hospital and community care in procedures for discharge

Prospective observational studies

Prospective studies by trained observers are not often reported. They are most easily undertaken in an acute care setting (for example in an emergency room[29] and in intensive care[30]) and show higher rates of adverse events than retrospective studies. For example Steel *et al* found that 38% of 815 consecutive patients admitted to a general medical service at a university hospital had an iatrogenic illness. Nine per cent suffered an adverse event which was life threatening or produced disability.[31]

Prospective studies are particularly useful for investigating the risks of giving drugs.[32] In the 1960s in both the US and the UK drugs were given from a ward stock. Direct observation showed that administration errors were of the order of 10–15%.[33,34] In the US introducing a dose dispensing system, run by pharmacists who delivered drugs to the ward every two hours, reduced the error rate to less than 2%.[34] In the UK the Gilles report[35] advocated the ward pharmacy system which is still used in nearly all NHS hospitals. This has an error rate of 3–4%.[36-38] In an interesting comparative study of a hospital in the US with one in the UK Dean *et al*[37] showed that the error rate was higher in the US and that the types of error between the two hospitals were different. In the UK ward pharmacy system the main error was omitting to give doses whereas in the US hospital with a modified unit dose system the principal errors were the giving of unordered and incorrect medication.

Summary

Risks in the practice of general medicine are diverse and often not readily apparent. Each of the methods of recognising and analysing adverse events has intrinsic values and weaknesses (Table 10.2). Clinical risk managers have to be flexible and should be prepared to use data both from observations within the Trust and from regional and national surveys.

How risks may be reduced

Reducing risks in the care of patients referred as medical emergencies

Several studies[7,29,39] have shown that serious adverse events occur commonly in the emergency room. Delays in diagnosis and in providing effective treatment appear to be related to inadequate input by fully trained and experienced doctors. Almost certainly, ensuring that a specialist with a major interest in general medicine is available full-time in the emer-

Table 10.2 Methods of investigating adverse events in the practice of general medicine in hospitals

	Applicability	Difficulties
Audit	Unit level: Assessment of management of specific disorders Trust level: Quality of case notes; discharge arrangements	Has proved difficult to maintain interest Audit cycles rarely completed
Critical incident reporting	Invaluable In practice used mainly for clear cut discrete events	Difficult to get open honest discussion Dependent on ethos in the Trust
Comparison of clinical and autopsy findings	Undoubted value in finding unexpected pathology	Clinical applicability a little uncertain Requires a regeneration of interest
"Closed" complaints and claims	Could be of great value if analysed openly Regional/national data may demonstrate important errors*	At present only a few small studies[17,26] Needs regional and national collection and analysis of data
External retrospective studies	Useful in determining the incidence of adverse events both locally and nationally	Expensive and time-consuming
Prospective reporting	Useful in assessing clearly defined procedures	Few studies but potentially useful
Prospective observational studies	Primarily of research interest	Very expensive Probably only of value in investigating specific circumstances

*Some adverse events occur so infrequently that an individual hospital trust is unlikely to see an isolated adverse event as a significant problem requiring a change in organisation. For example it is probable that several young adults die each year because of failure to recognise the "premonitory" bleed of a subarachnoid haemorrhage. This error occurs because inexperienced ward doctors are responsible for the assessment of acute headache. If the potential diagnosis is recognised and a CT scan (if available) is reported as negative (which may not be a true negative – subtle changes may be missed because few NHS hospitals have a neuroradiologist) then the clinician should undertake lumbar puncture and examination of cerebrospinal fluid. However a junior doctor may be required to do such a test only once or twice a year and often makes an error.[7] In an individual hospital if this happens only once every decade there would still be about 25 cases in England and Wales each year. One could make a good case for lumbar puncture to be performed only by or in the presence of a senior experienced clinician.

gency department to help assess patients and to teach junior staff would significantly reduce risks. Moreover there is evidence to show that such consultant input would lead to fewer hospital admissions and would expedite referral for specialist opinion when appropriate. In this way patient care could be improved and available beds could be used more effectively. An analysis of medical claims involving emergency care has led to the recognition of common organisational defects as summarised in Table 10.3.[7]

Table 10.3 Risk management in the care of medical emergencies admitted to hospital[7]

Organisational defects	Possible solutions
Assessment of emergencies by insufficiently experienced junior staff	Experienced clinicians available full-time in A&E departments
Inadequate systems for recording and assessing findings	Systems that follow clear lines for recording evidence, making differential diagnoses and planning appropriate action
Inadequate use of specialist opinion	Involvement of specialists in the training of staff Appreciation of the danger of junior staff taking opinions from one another
Inadequate reading of simple radiographs	Training of staff in the reading of radiographs[40] "On call" radiologists to assess films
Poor management of standard situations	Use of protocols with sensitivity
Inadequate assessment before discharge	Senior staff to take responsibility for discharges from A&E

Reducing risks in making a diagnosis

It is difficult to provide adequate guidelines for avoiding diagnostic error other than to stress the importance of an enquiring mind and eternal vigilance. As with the care of medical emergencies the amount of input by consultant staff is crucial. In specialist outpatients clinics set scenarios are repeated endlessly. Experienced staff become very adept at sorting the wheat from the chaff and try to pass on their skills to trainees. At present medical clinics are flooded with patients with functional disorders (such as irritable bowel syndrome in gastroenterology (which make up more than 50% referrals); palpitations in cardiology and overbreathing in respiratory medicine) and it is difficult to cope with the workload without cutting corners and inevitably running the risk of making an error. An analysis of adverse events in gastroenterological practice[26] has indicated some guidelines for diagnosis (Table 10.4) but these may be of limited use in preventing error. There seems to be a need for research into the value of educating the population on the nature of disease and how to cope with it; how best to improve the confidence of general practitioners in making straightforward diagnoses; and in determining how best to use specialist services. Although rarely mentioned, in present day practice, there is a risk of over-investigation of functional disorders. Patients with introspective personalities have their fears reinforced by inappropriate investigation and as a result may end up chronic invalids.

Reducing the risks of investigation

Investigation has become the centrepiece of medical practice. Indeed in some clinics the consultant will not see the patient before certain baseline

Table 10.4 Risk management in medical out-patients – reducing diagnostic error[27]

Potential errors	Possible avoidance of error
Failure to take a well-focussed case history	Concentrate on key elements in case history Better training
Failure to assess the evidence and make a differential diagnosis	Write down conclusions before making a plan Beware labelling an illness as psychological without excluding organic pathology
Inappropriate use of tests	Define specific questions to be answered by chosen tests With invasive tests consider risk:benefit ratios
Dismissing episodic disease – inappropriate discharge of patient from care	Arrange to assess the patient when symptomatic
Leaving the problem unexplained	Get a second opinion

investigations have been performed (e.g. blood count, ECG and chest radiograph in a cardiological clinic). Undoubtedly this sort of practice improves efficiency if one judges efficiency by the number of patients processed. But it is a practice that inhibits the thought processes and does not encourage good medical practice.[9]

The risks of misinterpreting tests have been analysed in Emergency Departments. For example most SHOs learn about ECGs from a simple manual and from listening to the opinions of more senior staff. Some may spend six months working with a cardiologist and become reasonably experienced but very few are tested formally. In an interesting study it has been shown that the number of serious errors made by senior house officers in interpreting ECGs was more than 10%. This could be reduced to less than 5% if the tracings were also read and reported by the cardiac technician at the time of recording.[41]

Similarly errors in the reading of emergency radiographs of acutely ill patients has not been adequately assessed. We know that casualty officers often make errors in reading films showing bone and joint injuries. In one study the overall error rate was around 2% of all films but more than 90% of films show no abnormality. Of those films showing an abnormality the error rate exceeded a third.[42] In acute general medicine a critical decision is often made on the basis of the appearance of a straight film of the chest or abdomen. Serious errors undoubtedly occur[/] and it is likely that such errors would be considerably reduced if the admitting clinician could discuss the clinical and radiological findings with an experienced "on call" radiologist.[40] The extent to which this would be cost-effective should be examined.[43]

It is also necessary to recognise the risks associated with an over-dependence on investigation as described in example 7. In this case the patient's disease (in the true sense of the word) could have been well-managed with minimal investigation but the specialist was determined to find organic pathology. As a result the patient was seriously and

Table 10.5 Reducing the risks of investigation

Error	Means of reducing the risk
Clinician misreads visual evidence e.g. *x* ray; ECG	Fully trained staff (not necessarily clinicians) to interpret and report on tests Doctors to interpret results of tests in the light of the clinical situation (especially for radiographs, scanning procedures and electrical traces for example ECG, EMG, EEG)
Clinician not aware of lab results	Clinically important results to be relayed to clinician urgently At weekends all reported results to be checked by clinicians
Clinician not aware of ward observation	Ward tests to be supervised and results discussed with clinicians for example TPR charts; urine tests; fluid balance charts; weights
Clinician fails to understand test result	Junior staff to be aware of the limits of their competence More senior staff to check repeatedly
Inappropriate use of tests	Careful supervision by senior staff Economic use of resources

irrevocably harmed. In reviewing this case a very experienced gastroenterologist thought that the management was "perfectly reasonable". This is a worrying feature of modern medical practice in which specialists work as technicians rather than as doctors.[44]

Reducing the risks of invasive procedures

When considering an invasive procedure that carries a significant risk the clinician should consider alternative means of management.

Reducing risks in association with interventional procedures

- Consider carefully the risk: benefit ratio.
- Discuss the procedure with the patient – its advantages, alternatives and risks. And whenever possible give the patient time to contemplate and ask questions.
- Allow sufficient time for carrying out the procedure including coping with potential difficulties.
- Ensure that the equipment is in good working order and that back-up equipment is available.
- If the procedure is not going well obtain help if possible. Otherwise be prepared to give up.
- Ensure that the operator has sufficient skill (especially important with the introduction of new techniques and working with trainees).
- When necessary ensure that the patient is adequately and safely sedated.[28]

Obtaining properly informed consent acts as an important safeguard. It is now impossible to escape the implications of informed consent in an increasing range of clinical endeavour from using patients in teaching to undertaking human research. It includes agreeing all invasive procedures and associated problems in anaesthesia, the use of drugs and blood transfusion, the order "not to resuscitate", medical interventions (or cessation of interventions) which may speed death, organ donation, screening for disease, and genetic testing. Informed consent is not about listing the risks, it does not mean that the patient should be provided with a comprehensive digest of information, nor does it mean that patients should be given information whether they want to hear it or not. A medical specialist should be first and foremost a physician who is there to advise his patients. And he should strive to give the impression that he has time to talk. Advising patients about options is much more important than obtaining a signature on a form.[45]

Reducing the risks of drug treatment

External retrospective review of case records provides a method of assessing drug-related adverse events (AE) but will miss most administration errors. The authors of the Harvard study showed that drugs were responsible for 14% AE.[10] Subsequently they sought to reduce risks by using computer physician order entry (POE) systems and team-based intervention directed by pharmacists. The POE system provided clinicians with a menu of medications and ranges of potential doses (with default values). Reminders to check drug levels, to consider drug allergies and to note potential drug–drug interactions appeared on the screen when appropriate. For some medications relevant laboratory results were displayed automatically (for example serum potassium when prescribing frusemide). POE decreased serious medication errors from 10·7 to 4·9 events per 1000 patient-days. Team intervention did not provide additional benefit[46] A less ambitious computer prescribing system to reduce the risks of drug treatment was used in Phoenix, Arizona. It was designed to recognise 37 potential drug-specific AE. Alerts were triggered at a rate of 64 per 1000 admissions. It was shown that 44% of potential drug-specific AE would have gone unrecognised by the prescribing clinicians.[37]

Critical incident reporting may be used to determine the incidence and consequences of medication errors. One such study on a paediatric unit in Cardiff [47] showed that incidents were most likely to be reported by nurses (61%) with pharmacists reporting 33%, and clinicians only 4%. There were 83 reported errors per 1000 in-patient days with errors seven times more likely in an intensive care setting. Two-thirds of errors were detected before the drugs were given. Twenty-four serious medication errors were not detected in advance (4·5 per 100 in-patient days) but only 4 had overt clinical consequences that in one case required specific treatment. The authors concluded that a non-punitive, multi-disciplinary approach to medication errors highlighted sources of recurrent error and led to improvements in drug policies and staff training. However the effects of intervention were not quantified.

The cause of prescribing errors and how these may be avoided in general terms was described in the first edition of this book.[27] More recent studies have provided more specific data. In a study from Albany, NY[48] over 2000 drug errors were identified in a year-long study (3·99 per 1000 medication orders). A third of these had the potential to cause AE. The most common specific factors are shown below.

Common specific factors associated with drug adverse events[48]

- Failure to take account of declining renal/hepatic function
- Failure to check for possible allergic responses
- Using the wrong drug name or means of administration
- Miscalculation of dosage
- Prescribing an unusual critical frequency of dose

It was suggested that risk management strategies should be concentrated on how to reduce such errors. It would seem that this is an area in which information technology can play a key role.[49,50]

Reducing the risks of ward care (management)

Most adverse events in ward care stem from inadequate supervision, poor teamwork and defective or incomplete case records. By reading the case notes, an experienced clinician should be able to construct a reasonably detailed and accurate history of the patient's illness, its progress, and the thought processes of the carers. This is probably the most effective way of assessing the work of junior staff and the efficacy of the ward team. It should be a routine part of the work of consultants.[51] Organisational risks are summarised in Table 10.6. Critical incident reporting is the most effective way of determining the nature of adverse events and analysing the causes. Regrettably this seems to be rarely undertaken in the practice of general medicine.

Reducing the risks of discharge back to community care

Good practice requires that patients are carefully assessed both with respect to their clinical condition and the appropriateness of therapy at

Table 10.6 Reducing the risks of ongoing ward care

Organisational risks	Means of minimising risks
Failure to monitor clinical progress adequately	Joint education of house officer, nurses, and other professional carers regarding appropriate monitoring (NB value of integrated note-keeping); recognising actual and potential problems; taking appropriate action
Failure to recognise that a patient is not making satisfactory progress	Regular supervision by experienced staff (for example consultants/specialist registrars; senior nurses)
Failure to provide appropriate and/or adequate treatment	As above plus the use of specialist staff – for example clinicians from appropriate units; nurse specialists; physiotherapists; occupational therapists and ward pharmacists
Shift working	Adequate handover both oral and written Senior staff to keep in touch regarding the care of patients at risk

the time of discharge and for the immediate future. GPs should be provided with a thoughtful summary not only of the consequences of the illness that led to the admission to hospital but also of the specialist's recommendations for future care. In addition the list of active problems at the front of the case notes should be updated (regrettably any such list seems to be a rarity in NHS records). As with the assessment of case notes in monitoring standards of ward management, repeated audit of summaries of patients' conditions and plans for their future care should be part of routine medical practice. In an ideal world this might best be done as a part of a weekly ward meeting of professional carers.

Conclusion

In writing this chapter I have attempted to identify the more important risks to patients in hospital for the management of a medical disorder. Most of the patients are elderly and so are more vulnerable than the general population. Complaints regarding the quality of medical care usually centre around delays in admission to a ward and insufficient nursing attention after admission. But the problems are much deeper than insufficient beds and too few nurses. Much could be done by managers paying closer attention to the quality of overall care. Unfortunately recent changes in the training of hospital doctors, through specialist registrar programmes, have diminished the length of general training for trainees after their house jobs. Moreover restriction in the working hours of hospital doctors (and nurses) has fragmented the clinical care of patients. It seems likely that the developing generation of hospital clinicians will be very good specialists, well-trained in using "high-tech" equipment but will have less interest in how best to provide optimal care for the "whole" patient. This may have important implications in the future for clinical risk management in general medicine.

References

1 Chantler C. The role and education of doctors in the delivery of healthcare. Hollister Lecture delivered at the Institute of Health Services Research, Northwestern University, Illinois, USA. October 1998. *Lancet* 1999;**353**:1178–81.
2 Department of Health. *Medical audit in the hospital and community services*. London: HMSO 1991. (HC 91(2).)
3 Lindgren O, Secker-Walker J. Incident reporting systems: early warnings for the prevention and control of clinical negligence. In: Vincent C, ed. *Clinical risk management*. London: BMJ Books 1995: 375–90.
4 Department of Health. *Report on confidential enquiries into maternal health in the United Kingdom*. London: HMSO 1994.
5 Department of Health. *Confidential enquiry into stillbirths and deaths in infancy (CESDI)* London: Department of Health, 1995.
6 Lunn JN. The National Confidential Enquiry into Peri-operative Deaths. *J Clin Monit* 1994;**10**:426–8.
7 Neale G. Risk management in the care of medical emergencies after referral to hospital. *J R Coll Physicians Lond* 1998;**32**:125–9.
8 Woloshynowych M, Neale G. Unpublished observations.
9 Hampton JR, Harrison MJ, Mitchell JR, *et al.* Relative contributions of history-taking, physical examination and laboratory investigation to diagnosis and management of medical outpatients. *BMJ* 1975;**270**:486–9.
10 Leape L, Brennan TA, Laird N, *et al.* The nature of adverse events in hospitalized patients. Results of the Harvard Medical Practice Study II. *N Engl J Med* 1991;**324**:377–84.
11 Runciman WB, Sellen A, Webb RK, *et al.* The Australian incident monitoring study. Errors, incidents and accidents in anaesthetic practice. *Anaesth Intens Care* 1993;**21**:506–19.
12 Beckman U, Baldwin I, Hart GK, *et al.* The Australian Incident Monitoring Study in Intensive Care: AIMS-ICU. The development and evaluation of a voluntary anonymous incident reporting system. *Anesth Intens Care* 1996;**24**:315–26.
13 Department of Health. *Working for patients*. London: Department of Health, 1989.
14 Earnshaw JH. Auditing audit: the cost of the emperor's new clothes. *Br J Hosp Med* 1997;**58**:189–92.
15 Hopkins A. Medical audit: a second report. A comment on the report. *J Roy Coll Phys (Lond)* 1993;**27**:131–1.
16 Miles A, Bentley P, Polychronis A, *et al.* Clinical audit in the National Health system: fact or fiction? *J Eval Clin Prac* 1996;**2**:29–35.
17 Lord J, Littlejohns P. Evaluating healthcare policies: the case of clinical audit. *BMJ* 1997;**315**:668–71.
18 Williams O. What is clinical audit? *Ann R Coll Surg Engl* 1996;**78**:406–11.
19 McIntyre N, Popper K. The critical attitude in medicine: the need for a new ethics *BMJ* 1983;**287**:1919–23.
20 Neale G. We should look at complaints again. *BMJ* 1997;**315**:434–5.
21 Editorial. The autopsy in the 1990s. *Br J Hosp Med* 1998;**58**:544–5.
22 McPhee SJ. Maximizing the benefits of autopsy for clinicians and families. What needs to be done. *Arch Path Lab Med* 1996;**120**:743–8.
23 Lundberg GD. Low-tech autopsies in the era of high-tech medicine: continued value for quality assurance and patient safety. *JAMA* 1998;**280**:1273–4.
24 Zaitoun AM, Fernandez C. The value of histological examination in the audit of hospital autopsies: a quantitative approach. *Pathology* 1998;**30**:100–4.

25 Neale G. Reducing risks in medical practice. In Vincent CA, ed. *Clinical risk management.* London: *BMJ Publishing Group*, 1995: 253–73.

26 Neale G. Reducing risks in gastro-enterological practice. *Gut* 1998;**42**:139–42.

27 Ferriman A. UK considers logging adverse incidents. *BMJ* 1999;**319**:212.

28 Quine MA, Bell GD, McCloy RF, *et al.* Prospective audit of upper gastro-intestinal endoscopy in two regions of England: safety, staffing and sedation methods. *Gut* 1995;**36**:462–7.

29 Brook RH, Berg MH, Schechter PA. Effectiveness of non-emergency care via an emergency room. *Ann Intern Med* 1973;**78**:333–9.

30 Andrews LB, Stocking C, Krizek T, *et al.* M. An alternative strategy for studying adverse events in medical care. *Lancet* 1997;**349**:309–13.

31 Steel K, Gertmann PM, Crescinzi C, Anderson J. Iatrogenic illness on a general medical service at a university hospital. *New Engl J Med* 1981;**304**:638–42.

32 Barker KN, McConnell WE. The problems of detecting medication errors in hospitals. *Amer J Hosp Pharm* 1962;**19**:360–9.

33 Barker KN, Heller WM, Brennan JJ. The development of a centralized unit dose dispensing system: Part six: The pilot study – medication errors and drug losses. *Amer J Hosp Pharm* 1964;**21**:609–25.

34 Barker KN. The effects of an experimental medication system on medication errors and costs: I. Introduction and errors study. *Amer J Hosp Pharm* 1969;**26**:324–33.

35 DHSS. *Central Health Services Council report of the joint sub-committee on measures for controlling drugs on the wards* (The Gilles Report) IIM(70)36. London: DHSS, 1970.

36 Ridge KW, Jenkins DB, Barber ND, Noyce PR. Medicines resource during hospital drug rounds. *Qual Health Care* 1995;**4**:240–3.

37 Dean BS, Allan EL, Barber ND, Barker KN. Comparison of medication errors in an American and a British hospital. *Amer J Health-System Pharm* 1995;**52**:2543–9.

38 Jenkins DB. *The evaluation of an automated drug distribution system using a health technology assessment approach.* PhD thesis, University of London, 1997.

39 Houghton A, Hopkins A. Acute medical admissions: results of a national audit. *J R Coll Physicians* 1996;**30**:551–9.

40 Espinosa JA, Nolan TW. Reducing errors made by emergency physicians in interpreting radiographs: longitudinal study. *BMJ* 2000;**320**:737–40.

41 Dudley M, Channer KS. Assessment of the value of technician reporting of electrocardiographs in an accident and emergency department. *J Accid Em Med* 1997;**14**:307–10.

42 Vincent CA, Driscoll PA, Audley RJ, Grant DS. Accuracy of detection of radiographic abnormalities by junior doctors. *Arch Em Med* 1988;**5**:101–9.

43 Lufkin KC, Smith SW, Matticks CA, Brunette DD. Radiologists' review of radiographs interpreted confidently by emergency physicians infrequently lead to changes in patient management. *Ann Emerg Med* 1998;**31**:202–7.

44 Booth CC. What has technology done to gastroenterology? *Gut* 1985;**26**:1088–94.

45 Neale G. Informed consent. *Gut* 2000;**46**:5–6.

46 Bates DW, Leape LL, Cullen DJ, *et al.* Effects of computerised order entry and a team intervention on prevention of serious medication errors. *JAMA* 1998;**280**:1311–16.

47 Wilson DG, McArtney RG, Newcombe RG, *et al.* Medication errors in paediatric practice: insights from a continuous improvement quality approach. *Eur J Pediat* 1998;**157**:769–74.

48 Lesar TS, Briceland L, Stein DS. Factors related to errors in medication prescribing. *JAMA* 1997;**277**:312–17.

49 Nightingale PG, Adu D, Richards ND, Peters M. Implementation of rules-based computerised bedside prescribing and administration: intervention study. *BMJ* 2000;**320**:750–3.

50 Bates DW. Using information technology to reduce rates of medication errors in hospitals. *BMJ* 2000;**320**:788–91.

51 McIntyre N. Evaluation in clinical practice: problems, precedents and principles. *J Eval Clin Pract* 1995;**1**:5–13.

11 Risk management in clinical oncology

GARETH REES

The practice of clinical oncology involves:

- giving opinions on the overall management of patients with cancer
- initiating and supervising non-surgical treatment with radiotherapy or drugs, with the aim of shrinking or eradicating cancers
- giving advice on the management of symptoms in ways other than those involving anti-cancer therapy, for example recommending other treatments to relieve or alleviate pain, nausea or depression. Anti-cancer therapy is not always successful or quick in relieving symptoms and for some patients it may not even be appropriate. A clinical oncologist should always endeavour to consider the whole patient, not just the cancer
- following up patients who have had treatment, with the aim of discovering any recurrent cancer at an early and treatable stage, dealing with any side effects of treatment, and providing reassurance

This chapter is concerned with the management of risks arising from radiotherapy and chemotherapy. As far as adverse outcomes are concerned, the main risks are unacceptable toxicity and an unacceptable failure to achieve benefit, particularly cure.

There are very many possible causes of these, but the chapter concentrates on those that are more important or common. A broad view is taken, in the belief that risk management is concerned not merely with obvious errors, but with improvement in the overall quality of care. Thus some discussion of aspects of clinical decision making is included: the scope for acceptable variation in clinical judgement has been reduced substantially in recent years.

197

Damage to normal tissues is as inevitable with radiotherapy and chemotherapy as it is with surgery. Thus side effects are apparent in the great majority of patients. In some circumstances they are minimal, but in others they can be severe and even fatal.

How radiotherapy and chemotherapy work

Both radiotherapy and chemotherapy work by damaging crucial structures in the nuclei of cancer cells. This results in loss or impairment of the ability of the cancer cells to divide. Cancer cells die naturally of old age. A cancer grows by virtue of its cells dividing to produce new cells more rapidly than the loss of cells from old age. Thus if cellular multiplication is inhibited a cancer will shrink. If the multiplication is inhibited sufficiently and over a long enough period, a cancer will be destroyed completely. However, cancer cells are often only slightly more susceptible to the effects of radiotherapy and chemotherapy than normal cells.

Radiotherapy involves beams of radiation, usually high energy x rays, being focused on a tumour. Radiotherapy is thus a localised treatment. If it is able to destroy a cancer completely and that cancer has not spread elsewhere via the blood stream or lymphatic vessels, then the patient will be cured.

For the treatment beams to get to the tumour they have to pass through normal tissue. If three or four beams are focused on a tumour from different angles it is possible to give the tumour a considerably higher dose than the surrounding normal tissues. If the aim is cure, it is important that a rim of apparently normal tissue immediately surrounding the tumour also receives a high dose because of the chance that it has been invaded microscopically by the cancer cells. The side effects seen with radiotherapy tend to be dominated by those resulting from damage to the normal tissues in close proximity to the tumour.

Chemotherapy, being a drug treatment, inevitably has effects on virtually the whole of the body. The drugs are usually administered by injection into a vein and they are then carried around the body by the blood stream. Chemotherapy thus tends to have more generalised side effects than radiotherapy.

Balancing the effects of treatment on cancer and host

In theory, all cancers could be destroyed by radiotherapy or chemotherapy if given in sufficiently high dosage. In practice this is not possible because exposing all the cancer cells present to sufficient dosages of radiotherapy or chemotherapy to destroy them would result in very many patients experiencing inevitably fatal damage to normal tissues.

Fundamental to the practice of clinical oncology is weighing up the likely effects of treatment against the cancer, and on the normal tissues, and arriving at a reasonable compromise which is believed to represent the right balance for a particular patient with a particular type and extent of cancer. The concept of the "therapeutic ratio" – the risk of damage to tumour cells versus that of damage to normal cells is enshrined within clinical oncology training and practice.

Deciding on treatment intent

If it is deemed that a cancer is incurable then the main aim of treatment will be to relieve symptoms and possibly achieve some prolongation of life. In these circumstances there is no point in replacing the symptoms of the disease by equally troublesome or even worse symptoms due to the effects of treatment on normal tissues. Thus "palliative" radiotherapy or chemotherapy is almost always less intensive and toxic than treatment aimed at achieving a cure.

If cure seems feasible it is usually felt that a higher risk of troublesome side effects is justified. Thus the intensity of potentially curative or "radical" treatment often leads to unpleasant symptoms, at least in the short term. Even very aggressive and highly unpleasant treatments will be accepted by most patients if they offer the only chance of restoring them to normal life expectancy. However, some older and frailer patients and those with other significant medical problems may be less able to cope with the effects of such treatments. It is sometimes appropriate to lessen somewhat the intensity of treatment, accepting that there will be a reduced chance of cure.

As well as palliative and radical treatments there is another treatment category. "Adjuvant" treatment is given in addition to the main treatment with the aim of increasing the chance of cure. This commonly involves giving radiotherapy or chemotherapy to try to destroy any residual microscopic traces of cancer that may have been left behind after surgery.

For example, both radiotherapy and chemotherapy given after surgery for breast cancer have been shown to improve the chance of cure. Similarly, a short course of radiotherapy prior to surgery for rectal cancer, and additional chemotherapy given during a course of radiotherapy for oesophageal cancer, have both been shown to improve the chance of cure.

Inevitability of side effects

It is usually accepted that some patients will get serious side effects from treatment, particularly treatment given with curative intent. If at least a small percentage of patients are not getting troublesome side effects, then as a group they are probably not receiving treatment that is sufficiently intensive to give them the best chance of cure. This acceptance of the inevitability of some severe side effects and the close linkage between the chance of side effects and the chance of success to a large extent sets clinical oncology apart from other specialties. The relationship between radiation dose and the chances of cure and serious side effects can be represented graphically (Figure 11.1).

Thus, at dose level A, for approximately a 70% chance of cure there is a 5% chance of severe side effects. However, if the dose is increased to level B the chance of cure rises to almost 90%, but the chance of a major complication rises proportionately greater to 30%. The graphs also show that the chances of both cure and side effects can be altered significantly by quite small changes in dose – the dose/effect curve is very steep in the dose range used in routine clinical practice.

Side effects occur both during and after treatment with radiotherapy and chemotherapy. Short term or "acute" side effects come on during or very shortly after treatment and last usually for a few days or a couple of weeks. Long term or "chronic" side effects are more common with radiotherapy than chemotherapy. They usually become manifest some time after treatment, sometimes only after many years.[1] It is these long-lasting, usually irreversible and sometimes slowly progressive effects which are likely to give rise to serious morbidity, complaints and litigation. However, the number of patients experiencing severe long-term side effects from radio-

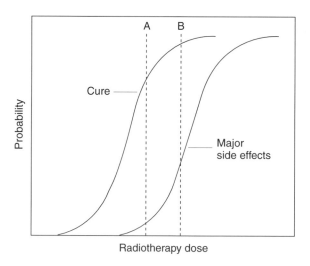

Figure 11.1 Relationship between radiation dose and chances of cure and side effects.

therapy is very small, especially bearing in mind that between 1990 and 2000 well over a million people received radiotherapy in the United Kingdom.[2]

In clinical oncology the famous aphorism *"Primum Non Nocere"* ("Above all do no harm") is particularly inappropriate. It is unusual to achieve benefit from anti-cancer treatment without some treatment toxicity. Indeed it is common for treatments to be given (and willingly accepted) when there is a probability that they will do more harm than good. Patients in serious and desperate situations will frequently find this type of risk acceptable, given the circumstances.[3]

Why complaints and litigation are rising

Approximately one in three people can expect to get cancer at some time during their lives. Overall, perhaps about 40% of cancer patients are cured. But many that are not cured can have their disease kept under control for long periods, often many years. Approximately 1 in 25 people have had treatment for cancer and many of these are in long-term remission or have been cured.

The converse, however, is that perhaps 60% of patients who develop cancer will eventually die from it. This combination of high mortality and almost inevitable treatment toxicity has implications for both complaints and litigation. Historically, patients have been so grateful to be alive that they have as a rule not been minded to complain, even when this would have been justifiable. Also, a significant proportion of patients who might have complained or resorted to litigation are unable to do so because they are dead.

However, the situation is changing. Anti-cancer treatments are becoming more successful and they are being given increasingly to patients who have good chances of long term survival, particularly adjuvant treatments. There are thus increasing numbers of long term survivors following anti-cancer treatment with radiotherapy and/or chemotherapy. The expectations of cancer patients have risen also. This, together with a general attitudinal change, is resulting in a considerable increase in the number of patients who are now prepared to consider complaint or litigation.

Delay in diagnosis is the commonest cause of litigation by cancer patients, but this concerns usually the quality of care offered by general practitioners or hospital specialists in medicine, surgery and diagnostic radiology. Almost all patients seen by clinical oncologists already have a diagnosis of cancer. Of these, those most likely to complain or litigate are those with long term side effects of treatment.

Types of risk

The main areas of risk are as follows:

1 **Incorrect diagnosis**, resulting in:

- anti-cancer treatment being given for a patient who does not have the disease
- anti-cancer treatment being given for a non-cancerous development in someone who has had cancer in the past
- treatment being given for the wrong type of cancer

2 **Treatment toxicity**, arising in:

- a patient who has been treated competently but who was not warned of the risk
- a patient who has been given treatment thought to be competent, but later found to be unsafe
- a patient who has been treated incompetently

3 **Inadequate treatment**, resulting in failure to cure or a reduced chance of cure.

These are the main possible adverse outcomes that would be of concern to patients. This chapter thus deals with various aspects of risk management under these headings. Some of the causes and strategies discussed will of course have a wider relevance than merely to the particular risk category in which they are included.

The practice of clinical oncology differs substantially from other areas of medicine in a further respect. Almost all treatment is administered not by doctors but by specially trained paramedical staff. The administration of radiotherapy and chemotherapy is a multidisciplinary exercise. Radiotherapy machines are operated by radiographers. Checking that the machines are operating correctly is the job of physicists. Most chemotherapy is now administered by specially trained nurses.

Incorrect diagnosis

Anti-cancer treatment given for a patient who does not have the disease

It is a fundamental rule of oncological practice that treatment should not proceed unless the diagnosis of cancer has been confirmed by examination of a specimen of tissue or fluid under the microscope by a pathologist, except under certain compelling circumstances. This is known as establishing a "tissue diagnosis".

There are occasions when a patient presents with an overall clinical picture for which the overwhelmingly most likely explanation is cancer and which is sufficiently serious to demand urgent treatment, when obtaining a tissue diagnosis is either not feasible or would involve an unacceptable delay. This can happen, for example, when lung cancer spreads to lymph glands in the centre of the chest causing obstruction to the veins and a potentially very unpleasant engorgement and swelling of the head and arms. It is often thought reasonable to proceed promptly with palliative radiotherapy in such circumstances.

It is of course important to explain and document the circumstances thoroughly and it should be made particularly clear in the notes that there has not been a tissue diagnosis. This may be relevant should the subsequent course be atypical for cancer. Very infrequently there can be "benign" causes for such obstruction, such as an enlarged extension of the thyroid gland from the neck to a position behind the breast bone, or a massive distension or aneurysm of the aorta, the main blood level leaving the heart.

Clinical oncologists are well aware of the potential pitfalls of proceeding to treat without a tissue diagnosis. In addition, it is very unusual for a pathologist to make an erroneous unequivocal diagnosis of cancer. Thus in practice, treating someone for cancer when they do not in fact have the disease is extremely rare. Nevertheless, continued vigilance is most important and it is a good rule for departments to demand that treatment should not proceed unless there is a copy of the original pathology report confirming the diagnosis in the oncology notes, except under certain fully explained and documented circumstances.

A significant proportion of those patients treated in the past for cancer and who were considered to have done "miraculously" well after treatment (or even no treatment) when deemed to have had virtually no chance of achieving a cure, never had a tissue diagnosis. Probably most of these patients never had cancer.

Anti-cancer treatment given for a non-cancerous development in someone who has had cancer in the past

This is a more frequent occurrence. The most common circumstance is when a patient who has had treatment for cancer in the past is thought erroneously to have developed a secondary cancer or "metastasis" as a result of spread of cells from the original cancer to another part of the body via the blood stream.

A variety of other conditions can mimic secondary spread, particularly a solitary metastasis. For example, an infection can mimic a metastasis in bone, a benign cyst can mimic a metastasis in the liver, and an area of inflammation can look just like a secondary growth in the lung on a scan or radiograph. An incorrect diagnosis of secondary spread can lead to potentially disastrous consequences, both physical and psychological. It can set in train totally inappropriate treatment, sometimes over several years, and during this time patients live with the immense mental burden of believing they have incurable disease which will kill them sooner or later.

Example 1

A private patient being followed up after surgery for breast cancer complained of arm pain. Although a bone scan was not reported as showing a metastasis the clinician in charge concluded that this was nevertheless the most likely explanation and arranged a course of radiotherapy intended to provide pain relief. Admittedly bone scans can give false negative results but the clinician failed to keep in mind, and to document, the fact that metastatic disease had not been confirmed beyond all reasonable doubt. When the patient subsequently developed back pains these too were assumed to be due to metastatic cancer and she received further courses of radiotherapy.

Over several years the patient not only received a considerable amount of radiotherapy to her back, but a variety of drug treatments, one of which led to a perforated duodenal ulcer and several weeks in intensive care. Only when the patient moved to another part of the country was it suspected that she had never had metastatic disease and that the problems in her bones had been due not to cancer but to degenerative weakening or osteoporosis. The radiotherapy had contributed to this process and the effect on the spine was to contribute to the loss of some inches in height and curvature.

This case shows also the potential danger that can arise when the specialist care of a patient is managed entirely by a single doctor who fails to question subsequently an initial assumption. The almost inevitable involvement of other medical staff in care and follow up in the National Health Service setting can help to prevent this type of mismanagement. The best protection against such a mistake is clinical competence and vigilance.

Clinicians should be particularly suspicious about diagnosing a solitary metastasis without confirmation by biopsy. If a decision to treat is made despite some doubt, sometimes because of apparent clinical urgency, then there should be good documentation of the circumstances to serve as a reminder to both the clinician concerned and to any others involved in future care. If the subsequent course is not typical for someone with secondary cancer this should prompt re-evaluation of the diagnosis. Without such documentation it is quite likely that a diagnosis of metastatic disease will be assumed subsequently by the same doctor and by others.

Treatment given for the wrong type of cancer

Different types of cancer are managed in very different ways and have very different prognoses. There have been considerable refinements in recent years in laboratory techniques and these have assisted pathologists greatly in making a precise diagnosis. Difficulties can still arise however in the precise classification of some tumours. Sometimes further laboratory investigation causes an initial diagnosis to be revised. If this happens it is vital that this information is passed on to whoever is responsible for the treatment. Diagnosing the wrong type of cancer is sometimes of little practical importance but on other occasions it can have major implications for management and prognosis. Fortunately it is very rare.

Example 2

A man in his sixties was discovered to have a growth in the space behind his nose. A biopsy from this was reported as showing a "nasopharyngeal carcinoma". He was told there was a very slim chance of cure but that this would be attempted with a course of radiotherapy which would be very unpleasant and which would last several weeks. The radiotherapy was given and seemed to be successful, but much later in the year the patient developed cancerous glands in a groin and an enlarged spleen. This would be most unusual for nasopharyngeal carcinoma.

It was decided to request a review of the original laboratory diagnosis and it was then discovered that this had been revised after only a short while, following further tests on the biopsy specimen. The correct diagnosis was "non-Hodgkin's lymphoma" – which can look very similar to nasopharyngeal carcinoma down the microscope. For some reason this had not been communicated to the cancer centre from the other hospital where the biopsy had been taken and analysed. The patient was cured eventually with the chemotherapy he should have received initially, but he experienced quite serious long-term side effects from the intensive radiotherapy which he should never have had, such as a dry mouth, cataracts and impaired hearing.

The original erroneous diagnosis had been communicated by word of mouth, with no indication that further tests were in progress. The later typewritten report from the pathology department gave the correct diagnosis of non-Hodgkin's lymphoma. The patient would not have been incorrectly treated had treatment been put on hold until a copy of the report was available. This might have been overlooked because of the wish to get treatment underway as quickly as possible, in view of the seriousness of the situation.

This case illustrates the importance of very good communication: the care of cancer patients very often involves specialists of different disciplines who may be based in different hospitals many miles apart. It shows also how the pressure for very urgent treatment can lead to some aspects of quality control being overlooked.

The examples given should help to illustrate that the risks associated with cancer treatment are enhanced considerably if diagnostic services are not of a high quality. It is important that cancer centres are served by departments of pathology of sufficient size and with sufficient expertise to elucidate the more difficult areas of cancer pathology, and served also by departments of clinical radiology with access to the full range of modern diagnostic techniques and appropriate expertise.[2]

Treatment toxicity

Competent treatment, but not warned of risk

All patients should give their written consent prior to treatment with radiotherapy or chemotherapy. Consent must be obtained by the doctor responsible for the treatment, or a delegated person who is suitably trained and qualified and who has sufficient knowledge of the proposed treatment and understands the risks involved.[4]

Radical treatment can result in very severe side effects in a small minority of patients, and moderately severe side effects in a larger proportion, even though it is given entirely competently. For example, radical radiotherapy for carcinoma of the cervix carries an inevitable risk of significant bowel damage. Approximately 5% of patients will have sufficiently severe damage to require surgery, sometimes a permanent colostomy. Patients being offered radical radiotherapy for carcinoma of the cervix must be informed of this risk, even though it is low. For patients with relatively early cancers that might be amenable to alternative treatment with surgery, knowledge of this risk and other side effects might influence some to opt for a radical hysterectomy (with its own risks), rather than radiotherapy.

Radiotherapy given for some cancers at the back of the mouth will cause permanent mouth dryness if the treatment beams have to pass through both parotid salivary glands. This can lead to tooth and gum disease. It is obvious that such an inevitable complication must be discussed fully with the patient.

Chemotherapy usually affects the bone marrow and carries a risk of causing a fall in the white blood cell concentration sufficient to render a patient more susceptible to an infection and less able to fight it. If an infection occurs prompt intravenous antibiotic treatment is required to prevent serious illness and a risk of death. Patients must be warned of this and told to report any evidence of infection, particularly a fever, very promptly. It is essential that adequate facilities are available for dealing with such complications wherever chemotherapy is administered. This includes the provision of emergency beds, appropriately trained medical and nursing staff and a departmental protocol for investigation and treatment of infection.[5]

Chemotherapy given to young men with testicular cancer is now highly effective and the majority of even those with advanced disease can expect to be cured. However, the treatment carries a significant risk of damaging permanently the remaining testicle, resulting in infertility. A risk such as this must be explained to patients and if appropriate they should be offered sperm storage, which may offer them the chance of fathering a child in the future. Failure to mention such a risk and/or to offer sperm storage has resulted in justifiable complaints and litigation.

Discussion of the side effects of anti-cancer treatment has become much more thorough in recent years. It is often supplemented by written information. It can, however, be time consuming. Understandable anxiety about possible adverse consequences can lead some patients to ask many questions and to require repeated reassurance that the proposed treatment is, overall, in their best interest.

It is common for a clinical oncologist in the United Kingdom to be required to see five or more new patients and 15 or 20 for follow up in a single 3½-hour clinic. A couple of unanticipated prolonged discussions, combined with the almost inevitable other disruptions arising, for example, from other colleagues telephoning to ask opinions or to request an urgent appointment for their patients, can result in a clinic overrunning substantially, and long delays for anxious patients. The very large workload of British oncologists is a powerful incentive to keep discussion to a minimum. On occasions patients may not be informed of risks that they should know about. Attempting to see most new patients in under half an hour is likely to lead to an increased risk from lack of information, and error.[2]

Treatment thought to be competent, but later found unsafe

Patients may be treated in a way that is deemed to be competent at the time, but which is subsequently shown to have been unsafe. This was the case for some patients with breast cancer treated with radiotherapy, mainly during the 1980s, at a number of different cancer centres in the United Kingdom. These patients had surgery and radiotherapy for the primary breast cancer, but in addition underwent radiotherapy to the armpit and lower neck with the intention of eradicating any cancer cells that might have spread to the lymph nodes from the breast. This treatment has subsequently been proven to increase the chance of cure, but a very small percentage (probably less than 1%) of patients developed severe injury to the nerves supplying the arm, resulting in weakness or paralysis, and severe pain. This damage is called brachial plexus neuropathy and it was identified in 48 patients in an independent review.[6]

This was shown later to be due substantially to an unsafe radiotherapy technique. When the lymph nodes were treated the arm was in a different position from when the breast or underlying chest wall had been treated. Although the radiotherapy beams appeared to abut each other on the surface, the arm movement resulted in the skin having an altered relationship to the underlying tissues such that the radiotherapy beams were in fact overlapping at depth. This resulted in a small amount of deeper tissue receiving a much higher radiation dosage than intended, causing severe damage, particularly to the nerves. The demonstration that this particular technique of radiotherapy was largely responsible for the brachial plexus neuropathy has resulted in its abandonment. No change in arm position is now allowed between treatments to the two areas.

The radiation damage experienced by these breast cancer patients was largely responsible for the establishment of Radiation Action Group Exposure (RAGE), an organisation of patients who were injured, or believed that they had been injured, by radiotherapy. It also led to litigation, but when two cases came to trial no negligence was found because the treatment was of a standard recognised as proper by a reasonable and competent body of professional opinion at the time it was given.[7]

Incompetent treatment

This may arise as a result of medical incompetence or due to deficiencies in the performance of other staff, including nurses, radiographers and physicists. When mistakes occur in treatment this tends to be due to the failure of other staff to detect an initial error made by a single individual. Clinician errors are likely to be picked up and questioned by other members of the team, for example radiotherapy or chemotherapy dosages.

Radiotherapy in particular is a multidisciplinary activity. When errors occur in radiotherapy they are more likely to affect a group of patients rather than individuals. It is important to recognise the essential role of the radiation physicist in ensuring quality and safety in radiotherapy departments.

Radiotherapy has become more accurate as a result of improved radiological assessment, for example by CT and MRI scanning, leading to a more accurate indication of the exact size and extent of cancers. Improved accuracy is also a result of considerable refinements in computerised treatment planning, and delivery. In the past radiotherapy was planned in a single plane through the centre of the tissue to be treated and the treatment beams that converged on the tumour were always square or rectangular shaped, but now three-dimensional planning is routinely available in most departments. This enables the use of specially shaped treatment beams aimed both at adequately covering the tumour and minimising unnecessary treatment of adjacent normal tissues, not just in one plane but at several planes throughout the volume of tissue being treated.

There have been improvements also in the process of verification that the planned treatment is in fact being delivered accurately. It is now possible to produce images on the treatment machine of the exact volume of tissue being irradiated by each treatment beam, and these can be correlated with images of the intended treatment volume generated on the planning computer.

The scope for maverick clinical decision making has been reduced greatly by "site specialisation". The increasing complexity of clinical management made it impossible for individual clinicians to develop and maintain appropriate expertise in the management of more than a limited number of different types of cancer. Most oncologists now specialise in the care of patients whose cancers have developed from a limited number of different organs or sites. For example, one oncologist may care for patients with breast, bowel, and skin cancer while another may care for those with head and neck, prostate, and bladder cancer.

The delivery of competent, "state of the art" care has also been helped by the development through consensus of evidence based guidelines for the management of patients, particularly those with the more common tumours. Litigation risk is also reduced if consultants collectively agree common treatment techniques and dosages. Another closely related initiative has been the increased emphasis on multidisciplinary management – clinical decision making by teams composed of representatives from different disciplines, rather than by individual clinicians working in isolation.

The increased emphasis on a consultant provided service has reduced the chance of treatment errors arising from inexperience in junior medical staff. A greater percentage of patients now have a consultant closely involved in their care than in the past but this, together with the increased requirements for training their junior staff as opposed to relying on them for service delivery, has entailed a further rise in workload for consultants.

Junior staff are of course still involved in treatment delivery and must have "hands on" experience in order to become consultants themselves in future. It is important, however, that their level of input is appropriate to their stage in training and experience. One example of unacceptable toxicity, arising from a failure of supervision or proper training of junior staff, is incompetent injection of chemotherapy by a senior house officer or registrar. This can result in leakage of drug into the tissues outside the vein, causing potentially severe and permanent tissue damage. This can be very painful and the injury may require plastic surgery. It is a not uncommon cause of litigation in oncology.

Another example, fortunately very rare, is erroneous injection of a drug into the lower spine via lumbar puncture. Injection of small amounts of the drug methotrexate into the cerebro-spinal fluid bathing the spinal cord and brain is an important part of treatment for some types of leukaemia. Deaths have occurred as a result of injection of the wrong drug or the correct drug in too high dosage, and doctors have been charged with manslaughter.

There have also been occasions when radiotherapy has been prescribed inappropriately by a trainee with insufficient experience or knowledge for the particular clinical situation. It is perfectly appropriate for trainees with appropriate experience and training to prescribe some types of radiotherapy, but departments should specify who can provide what and in what circumstances.

Example 3

A trainee prescribed radiotherapy to the front of the chest wall in someone who had recurrent breast cancer. The trainee did not realise that treating such a large area with a beam of an energy sufficient to make it quite penetrating would result in a radiation dose to the lungs which they would not tolerate. Serious inflammation of the lungs occurred about six weeks later, from which the patient died.

Incompetent treatment can occur also as a result of avoidable errors made by physicists, radiographers or nurses. There have been two major radiotherapy incidents in the United Kingdom in recent years. These were systematic errors, affecting large numbers of patients, that are discussed in more detail later. Most radiation treatment incidents are caused by "one-off" errors. It is not uncommon for there to be a number of contributory factors involved in either causation or in failure of recognition or both. It is particularly important that checking is not regarded as a rubber stamping procedure. Those involved in checking should never assume that someone else's documentation or calculation is correct.

Example 4

> *A middle-aged man with an inoperable brain tumour was offered a course of radical radiotherapy. An error was made by a radiographer in transferring the treatment planning data from the physics department to the treatment sheet used by the radiographers. This resulted in an excessive amount of treatment being administered on one of two radiotherapy beams. Although the data was checked by another radiographer the error was not detected. Inappropriate belief that the procedures used were safe also resulted in a radiation dose measurement that indicated that an overdose was being administered, not being taken seriously. It was concluded that it was the radiation dose measurement equipment that was faulty. In this incident the lack of a departmental procedure for dealing with an unexplained abnormal radiation dose measurement, combined with a lack of vigilance, resulted in severe radiation brain damage.*

The establishment of routine systems for treatment incident reporting is invaluable in providing information for risk management. Most radiotherapy incidents are minor and have little or no adverse clinical consequences, but identifiable trends in the occurrence of errors can lead to the redesign of working practice and a reduction in the incident rate. In addition it has been shown that the use of computerised verification systems for linear accelerators are valuable in reducing risk. However, verification systems are not infallible and strict systems of work should be adhered to in the input and checking involved with radiotherapy prescription data.[8]

Inadequate or insufficient treatment

Insufficient treatment may occur as a result of a failure of quality control in treatment delivery or as a result of inappropriate clinical judgement. The consequences of an underdose in either radiotherapy or chemotherapy, particularly when treatment is being given with curative intent, are potentially every bit as serious as those of an overdose. There has been one major systematic radiation incident involving underdosage that will be discussed separately.

Consensus development and site specialisation have both had an important part to play in helping to ensure that clinical advice offers patients the best chance of cure or the optimum balance between the chance of cure and the risk of serious adverse effects. In recent decades treatments have generally become more intensive. A far greater proportion of patients with cancer are now offered adjuvant treatments, increasing toxicity but increasing also the chance of long-term success.

If there is any systematic tendency to treat any category insufficiently, then it must be older patients who, as a group, are at greatest risk of being offered insufficient treatment. Treatment recommendations for the elderly are subject to considerable variation despite clinical management guidelines. Individual clinician philosophy and assessment of how a given patient is likely to cope with treatment have a large influence on what is offered. The results of most trials indicating the value of certain treatments are based on results in otherwise fit often relatively young patients. Many trials exclude patients above a certain age or those with other significant illnesses. The extent to which the conclusions of such trials are relevant to individual elderly patients will always be a matter of individual clinical judgement, but there is now a trend towards realising that many patients above the age of 75 have a very reasonable life expectancy and will cope well with carefully planned, delivered and monitored treatment with either radiotherapy or drugs.

Cancer treatment is becoming less ageist, but some elderly patients are missing out on chances of cure that they would have been offered had they been seen by another clinician. Many are not being referred for an oncological opinion in the first place. Some would benefit from further and franker discussions in an environment where they feel free to ask why they are not being offered something else. Perhaps their general practitioners should be more questioning on their behalf. Perhaps oncological departments should create systems of routine discussion of those patients who have not been offered potentially curative treatment on the grounds of age or other illness.

Major radiotherapy incidents

There have been two major radiotherapy incidents in Britain. Both involved systematic errors in the dose delivered to large numbers of patients. In 1988 207 patients were overtreated by a factor of 25%. The direct cause of the accident was an error in measuring the dose of radiation emitted from a new installation of radioactive cobalt in a treatment machine at Exeter. The Report of the Committee of Enquiry criticised the Department of Physics in not having a clear written procedure for the calibration (measurement) of sources of irradiation.[9]

When nurses began to notice excessive radiation skin reactions some three or four months after the replacement cobalt had been installed, this did not lead to a sufficiently thorough investigation of the possibility that there had been an error in calibration. The Exeter incident was a catalyst for establishing a Department of Health Working Party on Quality

Assurance. The Working Party's report took the form of a Quality Standard and all radiotherapy centres in the United Kingdom are now required to have a comprehensive quality assurance system that conforms to the requirements laid down in the Standard.[10,11] It has been argued that had current quality assurance standards been operating in Exeter the accident would have been avoided.[12]

For example, the ISO 9000 Standard would have required a quality manual containing clear work instructions for source calibration using a dedicated log-book, with independent checks of the work. An appropriate complement of staff, detailing the number of people available for checking as well as simply carrying out the work, would also have been specified. If the error had still been made the corrective and preventive action required by ISO 9000 would have ensured a full investigation of the calibration at the first mention of the nurses' observations. The Report of the Committee of Enquiry also emphasised the inadequate staffing level in the physics department and recommended an additional consultant in clinical oncology, given the number of patients being treated in the department.

The second major systematic radiation incident was the accident at North Staffordshire Royal Infirmary, Stoke on Trent. During the period 1982–1991, 1045 patients were underdosed by up to 25%. This happened because the physicist responsible acquiesced with radiographers concerning a newly acquired computer treatment planning system. In their view this did not make allowances for the reduction in dose with increased distance of the part of the body being treated from the source of the radiation beam in the treatment machine. This view was wrong and the error resulted in the allowance being duplicated, which led to the underdosing of all patients treated in a particular way until the discovery of the error in 1991.[13]

It has been argued that modern quality assurance would have prevented this accident also. The physicist did not have supervisory authority over the production of treatment plans, which made it difficult to monitor the effects of advice given. ISO 9000 would have required that the physicist had supervisory authority over the processes for which she was responsible, and this one factor would have reduced the likelihood of the error being committed, and increased the chance of early detection in the event that it might still have been committed. Other requirements of ISO 9000, such as the need to write down the advice given to the radiographers and to have it checked would similarly have reduced the possibility of the accident.[12]

The report of the independent enquiry concluded that the department had been operating with less physics staff, clinical oncologists and radiographers than recommended by the Institute of Physical Sciences in Medicine, the Royal College of Radiologists and the College of Radiographers.

Important requirements for safe and effective treatment

Non-surgical cancer treatment has become vastly more complicated in recent years. Planning, delivering, and monitoring optimal treatment are all much more time consuming than in the past. Treatment safety also depends crucially on there being sufficient time and on proper checking. Several components necessary to ensure a high quality service have already been mentioned, but this section discusses further some of the more important requirements.

Site specialisation and the consensus development of clinical practice guidelines have already been mentioned briefly. Advances in clinical and laboratory research have led to a staggering increase in new knowledge about the nature of cancer and how best to treat it. Only 15 years ago a clinical oncologist would have been expected to arrange treatment for patients with most types of cancer, but this is now considered unacceptable. It is impossible for a single oncologist to remain competent and up to date with the management of more than a very limited range of cancers. Site specialisation has undoubtedly resulted in a considerable reduction in the risk of incompetent medical management. Those providing care must be suitably qualified or trained in the relevant areas of clinical practice. Clinical oncologists should not normally offer care outside their subspecialty competence, except in unavoidable circumstances.[4]

Clinical oncologists should strive to establish uniform departmental treatment policies for patients with defined types and stages of cancer. Most if not all departments will by now have developed or adopted such guidelines. Keeping treatment variation to a minimum reduces the risk of error and facilitates the maintenance of high standards through audit of both process and outcome.[4]

The importance also of continuing professional development (CPD), continuing medical education (CME), and regular participation in audit in maintaining good practice cannot be overstated. The Royal College of Radiologists requires that clinical oncologists obtain 250 CME credits over a five-year period.[4] Risks occur when clinicians fail to keep abreast of new developments; when they retain an inappropriately broad spectrum of clinical work; if they advise on the management of cancers falling outside their own field of expertise – for example, when covering absent colleagues; or as a result of not taking sufficient care. Excessive patient workload is an important factor in any tendency to cut corners and to pay insufficient attention to detail.

Multidisciplinary management was strongly recommended in the Calman/Hine report on commissioning cancer services.[14] This involves consultants of the different disciplines involved in care, meeting regularly to discuss the diagnosis and management of individual patients. This creates extra demands on time and the logistic constraints are such that this is usually only feasible for patients with some of the more common cancers. As an example, weekly breast cancer multidisciplinary meetings are now held in almost all cancer centres and units. Those attending include oncologists, surgeons, radiologists, pathologists, breast care nurses and medical staff in training. Such meetings help further to ensure that clinical decision making for individual patients is entirely appropriate.

Radiotherapy should be initiated and clinically directed by doctors who are approved by their department as having the requisite competence for the particular clinical situation. Radical radiotherapy must be initiated and clinically directed by an accredited clinical oncologist and the planning and checking of treatment must conform to national and international recommendations.[4]

Ensuring the accuracy of radiotherapy is obviously vital, particularly given the potential for systematic errors to affect large numbers of patients. The need for radiotherapy departments to have a comprehensive quality assurance system has already been referred to. All cancer centres have regular checking programmes for treatment machines. Linear accelerators have their dose rate production and beam alignment checked daily. Regular safety checks are carried out on a weekly basis, and preventive maintenance servicing, monthly. Major dosimetry checking is carried out annually and centres are encouraged to establish mutual cross-checking of calibration and other physics data with other centres. There should also be a rolling programme of equipment replacement, and sufficient equipment to allow time for safety checks and preventive maintenance.[2] A centre serving a population of 1·25 million will require six linear accelerators.[15]

Radiotherapy departments must comply also with all current national radiation protection legislation and recommendations. The current Ionising Radiation Recommendations[16,17] and the associated Approved Code of Practice[18] provide a legal basis of safety standards to which all users of ionising radiation must conform. New regulations and a revised approved Code of Practice will come into force in the near future.[19]

Chemotherapy too must be initiated and supervised by clinicians who are appropriately accredited and experienced.[4] It is important also that all chemotherapy is undertaken in designated wards or outpatient clinics, staffed by clinical nurse specialists and medical staff with appropriate expertise.[5] Those giving the treatment must have undergone formal training in chemotherapy administration and they must be approved by their department as having the necessary competence.

Whenever possible chemotherapy should be administered in properly staffed units within normal working hours. There is evidence that the administration of chemotherapy outside normal working hours carries an increased risk, but the workload in many centres is so high that this increased risk becomes unavoidable. Finally, it is also important that chemotherapy regimens accord, whenever possible, to departmental protocol and that treatment is initiated and monitored by medical staff with appropriate training and expertise.

All common side effects should be discussed prior to treatment and also any potentially serious effects unless these are exceedingly rare. The nature and amount of information given remains a matter of clinical judgement, taking into account the clinical situation and the assessment of the individual patient. The need for written consent has already been mentioned.

Resources

Non-surgical cancer treatment is improving steadily as a result of laboratory and clinical research, greater uniformity of treatment, site specialisation and quality assurance. However, the numbers of patients being treated and the complexity and intensity of many treatments are also increasing. Very many patients do not receive state of the art treatment simply because it is impossible for this to be delivered safely by an oncological community that is the busiest in the western world.

For all the common cancers, British survival figures are well below the European average. If British survival figures could reach the average, 10 000 lives would be saved each year. If they reached the best then 25 000 lives would be saved. There is compelling evidence that the poor British figures are a result of inferior resources. In particular, Britain has fewer oncologists per head of population than almost all other European countries and many patients who could benefit from a specialist oncological opinion never receive one.[20]

Audit is a crucial aspect of risk management in clinical oncology, particularly the monitoring of treatment outcomes: cancer control rates and complication rates. Unfortunately, sufficiently detailed information is still not available to most cancer centres because the resources of information technology and manpower have generally been insufficient to meet the needs of the immediate clinical service.[2,4] The pressure of work has caused most departments to reduce substantially the follow up of patients who have been treated. Follow up is vital in the assessment of treatment outcomes and thus a reduction in follow up has important implications for risk management.

Adequate staffing levels are essential in cancer services if standards are to be maintained. The incidence of new cases of cancer is increasing at over 2% per year, and this, together with advances in treatment, translates to a workload increase of 4% per year in cancer centres.[2] Since cancer patients cannot wait for more than a week or two there is great pressure on staff to fit more work into a given time, with consequent danger to standards and increase in risk. An excessive patient workload is an important factor in any tendency to cut corners and to pay insufficient attention to detail.

In both Exeter and Stoke, deficiencies in staffing were recognised by the committees of inquiry as contributing to the risk of accident. The Royal College of Radiologists considers that the safe upper level of workload for a clinical oncologist is now 315 new patients per annum,[21] but many clinical oncologists have a workload substantially greater than this and there are some who are seeing more than double this number.

An important manifestation of insufficient resources is delay in starting treatment. Delay allows a cancer to grow and increases the chance of its spreading. It is inevitable that delay reduces the chance of success, and of course it can give rise to substantial additional anxiety. It has been recommended, for example, that radical radiotherapy should be started within two weeks of a patient first seeing a clinical oncologist, but unfortunately this is currently only being achieved for a minority of patients in the United Kingdom.[22]

The future

There has been a steadily increasing discrepancy between expectations and resource provision. Nevertheless there can be no doubt that the substantial changes in work practice and quality assurance seen during the last decade have resulted in a significant improvement in the safety of non-surgical anti-cancer treatment, as well as in its efficacy. The advent of clinical governance and regular appraisal offer, in theory, the prospect of a further reduction in risk.

However, the broad challenge for the next decade will be to maintain the quality of treatment delivery in the face of a further substantial increase in demand arising from a steadily growing number of cancer patients who stand to benefit from a rapidly growing number of new treatments. Specific aims to be given priority should be: to ensure that all patients who might benefit from an oncological opinion receive one; that all treatments start promptly; and that much better information on the process and outcomes of treatment is available for audit.

References

1 Consumers' Association. *Late complications of radiotherapy.* DTB. 1997;**35**:13–16.
2 Board of the Faculty of Clinical Oncology. *Risk Management in Clinical Oncology.* London: Royal College of Radiologists, 1995.
3 Brewin TB. Primum non nocere? *Lancet* 1994; **344**:1487–8.
4 Board of the Faculty of Clinical Oncology. *Good Practice Guide for Clinical Oncologists.* London: The Royal College of Radiologists, 1999.

5 Joint Council for Clinical Oncology. *Quality Control in Cancer Chemotherapy*. London: The Royal College of Physicians, 1994.
6 Bates T, Evans RGB. *Report of the Independent Review Commissioned by The Royal College of Radiologists into Brachial Plexus Neuropathy following Radiotherapy for Breast Carcinoma*. London: Royal College of Radiologists, 1995.
7 Dische S, Joslin CAF, Miller S, Bell NL, Holmes JC. The breast radiation injury litigation and the clinical oncologist. *Clin Oncol* 1998;**10**:367–71.
8 Walker SJ. The management of treatment incidents: an analysis of incidents in radiotherapy. In: Faulkner K, Harrison RM, eds. *Radiation incidents*. London: British Institute of Radiology, 1996.
9 Exeter District Health Authority. *The Report of the Committee of Enquiry into the Overdoses Administered in the Department of Radiotherapy in the Period February to July 1988*. Exeter: North and East Devon Health Authority, 1988.
10 Department of Health. *Quality Assurance in Radiotherapy. Report of a Working Party Chaired by Professor NM Bleehen of the Standing Subcommittee on Cancer of the Standing Medical Advisory Committee*. London: DoH, 1991.
11 Department of Health. *Quality Assurance in Radiotherapy. A Quality Management System for Radiotherapy*. London: DoH, 1994.
12 McKenzie AL. Would the two most serious radiotherapy accidents in the UK have occurred under ISO 9000? In: Faulkner K, Harrison RM, eds. *Radiation Incidents*. London: British Institute of Radiology, 1996.
13 West Midlands Regional Health Authority. *Report of the Independent Inquiry Commissioned by the West Midlands Regional Health Authority into the Conduct of Isocentric Radiotherapy at the North Staffordshire Royal Infirmary between 1982 and 1991*. Birmingham: West Midlands Regional Health Authority, 1992.
14 Department of Health and Y Swyddfa Gymreig. *Policy Framework for Commissioning Cancer Services: Guidance for Purchasers and Providers of Cancer Services*. London: HMSO, 1995.
15 Department of Health. *Report of an Independent Review of Specialist Services in London: Cancer*. London: HMSO, 1993.
16 Department of Health. *The Ionising Radiations Regulations*. London: HMSO, 1985.
17 Department of Health. *The Ionising Radiations (Protection of Persons Undergoing Medical Examination or Treatment) Regulations*. London: HMSO, 1988.
18 Department of Health. *The Approved Code of Practice, the Protection of Persons Against Ionizing Radiation Arising from any Work Activity, the Ionising Radiations Regulations*. London: HMSO, 1985.
19 Department of Health. *Draft Proposal for the Ionising Radiation (Medical Exposure) Regulations. Replacing the ionising Radiation (Protection of Persons Undergoing Medical Examination or Treatment) Regulations 1988*. London: HMSO, 1999.
20 Sikora K. Cancer survival in Britain. *BMJ* 1999;**319**:461–2.
21 Board of the Faculty of Clinical Oncology. *Consultant Workload in Clinical Oncology*. London: Royal College of Radiologists, 1998.
22 Board of the Faculty of Clinical Oncology. *A National Audit of Waiting Times for Radiotherapy*. London: Royal College of Radiologists, 1998.

12 Risk management in psychiatry

MAURICE LIPSEDGE

This chapter deals with suicide and violence to others, which constitute the topics of greatest current concern in risk management in the mental health services. Despite the recent plethora of sensational and stigmatising media reports, most acts of violence in the community are not committed by psychiatric patients. Conversely, the majority of people with psychiatric diagnoses do not commit serious violent acts.

It is self-evident that reduction of risk requires the accurate prediction of undesirable events. In clinical psychiatry the high rate of "false positives" might undermine a robust programme of risk management. Thus, suicide is a relatively rare event, although many people might carry identifiable risk factors.[1] Psychiatrists tend to greatly overestimate the likelihood of violent behaviour, with twice as many false positive predictions as true positives.[2] By the same token, psychiatric nursing staff can correctly identify the verbal and non-verbal antecedents of physically aggressive behaviour on their wards, but a high proportion of patients showing the same behavioural markers do not actually go on to commit violent acts.[3] The hazards associated with a high level of false positive predictions of self-destructive or violent behaviour include unnecessary restrictions on patients on the one hand, and a sense of demoralisation and futility among mental health staff on the other.

The Confidential Inquiry into Homicides and Suicides was informed that many of the cases were "totally unpredictable" or "had come as a complete surprise to the clinical team". In the present litigious ethos, staff will feel persecuted by the outcry over "false negatives" such as these. Oscar Hill, an experienced psychiatrist, has written: "In the present climate, if one of these patients whom I discharge, murders someone I will be publicly pilloried, with no account taken that my service would have long since been destroyed if I had not taken such risks".[4]

Furthermore, there is inevitably a degree of risk associated with caring for potentially suicidal or violent patients. The Department of Health and the Home Office have acknowledged the difficulties encountered when trying to make accurate judgements about future risks.[5] The aim of this chapter is to provide pointers to risk management while recognising that a state of total elimination of risk is Utopian in the literal sense, i.e. it does not exist anywhere. As a recent editorial in the *Lancet* emphasised: "Although negligence is unacceptable, the fact that risk assessment is not fool-proof must be recognised . . .".[2]

Psychiatric disorder and dangerous behaviour

Although violence by the severely mentally ill accounts for only a small proportion of the annual number of violent acts in the community,[6] psychiatric disorder, especially schizophrenia, is associated with a significant risk of violence before admission to hospital.[7] Patients with schizophrenia in one large scale longitudinal study committed four times as many violent offences as the general population.[8]

Cross sectional surveys also show an association between self-reported violent behaviour and either a diagnosis of schizophrenia or current psychotic symptoms.[9] In a large scale study which combined data from both a community survey and a clinical survey, violence was significantly associated with substance abuse comorbidity, specific psychotic symptoms (perceived threat, thought insertion and passivity), and loss of contact with community mental health services.[10] The risk of violence in mental illness is greatest when the patient has persecutory delusions, passivity experiences[11] and command hallucinations [12] and there is a well recognised association of violence with some other types of delusional belief, as in the "pathologies of passion" such as morbid jealousy and erotomania.[9] Persecutory delusions whose content implies a particular course of action is a high risk factor.[13] Thus violence is most likely to occur when patients have active symptoms of psychosis, and the risk significantly diminishes after treatment.[14] Among inpatients, those with schizophrenia are also disproportionately more likely to be violent.[15]

Schizophrenia is also over-represented among men remanded for homicide[16] and in a recent Finnish study[17] schizophrenia was found to increase the odds ratio of homicidal violence about 8 fold in men and 6·5 fold in women. Nevertheless much of the violence perpetrated by those with schizophrenia is fairly minor and homicide is uncommon.[18]

Predicting dangerous behaviour in any individual case is known to be an uncertain exercise, and psychiatrists tend to overestimate the likelihood of

Predicting dangerous behaviour

Antecedents:	A previous history of violence
	Poor impulse control/history of obtaining weapons
Diagnosis:	Schizophrenia
	Morbid jealousy and erotomania
	Illicit drug use or alcohol misuse, or both
Social or domestic factors:	Loss of family support and deterioration in personal relationships
	Concerns expressed by family/carers/relatives; access to potential victims
	Loss of accommodation
Clinical:	Patients declared intentions and attitudes to previous and potential victims
	Threats of violence
	Presence of active symptoms including delusions, especially regarding poisoning and sexual matters, passivity experiences, command hallucinations, jealousy, depression and angry outbursts
	Signs and symptoms of relapse
Management:	Loss of contact with mental health services
	Poor compliance with medication

Modified from Linford Rees W, Lipsedge M, Ball C, eds, *Textbook of Psychiatry*. London: Arnold 1997.

violence by patients considered for release from secure institutions.[19,20] Methodological problems have vitiated attempts to research the accuracy of psychiatrists' prediction of dangerousness. Difficulties include over-inclusive diagnostic groups, failure to recognise the importance of the situational context (for example, violence within the family), lack of data on aftercare arrangements and compliance with treatment, and failure to define violence clearly (for example, arrest rates, conviction rate, or self-reported antisocial behaviour).[21] A major problem lies in the design of studies purporting to validate risk assessment, since those patients predicted to behave violently will tend to be admitted to hospital to be given preventive treatment and only those considered unlikely to be violent in the near future will be released into the community.[22]

However, one study[23] in the United States has helped to validate the clinical prediction of violence in the community: male, but not female, patients who had been assessed in a hospital emergency room as potentially violent turned out to be significantly more violent over the next six months than comparison patients. Although these clinical judgements had low sensitivity and specificity,[23] it is likely that a more systematic and thorough assessment of a patient who might be at risk and a careful and detailed review of both the circumstances and the victim of any past violent behaviour will enhance risk assessment and management.[24,25]

Critical factors include the patient's declared intentions and attitudes to both previous and potential victims and to staff, as well as the patient's mental state, including delusions, command hallucinations, jealousy, depression and proneness to angry outbursts. Schizophrenic delusions, especially of poisoning or of a sexual nature, are more likely to lead to deliberate personal violence than imperative hallucinations.[7] Detailed discussion should be held with the patient about their thoughts and feelings at the time of any specific offences, supplemented by documentary evidence on these events from police depositions and witness statements.

Information about the patient's history, psychiatric condition, likely compliance with treatment, ability to take responsibility for his or her behaviour, and modes of responding to stress, as well as an assessment of relationships, provide a basis on which to predict those circumstances in which violence might occur[26] and permit interventions designed to modify these situations. While the patient is still in hospital, the clinician should ideally work with both the perpetrator and any family victim of aggression to review past patterns of violence and develop protective strategies.[27]

Knowledge about risk factors for violence will help to inform decisions about the timing of discharge and the planning of aftercare.[28] However, although clinical judgement adds to predictive accuracy,[26] Gunn warns that predictions about violent behaviour can be safely made only for fairly short periods, hence the need for careful supervision, vigilant monitoring, and the development of supportive therapeutic relationships. Those providing such support require their own supervision and support and an awareness of transference issues.[26]

Transference refers to the way a patient's relationship with mental health professionals is coloured and shaped by their own earlier relationships and by the projection of images derived from the formative experience of close contact with others in the past. A specific factor associated with danger can be the patient's unrealistic perception of a special relationship with a particular mental health professional.[29] The latter may inadvertently collude with this process and the counter-transference might contribute to the transgression of professional boundaries and an increased risk of violence, especially from patients with borderline personality disorder.[30]

The predictive power of decisions based on actuarial data can be substantially increased by using a more realistic, shorter time frame[12] and by considering the environment into which a patient with a history of violence is to be discharged, since violent acts by psychiatric patients are known to be more likely to occur within a family setting. Although the view that the best predictor of future violence is a history of physically aggressive behaviour[31] has become axiomatic, the individual person's mental state is a crucial variable, which, surprisingly, has often been omitted from predictive research on violence.

Gunn has enumerated the important variables involved in predicting dangerous behaviour.[26] He emphasises the significance of those elements which are subject to change, such as family support and personal relationships and the availability of potential victims.

The targets of violent acts by psychiatric patients tend to be family members or other intimates rather than strangers[32,33] and those patients who are violent just before admission tend to be the most violent after discharge and to attack the same person within two weeks of leaving hospital.[28] The report of the confidential inquiry[34] into homicide also found that most of the victims were family members or were already acquainted with the attacker.

Comorbidity and violent behaviour

Comorbidity is now recognised as a key factor in violence.[35,36] (Comorbidity or dual diagnosis refers to individuals who meet criteria for the diagnosis of both a severe mental illness and of an alcohol or drug misuse disorder.) The combination of poor adherence to medication and alcohol or other drug abuse problems is significantly associated with serious violent acts in the community among patients with severe mental illness.[37] A recent inner-London study demonstrated that the dual diagnosis of severe mental illness and substance misuse has a highly significant association with aggressive and hostile behaviour, a lifetime history of committing an offence and a recent history of assault.[38]

A prospective study of physical assaults in a psychiatric intensive care unit has shown that both a criminal record and prior drug misuse have predictive value, so that a urine test for drugs and attention to forensic history and previous mental health problems will help to identify those patients who are most likely to become aggressive.[39] Substance abuse also significantly raises the level of violence in patients discharged from acute psychiatric inpatient units.[32] One way of attempting to reduce this risk would be closer integration of mental health and substance abuse treatment programmes.[40]

Managing potentially dangerous psychiatric patients

The Ritchie inquiry into the care of Christopher Clunis, a young man with schizophrenia who killed a stranger in 1992, concluded that this patient's care and treatment "was a catalogue of failure and missed opportunity" over the five years of hospital and community care before he stabbed his victim.[41]

Like Clunis, most mentally abnormal offenders who commit serious offences are already well known to the psychiatric services.[23] Since 1992 there have been further incidents of grave acts of violence committed by patients with severe mental illness.[42]

The Ritchie inquiry found a significant failure in passing on information between psychiatrists, nurses, general practitioners, social workers, hostel staff and Christopher Clunis's family. Other deficiencies in care, which might have ultimately contributed to the death of his victim Jonathan Zito, include failure to obtain an accurate history and to consider Christopher Clunis's history of violence and to assess his propensity for further violence. Doctors, nurses, and social workers failed to make adequate contemporaneous records of important events, and violent incidents were either minimised or even omitted from records, correspondence, and discharge summaries and were not picked up by clinicians and social workers from the nursing notes.[41]

In considering all of the violent incidents which had occurred three years before the fatal stabbing, the inquiry concluded that the medical professionals had tended to minimise the gravity of a series of attempts by Christopher Clunis to stab people, on the grounds that little actual physical damage was caused in that particular cluster of incidents: "We feel there is a real danger of looking too much at the consequences of an action without looking at the action itself".[41]

The same inquiry also disclosed a failure to provide and co-ordinate adequate aftercare according to section 117 of the Mental Health Act 1983 (MHA) by both medical and social services and a failure to act on warning signs to prevent a relapse. (Section 117 of the Act requires health services and social services to provide aftercare for patients on discharge from hospital after compulsory detention under Section 3 of the MHA). Throughout, the report refers to a tendency to overlook or minimise violent incidents, to ignore reports of violence made by members of the public, and a failure to ensure continuity of care when the patient had left a particular health district (paragraph 109).[41]

The report of the Independent Panel of Inquiry examining the case of Michael Buchanan, a man with chronic schizophrenia and personality disorder who abused cocaine and who murdered a stranger in 1992, found many failures of care which resemble those in the Clunis case.[42] These included inadequate aftercare planning, failure to allocate a keyworker according to Section 117, lack of recording of numerous violent episodes, failure to assess risk of dangerousness, and premature removal of the patient from the caseload of the community psychiatric nurse. As with Clunis, these failures led to a potentially dangerous patient slipping out of the aftercare system.

To prevent patients with serious mental illness falling through the net of care in this way the Ritchie inquiry reiterates the need for implementation of Section 117 of the MHA and of the care programme approach (CPA) so that the aftercare needs of each patient are systematically assessed by both health and social services before discharge and an individual plan of care is formulated by the multidisciplinary team[43]. This comprehensive plan should be discussed with and given to the patient and to all team members. The consultant psychiatrist and the team must assess the risk of the patient harming himself or herself, or others. A keyworker or "care co-ordinator" has to be appointed and a regular review of the patient arranged. The keyworker should have direct access to the responsible medical officer. There should be contingency plans if the patient fails to engage in treatment and an assertive approach to maintaining patient contact. If a crisis develops and a request is made for an urgent Mental Health Act assessment, this should be carried out within three hours. Non-urgent requests should be met within three working days. The foreword to the 1993 Revised Code of Practice emphasises that the MHA can be used to admit patients not only to prevent harm to self or to others but also to forestall deterioration in a patient's health.[44]

All team members should be aware of the likely signs of an impending relapse and react promptly. The Confidential Inquiry into Homicide and Suicide of Mentally Ill People[34] states that in over half the cases some reduction in attendance for treatment or some failure to take prescribed medication had occurred. Non-compliance with treatment is often an important pointer to relapse.[45] Other circumstances which increase the risk of dangerous behaviour include drug or alcohol misuse in a patient with major mental disorder,[45] as in the case of Michael Buchanan,[42] the occurrence of a potentially dangerous personal situation, such as marriage, in a patient with a history of morbid jealousy; or disappearance from hostel or bed and breakfast accommodation, as in the case of both Buchanan and Clunis. Identifying all relevant factors in past violent behaviour is essential.[43]

The Royal College of Psychiatrists' guidelines also recommend a period of trial leave under Section 17 of the Mental Health Act to test out uncertainties about the patient's ability to cope in the community and to permit staff to monitor the patient's progress. While on leave the patient's general practitioner should be informed in anticipation of possible problems.[46]

Passing on confidential information

When a patient who is subject to aftercare under section 117 moves out of his or her area, responsibility remains with the multidisciplinary team until the aftercare has been effectively transferred to a new team. If there is a risk of harm to self or others, all those providing a service to the patient in terms of housing or occupational therapy need to be informed of the risk. Information about any violent or potentially violent incident and a thorough assessment of the risk of dangerousness should be included in the discharge summary. The Ritchie inquiry seems to recommend (paragraph 48) that the need to transmit information about the risk of dangerousness transcends considerations of professional confidentiality.[41] This is supported by the judgement in *W* v *Egdell and others*,[47] which prompted a legal comment that "whenever a doctor perceives a patient to be a serious danger to his family or the public at large, his duty of confidence to that patient will be reduced".[48] The guidelines of the Royal College of Psychiatrists on the aftercare of potentially violent or vulnerable patients indicate that considerations of public safety should give exemption from absolute professional confidentiality, but recommends (paragraph 44) that when such a disclosure occurs the reasons for the decision should be documented.[46] The clinician should also record the steps taken before disclosure, such as attempting to persuade the patient to authorise the disclosure, and advice might be sought from medical colleagues and defence organisations.

To justify disclosure of personal information about patients to agencies outside the National Health Service such as housing association staff or the police, it is important to be clear precisely what and how much information should be disclosed and to whom, and for what purpose the confidential material is being passed on.[49]

Summary of review of 11 homicide inquiries into homicide by psychiatric patients

1 Failure to obtain, heed or pass on information about risk;
2 under-reporting and downgrading of previous violent incidents;
3 failure to meet the needs of carers – the majority of victims were family members;
4 lack of resources, especially shortage of acute hospital beds and supervised hostels;
5 Failure to monitor risk in the community;
6 Failure to use the Mental Health Act both to admit deteriorat-ing patients and to apply Section 117

See also Petch, E and Bradley, C.[94]
Modified from *Review of 11 independent inquiries into homicide by psychiatric patients.*[33]

Violence in psychiatric units

Violence is the result of the interplay between the individual, the institution and structural factors rather than simply the expression of individual psychopathology.[50]

The following are predictive factors for inpatient violence.[51]

Individual factors

- The acute phase of a psychotic illness[52] especially if exacerbated by drug abuse,[36] particularly with psychostimulants or alcohol
- young people with a history of violent behaviour
- a minority of patients are responsible for the majority of incidents[53,54]
- low self-esteem and lack of verbal fluency are also associated with violent outbursts, both expressive and instrumental.

In an important American study[55] of the correlates of accuracy in the assessment of psychiatric inpatients' risk of violence, it was found that schizophrenia, mania or an organic psychotic condition (generally drug-induced), a high level of hostile suspiciousness, and a recent history of violent behaviour accurately predicted the likelihood of physically assaulting others during the first week of hospitalisation. However, clinical judgements that emphasised gender and "race"/ethnicity were associated with predictor errors: the risk of violence was over-emphasised in both men and any persons who were "non-white".[56]

Institutional factors

These include:

- over-crowding
- lack of privacy and inactivity
- provocation from other patients
- staff expectations and/or lack of experience
- under-involvement of medical staff.

Patients, visitors and psychiatric staff might all be at risk. Although physical assaults by patients tend to be under-recorded,[54] it has been estimated that half of all mental health professionals will be assaulted at some point in their careers[57] and nurses are the most likely targets of assault.[58]

Wards with high levels of incidents are characterised by limited and hostile communication between staff and patients, irregular and unscheduled activities and meetings, poorly defined staff responsibilities and patients not knowing whom to approach about their problems and requests.[59] The quality of the relationship between patients and staff (the initial therapeutic alliance) can be a strong predictor of violence.[60] It follows that psychiatric teams should not only carry out regular risk assessments but should also have regular routines and activities, and staff should have clear roles and responsibilities so that patients know whom to approach for help.[60]

Structural factors

These include:

- the rising level of violence in society in general
- the concentration on dangerousness as a criterion for admission
- the lack of beds and of community resources resulting in the admission of patients whose condition has deteriorated outside hospital and who have become more conspicuously disturbed.

Reducing violence in psychiatric units

There is a tendency to concentrate disproportionately on strategies to contain violence on psychiatric wards (with control and restraint and alarm systems) while neglecting any systematic attempt to reduce the frequency of violent incidents.[61]

In a radical challenge to the widespread use of physical restraint and enforced sedation, McDougall[62] points out that these coercive interventions are not only distressing for both patients and staff but they convey a message that force is an acceptable way of solving problems, so that the patient might feel absolved of the need to take responsibility for their own aggression. After all, the expression of anger and aggression in patients who are compulsorily detained is not always a clinical problem. Other hazards of using restraint and sedation as an early intervention include the risk of escalating a cycle of violence and the retraumatisation of patients who have been abused.[62]

An alternative approach uses proactive interventions including de-escalation, diversion and engagement. Techniques based on interpersonal skills, negotiation and collaboration do, of course, require intensive training and adequate staff levels. Professional actors who have a detailed knowledge of disturbed behaviour are an invaluable resource in training staff in negotiation and de-escalation skills.[63]

Assessing risk of suicide

Suicide occurs far more commonly than homicide committed by psychiatric patients, with over five and a half thousand cases in England in 1992[64] compared with 39 homicides over a 33 month period committed by people who had had contact with the mental health services in the preceding year.[34]

Deliberate self-harm (DSH) leads to 100 000 hospital admissions in England and Wales every year and its incidence is increasing.[65] Suicide accounts for at least 1% of all deaths annually, with a male: female ratio of over 2:1. The highest suicide rates occur in people aged over 75 but the past 15 years have seen an alarming increase in the suicide rate among young men.[66] The commonest means of suicide used by men include asphyxiation with car exhaust fumes and hanging, whereas self-poisoning with drugs is the preferred method of committing suicide among women.

In addition to age and sex, the socio-demographic and personal factors showing a positive statistical correlation with suicide include divorce, loss of job, unemployment, or retirement; social isolation, recent bereavement, chronic, painful or terminal illness; a history of mood disorder, alcoholism or attempted suicide; loss of a parent in childhood; and being in either social class I or V. In addition, most people who commit suicide have a psychiatric disorder, most commonly depression, schizophrenia, and alcohol addiction.[67]

High risk clinical factors for suicide-associated illness include severe insomnia, self-neglect, memory impairment, agitation, and panic attacks. In patients with schizophrenia the risk of suicide is known to be greater in young and unemployed men with a history of depression, loss of appetite and weight, recurrent relapses, and a fear of deterioration.[68] (Clozapine has recently been shown to significantly reduce suicidality in patients with treatment-resistant schizophrenia by suppressing both positive and negative symptoms, improving mood and reducing extrapyramidal symptoms and tardive dyskinesia.[69])

A previous history of self-harm greatly increases the risk of subsequent suicide, to 30-fold higher than that expected during the 10 years after an episode of deliberate self-harm (DSH), the first six months being the period of greatest risk. One per cent of patients kill themselves in the year after an episode of deliberate self-harm[65] and between one fifth and one quarter of patients who die by suicide have presented to a general hospital after episodes of DSH in the year before their death.[70] Eventual suicide in such patients is significantly commoner among unemployed men of social class V who misuse alcohol or drugs and who have a history of psychiatric disorder.[1]

The *Health of the Nation* document on suicide[71] is a model practical manual which provides an effective strategy for reducing the risk of suicide. This section draws extensively on its procedures and recommendations.

In the clinical evaluation of a particular person who might be at risk of suicide, the statistical correlates of suicide enumerated above have low specificity and sensitivity so that screening for at-risk cases results in high numbers of both false positives and false negatives.[1] In one study, risk factors for suicide combined had a sensitivity of 60% and a specificity of 61%.[72] Although risk factors are not especially helpful in the clinical assessment of short-term risk, they can contribute to the overall assessment of risk.[1] Rather than relying too heavily on actuarial risk factors, the evaluation of short-term risk should be based on assessing the person's state of mind, recent adverse life events, relationships and degree of available support[38], which requires a detailed history of the present illness, an assessment of mental state, and a diagnostic formulation.[1,72] These factors are summarised below.

Factors predicting risk of suicide: summary

- Declared intent
- Preparation, including hoarding of tablets, settling financial affairs or leaving a note, or both
- Past history of deliberate self-harm, especially in the previous six months
- Severe depressive illness, schizophrenia, and substance abuse
- Depression in young unemployed men with schizophrenia, with frequent relapses and fear of deterioration
- Pessimism, anhedonia, despair, morbid guilt, insomnia, self-neglect, memory impairment, agitation, and panic attacks
- Recent adverse life events and lack of supportive relationships or failure to establish a working alliance with a mental health professional (malignant alienation), or both
- First few weeks after discharge from hospital are particularly risky.

Modified from Linford Rees W, Lipsedge, M, Ball C, eds, *Textbook of Psychiatry*, London: Arnold 1997.

In addition to establishing whether the person has shown evidence of suicidal intent by leaving a note or making a will, the extent of his or her pessimism and anhedonia, despair, and morbid guilt should be assessed since hopelessness and helplessness are known precursors of suicidal behaviour.[73]

Has the person seriously considered possible methods of suicide? What circumstances might increase the risk? Is there a risk to others? Information should also be obtained from previous medical and psychiatric records, from relatives, and from other key informants.

The degree of suicidal intent can fluctuate, and apparent improvement may occur in the patient on being removed from a stressful environment, with a risk of relapse on discharge.

Furthermore, while one gravely suicidal person may deliberately conceal their lethal intentions, another may appear calm and even serene to the interviewer after they have made an undisclosed but firm decision to kill themselves. Guidelines produced by the Department of Health and the Royal College of Psychiatrists recommend a specialist psychosocial assessment and aftercare plan that can be carried out by a trained and supervised psychiatric nurse. However, only about 50% of those who present after DSH receive such an assessment.[74]

The assessment and management of deliberate self-harm undertaken by accident and emergency medical staff might be inadequate. A recent review of the records of one accident and emergency department covering a period of one year[75] showed that while nearly a third of the patients were discharged directly home by accident and emergency staff, less than a quarter had had an assessment of risk of further deliberate self-harm and little information concerning alcohol or substance misuse was recorded (the use of alcohol is known to be associated with repetition of DSH).[76,77] A south London study[78] showed that patients who discharged themselves from an accident and emergency department before completion of the initial assessment have three times the rate of repetition of self-harm compared with those who complete the initial psychosocial screening.

Some patients who are at risk of suicide may be cared for in the community (see below). Patients who present a more serious risk will have to be admitted to hospital. This might be as a voluntary patient or under the Mental Health Act 1983 for those who seem to be at severe and immediate risk of suicide but who refuse admission.

Managing suicidal patients[71]

Community management

The advantages of the community care of suicidal patients include avoiding the stigma associated with admission to a mental hospital and maintaining contact with the patient's usual social environment. This permits retention of personal autonomy and the deployment of coping skills with the back up of a supportive and understanding therapeutic relationships. The disadvantages include lack of close supervision of the patient's safety and of compliance with treatment, and, at times, the imposition of excessive strain on the family or carers. Young men can be difficult to engage in treatment and an aggressive outreach approach might be needed.[79]

Community management is not indicated when there is a grave risk of suicide or lack of adequate support, or both, or failure to establish a good working alliance with the patient. The risk is significantly increased by a history of self-destructive impulsive behaviour, current substance misuse, and failure to set up a therapeutic rapport. Valuable information can be obtained by a domiciliary visit, which might disclose a cache of medication, evidence of alcohol misuse, or the proximity of a railway line or other hazardous local factors.

Community management requires a care plan that states the type of support and the names of key care staff. The plan should be discussed and agreed by the patient and the professionals involved. There should be regular systematic reviews of suicide risk, with frequent reassessment of mental state, in the first instance. These reviews should be recorded and the management plan modified when necessary. Hospital admission may become the only safe option if the patient's condition deteriorates. Communication between general practitioners, carers, and other agencies must be thorough. The patient and carer should be given a contact number to use in a crisis (the emergency access card system with information on available sources of help introduced by Gethin Morgan et al [80]) as well as a specific appointment for the next review. Drug treatment should be prescribed only in limited quantities. The selective serotonin re-uptake inhibitor antidepressants are generally regarded as less toxic if taken in an overdose.[81] Ideally, storage and dispensing of drugs should be delegated to a responsible carer. In addition to the drug treatment of depression, the risk of repetition of deliberate self-harm can be reduced by training in a cognitive-behavioural problem-solving technique.[82] Cognitive-behaviour therapies that specifically focus on interpersonal problem-solving skills can reduce the repetition of suicide attempts even in moderate to high risk patients.[83]

Some patients will require long-term community support for a persistent but relatively mild suicide risk. Patients who can eventually be discharged from follow up require gradual and planned termination of contact rather than an abrupt ending, whereas patients whose care is to be transferred to another service should be "handed over" in a measured fashion to allow their familiarisation with the new team.

Hospital management

The period shortly after admission carries a high risk of self-harm, and when the suicide risk is particularly high patients are initially nursed in bed, and belongings such as ties, belts, and scissors are removed. The patient should remain continuously visible to the staff and should not be allowed to leave the ward. The staff should carefully supervise smoking and the patient's use of matches and lighters. Patients should be examined as soon as possible after admission by the ward doctor. The treatment plan and the level of observation need to be agreed jointly by medical and nursing staff and recorded and communicated to all ward staff and the patient.

The wards where patients at high risk of suicide are nursed must be physically safe. There should be no access to high windows or staircases, curtain rails should not be able to bear heavy weights, and exit from the ward must be controlled. A guaranteed quota of staff is essential to provide intensive levels of supervision. A keyworker and a deputy should be designated to the patient to try to establish an effective therapeutic rapport, and, in general, the patient should be encouraged to approach staff when feeling distressed and to discuss suicidal ideas freely.

Staff should be aware of the possibility of a misleading short-lived improvement due to respite from a stressful home situation, which will cause a later recrudescence of suicide risk if unresolved. They should also be able to recognise "malignant alienation" which is a potentially lethal distancing of the patient from staff and from carers caused by challenging behaviour or repeated relapses, or both.[84] Another risky clinical situation is the period of recovery of drive and energy in a depressed patient who retains suicidal ideas.

Home leave from the ward presents a period of high risk in recently suicidal inpatients.[85] Patients should be encouraged to return to the ward at any time of the day or night if they feel unable to cope at home. If a patient goes absent without leave the nurse in charge and the resident medical officer should be informed immediately, the hospital and its grounds should be searched, and both the carers and the police should be informed. After an absence without leave or an incident of deliberate self-harm within the hospital or while on leave, the level of observation and the management plan should be reviewed, leading to a higher level of surveillance.

An appropriate level of supportive observation is decided after discussion between the medical and nursing staff and may be intensified unilaterally by the nursing staff. It should be reviewed at every change of nursing shift and confirmed by the patient's ward doctor and also reviewed periodically by the consultant. Intensive supportive observation permits close monitoring of the patient's behaviour and mental state.

The first few weeks after discharge represent a period of greatly increased risk of suicide.[86] The risk can be reduced by careful planning for discharge in accordance with the Care Programme Approach (CPA)[43] by prescribing medication in safe amounts, by arranging for an early review, and by ensuring that the patient and carers know how to obtain help rapidly if the patient's condition deteriorates.

Successful litigation against hospitals in connection with self-harm and suicide has highlighted contributory factors for which the hospital and its staff might be regarded as responsible:[87]

- Unsafe design
- Failure to monitor patient
- Failure to remove dangerous objects
- Failure to use a locked ward
- Failure to supervise staff

233

- Failure to obtain past records
- Poor communication between staff
- Failure to treat psychiatric disorder adequately
- Negligent discharge.

In a survey of litigation claims against hospitals in Australia from 1972 to 1992, in which 20 cases claiming failure to prevent suicidal behaviour were identified,[88] all but one case involved inpatients, and failure to supervise was the leading basis of the claims. Jumping from heights accounted for 13 of the 20 incidents, seven of which were jumping through hospital windows. The claims of alleged failure to provide a suitable degree of observation and supervision resulted most commonly in settlement in favour of the plaintiffs. The high frequency of suicide jumps has implications for the architectural design of psychiatric units. Death due to jumping as an act of suicide is well recognised in severe depression but the risk of violent self-harm in patients with delusions of persecution is often under-estimated. Paranoid patients may leap from windows to escape imaginary persecutors or commit suicide because they believe that instant death is preferable to torture by their imaginary enemies.

The care programme approach

The purpose of the Care Programme Approach (CPA)[89,90] is to set up and monitor an individualised system of support for mentally ill people in the community, thereby minimising the possibility of their losing contact with services and maximising the effect of any therapeutic intervention. The essential elements of the programme include:

- systematic assessment of both health and social care needs
- preparing a written care plan agreed between professional staff, the patient and carers
- allocating a keyworker to keep in close contact with the patient, to monitor that the programme of care is delivered, and to take immediate action if it is not
- implementation of the CPA ensured by regular reassessment and review of the patient's progress. This policy emphasises the importance of ensuring continuity of care and of staying in touch,[64] with specific guidelines on how to reduce the risk of patients "falling through the net" when they move from one area to another.

The NHS Management Executive's guidance on discharging mentally disordered patients[43] includes practical advice on carrying out an assessment of risk in potentially violent patients and emphasises the need to take into account the patient's history, their own self-reporting, their behaviour and mental state, and any discrepancies between what is reported and what is observed. Effective risk assessment must identify relevant factors involved in previous violent behaviour including:

- the personal and domestic circumstances which might lead to a recurrence
- loss of a supportive relationship
- loss of accommodation
- ceasing to take medication.

Risk assessment should be accompanied by a risk management strategy with a clear action plan to be implemented in response to early warning signs of deterioration.

It might be thought that there is an undue reliance in the CPA on pro-phylactic antipsychotic treatment, but there is well-documented evidence that regular neuroleptics greatly reduce the risk of both relapse and violent incidents in mentally disordered offenders.[91]

Why do things go wrong?

The concluding points below summarise the factors contributing to clinical risk in psychiatry.

1 Professional arrogance combined with a reckless tolerance of defiance can lead to failure by mental health professionals to heed reports by carers and members of the public about disturbed behaviour.[41,92]
2 Undue emphasis on the civil liberties of psychiatric patients at the expense of tolerating grave suicidal risk and the danger of violent behaviour.
3 Failure to implement the 1993 Revised Mental Health Code of Practice (paragraph 2.6) recommendation that compulsory admission is indicated to prevent deterioration and not just when the patient is regarded as a danger to self or others;
4 Belief that compulsory admission under the Mental Health Act cannot be implemented "until a patient actually does something dangerous". Formerly this was a widely held view among mental health professionals, but since the publication of the Ritchie report they are now prepared to be somewhat more proactive. Mental health professionals have to accept that the practice of psychiatry is essentially a paternalistic activity and that imposing treatment against a patient's will is justified when they believe that the patient's life or health would be at risk if coercion were not applied and the condition were allowed to deteriorate.[93]
5 A tendency, especially among approved social workers, to take a "snapshot" cross sectional view of the potentially suicidal or violent patient's mental state and behaviour and to ignore both previous episodes and

any recent history of deterioration. Social workers routinely take a "longitudinal" view when assessing a case of alleged child abuse, but, paradoxically, often insist on minimising the importance of both past and recent history when making mental health assessments.

6 Failure to pass on information about potential dangerousness to other professionals, such as hostel staff, for reasons ranging from inertia, inefficiency, or overwork to a misguided overprotective view of the patient at the expense of the safety of potential victims.

Lack of resources, in terms of staff and inpatient facilities. There is a grave shortage of general adult psychiatric beds and of beds on closed wards. With an increasing awareness of the risks of both suicide and violence within the community, there is a greater demand for admission. However, the beds tend to be occupied for longer because of staff reluctance to discharge potentially dangerous or suicidal patients into the community, where hostel accommodation and support services are inadequate. The shortage of beds places psychiatric staff in a difficult position if they try to follow the Department of Health's guidance on the discharge of mentally disordered people This seeks to ensure that psychiatric patients are discharged "only when and if they are ready to leave hospital", and, "any risk to the public or to patients themselves is minimal and is managed effectively . . ." The Threshold Assessment Grid (TAG) is a user-friendly scoring-system for identifying the priority group in the community with severe mental illness. It is likely to provide a constructive way of reducing risk.

I am grateful to Dr John Reed, Professor E Murphy, and Dr John Bradley for helpful advice and comments, and to the late Mrs Marcia Andrews for typing the original manuscript.

The following provided helpful information for the second edition: Anne Benson, Roland Dix, Sharon Dennis, Samantha Rudderham Bland and Sharon Cahill.

References

1 Hawton K. Assessment of suicide risk. *Br J Psychiatry* 1987;**150**:145–53.
2 Detention of potentially dangerous people. Editorial. *Lancet* 1998;**352**:1641.
3 Whittington R. Verbal and non-verbal behaviour immediately prior to aggression by mentally disordered people: enhancing the assessment of risk. *J Psychiatr Ment Health Nurs* 1996;**3**:47–54.
4 Hill O. Detention of potentially dangerous people. *Lancet* 1998;**352**:1641.
5 Department of Health/Office. *Review of services for mentally disordered offenders*. Final Summary Report, Cm 2088. London: HMSO, 1992.
6 Coid J, Cordess C. Compulsory admission of dangerous psychopaths: psychiatrists are damned if they do and damned if they don't. *BMJ* 1992;**304**:1581–2.
7 Humphreys MS, Johnstone EC, MacMillan JF, Taylor PJ,. Dangerous behaviour preceding first admissions for schizophrenia. *Br J Psychiatry* 1992;**161**:501–5.
8 Lindqvist P, Allebeck P. Schizophrenia and crime. *Br J Psychiatry* 1990;**157**:345–50.
9 Link B, Andrews J and Cullen F. The violent and illegal behaviour of mental patients reconsidered. *Am Sociol Rev* 1992;**57**:275–92.
10 Swanson J, Estroff S, Swartz M, *et al.* Violence and severe mental disorder in clinical and

community populations: the effects of psychotic symptoms, comorbidity, and lack of treatment. *Psychiatry* 1997;**60**:1–22.

11 Addad M, Benech M, Bourgeois M, Yesevage J. Criminal acts among schizophrenics in French mental hospitals. *J Nerv Ment Dis* 1981;**169**:289–93.

12 Buchanan A. The investigations of acting on delusions as a tool for risk assessment in the mentally disordered. *Br J Psychiatry* 1977;**170**(32):12–16.

13 Junginger J. Psychosis and violence: the case for a content analysis of psychotic experience. *Schizophrenia Bull* 1996;**22**:91–103.

14 Krakowski M, Jaeger J, Volavka J. Violence and psychopathology: a longitudinal study. *Compr Psychiatry* 1988;**29**:174–81.

15 Noble P, Rodger S. Violence by psychiatric inpatients. *Br J Psychiatry* 1989;**155**:384–90.

16 Taylor PJ. Motives for offending among violent and psychotic men. *Br J Psychiatry* 1985;**147**:491–8.

17 Eronen M, Hakola P, Tiihonen J. Mental disorders and homicidal behaviour in Finland. *Arch Gen Psychiatry* 1996;**53**:497–501.

18 Steering Committee of the Confidential Inquiry on Homicides and Suicides by Mentally Ill People. *Report of the Confidential Inquiry into Homicides and Suicides by Mentally Ill People.* London: Royal College of Psychiatrists, 1996.

19 Coccozza J, Steadman H. Failure of psychiatric predictions of dangerousness. *Rutgers La Revie* 1976;**29**:174–81.

20 Monahan J. The prediction of violent behaviour: toward a second generation of theory and policy. *Am J Psychiatry* 1984;**141**:10–15.

21 Monahan J. Risk assessment of violence among the mentally disordered: generating useful knowledge. *Int J Law Psychiatry* 1988;**11**:249–57.

22 Monahan J, Steadman HJ. Toward a rejuvenation of risk assessment research. In: Monahan J, Steadman, HJ eds. *Violence and mental disorder.* Chicago: University of Chicago Press, 1994.

23 Lidz CW, Mulvey EP, Gardner W. The accuracy of predictions of violence to others. *JAMA* 1993;**269**:1007–11.

24 Chiswick, D. Dangerousness. In: Chiswick D, Cope R, eds. *Seminars in practical forensic psychiatry.* London: Royal College of Psychiatrists, 1995.

25 The Royal College of Psychiatrists Special Working Party on Clinical Assessment and Management of Risk. *Assessment and clinical management of risk of harm to other people.* London: Royal College of Psychiatrists, 1996.

26 Gunn J. Dangerousness. In: Gunn J, Taylor PJ, eds. *Forensic psychiatry.* Oxford: Butterworth-Heinemann, 1993.

27 Tardiff K. *Assessment and management of violent patients,* 2nd edition, Washington, DC: American Psychiatric Press, 1996.

28 Tardiff K, Marzuk PM, Leon AC, Portera L. A prospective study of violence by psychiatric patients after hospital discharge. *Psychiatr Serv* 1997;**48**:(5):678–81.

29 Vincent M, White K. Patient violence toward a nurse: predictable and preventable? *J Psychosoc Nurs* 1994;**32**:(2):30–2.

30 Dubin WR. The role of fantasies, countertransference, and psychological defenses in patient violence. *Hosp Commun Psychiatry* 1989;**40**:1280–3.

31 Scott PD. Assessing dangerousness in criminals. *Br J Psychiatry* 1977;**131**:127–42.

32 Steadman HJ, Mulvey EP, Monahan J, *et al.* Violence by people discharged from acute psychiatric inpatient facilities and by others in the same neighbourhoods. *Arch Gen Psychiatry* 1998;**55**:393–401.

33 Lipsedge M, Rudderham Bland S. Review of 11 independent inquiries into homicide by psychiatric patients. *Clin Risk* 1997;**3**:1–7.

34 Confidential Inquiry into Homicides and Suicides. *Report of the Confidential Inquiry into Homicides and Suicides by Mentally Ill People.* London: Royal College of Psychiatrists, 1996.

35 Mulvey E, Shaw E, Lidz C. Why use multiple sources in research on patient violence in the community? *Crim Behav Mental Health* 1994;**4**:253–8.

36 Johns A. Substance misuse: a primary risk and a major problem of comorbidity. *Int Rev Psychiatry* 1997;**155**:227–31.

37 Swartz MS, Swanson JW, Hiday VA, *et al.* Violence and severe mental illness: the

effects of substance abuse and nonadherence to medication. *Am J Psychiatry* 1998;**155**: 227–31.

38 Scott J, House R, Yates M, Harrington J. Individual risk factors for early repetition of deliberate self-harm. *Br J Med Psychol* 1997;**70**:387–93.

39 Walker Z, Seifert R. Violent incidents in a psychiatric intensive care unit. *Br J Psychiatry* 1994;**164**:826–8.

40 Johnson S. Dual diagnosis of severe mental illness and substance misuse: a case for specialist services? *Br J Psychiatry* 1997;**171**:205–8.

41 Ritchie JH, Dick D, Lingham R. *Report of the inquiry into the care and treatment of Christopher Clunis.* London: HMSO, 1994.

42 Heginbotham C. *Report of the Independent Panel of Inquiry Examining Case of Michael Buchanan.* London: North West London NHS Mental Health Trust, 1994.

43 NHS Management Executive. *Guidance on the discharge of mentally disordered people and their continuing care in the community.* Leeds: NHSMME (HSG 94 27), 1994.

44 *Revised Code of Practice, Mental Health Act 1993.* London: HMSO, 1993.

45 Swanson JW, Holzer CE, Ganju VK, Jono RT. Violence and psychiatric disorder in the community: evidence from the epidemiological catchment area surveys. *Hosp Commun Psychiatry* 1990;**41**:761–70.

46 Royal College of Psychiatrists. *Good medical practice and the aftercare of potentially violent or vulnerable patients discharged from inpatient psychiatric treatment.* London: Royal College of Psychiatrists (Council report CR 12), 1991.

47 *W* v *Egdell and others* (1988) 2WLR, 689.

48 Brahams D. Psychiatrist's duty of confidentiality. *Lancet* 1988;**ii**:1503–4.

49 Harbour A. Limits of confidentiality. *Adv Psychiatr Treat* 1998;**4**:66–9.

50 Davis S. Violence by psychiatric inpatients: a review. *Hosp Commun Psychiatry* 1991;**42**: 585–90.

51 Owens R, Ashcroft J. *Violence: a guide for the caring professions.* London: Croom Helm, 1985.

52 Kay S, Wolkenfeld F, Murrill L. Profiles of aggression among psychiatric patients: nature and prevalence. *J Nerv Ment Dis* 1988;**176**:539–46.

53 Barber J, Hundle P, Kellogg E *et al.* Clinical and demographic characteristics of fifteen patients with repetitively assaultive behaviour. *Psychiatr Quart* 1988;**59**:213–24.

54 Cheung P, Schweitr I, Tuckwell V, Crowley KC. A prospective study of assaults on staff by psychiatric inpatients. *Med Sci Law* 1997;**37**:46–52.

55 McNiel DE, Binder RL. Correlates of accuracy in the assessment of psychiatric inpatients' risk of violence. *Am J Psychiatry* 1995;**152**:901–6.

56 Lipsedge M. Dangerous stereotypes. *J Forensic Psychiatry* 1994;**5**:14–19.

57 Blair DT, New SA. Patient violence in psychiatric settings: risk identification and treatment as provocation. In: Smoyak SA, Blair DT, eds. *Violence and abuse*, 36–53. Thorofare, NJ: Slack, 1992.

58 Owen C, Tarantello C, Jones M, Tennant C. Violence and aggression in psychiatric units. *Psychiatr Serv* 1998;**49**:1452–7.

59 Katz P, Kirkland F. Violence and social structure on mental hospital wards. *Psychiatry* 1990;**53**:262–77.

60 Beauford JE, McNiel DE, Binder RL. Utility of the initial therapeutic alliance in evaluating psychiatric patients' risk of violence. *Am J Psychiatry* 1997;**154**:1272–6.

61 Warren J, Beadsmore A. Preventing violence on mental health wards. *Nurs Times* 1997;**93**:47–8.

62 McDougall T. Coercive interventions: the notion of the "last resort". *Psychiatric Care* 1997;**4**:19–21.

63 Doulton P, personal communication.

64 Reed J. Risk assessment and clinical risk management: the lessons from recent inquiries. *Br J Psychiatry* 1997;**170**(32):4–7.

65 Hawton K, Fagg J, Simkin S, *et al. Attempted suicide in Oxford 1995.* Oxford: University Department of Psychiatry, 1996.

66 Hawton K, Fagg J, Simkin S, *et al.* Trends in deliberate self-harm in Oxford, 1985–1995. *Br J Psychiatry* 1997;**171**:556–60.

67 King E. Suicide in the mentally ill: an epidemiological sample and implications for clinicians. *Br J Psychiatry* 1994;**165**:658–63.
68 Drake RE, Gates C, Cotton PG. Suicide among schizophrenics: who is at risk? *J Nerv Ment Dis* 1984;**172**:613–17.
69 Meltr HY. Suicide in schizophrenia: risk factors and clozapine treatment. *J Clin Psychiatry* 1998;**59**(3):15–20.
70 Foster T, Gillespie K, McLelland R. Mental disorders and suicide in Northern Ireland. *Br J Psychiatry* 1997;**170**:447–52.
71 Morgan HG, Williams R. Suicide prevention: the challenge confronted. London: HMSO, 1994.
72 Goldstein RB, Black TW, Nasarallah A, Winokur G. The prediction of suicide. *Arch Gen Psychiatry* 1991;**48**:418–22.
73 Beck AT, Resink HLP, Lettieri D. *The prediction of suicide.* Bowie, Maryland: Charles Press, 1974.
74 Melville A, House A. Understanding deliberate self-harm. *Nurs Times* 1999;**95**:46–7.
75 Dennis M, Beach M, Evans PA, *et al.* An examination of the accident and emergency management of deliberate self-harm. *J Accid Emerg Med* 1997;**14**:311–15.
76 Buglass D, Horton J. The repetition of parasuicide: a comparison of three cohorts. *Br J Psychiatry* 1974;**125**:168–74.
77 Hawton K, Fagg J, Platt S, Hawkins M. Factors associated with suicide after parasuicide in young people. *BMJ* 1993;**306**:1641–4.
78 Crawford MJ, Wessely S. Does initial management affect the rate of repetition of deliberate self-harm? Cohort study. *BMJ* 1998;**317**:985.
79 Van Heeringen C, Jannes S, Buylaert W, *et al.* The management of non-compliance with referral to outpatient after-care among attempted suicide patients: a controlled intervention study. *Psychol Med* 1995;**25**:963–70.
80 Morgan H, Jones E, Owen J. Secondary prevention of non-fatal deliberate self-harm. The Green Card Study. *Br J Psychiatry* 1993;**163**:111–13.
81 Anon. Selective serotonin reuptake inhibitors for depression? *Drug Therapies Bull* 1993;**31**:57–8.
82 Salkovskis PM, Atha C, Storer D. Cognitive-behavioural problem solving in the treatment of patients who repeatedly attempt suicide. *Br J Psychiatry* 1990;**157**:571–6.
83 Linehan MM, Armstrong HE, Suarez A, *et al.* Cognitive-behavioural treatment of chronically parasuicidal borderline patients. *Arch Gen Psychiatry* 1991;**48**:1061–4.
84 Watts D, Morgan HG. Malignant alienation. *Br J Psychiatry* 1994;**164**:11–15.
85 Morgan HG, Priest P. Suicide and other unexpected deaths among psychiatric patients. *BMJ* 1991;**158**:308–74.
86 Goldcare M, Seagrott V, Hawton K. Suicide after discharge from psychiatric care. *Lancet* 1993;**342**:283–6.
87 Amchin J, Wettslein RM, Roth LH. Suicide, ethics and the law. In: Blumenthal SJ, Kupfer DJ, eds. *Suicide over the life cycle,* 637–63. Washington DC: American Psychiatric Press, 1990.
88 Cantor CH, McDermott PM. Suicide litigation: an Australian survey. *Aust NZ J Psychiatry* 1994;**28**:426–30.
89 Department of Health. *The Care Programme Approach for People with a Mental Illness Referred to the Specialist Psychiatrist Service.* HC(90)23/LASSL(90)11. London: DoH, 1990.
90 Department of Health. *Health of the Nation. Building Bridges: a guide to inter-agency working for the care and protection of severely mentally ill people.* London: DoH, 1995.
91 Wessely SC, Castle D, Douglas AJ, Taylor PJ. The criminal careers of incident cases of schizophrenia. *Psychol Med* 1994;**24**:483–502.
92 Hogman G. *The silent partners.* National Schizophrenia Fellowship, 1995.
93 Lipsedge M. Choices in psychiatry. In: Dunstan GR, Sinebourne EA, eds. *Doctors' decisions: ethical conflicts in medical practice.* Oxford: OUP, 1989.
94 Petch E, Bradley C. Learning the lessons from homicide inquiries: adding insult to injury? *J Forens Psychiatry* 1997;**8**:161–84.

Further reading

Reports giving practical advice on reducing risk

Assessment and clinical management of risk of harm to other people. Council Report CR53. The Royal College of Psychiatrists Special Working Party on Clinical Assessment and Management of Risk. London: Royal College of Psychiatrists, April 1996.

Management of imminent violence: clinical practice guidelines to support mental health services. Occasional Paper OP41. London: Royal College of Psychiatrists, March 1998.

Morgan HG, Williams R. *Suicide prevention: the challenge confronted.* NHS Health Advisory Service Thematic Review. London: HMSO, 1994.

Slade M, Powell R, Strathdee G, Kelsey W. *The Threshold Programme.* Bethlem Royal Hospital.

13 Risk management in general practice

STEPHEN ROGERS

The majority of contacts in general practice are for minor, self limiting illnesses, but practitioners also provide ongoing care to chronically ill patients with complex needs, diagnose serious disease at first presentation, respond to calls for assistance in life threatening situations, and manage preventive care. They have an important role in liaising with other professionals in primary and secondary care and are responsible for managing premises and employed staff who support and/or complement their activities.[1] Recent years have witnessed unprecedented changes in the environment of primary care, with raised patient expectations and demand, increasing responsibility for providing a wider range of services, and greater accountability to patients, professional groups, and to Health Authorities.[2-4] Primary Care Groups (PCGs) have been in place since April 1999. These comprise groups of local healthcare professionals (including general practitioners, nurses, and social service staff) who are vested with a responsibility to improve the health of their communities, to develop primary care and community services, and to advise on the commissioning of hospital services. In this context, PCGs will be required to assure the quality of clinical care by making individuals and organisations accountable for setting, maintaining, and monitoring performance standards.[5] Each PCG has a clinical governance lead whose goal will be to promote a number of inter-linked activities; clinical audit, clinical effectiveness, risk management, quality assurance, together with professional and organisational development.[6]

The Royal College of General Practitioners and Medical Audit Advisory Groups have done important groundwork in promoting quality in general practice, with the last decade witnessing more demanding education and training requirements for general practice, widespread acceptance of audit, and increasing use of clinical guidelines as tools to improve the quality of care.[7] The risk of litigation or complaints has also featured as a consistent and important influence on the care which practitioners provide to their patients.[8] What is new to general practice however, is the thinking that safety, like effectiveness, needs to be explicitly managed and monitored. This chapter begins by presenting information on adverse events associated with medical management in the general practice setting. Then factors which might explain the occurrence of such events are explored, before moving on to a discussion of approaches which might be adopted by individuals, or by organisations, to help avert their occurrence.

Adverse events in the general practice setting

There is no single source of data that can provide information on the incidence of adverse events in the general practice setting. The principal sources of information are medical negligence claims, reviews of primary care deaths, significant event audits, experimental reporting systems, and the literature on adverse drug events. Each of these sources provides a selective view, but together they paint a picture of the kinds of things that can go wrong.

Analyses of completed claims

Medical negligence is proven when a patient suffers harm and it is shown that the harm has resulted from failure on the part of the defendant to act in a manner consistent with that of a "responsible body" of colleagues.[9] The most serious cases of misadventure associated with clinical care in general practice are represented in the claims databases of the medical defence agencies. Delays in diagnosis and treatment account for the majority of completed claims against general practitioners, with adverse outcomes from prescribing errors, or other treatments, appearing less often. Sixty-six per cent of completed claims were attributed to delays in diagnosis and treatment in a series published by the Medical Defence Union,[10] and only 25% to prescribing errors.[11] The medical conditions for which diagnoses were delayed, will be of no surprise to practising doctors. Serious infections (meningitis, pneumonia, epiglottitis and malaria) were the most common group (15%), then orthopaedic conditions including missed fractures, slipped epiphyses, and disabling vertebral disc lesions (14%). Delays in diagnosing common cancers was next (11%), followed by delays in diagnosing appendicitis, pregnancy (ectopic or intra-uterine), diabetes, and myocardial infarction. The drug groups most frequently associated with claims were steroids, antibiotics, contraceptives, anti-coagulants, non-steroidal anti-inflammatory drugs, and opiates, with the last three drug classes associated with 53% of the deaths attributed to prescribing.

Reviews of primary care deaths

Hart and Humphreys[12] examined the medical records of 500 deaths occurring in a defined population served by a single general practice over a 20-year period and found avoidable causal factors in 223 deaths (45%). Avoidable factors attributable to the patient were evident in 26% of all deaths, to the general practitioner in 9% and to the hospital in 2%. A similar exercise is described by Holden et al.[13] In their series of 1263 deaths, avoidable causal factors were found in 682 (54%). As in the earlier study, avoidable factors attributed to patients were the most important (40% of all deaths), with factors attributable to general practitioners in 5%, and factors attributable to the hospital in 6% of all deaths. These studies have methodological limitations; information is likely to be incomplete and the criteria for avoidable factors are "neither standardised nor reproducible", but they provide a useful overview of the scope for clinical risk management in primary care.

Analyses of significant events

Significant event auditing is an approach in which individual cases are discussed by health care staff, with a view to identifying factors which can lead to improvements in the delivery of care.[14] The cases are selected on account of an occurrence which is considered to be significant (usually, but not necessarily adverse) and would include patients dying in the primary care setting, and other adverse incidents or outcomes.[14-16] Pringle et al[14] describe a study involving some ten practices in Lincolnshire or Manchester, participating in significant event audits over a year. 489 clinical events (50 events per practice per year) were recorded, with 177 selected for review. These included 41 cases with cardiovascular disease events, 35 concerned with care of chronic diseases, 31 events in the care of patients with cancer (mainly around diagnosis); 15 related to contraception and women's health; 12 to suicide, attempted suicide, violent deaths and trauma, and 13 related to infections including 4 of meningitis. Delays in diagnosis and treatment were represented in this series, a number of acute medical conditions where preventive care was questioned, cases where there were evident communication difficulties, and some medication errors. Action points for improving care were identified for over half of the cases reviewed, and ranged from exhortations to be more careful and plans for educational activity, through to the drafting of new practice protocols and policies.

Incident reporting systems

Britt *et al*[17] set up a monitoring system for documenting adverse or potential adverse events in Australian general practice. Five hundred and ten GPs from membership lists of research and professional groups were invited to participate and 297 (42%) agreed. General practitioners were sent incident reporting forms and asked to provide details of "any unintended event, no matter how seemingly trivial or commonplace, that could have harmed or did harm a patient". The findings are interesting, in that of the first 805 reports received, 51% of reported incidents were related to pharmacological treatments, 42% due to other treatments and 34% due to diagnostic errors. The reason for this relative over-representation of incidents related to pharmacological treatments (compared to other data sources) is open to speculation, but factors might include selective reporting and familiarity with surveillance systems for reporting adverse drug reactions. The pattern does not seem to be due to increased reporting of "near misses" with pharmacological therapy, as 18% of incidents were associated with serious adverse consequences for patients (compared to 21% in the series overall).

Adverse drug reactions and prescribing errors

In its broadest sense, an adverse drug reaction is an undesirable effect caused by a drug, usually excluding intentional or accidental poisoning and drug abuse. It is notoriously difficult to establish that an adverse event is the effect of a drug and of those adverse reactions which do occur, the majority are known, often mild and might even be considered trivial in the context within which they occur. For example, in one general practice-based study, Martys[18] found that 41% of his patients reported some sort of adverse reaction (mainly effects on the gastro-intestinal tract and central nervous system) when interviewed one week after starting a new drug. In contrast, Mulroy[19] documented a patient initiated consultation rate of closer to 3% in a study of follow up consultations for iatrogenic illness (mainly drug associated). This series includes patients with more serious adverse effects including acute glaucoma with tricyclic antidepressants, gastrointestinal bleeding with aspirin, intrahepatic obstruction with chlorpromazine, and severe facial herpes simplex in a patient on steroids. Some might have been preventable, though the degree to which this may have been the case was not formally assessed.

In another study, Shulman *et al*[20] worked with local pharmacists to monitor potential adverse drug reactions (ADRs) and prescription errors. During the three-year study, a total of 64 406 items were dispensed on 33 593 NHS prescriptions and 86 potential ADRs were picked up. Again this approximates to about 3% of patients for whom prescriptions were offered, and while these errors were relatively rare, some could have had serious consequences (for example one asthmatic patient was prescribed propranolol and two patients on monoamine oxidase inhibitors were prescribed sympathomimetics).

A number of other studies using a similar approach have since been published and rates of potential adverse drug reactions and/or prescribing errors for scripts issued in primary care and presented at community pharmacies have been in the range 0·5–6%.[21-23]

Determinants of adverse events in general practice

The reasons why avoidable adverse events occur to patients are always complex. A short consultation with a patient might involve a number of decisions being taken, and the consultation itself is a mere segment of a patient care pathway which could involve diagnostic testing, follow up, initiation and maintenance of treatment, referral, and liaison with secondary care. At every point there is a risk of error, and a variety of factors can have implications for the safety of the patient. Such factors may operate at the level of the individual health professional, in relation to the particular healthcare process, or as a feature of the organisation in which care is delivered.

Doctors' characteristics

The General Medical Council now emphasises the importance of the quality of professional relationships with patients alongside more traditional expectations of doctors to provide high quality care, and to maintain proberty in professional matters.[24] Similarly, in *Tomorrow's Doctors*,[25] the importance of acquiring appropriate clinical knowledge and practical skills appears cheek by jowl with the need for proficiency in communication skills. It is interesting to speculate on the relationship between these aspects of clinical competence and of safety in medicine.

Sloan et al [26] published an important study in which the characteristics of doctors with favourable and unfavourable claims were compared. Doctors with more prestigious credentials did no better than those with less prestigious credentials in any speciality, and there was no association with country of qualification, solo or group practice, or involvement in research or teaching. Levinson et al [27] studied the relationship between communication skills and malpractice claims amongst primary care doctors and surgeons. Although no relationships were noted amongst the surgeons, primary care physicians with claims were characterised by shorter clinic visits and particular modes of communication. In particular "claims" physicians used less orienting statements (for example explaining what was

245

going to happen next), and less facilitating comments (asking opinions and checking understanding).

The literature is consistent in the respect that complaints about doctors are more usually about communication problems rather than issues around technical competency. While there is no study, which directly addresses doctor–patient communication and safety, there is good evidence that particular aspects of communication skills can effect patient satisfaction, adherence and co-operation with management plans and it seems likely that doctors with appropriate communication skills are likely to be safer as well as more popular.[28]

Factors influencing doctors' decision making

There is a large literature on medical decision making[29] and a selection of studies that enquire into factors which can lead to physician error. Two studies of primary care doctors, bring out some common themes.

Ely et al[30] interviewed 53 family doctors in Iowa, USA. The data is based on in-depth interviews in which physicians were asked to describe their most memorable error and the perceived causes. The investigators developed a classification of perceived causes and found these to fall within one of four groups: physician stress (being hurried or distracted), process of care factors (for example premature closure of the diagnostic process), patient related factors (for example misleading or normal findings), and physician characteristics (for example lack of knowledge). Often these were acting together, with physician stress relevant in 91% of errors, process of care factors in 91%, patient-related factors in 72% and physician characteristics in 62%.

Bradley[31] carried out another qualitative study, this one focused on uncomfortable prescribing decisions in UK general practice. Seventy-four doctors provided details of 307 incidents in which they had felt uncomfortable with their prescribing. Antibiotics, tranquillisers or hypnotics were the drugs most often involved. Reasons given for decisions taken were patient expectation, clinical appropriateness, factors related to the doctor–patient relationship, and being led by preceding events. Logistic problems such as lack of time, a wish to avoid drug toxicity, a need to close the consultation, drug costs, and seeking to avoid extra work also appeared, if less frequently.

As these studies are based on physicians' perceptions they cannot provide a basis for assessing the relative importance of various factors. However, they do show the importance of social and logistic influences on decisions taken in primary care. In particular, the environment in which the doctor works and the nature of the doctor–patient relationship can have a capricious influence on the decision making process.

Practice procedures

Practice policies and procedures for arranging appointments and follow up consultations, emergency care and home visits, communications with secondary care providers, the review of test results, and the management of repeat prescriptions can have a direct influence on the risk of adverse events occurring to patients. Such problems were frequently identified as contributory factors to adverse events in significant event audit data[14] and in the Australian incident reporting study[32].

Apparent failures of practice procedures also feature prominently in data on complaints made about general practitioners and the service they offer. Owen[33] describes a series of 1000 complaints notified to the Medical Protection Society during 1976–88. About 50% of complaints arose in situations where complainants felt there had been inappropriate delay in diagnosis, treatment or referral, and 30% of these occurred specifically as a result of a failure to carry out a home visit. A further 8% of complaints were precipitated by errors in prescribing. Delays may result from poor communication with patients, or errors of judgement, but can also be introduced by poor administrative systems within practices (for example referral letters or test results being mislaid). The issue of dealing with requests for home visits continues to exercise the profession. General practitioners no longer have a contractual obligation to conduct home visits "unless medically indicated" but the effectiveness of assessment procedures used and the threshold for visiting could determine whether patients are put at risk.[34] Wrongly written prescriptions which could not be dispensed accounted for some of the prescribing errors in this series, but more serious errors of dosage and drug and the prescription of contraindicated drugs were also represented.

Practice characteristics

There are considerable variations in the levels of development of practices in the United Kingdom and elsewhere.[36,37] Baker[36] devised a development score based on a questionnaire assessment of equipment, staff, clinical activities, records, organisation, premises, availability and clinics and found a wide variation across three counties in England. In a multiple regression analysis he found that being a training practice, having a practice manager, a larger total number of patients, and a lower Jarman score for underprivileged areas was associated with higher levels of practice development.

However, research to date has shown no clear relationships between practice characteristics, their level of development and the quality of care they offer. For example, Ram et al [37] carried out a study of 93 GPs, who agreed to submit videotapes of their consultations. A range of practice characteristics were assessed and a validated instrument was used to assess physician performance (competence and communication skills). The authors of this study concluded that practice structure and clinical performance were not related and suggested that although each might effect particular patient outcomes, they need not be associated within individual practices. In another study, lower patient satisfaction was associated with increasing list size, shared patient lists and being a training practice, which suggests an inverse relationship between practice development and some aspects of quality of care.[38]

Lower admission rates for asthma are to be found in practices whose prescribing rates suggests better preventive care and lower admission rates for diabetes in practices with better organised diabetic care[39,40] but no clear links have been demonstrated between admission rates and practice characteristics such as the number of partners, list size or staffing patterns. Another study of admission rates for chronic diseases also draws attention to the importance of socio-demographic and hospital, rather than general practice, factors as determinants of hospital admissions,[41] and similar conclusions are drawn in a third study of admissions from 120 general practices in South London.[42]

Inevitably there will be relationships between some aspects of practice structure and whether the care offered is safe and effective. However, the huge variations in the way practices are organised, and the effects of individual as well as organisational factors on the quality of care make it hard or impossible to elucidate the relevance of individual practice characteristics in simple quantitative studies.

Preventing adverse events in general practice

A number of strategies might be adopted to help reduce the occurrence of unintended adverse events in primary care. Some of these would operate at the level of the consultation between doctors and patients, while others would relate more to the organisation and management of the practice. Some would be managed and promoted on a locality basis, for example at PCG level, while others require promotion through medical school curricula or national frameworks.

The consultation

The consultation is central to the experience of general practice.[43-45] The consultation as the setting for risk management is a new focus, but current developments in a number of areas are relevant and growth in the literature on this important issue is to be expected.

Clinical guidelines

Clinical guidelines are "systematically developed statements to assist practitioner and patient decisions about appropriate health care for specific clinical circumstances".[46] The potential for guidelines to affect the quality of patient care is considerable[47] and the acceptance of, and familiarity with, clinical guidelines is growing.[48,49] In a systematic review of the 59 published evaluations of guidelines implemented by a variety of means, all but four detected significant improvements in the process of care.[50]

High quality, evidence-based guidelines are now available for many of the common conditions which are managed in primary care.[51-54] Their implementation might be expected to reduce acts of omission on the part of general practitioners, and to help prevent associated adverse outcomes for patients. Evidence-based materials on the predictive value of various diagnostic manoeuvres are also important to the practising physician, who needs to make rational choices about test ordering or changing referral thresholds, and to avoid missing important diagnoses. A series of papers appearing in the *Journal of the American Medical Association* provide an excellent overview of the issues.[55-58]

Decision analysis

Formal decision analysis has typically been used in research settings, to combine data from various studies, in order to determine optimal strategies for particular clinical situations. In formal decision analysis different diagnostic and management options are drawn out like the branches of a tree, with branches allocated numerical values corresponding to the likely benefits and risks of pursuing a particular course of action.[59] The approach is becoming more well known[60-63] and optimists hope that eventually there might be a library of computerised decision trees which could be linked up with diagnostic codes in electronic records.[64] Greenhalgh and Young[65] show how decision analysis can contribute to the consultation with individual patients, but point out that the relevant information is often not readily accessible, and that skills at assessing the values and perspectives of individual patients remain paramount. For example, it is notoriously difficult to portray the risks and benefits of even commonly met problems and the way the information is presented (verbal, tabular or graphical presentations, leaflets, videos, web pages etc.) can have a very significant effect on its meaning and impact.[66]

Computerised decision support

Various computer systems have been described which might aid clinical decision making, and some have been evaluated in research studies.[67] Systems which provide prompts to encourage doctors to perform preventive

249

procedures have delivered demonstrable benefits in the care of hypertension[68,69] and in cervical screening[70]. Systems to improve the safety of prescribed drugs also show great potential. For example, in an American trial, a computer system designed to give advice on warfarin dosage was shown to lead to better control than usual care,[71] and systems for supporting use of digoxin might reduce the risk of digoxin toxicity.[72] Computerised decision support to aid diagnoses have been more disappointing, though their low impact has largely been attributed to a failure to utilise the systems rather than to the quality of the systems as such.[73,74]

Computers are widely used in general practice, though mainly to store and retrieve information and to simplify administrative processes like the organisation of appointments and the printing of repeat prescriptions.[75] General practice computer software systems are now becoming increasingly sophisticated and a fully developed prescribing system will check the name of a drug against previous drug idiosyncrasies held in the patient record, against possible interactions with current medications, and against conditions in the patient record for which the drug is contraindicated. Many systems will carry out simple calculations and compare individual measures with standards, or calculate risk scores from combinations of variables and computerised decision support in primary care may be an area due for further growth.[76]

Shared decision making

Consumerism and increasing availability of information has shifted the emphasis of doctor–patient decision making away from paternalistic transfer of information from doctor to patient.[77] Shared decision making is said to sit somewhere between paternalism and informed choice and is increasingly advocated as the ideal model for treatment decision making in the medical encounter.[66,78,79] Five steps are described: understanding patients' views on treatment options, eliciting patients' preferences, transferring technical information, weighing up risks and benefits then sharing the recommendation and/or affirming the treatment preferences.[66]

It has been argued that the key dimensions of communication represented in the shared decision making model, are the same as those which have been associated with positive outcomes in empirical studies.[66] As yet there is no information to suggest that shared decision making will be associated with safer care, though it seems likely that the information sharing process and the associated patient empowerment could have a positive effect on risk avoidance. The ethical and medico-legal issues associated with the shared decision making model are not straightforward, and experience and expertise are required to ensure balance between opposing positions (consumers versus passive recipient) which patients might wish to adopt in different situations and at different times. It has been argued a move towards "informed choice" could be a consequence of doctors behaving defensively. However the model provides more than a medico-legal defence in the event a patient suffers harm, as the communication strategies adopted are also those more likely to be associated with constructive mediation between the parties.[28]

Quality assurance in the practice

It is argued that the most appropriate model for assuring quality in general practice is one which is managed by individual practices on behalf of the patients they serve.[7] Risk management is explicitly one of the components of quality assurance activity in health services[80] and this section focuses on approaches advocated to assure the safety of the organisational systems in the primary care setting.

Addressing complaints

A general practitioner who is a principal on the list of a health authority is subject to statutory obligations to "render to his patients all necessary and appropriate services of the type usually provided by medical practitioners" under their terms of service. In a survey carried out by Summerton[8] in 1994, 98% of general practitioners reported having made changes to counter the risk of patients lodging complaints or taking legal action in response to perceived inadequacies in care. Such changes included lowering thresholds for referral, avoiding treating certain conditions, increased diagnostic testing and follow-up, reduced prescription of unnecessary drugs, increased screening, increased audit, more detailed note taking, and more detailed explanations to patients.

Following the Wilson Report,[81] the highly adversarial complaints system involving service committee hearings was replaced by a two stage system, in which the first stage is an in-house reconciliation procedure. The vast majority of complaints are now defused at the level of the practice.[82] Such complaints can still provide a good source of data for quality improvement activities.[83] For example, complaints can provide information on issues which are relevant to patient satisfaction, and to the functioning of practice systems such as message taking and appointments.[11] The analysis of complaints has recently been advocated as a core component for clinical governance.[6]

Death registers

Hart and Humpherys[12] argued that "A retrospective search for avoidable factors in individual deaths is perhaps the most stringent form of self criticism available to any clinical team". In a similar exercise, Holden *et al*[13]

251

developed a protocol that was shared across four practices. This group emphasised the educational value of the exercise and participating practices are examining deaths on an ongoing basis. The efficacy of the approach in making practice safer is as yet unknown. One of the barriers to the systematic analyses of deaths is the lack of routine data on deaths occurring in practice, though providing a death register will not, on its own, result in improvements in the organisation of care.[84]

Significant event auditing

The approach draws on the philosophy of the critical incident technique, originally developed and applied to the analysis of accidents in the aviation industry,[85] though a key difference between significant event auditing in general practice and the critical incident technique as originally described, is the emphasis given to drawing on the experience of a group of informants.[14,16] Particular attention is given to managing the dynamics of the group, so that individuals can openly discuss inadequacies in care. An external facilitator may be employed to good effect or the participants themselves may run the process. "Individual cases in which there has been a significant occurrence" are analysed in a detailed way to ascertain what can be learned about the overall quality of care and to indicate changes which might lead to future improvements".[14] Some commentators advocate a structured enquiry into various areas including the immediate management of a case, preventive care, arrangements for follow up, interface and team issues, and action points arising.[14] Alternatively, the discussion is deliberately kept open and far reaching, with post hoc classification of findings into various categories.[15] Whichever approach is taken, there is an assumption that the emotional engagement with issues of concern is an important motivating factor in subsequent delivery of change.

Audits of clinical care and administration

Medical audit as a strategy for quality assurance is well established in primary care.[86] A systematic review of the effect of audit and feedback on professional behaviour has demonstrated that the approach can lead to improvements in performance, especially with respect to prescribing and test ordering.[87,88] Of course, audit and feedback should not be used generally for all problems, but should be targeted towards areas where the approach is likely to generate change.[88] Pringle et al[14] attempted to compare the effect of conventional audit and significant event audit in 20 practices. Practices using conventional audit covered fewer areas of clinical care, but areas covered were done in greater depth. In their conclusions, the researchers suggest that conventional audit and significant event auditing should in fact be used as complementary approaches. Other advocates of significant event auditing now explicitly link the information gathering process, inherent to the significant event audit, to a conventional audit which serves as the implementation phase in a "double loop audit cycle".[16]

Continuous quality improvement

Continuous quality improvement is an approach to quality assurance which is underpinned by a focus on the improvement of the systems required to deliver quality care. Positive outcomes are achieved by involving key organisational members, and by the application of a range of tools and techniques for studying health systems. Cycles of improvement are envisaged and measures are identified such that improvements can be monitored.[89] The approach has been applied both to administrative and clinical problems, and the approach is particularly suited to problems where the two overlap. As continuous quality improvement is specifically directed towards systems improvement, there are many examples where its application has implications for risk management. For example, Kibbe et al [90] used the approach to address continuity of care issues in a University based family practice, Pachclartz et al [91] overhauled a cervical screening service, and Rawes[92] used the approach to engineer "the perfect prescription procedure". Specific skills and a high degree of motivation are required to apply continuous quality improvement methods, but a particular strength is that the approach integrates the investigative features of approaches like significant event auditing, then explicitly identifies and addresses health systems problems that get in the way of desirable outcomes.[93]

Undergraduate and postgraduate medical education

The training of competent doctors with good communication skills and the reinforcement of appropriate attitudes and practice during undergraduate medical education set important precedents which will apply throughout the career of a doctor.[25] Many of these attributes are emphasised during vocational training for general practice.[94] It is hoped that new initiatives to promote and support continuing professional development will provide opportunities for busy general practitioners to take time out of practice to address their educational needs, to reflect on their practice and to address quality issues within the organisations they manage.[95]

Undergraduate education

Attitudinal objectives are given much greater emphasis in modern medical school curricula[25] than was previously the case and a move towards teaching these in a general practice setting is a recognition of the importance of these in the primary care setting, and the abilities of general practitioners to teach them.[94] All doctors need to be able to recognise acute serious illness. For the medical generalist the exclusion of acute serious illness is a key function in any consultation, and diagnostic skills learned at medical school will be brought to bear to assess a range of more or less specific presentations: abdominal pain, headache, chest pain, fever and so on. While these conditions are likely to be included in the core curricula of all medical schools, the clinical epidemiology of these conditions, and the issue of diagnostic uncertainty should also be represented. Likewise, the principles of screening and case finding are important in the detection of treatable chronic illness and the integration of public health principles into the teaching of undergraduates will make an important contribution.[25]

Vocational training for general practice

Communication skills and attitudinal objectives are perhaps given more explicit attention in the training of the medical generalist than in the training of any medical specialist. The consultation is the focus of much of the work during vocational training and consultation skills include not only communication skills, but also the ability to assimilate information from various sources, note keeping and summarising records, issues around safe prescribing and mechanisms for ensuring appropriate follow up and continuity of care.[96,97] Summative assessment for training in general practice was introduced on 1 September 1996. A year later an Act of Parliament was to make satisfactory completion of vocational training a legal requirement for doctors wishing to work as general practitioners in the National Health Service.[98] Professional training in other specialities depends on completion of professional examinations and accredited training posts but summative assessment for general practice includes not only written papers, but also videotaped assessments of consultation skills, satisfactory completion of a practice based audit and a trainers' report which would cover clinical competence, professionalism, reliability and organisational skills.[99]

Continuing professional development

The old system for the continuing medical education (CME) of general practitioners in the United Kingdom is due to be swept away with the introduction of professional practice development plans. It is proposed that the professional practice development plan will be a vehicle by which the educational activities of individual members of healthcare staff will be explicitly linked to their professional development needs and to the overall development needs of their practices.[95] Although there is little detail as to how all this will work, the approach does provide an opportunity to develop multi-professional working and to link education and quality improvement activities.[100,101] Primary care groups are beginning to insist on practices constructing practice professional development plans as a clinical governance activity[6] and it is likely that they will be a requirement when reaccreditation is introduced into general practice.[102] As yet, there is little experience with the approach in the health sector, but this experience is likely to grow rapidly in the future.[103]

Summary and conclusions

Avoidable adverse incidents occur to patients in primary care as in any other sector of healthcare. Errors of omission may be more important in this sector than is the case for inpatient care, although adverse effects relating to drug use also remain important. The absolute numbers of adverse events are not known, but because of the large numbers of contacts in primary care, even very low rates can generate large numbers of cases.

Communication skills are likely to be important both in avoiding adverse outcomes and in avoiding litigation, and social and logistic influences in the general practice setting, as well as clinical evidence, are important influences on clinical decisions taken. There does not seem to be any clear association between the risk of adverse events and the size or level of services offered by practices, but the integrity of various practice systems might have a bearing on the risk of adverse events occurring. Clinical guidelines are gaining acceptance in general practice, and in the context of shared decision making might be expected to make an important contribution to risk management in the consultation. Audit work is well established as an integral function of modern general practice and systems thinking, as represented in continuous quality improvement, is becoming better known. The educational framework for training young doctors, and especially for the postgraduate training and continuing professional development of general practitioners, is a positive force for insuring that general practitioners and the organisations they run are both safe and effective.

Further work is required to establish the frequency of adverse events in the primary care sector and the underlying factors that account for them. Aids to support shared decision making in the consultation are required and further experimentation with continuous quality improvement techniques in the primary care setting could be fruitful.

References

1 Fry J. *General practice. The facts.* Oxford: Radcliffe, 1993.
2 NHSE. *Primary care. The future.* London: HMSO, 1996.

3 NHSE. *The New NHS. Modern, dependable.* London: HMSO, 1997.

4 HHSE. A first class service: quality in the new NHS. HSC(98)113. London: DoH, 1998.

5 Butler T, Roland M. How will primary care groups work? *BMJ* 1998;**316**:214.

6 Roland M, Baker R. *Clinical governance. A practical guide for primary care teams.* Manchester: University of Manchester, 1999.

7 Irvine D. *Managing for quality in general practice.* London: Kings Fund, 1990.

8 Summerton N. Positive and negative factors in defensive medicine: a questionnaire study of general practitioners. *BMJ* 1995;**310**:27–9.

9 Scott W. *The general practitioner and the law of negligence.* 2nd edition. London: Cavendish, 1995.

10 Green S, Lee R, Moss J. *Problems in general practice. Delay in diagnosis.* Manchester: Medical Defence Union, 1998.

11 Green S, Goodwin H, Moss J. *Problems in general practice. Medication errors.* Manchester: Medical Defence Union, 1996.

12 Hart JT, Humphreys C. Be your own coroner: an audit of 500 consecutive deaths in a general practice. *BMJ* 1987;**294**:871–4.

13 Holden J, O'Donnell S, Brindley J, Miles L. Analysis of 1263 deaths in four general practices. *Br J Gen Pract* 1998;**48**:1409–12.

14 Pringle M, Bradley CP, Carmichael CM, *et al.* Significant event auditing. A study of the feasibility and potential of case-based auditing in primary medical care. Occasional Paper 70. London: Royal College of General Practitioners, 1995.

15 Berlin A, Spencer JA, Bhopal RS, van Zwanenberg TD. Audit of deaths in general practice: pilot study of critical incident technique. *Qual Health Care* 1992;**1**:231–5.

16 Robinson LA, Stacy R, Spencer JA, Bhopal RS. Use of facilitated case discussions for significant event auditing. *BMJ* 1995;**311**:315–18.

17 Britt H, Miller GC, Steve ID, *et al.* Collecting data on potentially harmful events: a method for monitoring incidents in general practice. *Fam Pract* 1997;**14**:101–6.

18 Martys CR. Adverse reactions to drugs in general practice. *BMJ* 1979;**2**:1194–7.

19 Mulroy R. Iatrogenic disease in general practice: its incidence and effects. *BMJ* 1973;**2**:407–10.

20 Shulman JI, Shulman S, Haines AP. The prevention of adverse drug reactions – a potential role for pharmacists in the primary care team? *J R Coll Gen Pract* 1981;**31**:429–31.

21 Caleo S, Benrimoj S, Collins D, *et al.* Clinical evaluation of pharmacists' interventions. *Int J Pharm Pract* 1996;**4**:221–7.

22 Stevens RG, Balon D. Detection of hazardous drug/drug interactions in a community pharmacy and subsequent intervention. *Int J Pharm Pract* 1997;**5**:142–8.

23 Westerlund T, Almarsdottir AB, Melander A. Drug related problems and pharmacy interventions in community practice. *Int J Pharm Pract* 1999;**7**:40–50.

24 General Medical Council. *Maintaining good medical practice.* London: GMC, 1998.

25 General Medical Council. *Tomorrow's doctors. Recommendations on undergraduate medical education.* London: GMC, 1993.

26 Sloan FA, Mergenhagen PM, Burfield WB, *et al.* Medical malpractice experience of physicians. *JAMA* 1989;**262**:3291–7.

27 Levinson W, Roter DL, Malloly JP, *et al.* Physician–patient communication. The relationship with malpractice claims among primary care physicians and patients. *JAMA* 1997;**277**:553–9.

28 Stewart M, Brown JB, Boon H, *et al.* Evidence on patient–doctor communication. *Cancer Prevent Control* 1999;**3**:25–30.

29 Dowie J, Elstein A. *Professional judgement. A reader in clinical decision making.* Cambridge: CUP, 1988.

30 Ely JW, Levinson W, Elder W, *et al.* Perceived causes of family physicians' errors. *J Fam Pract* 1995;**40**:337–44.

31 Bradley CP. Uncomfortable prescribing decisions: a critical incident study. *BMJ* 1992;**304**:294–6.

32 Bhasale AL, Miller GC, Reid SE, Britt HC. Analysing potential harm in Australian general practice – an incident monitoring study. *Med J Aust* 1998;**169**:73–6.

33 Owen C. Formal complaints against general practitioners: a study of 1000 cases. *Br J Gen Pract* 1991; 113–15.

34 Norwell N. Visits revisited. *J Med Def Union* 1999;**15**(3);15–17.
35 Neville RG, Robertson F, Livingstone S, Crombie IK. A classification of prescription errors. *J R Coll Gen Pract* 1989;**39**:110–12.
36 Baker R. General practice in Gloucestershire, Avon and Somerset: explaining variations in standards. *Br J Gen Pract* 1992;**42**:415–18.
37 Ram P, Grol R, van den Hombergh P, *et al.* Structure and process: the relationship between practice management and actual clinical performance in general practice. *Fam Pract* 1998;**15**:354–62.
38 Baker R. Characteristics of practices, general practitioners and patients related to levels of patients' satisfaction with consultations. *Br J Gen Pract* 1996;**46**:601–5.
39 Aveyard P. Monitoring the performance of general practices. *J Eval Clin Pract* 1997;**3**:275–81.
40 Farmer A, Coulter A. Organisation of care for diabetic patients in general practice: influence on hospital admissions. *Br J Gen Pract* 1990;**40**:56–8.
41 Giuffrida A, Gravelle H, Roland M. Measuring quality of care with routine data: avoiding confusion between performance indicators and health outcomes. *BMJ* 1999;**319**:94–8.
42 Reid FDA, Cook D, Majeed A. Explaining variation in hospital admission rates between general practices: cross sectional study. *BMJ* 1999;**319**:98–103.
43 Sullivan FM, McNaughton RJ. Evidence in consultations: interpreted and individualised. *Lancet* 1996;**348**:941–943.
44 Byrne PS, Long BFL. *Doctors talking to patients.* London: HMSO, 1976.
45 Pendleton D, Schofield T, Tate P, Havelock P. *The consultation: an approach to learning and teaching.* Oxford: OUP, 1987.
46 Field MJ, Lohr KN. *Clinical practice guidelines: direction of a new program.* Washington DC: National Academy Press, 1990.
47 Effective Health Care. *Implementing clinical practice guidelines.* University of Leeds, 1994.
48 Siwardena AN. Clinical guidelines in primary care: a survey of general practitioners' attitudes and behaviour. *Br J Gen Pract* 1995;**45**:643–7.
49 Newton J, Knight D, Woolhead G. General practitioners and clinical guidelines: a survey of knowledge, use and beliefs. *Br J Gen Pract* 1996;**46**:513–17.
50 Grimshaw JM, Russell IT. Effect of clinical guidelines on medical practice: a systematic review of rigorous evaluations. *Lancet* 1993;**342**:1317–22.
51 Scottish Intercollegiate Guidelines Network. *The care of diabetic patients in Scotland. Prevention of visual impairment.* Edinburgh: SIGN, 1996.
52 Scottish Intercollegiate Guidelines Network. *Helicobacter pylori. Eradication therapy in dyspeptic disease.* Edinburgh: SIGN, 1996.
53 North of England Evidence based Guideline Development Project. Guideline on the use of aspirin as secondary prophylaxis for vascular disease in primary care. *BMJ* 1998;**316**:1303–9.
54 North of England Evidence based Guideline Development Project. Guideline for ACE inhibitor use in primary care management of adults with symptomatic heart failure. *BMJ* 1998;**316**:1369–75.
55 Sackett D. A primer on the precision and accuracy of the clinical examination. *JAMA* 1992;**267**:2638–44.
56 Badgett RG, Lucey C, Mulrow C. Can the clinical examination diagnose left sided heart failure in adults? *JAMA* 1997;**277**:1712–19.
57 Margolis P, Gadomski A. Does this infant have pneumonia? *JAMA* 1998;**279**:308–13.
58 Anand SS, Wells PS, Hunt D, *et al.* Does this patient have deep vein thrombosis? *JAMA* 1998;**279**:1094–9.
59 Thornton JG, Lilford RJ, Johnson N. Decision analysis in medicine. *BMJ* 1992;**302**:1099–103.
60 Pauker SP, Pauker SG. Prenatal diagnosis: a directive approach to genetic counselling using decision analysis. *Yale J Med Biol* 1977;**50**:275–89.
61 Tomkins RK, Burnes DC, Cable WE. An analysis of the cost-effectiveness of pharyngitis management and acute rheumatic fever prevention. *Ann Int Med* 1977;**84**:481–92.
62 Tsevat J, Weinstein MC, Williams LW, Tosteson AN, Goldman L. Expected gains in life expectancy for various coronary heart disease risk factor modifications. *Circulation* 1991;**83**:1194–201.

63 Naimark DM, Naglie G, Detsky AS. The meaning of life expectancy: what is a clinically significant gain? *J Gen Intern Med* 1994;**9**:702–7.
64 Doubilet P, McNeil BJ. Clinical decision making. In: Dowie J, Elstein A, eds. *Professional judgement. A reader in clinical decision making.* Cambridge: CUP, 1988.
65 Greenhalgh P, Young G. In: Silagy C, Haines A, eds. *Evidence based practice in primary care.* London: BMJ Publications, 1998.
66 Elwyn G, Edwards A, Kinnersley P. Shared decision making in primary care: the neglected second half of the consultation. *Br J Gen Pract* 1999;**49**:477–82.
67 Hunt DL, Haynes RB, Hanna SE, Smith K. Effects of computer based clinical decision support systems on physician performance and patient outcomes: a systematic review. *JAMA* 1998;**280**:1339–46.
68 Barnett GO, Winickoff RN, Morgan MM, Zielstorff RD. A computer based monitoring system for follow up of elevated blood pressure. *Med Care* 1983;**21**:400–9.
69 McAlister NH, Covvey HD, Tong C, *et al.* Randomised controlled trial of computer assisted management of hypertension in primary care. *BMJ* 1986;**293**:670–4.
70 McDowell I, Newell C, Rosser W. Computerised reminders to encourage cervical screening in family practice. *J Fam Pract* 1989;**28**:420–4.
71 White RH, Hong R, Venook AP, *et al.* Initiation of warfarin therapy: comparison of physician dosing with computer-assisted dosing. *J Gen Intern Med* 1987;**2**:141–8.
72 White RH, Lindsay A, Pryor TA, *et al.* Application of a computerised medical decision-making process to the problem of digoxin intoxication. *J Am Coll Cardiol* 1984;**4**:571–6.
73 Pozen MW, D'Agostino RB, Selker HP, *et al.* A predictive instrument to improve coronary care unit admission practices in acute ischaemic heart disease. A prospective multi-centre trial. *New Engl J Med* 1984;**310**:1273–8.
74 Wellwood J, Johannessen S, Spiegelhalter DJ. How does computer aided diagnosis improve management of acute abdominal pain? *Ann R Coll Surg Engl* 1992;**74**:40–6.
75 Social Surveys (Gallop Poll) Limited. *Computerisation in GP practices. 1993 survey.* London: DoH, 1993.
76 Preece. J. *The use of computers in general practice.* London: Churchill-Livingstone, 1990.
77 O'Connor AM. Consumer/patient decision support in the new millennium: where should our research take us? *Can J Nurs Res* 1997;**29**:7–12.
78 Deber RB. Physicians in health care management: 8. The patient–physician partnership: decision making, problem solving and the desire to participate. *Can Med Assoc J* 1994;**151**:423–7.
79 Charles C, Gafni A, Whelan T. Shared decision making in the medical encounter: what does it mean? (or it takes at least two to tango). *Soc Sci Med* 1997;**44**:681–92.
80 World Health Organization. The principles of quality assurance. *Qual Assur Health Care* 1989;**1**:79–95.
81 NHSE. *Being heard: the report of review committee on National Health Service complaints procedures.* London: DoH, 1994.
82 McKee L. GPs getting more trivial complaints. *Pulse* 1996 (October), 20.
83 Pietroni PC, de Uray-Ura S. Informal complaints procedure in general practice: first year's experience. *BMJ* 1994;**308**:1546–9.
84 Stacy R, Robinson L, Bhopal R, Spencer J. Evaluation of death registers in general practice. *Br J Gen Pract* 1998;**48**:1739–41.
85 Flanagan JC. The critical incident technique. *Psychol Bull* 1954;**51**:327–58.
86 Lawrence M, Schofield T. *Medical audit in primary health care.* Oxford: OUP, 1993.
87 Balas EA, Boren SA, Brown SA, *et al.* Effect of physician profiling on utilisation. Meta-analysis of randomised clinical trials. *J Gen Intern Med* 1996;**11**:584–90.
88 Thomson MA, Oxman, AD, Davis DA, *et al.* Audit and feedback to improve health professional practice and health care outcomes. In: *The Cochrane Library*, Issue 1. Oxford: Update Software, 1999.
89 Berwick DM, Enthoven A, Bunker JP. Quality management in the NHS: the doctor's role. *BMJ* 1992;**304**:235–9.
90 Kibbe DC, Bentz E, McLaughlin CP. Continuous quality improvement for continuity of care. *J Fam Pract* 1993;**36**:304–8.
91 Pachclarz JA, Abbott MI, Gorman B, *et al.* Continuous quality improvement of Pap smears in an ambulatory care facility. *QRB* 1992;July:229–35.

92 Rawes GD. The perfect prescription procedure. *JAQH* 1994;**2**:55–62.
93 Shortell SM, Bennett CL, Byck GR. Assessing the impact of continuous quality improvement on clinical practice: what it will take to accelerate progress. *Milbank Quart* 1998;**76**:593–624.
94 Whitehouse C, Roland M, Campion P. *Teaching medicine in the community.* Oxford: OUP, 1997.
95 Elwyn GJ. Professional and practice development plans in general practice. *BMJ* 1998;**316**:564–6.
96 Royal College of General Practitioners. *The future general practitioner.* London: RCGP, 1972.
97 JCPTGP. *Assessment and vocational training for general practice: final report of a working party.* (1987/JCPTGP/5). London: JCPT, 1987.
98 Peirara-Gray D. Summative assessment of vocational training: to be required by law. *Br J Gen Pract* 1997;**423**:608–10.
99 Campbell LM, Murray TS. Summative assessment of vocational trainees: results of a 3-year study. *Br J Gen Pract* 1996;**408**:411–14.
100 Field S. Continuing professional development in primary care. *Medical Education* 1998;**32**:564–6.
101 Headrick LA, Wilcock PM, Batalden PB. Interprofessional working and continuing medical education. *BMJ* 1998;**316**:771–4.
102 Parboosingh J. Revalidation for doctors. *BMJ* 1998;**317**:1094–5.
103 Pitts J, Curtis A, While R, Holloway R. "Practice professional development plans": perspectives on proposed changes in general practice education. *Br J Gen Pract* 1999;**49**:959–62.

PART III: THE CONDITIONS OF SAFE PRACTICE

14 Communicating risk to patients and families

JAMES W PICHERT, GERALD B HICKSON

Britain's "Bristol Case" involves the deaths of 29 of 53 babies and young children undergoing two types of cardiac surgery (15 AVSD repairs, 38 arterial switches) between 1988 and 1995 at Bristol Royal Infirmary. A parent of one of four children who survived but suffered brain damage during surgery lamented, "If we had been informed of the mortality rates, we would never have consented to surgery and Ian could be running around like any normal 6-year-old today." The United Bristol Healthcare Trust admitted breaching its duty to Ian "in that it failed to provide accurate information to his parents".[1] In fact, the Bristol inquiry panel found the surgeons to have misled parents about their success rates, thereby denying the parents the facts on which to base truly informed consent.[2] Addressing these surgeons, the General Medical Council's president lectured, "A parent placing a child in a doctor's care must have confidence that the doctor will put the child's best interests before any other. A doctor who fails to live up to that expectation will seriously undermine not only his or her relationship with that particular patient or parents, but the confidence of all patients in doctors".[2,3]

The Bristol case demonstrates the understandable frustration and fury felt by patients and family members when they experience an adverse outcome and a breach of trust, i.e. they believe that they were not informed, that information was withheld, or that they were intentionally misled.[4] Such communication failures not only encourage claims of medical negligence in the face of dramatic adverse events as in the Bristol case, but also contribute to patient non-adherence to medical recommendations and doctor-shopping.[5] The converse is also true. Patients satisfied with physician communications tend to be more compliant and less likely to file suits. Therefore, the imperative recognised by most health professionals is to honestly discuss diagnostic and therapeutic alternatives in ways that appropriately convey medical uncertainties and risks.[6]

263

From Britain's *Patient Charter*:

- You have the right to have any proposed treatment, including any risks involved in that treatment and any alternatives, clearly explained to you before you decide whether to agree to it;

and similarly,

From the *Patient's Bill of Rights* used in many medical centers in the USA:

- You have the right to: Full disclosure from the provider of care about your condition, treatment, prognosis, significant complications, risks, benefits, alternative treatments available, and any additional information required to give informed consent prior to procedures.

Unfortunately, such conversations appear to be relatively rare in practice[7] or otherwise go awry, as illustrated by complaints recorded by various medical centres' patient advocates:

- "The surgeons didn't want to spend time giving my father all the reasons he should have surgery, so [rather than explain the pros and cons] they just said 'take it or leave it'."
- Ms. N complained that when she asked whether there were side effects of the recommended treatment, the doctor was patronising and dismissive, saying, "Now don't you worry your little head about that . . . just keep doing what we told you."
- Mrs. L says that the doctors "scared me to death by telling me about all the things that could go wrong regardless of which option I chose. I've been working hard to have a positive outlook about my illness, and in ten minutes Dr. G destroyed everything I've done to improve my attitude."

Patients, families, and doctors must routinely make therapeutic choices made difficult by the potential for unwanted consequences – the risks – associated with each decision to act or not.[8] Unfortunately, despite promulgation of research, editorials, guidelines, and even legislation, discussing medical risk is subject to many perils, even under ideal circumstances.[9-11] In this chapter we describe the conceptual issues that make risk discussions problematic, discuss common practical barriers that interfere with such discussions, provide a framework for thinking about risk communications, and suggest strategies that may aid risk communications between health professionals, patients and patients' families. We conclude with comments regarding communications following adverse outcomes. Case examples drawn from news reports, journal articles, closed claims of several malpractice insurers, and a patient complaint database[12,13] are used throughout to highlight the practical and philosophical issues faced in one way or another by all who participate in risk communications.

Challenges in risk communications

In their review of the literature on talking about medical risk, Bogardus *et al* make the case that doctors face at least three major conceptual challenges in discussing risks with patients.[8] These include issues associated with describing risks, conveying their probabilities, and choosing which risks to discuss. A fourth challenge involves accurate discernment of patients' widely varying preferences for involvement in decision making.

Describing the risks

The first communication challenge revolves around the risks themselves: identifying the pertinent unwanted outcomes and their relative permanence, severity (e.g. death, disability, minor pain), immanence, probability of occurrence, and personal meaning for the patient.[8] Unfortunately, identifying the specific risks associated with any particular case is not always straightforward. Some or all of the risks may not be known or fully understood. Discussing the relative permanence of injury adds to the burden. To gain a hoped-for benefit, some patients may accept high risk of a severe, but transient impairment, but they may decline a procedure accompanied by relatively low risk of permanent impairment (as with radiation oncology or surgery for lower back pain).[11]

The timeline for the unwanted outcome and age of the patient pose other challenges to effective risk communications. For example, a middle-aged person might perceive the perioperative risks associated with use of anaesthesia during an upcoming surgery quite differently from the potential long-term complications of uncontrolled diabetes. The surgery may improve life expectancy, but complications may result in immediate morbidity or mortality. Lifestyle and medication adjustments to control diabetes may reduce the ultimate risk of retinal disease, but may be perceived as impractical in the near term. The same person may calculate the risk equations very differently if the decisions apply to her toddler. Individuals vary widely with respect to the values they place on present and future outcomes, so discussions about average values are essentially meaningless.[15]

> *CY was a 9-month-old patient of Dr. N, who recommended a new vaccine to prevent rotaviral infections (most common cause of viral gastroenteritis). CY's mother agreed. Five days later CY presented with intense abdominal pain and was diagnosed with intussusception (a bowel obstruction in which one segment of the bowel becomes enfolded within another segment, potentially compromising blood flow and the integrity of the bowel wall) for which surgical correction was required. In pre-licensure studies, very few cases of intussusception occurred, so the vaccine was approved for use. Subsequent widespread use, however, revealed a higher-than-expected prevalence of this complication, prompting recall of the vaccine.*[16]

265

It's one thing to name a risk and quite another challenge to convey the probability that it will befall a particular patient. The numbers are known with varying degrees of certainty depending on the medical issue, the quality of the underlying epidemiological research, and, for many procedures, the match between the patients, the case mix and the doctors on whom the data is based.[17] Even if objective numbers were known for every condition, physicians would be hard pressed to remember or retrieve them. Moreover, compared with single surgeries or treatments, risks from multiple exposures may be even more challenging to convey. Explaining the probability of an unwanted outcome from a single dose of a new vaccine, though challenging enough, seems straightforward compared with gauging the risks associated with, for example, episodic use of non-steroidal anti-inflammatory drugs over many years.

Finally, even if the doctor capably conveys a particular risk's probabilities, another difficult communication issue involves the patient's or family's subjective determination of its meaning. An adverse outcome of orthopaedic hand surgery might be the concert pianist's catastrophe, the clerk's impediment and the World Cup football player's minor inconvenience.

Mr. Z was devastated over his loss of erectile function and bladder control following prostate cancer surgery. "Dr. D told me the chances of this were very low. But it's 100% for me. If I'd known how common these problems are, I'd have kept the cancer."

Conveying risk probabilities

The second major issue involves how risks are most effectively discussed. Patients vary considerably in their understanding of statistical probabilities (or words like "very low" intended to convey probability) and are greatly influenced by the manner and type of their presentation.[15,17] Physicians' choices of words and graphics to convey risk probabilities can jeopardise the goal of presenting unbiased information for unbiased decision-making. Even the physician's body language and tone of voice can affect the outcome of the discussion.[18,19]

DC was a 73-year-old male with pulmonary hypertension and fibrosing mediastenitis who agreed to undergo catheterisation and stenting of the right pulmonary vein. He understood that for him it was an exceedingly high-risk medical procedure, but he wanted to give it a try "if there's any chance it will allow me to get out of this wheelchair and take my grandsons fishing before I die." After anaesthetic induction and transseptal puncture were completed, all fluoroscopy was lost, then temporarily restored, only to fail again. The cardiologists chose to stop the case and explained their decision to DC's family. The patient died before the procedure could be attempted again. The family wanted to know how often fluoroscope equipment failed and why no one had warned DC that this could happen.

Which risks?

As DC's case suggests, the third major challenge associated with risk communications involves choosing which risks to discuss. At least three standards apply. The first, the "professional standard," requires doctors to share any risks generally disclosed by others in the medical peer community.[20] The problem is that professional standards may be perceived as paternalistic and self-serving. It is therefore no surprise that the "reasonable person standard," in which the risks that a reasonable person in the patient's position would want to know, has become increasingly recognised by most state courts in the USA.[20] Ultimately, both standards imply that physicians must understand what people generally want and need to know in order to make informed choices. Therefore, some courts have taken the next step and applied the "subjective standard," in which the correct amount of information disclosure is determined by the information needs considered relevant by a particular patient.[21] The subjective standard is consistent with the view that the aim of informed consent and risk communication is to foster individual patients' participation in shared decision-making.[22]

Which circumstances?

Kassirer has suggested the types of situations in which known risks should be presented and patient's preferences assessed.[6] These include circumstances when:

- Outcomes may differ dramatically depending on choice of treatment
- Treatments vary in likelihood and severity of complications
- Choices involve trade offs between short- and long-term outcomes
- One choice poses a grave outcome, even when its probability is low
- The patient is particularly risk averse or
- Certain outcomes have great importance for the particular person.

To complicate things further, many jurisdictions place responsibility on the doctor to assure patients' understanding of their communications.[23] Adding still more to the burden, we live in a time when the public's trust in authorities and ability to understand scientific uncertainty has ebbed, while, as the next case illustrates, the media have dramatised the promise of new treatments.

SW was a 26-year-old pregnant woman whose fetus had a neural tube defect (spina bifida). SW was referred to a regional perinatal center where pioneering fetal surgery to cover the defect was performed. SW hung on every word of intense media coverage that trumpets this experimental "breakthrough" even though no child receiving the procedure had yet reached the first year of age. Despite the lack of guarantees, SW was "determined to give my baby a normal life," and she insisted that surgery be performed. Unfortunately, SW's child was born premature and ultimately had no control of his bowel, bladder or lower extremities. The tearful mother cried, "All I could remember was the child and the happy parents in the TV interview. I guess they told me the procedure was experimental, but . . . someone must have thought it was a good idea . . . How could this happen?"

Patient preferences

Research and experience clearly indicate a wide range of patient preferences for involvement in medical decision making. In one formulation, "deferrers" simply accept whatever their doctors recommend, "delayers" briefly and superficially consider the options, then state a preference, and "deliberators" seek complete information (including the doctor's recommendation) with which to calculate their most satisfying alternative.[24] Variations on this formula include the "decision-averse" patient who cannot make a choice[25] and those, like SW, the mother described above, who are "determined" to obtain a particular treatment.

Typing patients according to their manifest preferences has both pros and cons for the treating physician.[26] On the one hand, the initial impression may allow respectful tailoring of messages and styles. However, the initial impression may be wrong, physicians may not attempt to "read" the patient's subsequent preferences, and/or the doctor may be unable or unwilling to adapt. As a result, problems may arise if the physician subsequently fails to offer other levels of involvement to those who, for whatever reasons, were initially reluctant. Problems may also arise if patients who usually wish to be actively involved in decision making feel a psychological need to defer to the doctor's judgement about a procedure they hoped to avoid.[27]

Specific barriers to risk communications

Besides the conceptual challenges associated with risk communications, research and experience suggest a host of other obstacles that can interfere. These barriers may be organised around those inherent to doctors, patients, and their families, and/or the external environment in which care is provided.

Barriers posed by physicians

MW complained to the patient advocate that her first visit with Dr. S, an orthopaedic surgeon, was very stressful. During her interview, she twice asked Dr. S about the status of a particular bone, her treatment options and the long-term prognosis for each. She reported that Dr. S was "vague, confrontational, got in our faces, and yelled at us." The patient, a nurse, said, "I go to doctors for their medical expertise and not their personalities, but . . . I don't know how I can continue with a doc-

tor for fear of his reaction." MW decided to seek another specialist, but asked the patient advocate, "please do not report this [complaint] to Dr. S in case our best option is to return to him."

Physicians themselves may pose or create barriers to good risk communications or guidelines of any kind.[28] While the intimidating tactics of Dr. S are certainly extreme, they are not uncommon and serve to highlight the unequal relationship between doctors and even sophisticated patients. Such behaviours are also associated with high risk of claims of medical negligence.[29-32] Other barriers are purely cognitive. Doctors may lack familiarity with treatment options or risk-related data due to limited exposure during training, the sheer volume of information and time needed to stay current, and/or not knowing how to access particular bits of data.[33]

Moreover, doctors may disagree with the value of communicating, rationalising "this treatment option isn't the best (or most cost beneficial) one for this patient." Some doctors disclose options and risks not on the basis of patient preference, but based purely on their subjective impression of characteristics like patient age, intelligence, relatives' wishes, and other factors.[34] Others may fail to discuss options because they lack confidence in the data or feel that presenting it challenges their authority. Other barriers involve low levels of physician self confidence ("I'm not good at discussing risks"), low confidence in patient ability ("I don't think I can make this patient understand the issues"), and arrogant underestimation of patient desire for information ("this patient doesn't need to know and wouldn't understand, anyway").[35] Similarly, outcome expectancies may interfere. For example, the prideful physician might think, "My patients have never experienced this adverse outcome, so why discuss it." And the patronising doctor thinks "Discussing the risk won't help this patient, may cause him unnecessary worry, or lessen his confidence in me and my skills".[36] Less often cited, but nonetheless important, is the physician's ability to overcome the inertia of previous practice (i.e. habit, "I've never done it this way before").

While the desire to serve patients generally exerts the greatest influence on physician decision making, doctors may be tempted to influence patients' choices in ways that are, unfortunately, but understandably, self-serving.[37,38] After all, doctors are motivated to seek income, a certain type and style of practice, leisure time, diagnostic certainty, and protection from litigation.[38] For some physicians (and patients), intolerance of ambiguity and desire for medical certainty lead to apprehension and, perhaps, fear of litigation which, in turn, may dispose them to evaluate or treat more than is necessary.[38-40]

Barriers in patients and their families

LB was an 83-year-old male with sudden onset of intense epigastric pain and diaphoresis. An initial EKG was normal, but cardiac enzymes were mildly elevated the second day, so a consulting cardiologist recommended a catheterisation. While attempting to provide informed consent, the patient's spouse interrupted, "I am worried enough and don't want to hear any more. He has to have the cath anyway and I know everything has complications. Just do the procedure. All this discussion is worrying me." The cardiologist attempted to continue, but was told, "Look, I trust you. No further information is necessary." Following the procedure, however, the spouse sought detailed information about the new medication regimen. The cardiologist reacted to the questions with some surprise. The spouse replied that for her to help provide good care, she wanted more education about the medicines and their potential side effects.

Patients and families also pose challenges to effective risk communications. As we discussed earlier, preferences for information and involvement vary widely across persons and, as seen above, may vary within individuals across circumstances. Unlike LB's spouse, some are so intimidated by their unequal relationship with health professionals that they find themselves unable to ask questions or state preferences unless the doctor is particularly warm and inviting.[41]

Another very challenging patient type are the hypochondriacal "worriers" who, concerned about a potential risk or complication, fail to be reassured by normal follow-up test results.[42] Dealings with such persons may dissuade some physicians from discussing risks with others. For example, the day after LB's MI (see case above), his 76-year-old sister went to her doctor complaining of chest pain and demanded a complete evaluation. Cardiac enzymes, EKG and exercise tolerance tests were all normal, but she demanded an arteriogram "just to be sure." She was referred to a cardiologist who performed the procedure after thoroughly and graphically contrasting its risks with the hoped-for benefit of anxiety reduction. The results indicated no heart problems. LB's sister was not reassured by this and remained concerned that "something is wrong, and now I think the arteriogram made it worse, but they're just not finding it."

Patients may simply not hear or recall risks, even when they are presented well. Stress, psychological overload, anxiety, and/or repression/denial may interfere, as when a patient repeatedly says things such as, "I just want to know how soon you are going to start the procedure," or "Do whatever you need to do". Or patients may not fully understand risks that are explained using technical language, euphemisms, or medical shorthand. Such instances highlight the importance of asking patients or family members to articulate their understanding of each alternative and its attendant risks and benefits, then thoroughly documenting both the decision and the discussion.

Bias, culture, and language

BB was an irritable 6-week-old infant who presented to the emergency department with a fever to 39·4°C (103°F), tachycardia, delayed capillary refill and "fussy" behaviour. Dr. A, the female ED physician from a different racial group from the 18-year-old mother, explained the importance of early detection of meningitis and concluded by recommending a spinal tap. The mother refused. After lengthy discussion, Dr. A called the child's general physician, Dr. J, who came into the facility and conducted his own examination. After a short discussion, the family agreed to the tap so long as Dr. J performed the procedure. Dr. J said, "I haven't said anything different from what Dr. A told you. Why are you now willing for me to do the tap?" The young mother responded, "I just don't trust lady doctors."

Cultural and language issues can be as challenging as bias, as in the next case.

GW was a 37-year-old Nigerian woman who spoke very broken English and was admitted for a C-section delivery of her second child. Before the procedure, a nurse discussed birth control alternatives, and GW made it very clear that she wanted no more children. The possibility of a tubal ligation was presented, and GW consented to have it performed. Her husband filed suit for battery, alleging that the tubal ligation was performed without consent. GW declared that she never understood what she and the staff were talking about.

Social, cultural and language factors may be barriers to putting shared decision making into practice, but if these represent more than a very small minority of a physician's encounters, remedies must be sought.[43] Finally, patients pose serious problems for their doctors when they use information provided in risk communications to set the stage for malingering. For example, some individuals intent upon securing disability income, like EM in the case that follows, have used pre-surgical risk information to feign injuries later.

EM was a 52-year-old with low back pain subsequent to a workplace injury. A myelogram revealed a large central disc defect at L3–L4. Her orthopaedic surgeon offered conservative treatment without success. He therefore presented two additional options, laminectomy or chemonucleolysis of the disc and documented his discussion of the attendant benefits and risks, including nerve root irritation and paraplegia. Three weeks following chemonucleolysis, EM presented complaining of increasing bilateral leg weakness and inability to walk, making her unable to work. A neurologist diagnosed paraplegia and parasthaesia caused by transverse myelitis secondary to the chemonucleolysis procedure. One year later, another neurologist noted that EM's reflexes were good and that there were no motor defects, even though she still could not work. As part of an investigation, EM was videotaped ambulating well. In fact, her friends testified that she was routinely "out on the town," and "loved to dance."

External barriers to risk communications

MLH was a 33-year-old female whose nasal reconstruction surgery required revision, which was unsuccessful. Shortly thereafter, a malpractice claim was filed alleging, among other things, the surgeon's failure to discuss the risks. During a

271

deposition, the operating surgeon declared that he did not personally conduct informed consent discussions with his patients, but left that to his office manager. When it was her turn, the office manager testified – to the surgeon's surprise – that while she discussed scheduling and wound care, she would never tell patients about the possibility of surgical failures, potential risks or complications. Declaring that he was very busy, the surgeon stated, "patients who want a nose job are going to get one regardless of any discussion of risks." And, he said, "except for this case, my results are outstanding."

External barriers such as poorly articulated policies and procedures can make it seem impossible to effectively communicate risks to patients. Environmental obstacles may also include lack of time and resources, misleading statements in patient education materials,[33] organisational constraints, lack of reimbursement, and inadequate staffing. The ways in which medical services are organised may also interfere. For example, while a patient may trust her general practitioner to provide satisfactory risk communications, that doctor may not always be available for consultation.[44] Nor can the patient count on a consulting specialist to offer the same kind and quality of information.

Perhaps the most pernicious external barriers involve financing and availability of healthcare. How physicians are paid may profoundly affect their behaviours and recommendations.[24,45,46] Wherever healthcare is rationed, physicians may feel they operate under written or unwritten "gag clauses," i.e. constrained from prescribing alternatives for which there may be high costs and/or long waits either for the service itself or an authorisation from "higher up" to allow it. Patients must be protected and their preferences assiduously sought whenever resource allocations may influence doctors' decisions.[6]

Heuristics for understanding and guiding effective risk communications

Most patients seem to want to know the full picture regarding risks and side effects of treatments so long as they are presented in a non-alarmist, "balanced" fashion that includes a careful and honest assessment of the pros and cons of treatment.[33,47] If the outcome probabilities are unknown, they want to know that, too.[48] Given the significant challenges, how might doctors and their patients arrive at therapeutic decisions? This section outlines one framework and a series of heuristics for understanding and guiding risk communications.

A framework for discussing risks

Helping patients make therapeutic decisions entails far more than obtaining a signature on a legal document. Rather, risk communications for truly informed decision-making require negotiating and consensus building, processes that emphasise the interests or concerns that underlie each party's position regarding a therapeutic decision.[49] Failures to understand each party's interests may complicate satisfactory decision-making. For example, a doctor may take the position that a patient needs to undergo a particular procedure or course of treatment and explain why, yet be baffled or frustrated by the patient's reluctance to pursue it. Patients may similarly be baffled and frustrated if they perceive themselves caught in a battle of wills with a physician who seems uninterested in their point of view. Therefore, parties involved in such discussions increase the chances of satisfactory outcomes if they:

- Identify, discuss and address interests to learn why the doctor, patient, or family member is asserting a particular position. Considering the range of each party's potential interests (see Table 14.1), this task may – but does not usually – require substantial time. The investment may be worthwhile, however, because interests may be discovered early and met in several ways, averting time-consuming problems and miscommunications later.
- Appreciate interpersonal dynamics in risk communications and help people move on. Emotions may play a large role in medical decision making, but feelings must not be allowed to shortchange discussion of each option and its merits. All parties' prejudices and experiences need to be understood, especially if they constitute barriers to decision making. For example, no party to the discussion should let negative interpersonal feelings about the others override their better judgement. In other words, "separate the people from the problems."
- Consider every alternative, minimising judgements at first. The goals are to ensure that patients understand the options and that doctors understand patients' wishes. One by-product is that patients may sense that they are valued and that their doctor is open and honest.
- Agree on criteria and principles by which to judge each option. Naming the basis for making judgements maintains a sense of common endeavour by legitimising each party's interests. Identifying the criteria may also help break impasses – or at least help everyone understand why they occur. When an impasse occurs, some criteria will have to take precedence. For example, for many patients (and juries), the principles of honesty and full disclosure will override a physician's preference for corporate efficiency and paternalism.[50]

Note that this framework can work equally well for patients who desire paternalistic physicians who control the decisions, autonomous patients who wish to use their physicians largely for consultation, and persons who want to share responsibility and decision making. To work, the framework simply requires discussion of each party's interests. It does not presume what the outcome should be.

Table 14.1 Variables representing potential interests of physicians, patients and family members. All parties may rate on a scale (e.g. from 1–5) the strength of their personal interest, perhaps helping them come to understandings that lead to satisfactory decisions.

Potential Interests	Patient Rating	Family Rating	(Physician Rating)
Restore health			
Lengthen life			
Reduce pain, suffering			
Achieve death with dignity			
Meet personal, legal obligations			
Obtain acceptable diagnostic certainty			
Save money, resources			
Understand what's happening medically			
Avoid worries, hassles, burdens of care			
Be respected			
Preserve values, maintain integrity, be honest			
Involvement in decision making			
Be satisfied that the "best" medical care was provided			
Participate in training of novice health professionals			
Contribute to society, help others			
Maintain good relationships with other members of healthcare team			
Avoid bad press			
Satisfy payers, regulators, avoid litigation			
Others:			

Special communication skills for risk discussions

Risk discussions require special communication skills not routinely taught in medical schools. Fortunately, such skills can be learned and do not lengthen interview time.[51,52] The following physician competencies are supported by research, law and clinical experience:[7,36]

- Establish the patient's preferences for amount and format of information and role in decision making

- Assess and respond to patient's ideas, concerns and expectations
- Discuss the clinical issue and nature of the decision to be made
- Identify all treatment alternatives, including those brought forward by the patient
- Evaluate the research evidence as it applies to the particular patient
- Present the evidence consistent with the patient's preferences
- Discuss the pros (or benefits) and cons (or risks) and help the patient assess impacts of alternatives on his/her values and lifestyle
- Discuss the uncertainties associated with the decision
- Assess the patient's understanding of the alternatives and their potential impacts
- Ask the patient to express a preference, resolve any conflicts, and make or negotiate a final decision
- Agree on an action plan and make arrangements for follow up and
- Document the nature of the discussion and the resulting plan.

Using decision aids

Adjuncts to personal communication such as decision aids may help with several of these steps. Research generally supports the use of videos, scripts, group discussions, patient education brochures and handouts, interactive videos, audio-guided workbooks, video imaging (for facial reconstruction), decision analysis tools, and computer-guided assessments for assisting with risk communications.[41,53,54] But not always.[55] Nevertheless, major reviews conclude that decision aids, so long as they are carefully prepared, can improve patient/family knowledge and involvement in decision making without increasing anxiety.[56] Decision aids had little effect, however, on satisfaction, and they had varied effects on actual decisions and outcomes. For example, decision aids significantly reduced patients' wishes for prostate specific antigen, but did not change preferences for newborn circumcisions.[56] For the increasing numbers of health professionals who correspond with patients via the internet and email, these communication tools should be used only as an adjunct to personal discussions, if at all, for communicating alternatives and their risks.[57]

Decision tools

In addition to "canned" decision aids, what other tools may help doctors and patients discuss risks both effectively and efficiently? For doctors who do not already have a method, the trick is to find one that seems like it might help, adopt it, adapt it to their individual talents and situations, and refine it until it becomes habitual. Consider, then, several strategies succinctly summarised by Worthley:[50]

275

- **Checklists.** The bulleted list above offers a flexible outline that may help keep risk communications on track during particularly complicated or vexing discussions.
- **Guiding questions.** For some, well-learned guiding questions, like the "reporter's questions" of who, what, when, where, why and how, are preferable to checklists. Such questions move from establishing the facts and the alternatives to illuminating the parties' styles, purposes, interests and motives.
- **Guiding principles.** Decide in advance what principles take precedence in decision-making. Recommended guides include the well-known "utilitarian principle" (acting to generate the greatest good with the least harm) and the "golden rule" (doing with/to others as you prefer to be treated). When these don't apply, one might consider using the "distributive justice" principle (acting so that those with the fewest resources are benefitted), or the "personal liberty" principle (acting to enhance the dignity in others' lives).
- **Decision science.** Persons who tend to base decisions on numbers might benefit from assigning subjective weights to various aspects of each therapeutic option. For example, Table 14.1 provides a matrix for helping the parties involved in decision making understand the value they assign to various interests. More formally, given the means for doing so, patients are sometimes capable of making complex "utility" judgements that can aid their understanding of the "value" they place on each alternative.[58,59]
- **Consequences table.** The simplest strategy might be to make short lists of the "pros" and "cons" associated with each alternative and then sort the items from "remotely possible" to "certain" (or similar) according to each item's likelihood. Unfortunately, specifying potential adverse outcomes and their probabilities in advance is not always possible.

Communications following unexpected or adverse outcomes

JL was a 57-year-old white male who received a cardiac transplant secondary to ischaemic cardiomyopathy. As a part of routine follow-up, JL consented for Dr. B to perform catheterisation and cardiac biopsy. Dr R, who started the procedure, had difficulty cannulating the right-side arteries due to significant scar tissue, so he asked Dr. B to assist. After another time-consuming attempt, a smaller catheter was utilised to complete the procedure successfully. Nine days later, JL presented to a local ER with pain in his right groin and a low haematocrit. An abdominal CT scan revealed a retroperitoneal haematoma, so he was hospitalised for evaluation. Throughout his hospitalisation, JL raised several issues with staff members: "Why didn't I see a doctor either before or after the cath procedure? I discovered that the doctor named on the consent form did not perform the cath procedure. Was it done by one of those student doctors? As I look there are 3–4 sticks that were made in my groin area. Doesn't this indicate that the doctor didn't know what he was doing? The procedure took four hours, and usually I am in and out in an hour. I think somebody owes me an explanation, but no one will tell me what happened. I want some answers."

Despite everyone's best efforts, not every patient recovers completely, and some experience unwanted outcomes. Sometimes the adverse outcome is associated with medical error.[60] Telling patients or their families about disappointing results and dealing with their reactions is not easy. Nevertheless, with care and compassion, such communication maintains the climate of concern that characterises quality care.[61-63] And, for the health professionals involved, accepting responsibility and engaging in problem-solving may lead to positive changes in practice and increased interest in continuing education.[64] Conversely, failing to communicate concern after an adverse outcome is a leading cause of malpractice claims. Patients commonly seek legal counsel because their health professional(s) showed "no concern, no warmth," and "wouldn't listen, wouldn't talk, wouldn't answer questions".[29,31] Then, when patients or family members related their experience to others, including other health professionals, they were often empowered to pursue legal action because those significant others recommended it.[29,65]

Explaining adverse outcomes and errors

When the outcome is less than optimal, doctors should take the initiative to seek out the patient and/or family and face the situation openly and honestly. Doctors should NOT avoid this task because delays suggest that they may have something to hide and are attempting a cover-up. Although one should never assume that the meeting would go as expected, the general outline that follows may help with difficult conversations.[66,67]

- If time permits, alert the institution's risk manager to the adverse outcome and seek his or her counsel regarding how to proceed.
- Select a setting that will preserve dignity and confidentiality. Give bad news in a private place where the patient and/or family may react and you can respond appropriately.
- Set the stage. "Mr. Jackson, I know you are aware that there were several risks associated with your therapy/procedure . . ."
- Clearly deliver the message. The adverse outcome must be understood. "I'm sad to report that the procedure resulted in ____ and, as you may recall, that means ____."
- Discuss transition support. Tell the patient/family what steps might come next to provide medical, social, or other forms of support.
- Wait silently for a reaction. Give the patient/family time to consider what has happened and formulate their questions.

- Deal with the reaction(s). The usual reaction to bad news is a mixture of denial, anger, resignation, shock, etc. Listen. Acknowledge feelings. Resist the urge to blame or appear to blame other health professionals for the outcome. Discuss next steps. Afterward, document a summary of the discussion.
- Express empathy, but be careful that it's not misinterpreted as an admission of negligence. Instead, be specific, "It's always sad when someone like you experiences a known risk of this treatment. You and your family have my sincere sympathy."
- Conclude the interaction. Be sure, near the end of the discussion, to acknowledge that you have talked about a lot of things and want to be sure that you have been clear. Then, saying that you ask all your patients to do so, ask the patient/family to summarise in their own words what has happened, what the next steps/decisions might be, where they can get help, and what, if anything, will be done by you or the medical centre. Finish by reassuring them about your continued willingness to answer any questions they might have. Afterwards, document a summary of the discussion.
- Consider scheduling a follow-up meeting. Some patients will want to talk only after the crisis has subsided. Be prepared for such a meeting and bring along a copy of the medical record if you'll need it to help explain anything that transpired.
- If the risk managers conduct an investigation, a part of a follow-up meeting should be devoted to sharing the findings. The doctor, risk manager and others should consider the best person(s) and means for discussing the results.

Finally, physicians who do not routinely carry out these practices effectively may be the subjects of disproportionate numbers of patient complaints. These physicians may thus be identified by the institutions in which they work and, given appropriate feedback, may be able to change their interaction styles or the systems that dissatisfy their patients.[12,68]

Conclusions

Communicating risks to patients and their families is an extremely important and equally challenging task routinely faced by doctors and other health professionals. The literature on the subject is extensive, revealing conceptual, behavioural, and environmental issues and obstacles. Guidelines for conducting effective risk-related discussions tend to reflect lofty ideals. These ideals may not be routinely achieved in daily practice, understandably frustrating some doctors. As we like to say, however, "Perfection must not be the enemy of the good." Doctors who care, who strive to earn and maintain the trust of their patients, can continue improving their risk communication skills, perhaps by using some of the strategies and techniques presented here and throughout this book (especially[69,70]). By doing so, they will increase patient satisfaction, foster patient involvement in self-care, improve compliance with therapy, and, perhaps, reduce the risk of unmerited charges of medical negligence when unwanted outcomes occur.

Acknowledgement

Support for this work was provided in part by the Vanderbilt University Risk Management Education Program and grants from The Robert Wood Johnson Foundation.

References

1 Dyer C. Bristol trust admits liability in baby heart surgery case. *BMJ* 1999;**319**:213.
2 Dyer C. Bristol doctors found guilty of serious professional misconduct. *BMJ* 1998;**316**: 1924.
3 Goldsmith LS. The myth about informed consent. *J Legal Med* 1975;**3**:17–20.
4 Hickson GB, Clayton EW, Miller CS, *et al.* Obstetricians' prior malpractice experience and patients' satisfaction with care. *JAMA* 1994;**272**:1583–7.
5 Anderson LA, Zimmerman, MA: Patient and physician perceptions of their relationship and patient satisfaction: A study of chronic disease management. *Pt Educ Counsel* 1993;**20**:27–36.
6 Kassirer JP. Incorporating patients' preferences into medical decisions. *N Engl J Med* 1994;**330**:1895–6.
7 Braddock CH, Fihn SD, Levinson W, *et al.* How doctors and patients discuss routine clinical decisions – informed decision making in the outpatient setting. *J Gen Intern Med* 1997;**12**:39–45.
8 Bogardus ST Jr, Holmboe E, Jekel JF. Perils, pitfalls, and possibilities in talking about medical risk. *JAMA* 1999;**281**(11):1037–41.
9 Braddock, CH III. Advancing the cause of informed consent: moving from disclosure to understanding [editorial]. *Am J Med* 1998;**105**:354–5.
10 Coulter A. Paternalism or partnership? *BMJ* 1999;**319**:719–20.
11 Smith R. All changed, changed utterly. *BMJ* 1999;**316**:1917–18.
12 Hickson GB, Pichert JW, Federspiel CF, Clayton EW. Development of an early identification and response model of malpractice prevention. *Law Contemp Problems* 1997;**60**: 7–29.
13 Pichert JW, Federspiel CF, Hickson GB, Miller CS, Gauld-Jaeger J, Gray C. Identifying medical centre units with disproportionate shares of patient complaints. *Joint Commission J Qual Improve* 1999;**25**:288–99.
14 Amols III, Saidei M, Hayes MK, Schiff PB. Physician/patient-driven risk assignment in radiation oncology: reality or fancy? *Int J Radiat Oncol* 1997;**38**:455–61.
15 Calman K. Cancer: science and society and the communication of risk. *BMJ* 1996;**313**: 799–802.
16 Rennels MB, Parashar UD, Holman RC, *et al.* Lack of an apparent association between intussusception and wild or vaccine rotavirus infection. *Pediat Infect Dis J* 1998;**17**: 924–5.
17 Rothwell PM, Slattery J, Warlow CP. Clinical and angiographic predictors of stroke and death from carotid endarterectomy: systematic review. *BMJ* 1997;**315**:1571–7.
18 Mazur DJ, Merz JF. How age, outcome severity, and scale influence general medicine clinic patients' interpretations of verbal probability terms. *J Gen Intern Med* 1994;**9**(5): 268–71.

19 Forrow L, Taylor WC, Arnold RM. Absolutely relative: how research results are summarised can affect treatment decisions. *Am J Med* 1992;**92**(2):121–4.

20 Mazur DJ. *Medical risk and the right to an informed consent in clinical care and clinical research* Tampa, FL: American College of Physician Executives, 1998.

21 Braddock, CH. Advancing the cause of informed consent: Moving from disclosure to understanding. *Am J Med* 1998;**105**:354–5.

22 President's Commission for Ethical Issues in Biomedical and Clinical Research. *Making Health Care Decisions. Vol. 1.* Washington, DC: US Government Printing Office; 1982.

23 Miller DS, Butler E. Legal aspects of physician–patient communication. *J Fam Pract* 1982;**15**:1131–4.

24 Pierce PF. Deciding on breast cancer treatment: A description of decision behaviour. *Nurs Res* 1993;**42**:22–8.

25 Degner LF, Sloan JA. Decision making during serious illness: What role do patients really want to play? *J Clin Epidemiol* 1992;**45**:941–50.

26 Guadagnoli E, Ward P. Patient participation in decision-making. *Soc Sci Med* 1998;**47**: 329–39.

27 Lidz CW, Meisel A, Osterweiss M, *et al.* Barriers to informed consent. *Ann Intern Med* 1983;**99**:539–43.

28 Cabana MD, Rand CS, Powe NR, *et al.* Why don't physicians follow clinical practice guidelines? *JAMA* 1999;**282**:1458–65.

29 Hickson GB, Clayton EW, Githens PB, Sloan FA. Factors that prompted families to file medical malpractice claims following perinatal injuries. *JAMA* 1992;**267**:1359–63.

30 May ML, Stengel DB. Who sues their doctor? How patients handle medical grievance. *Law Soc Rev* 1990;**24**:105–20.

31 Vincent C, Young M, Phillips A. Why do people sue their doctors? A study of patients and relatives taking legal action. *Lancet* 1994;**343**:1609–13.

32 Levinson W, Roter D, Mullooly J, *et al.* Physician–patient communication: The relationship with malpractice claims among primary care physicians and surgeons. *JAMA* 1997;**277**:553–9.

33 Coulter A, Entwistle V, Gilbert D. Sharing decisions with patients: is the information good enough? *BMJ* 1999;**318**:318–22.

34 Carnerie F. Crisis and informed consent: analysis of a law–medicine malocclusion. *Am J Law Med* 1986;**12**(1):55–96.

35 Edwards A, Matthews E, Pill R, Bloor M. Communication about risk: diversity among primary care professionals. *Fam Pract* 1998;**15**:296–300.

36 Cockburn J, Pit S. Prescribing behaviour in clinical practice: patients' expectations and doctors' perceptions of patients' expectations – a questionnaire study. *BMJ* 1997;**315**: 520–3.

37 Wennberg JE, Barnes BA, Zubkoff M. Professional uncertainty and the problem of supplier-induced demand. *Soc Sci Med* 1982;**16**:811–24.

38 Eisenberg JM. Physician utilisation: The state of research about physician practice patterns. *Med Care* 1985;**32**:461–83.

39 Eddy DM. Variations in physician practice: The role of uncertainty. *Health Affairs* 1984;**3**: 774–89.

40 Hickson GB, Clayton EW. Parents and their children's doctors. In: Bornstein MH, ed. *Handbook of parenting.* Mahwah, NJ: Lawrence Erlbaum Associates. 1995;163–85.

41 O'Connor AM, Tugwell P, Wells GA, *et al.* A decision aid for women considering hormone therapy after menopause: decision support framework and evaluation. *Pt Educ Counsel* 1998;**33**:267–79.

42 McDonald IG, Daly J, Jelinek VM, *et al.* Opening Pandora's box: the unpredictability of reassurance by a normal test result. *BMJ* 1996; **313**(7053):329–32.

43 Towle A, Godolphin W. Framework for teaching and learning informed shared decision making. *BMJ* 1999; **319**(7212):766–71.

44 Gambrill J. Commentary: proposals based on too many assumptions. *BMJ* 1999: **319**: 771.

45 Hickson GB, Altemier WA, Perrin JM. Physician reimbursement by salary or fee-for-service: Effect on physician practice behaviour in a randomised prospective study. *Pediatrics* 1987;**80**:344–50.

46 Ransom SB, McNeeley SG, Kruger ML, *et al.* The effect of capitated and fee-for-service remuneration on physician decision making in gynaecology. *Obstet Gynecol* 1996;**87**(5 Pt 1):707–10.

47 Makoul G, Arntson P, Schofield T. Health promotion in primary care: physician–patient communication and decision making about prescription medications. *Soc Sci Med* 1995;**41**:1241–4.

48 Coulter A. Partnerships with patients: the pros and cons of shared clinical decision making. *J Health Serv Res Policy* 1997;**2**:112–21.

49 Fisher R, Ury W. *Getting to yes: negotiating agreement without giving in* (2nd edition). New York: Penguin Books, 1991.

50 Worthley JA. The ethical dimension of ordinary professional life. *Healthcare Executive* 1999; Sept/Oct: 6–10.

51 Roter DL, Hall JA, Kern DE, *et al.* Improving physicians' interviewing skills and reducing patients' emotional distress. A randomised clinical trial. *Arch Intern Med* 1995;**155**: 1877–84.

52 McManus IC, Vincent CA, Thom S, Kidd J. Teaching communication skills to clinical students. *BMJ* 1993;**306**:1322–7.

53 Edwards A, Elwyn G, Gwyn R. General practice registrar responses to the use of different risk communication tools in simulated consultations: a focus group study. *BMJ* 1999; **319**:749–52.

54 Flood AB, Wennberg JE, Nease RF, *et al.* The importance of patient preference in the decision to screen for prostate cancer. *J Gen Intern Med* 1996;**11**(6):342–9.

55 Clark SK, Leighton BL, Seltzer JL. A risk-specific consent form may hinder the informed consent process. *J Clin Anesth* 1991;**3**:11–13.

56 O'Connor AM, Rostom A, Fiset V, *et al.* Decisions aids for patients facing health treatment or screening decisions: systematic review. *BMJ* 1999;**319**:731–4.

57 Spielberg A. On call and online: The sociohistorical, legal and ethical implications of email for the patient–physician relationship *JAMA* 1998;**280**(15):1353–9.

58 Handler RM, Hynes LM, Nease RF Jr. Effect of locus of control and consideration of future consequences on time trade off utilities for current health. *Qual Life Res* 1997;**6**: 54–60.

59 Fleming C, Wasson JH, Albertsen PC, *et al.* A decision analysis of alternative treatment strategies for clinically localised prostate cancer. *JAMA* 1993;**269**: 2650–8.

60 Kohn L, Corrigan J, Donaldson M, eds. *To err is human: Building a safer health system.* New York: Committee on Quality of Health Care in America, Institute of Medicine, National Academy Press, 2000. (see: http: //books.nap. edu/catalog/9728.html))

61 Wu AW, Cavanaugh TA, McPhee SJ, *et al.* To tell the truth: ethical and practical issues in disclosing medical mistakes to patients. *J Gen Intern Med* 1997;**12**:770–5.

62 Lape CP. Disclosing medical mistakes [letter]. *J Gen Intern Med* 1998;**13**:283–4.

63 Finkelstein D, Wu AW, Holtzman NA, Smith MK. When a physician harms a patient by a medical error: ethical, legal, and risk-management considerations. *J Clin Ethics* 1997;**8**: 330–5.

64 Meurier CE, Vincent CA, Parmar DG. Learning from errors in nursing practice. *J Adv Nurs* 1997;**26**:111–19.

65 Moran SK, Sicher CM. Interprofessional jousting and medical tragedies: strategies for enhancing professional relations. *AANA Journal* 1996;**64**:521–4.

66 Vincent C. Caring for patients harmed by treatment. In Vincent C, ed. *Clinical risk management*, pp. 433–52. London: BMJ Publishing Group, 1995.

67 Pichert JW, Hickson GB, Trotter TS. Malpractice and communication skills for difficult situations. *J Gen Commun Pediatr* 1998;**4**:213–21.

68 Hickson GB, Pichert JW, Federspiel CF, Miller CS. *Initial results of implementing an early identification and response model of malpractice prevention.* Proceedings of the American Medical Association Patient Safety Conference, 1999.

69 Allsop J, Mulcahy L. Dealing with clinical complaints. This volume, Chapter 26.

70 Vincent C. Caring for patients harmed by treatment. This volume, Chapter 24.

15 Guidelines and pathways

ROBBIE FOY, JEREMY GRIMSHAW, MARTIN ECCLES

A 74-year-old woman collapses three days following an operation for a hip replacement. Efforts at resuscitation are unsuccessful and she dies. Post-mortem findings reveal a massive pulmonary embolus and deep vein thrombosis in her right calf. Would the availability of a guideline for thromboprophylaxis have prevented this death? Were clinical staff aware of the existence of such a guideline? Were they in agreement with it? Was any system in place to support implementation of the protocol? Did the guideline offer clear and evidence-based advice on the prevention of thromboprophylaxis? How much of a difference would following a good guideline have made on reducing the risk of embolism? Does non-adherence to such a guideline render clinical staff more vulnerable to litigation? These are key questions regarding the potential impact of any clinical guideline.

Guidelines and pathways have their supporters and detractors. Extreme positions tend to result from naive expectations of their impact and the over-simplification of the processes required for their development and implementation. Guidelines are sometimes castigated as "cookbook" medicine, compromising clinical autonomy and reducing the role of clinical judgement in patient care. However, anyone who has tested cookbook recipes realises that cooking is messier in practice than on paper. It requires some degree of judgement and following a recipe does not necessarily guarantee a successful outcome. It also is unwise to assume that learners already possess the basic skills, knowledge and experience to follow a recipe.[1]

The development and implementation of guidelines carry potential costs and benefits, of which some are predictable whilst others may be unanticipated. Clinicians and managers need to decide whether their introduction is likely to lead to improvements in quality of care at an acceptable cost.

What are clinical guidelines and pathways?

Clinical guidelines have been defined as "systematically developed statements to assist practitioner and patient decisions about appropriate healthcare for specific clinical circumstances".[2] They may address specific clinical issues, such as the diagnosis or treatment of a defined disease or clinical problem, or the organisation of healthcare, such as the provision of diagnostic or therapeutic facilities.

Care pathways (also referred to as critical pathways or protocols) are "structured multidisciplinary care plans, which detail essential steps in the care of a patient with a specific clinical problem".[3] By mapping out processes along the expected course of clinical care, they can support decision-making and help identify where and why practice does not meet adopted standards. Care pathways therefore represent a systematic approach to the local application of guidelines.

Rationale for clinical guidelines

Appropriateness of healthcare

The availability of good research evidence does not guarantee its timely or widespread integration into routine clinical practice. For example, there is an extensive evidence base supporting the long-term use of ß-blockers following acute myocardial infarction. However, the adoption of this life-saving treatment has varied significantly between regions and many patients with no contraindications, particularly women and elderly people, still fail to receive it. [4] Inappropriate healthcare is more likely to continue without the effective delivery of knowledge to the clinical interface. Clinical guidelines represent one of several approaches to quality assurance that can improve the quality of care.[5]

Coping with information

Health professionals work in an age of information overload and increasing complexity of healthcare. Questioning practice and searching for and appraising evidence are becoming pivotal skills in professional development.[6] However, the production rate of new clinical evidence can overwhelm even the most committed professional in any field.[7,8] Guidelines can help meet healthcare professionals' need for relevant and reliable summaries of clinical evidence. By highlighting areas where the evidence is weak or unreliable, guidelines can help discriminate between actions which are based upon sound evidence and those which depend more upon clinical judgement and patient preference. Guidelines can also reinforce good practice, especially where clinicians are uncertain of potential benefits.

Shared information and decision-making

There is a growing emphasis on enhanced patient involvement in decisions relating to their care. Some guidelines are produced with "lay" versions to promote more consistent patient education, especially in chronic conditions which require a substantial degree of self care. In addition, patients can use guidelines to prompt their doctors to reconsider or change aspects of their care. The increasing availability of information and guidelines from the internet offers both an opportunity and a threat to shared decision-making. Like any guideline, the utility of such information depends greatly upon its validity and relevance to the healthcare system and to the patient's clinical and personal circumstances.

Care pathways can provide patients with a clearer idea of what to expect during their admission, investigation or treatment.[9] This may reduce the likelihood of misunderstandings and complaints arising from communication failures caused by differing expectations or failures of care.

Avoidance of litigation

Guidelines can help professionals reduce or cope with clinical uncertainty by explicitly balancing known benefits and risks. Whilst the avoidance of litigation is often associated with taking additional actions (e.g. an investigation), it is often necessary to define thresholds below which action is unlikely to produce clinical benefit. Defensive medicine is rooted in the syndrome of "nominators looking for denominators".[10] Recent experience in practice of a stillbirth may inappropriately but understandably lower the threshold at which an obstetrician would advise caesarean section in subsequent deliveries. Guidelines can help reduce inappropriate practice without compromising standards of care. In a high risk specialty, such as obstetrics, guidelines can aim to reduce the caesarean section rate by promoting a trial of labour in women with a previous caesarean section[11] or reduce inappropriate investigations and hospital admissions associated with mild, non-proteinuric hypertension.[12]

The local development and implementation of care pathways can help identify systematic faults in the delivery of care.[13] This informs the use of further steps to be taken locally to improve the process of care. At the level of the individual, pathways can alert staff to a patient's failure to progress satisfactorily.

Efficiency

It has been suggested that care pathways may contribute to reduced length of hospital stays and increased efficiency by minimising duplication of tasks and inappropriate interventions.[3] However, there are several concerns associated with care pathways, including the time and opportunity costs of their implementation and the work required to overcome staff scepticism. The foremost is the lack of evidence supporting their purported benefits. There is a large amount of literature reporting improved efficiency and quality of care but this is almost entirely, with the exception of one randomised controlled trial,[14] based on case and observational studies. Further, more rigorous evaluations are required to assess the impact of pathways upon efficiency.

Resource allocation

Resources available for healthcare are limited. Policymakers, managers and clinicians need relevant and reliable information to inform resource allocation. Rigorously developed guidelines may help in this process by highlighting under or over provision of certain services. However, this not infrequently results in guidelines being used as political instruments. Specialist, patient or pressure groups sometimes use guidelines (of variable quality) as a basis to lobby for the improved or more equitable provision of services.

Clinical guidelines may therefore help deliver improved healthcare at greater safety margins. However, clinicians and managers should be aware of avoidable pitfalls and the need for carefully planned and executed development, dissemination and implementation in order to realise these potential benefits.

What is the evidence that guidelines work?

Two critical conditions are necessary if any of the aforementioned benefits from clinical guidelines are to be realised. Firstly, the guideline itself must be valid, i.e. if "when followed they lead to the health gains and costs predicted for them".[15] Secondly, the guideline must be introduced using effective dissemination and implementation strategies.[5] A systematic review of rigorous evaluations, including randomised controlled trials, indicates that the use of clinical guidelines improves both clinical practice and the outcomes of care.[16] Out of 87 evaluations that examined effects on the process of care, all but six detected significant improvements. However, the size of such changes varied markedly and, in a minority, their clinical relevance was doubtful. Twelve out of 17 studies that assessed patient outcomes reported significant improvements. Guidelines developed internally, within the target groups of clinicians, appeared more likely to be effective than those developed externally. As will be discussed later, the effectiveness of guidelines is heavily influenced by the methods of their dissemination and implementation. Two illustrative examples of successful interventions are provided below.

Illustrative examples of evaluations testing strategies to implement clinical guidelines

"Corollary orders" to prevent errors of omission.

Clinicians often fail to order tests or treatments required to monitor or ameliorate the effects of other tests or treatments. Overhage *et al* randomised general medical teams, already familiar with using computer workstations, to intervention and control groups.[17] As the intervention physicians ordered certain tests or treatments, the computer automatically suggested "corollary" orders needed to detect or prevent associated adverse reactions. For example, an order for insulin triggered an order for four times daily blood glucose testing. During the trial, intervention physicians ordered the suggested corollary orders twice as often as control physicians (46% versus 22%). The intervention group also led to fewer interventions from hospital pharmacists to deal with errors considered to be life threatening, severe or significant.

Continuing medical education (CME) and quality assurance (QA) program to improve use of prophylaxis for venous thromboembolism.

Following the publication of a National Institutes of Health consensus guideline on prophylaxis and audits demonstrating the need for improvement, fifteen hospitals entered a randomised trial to evaluate methods of improving practice.[18] One third were allocated to CME (including lectures, mailings and general feedback on clinical performance), one third to CMA and QA (including feedback of general and individual clinical performance relating to compliance with agreed standards) and one third to controls. Prophylaxis use increased across all groups over time – but significantly more so in both the intervention groups. However, in this study, there appeared to be no additional benefit from participation in QA.

Do we need a guideline or pathway?

Both the development and implementation of guidelines carry resource implications. Therefore, appropriate clinical topics need to be identified and prioritised, preferably according to explicit criteria, so that the likely benefits of implementation outweigh probable costs.[19] Focused clinical questions are more likely to enhance the identification of relevant evidence and lead to practical recommendations.[6] There should be evidence of inappropriate clinical care and scope for preventing mortality and morbidity. Supporting valid and relevant research evidence should be available to inform the formulation of recommendations – although the depth (or even paucity) of this may not become apparent until development of the guideline. The financial costs and benefits of implementation require careful consideration, especially as professionals advocating a guideline may have an optimistic view of potential cost savings. Guideline implementation may result in additional resource use from greater clinical activity or the adoption of new, more costly practices. Finally, the selected topic should preferably be one likely to sustain the interest of those responsible for development and implementation.[20]

Once a topic has been agreed, local clinicians and managers have the option of either developing a new guideline themselves or adapting a guideline that has already been developed, usually at a national level. As most healthcare organisations lack the resources (especially in terms of professional time) required to develop new guidelines from scratch, it is usually expedient and probably more efficient to draw upon pre-existing guidelines. There may also be some advantages to promoting the adoption of national guidelines amongst different hospitals or healthcare teams, especially given the transience of parts of the healthcare workforce (e.g. professionals in training rotating around different units, or providing agency or locum cover). However, local adoption is more likely to succeed if guidelines are considered in detail by stakeholders and adapted, if necessary, to reflect local circumstances (such as the availability of services or patient characteristics).[5] For guidelines that cross care interfaces, such as those between different disciplines or between primary and secondary care – and many do in some way – it is particularly important to identify and seek agreement from all potential stakeholders, such as general practitioners, at an early stage.

Care pathways were initially employed for more predictable courses of clinical management, such as elective surgical procedures. Medical conditions have a lower predictability but those following common patterns are more likely to be eligible.[9] This may cover clinical presentations (such as chest pain) or diagnosed illness (such as acute myocardial infarction). Care pathways are presently largely hospital based but might also be appropriate for extension into primary or community care settings for the management of conditions such as asthma or depression.

How trustworthy and relevant is this guideline?

Guideline users need to be confident of their validity (trustworthiness) and relevance to clinical problems and circumstances but selecting the right guideline can be problematic. Forty-five different guidelines for the management of depression in primary care were identified within the United Kingdom.[21] There was a considerable range in the quality of a subset of guidelines appraised in detail. Therefore, rather than promote uniform standards of care, the proliferation of guidelines may perpetuate (or even augment) variations in practice.

Guidelines are more likely to be valid if produced by national or regional guideline development groups according to rigorous and explicit methods. Within the UK, the Scottish Intercollegiate Guidelines Network (SIGN) has been developing expertise and experience in guideline development. The recently established National Institute for Clinical Excellence (NICE) in England and Wales is undertaking a similar role. Elsewhere, internationally, several other initiatives are under way to improve the quality and dissemination of clinical guidelines (see below).

Electronic guideline resources

Canadian Medical Association Clinical Practice Guidelines Infobase – index of clinical practice guidelines includes downloadable full text versions or abstracts for most guidelines (http://www.cma.ca/cpgs/index.html)

National Institute of Clinical Excellence – Web site of UK organisation with responsibility for commissioning guidelines (http://www.nice.org.uk)

New Zealand Guidelines Group – full text versions of some guidelines, other useful guideline related resources (http://www.nzgg.org.nz/index.htm)

Medical Matrix (http://www.slackinc.com/matrix/index.html) – an index to medical resources available on the internet, includes section on guidelines (http://www.slackinc.com/matrix/clinprac.html)

National Guidelines Clearing house – US Agency for healthcare Policy and Research funded site which includes index of clinical practice guidelines, structured abstracts of guidelines and comparisons of guidelines for same clinical topic (http://www. guidelines. gov)

Scottish Intercollegiate Guidelines Network – full text copies of SIGN guidelines (http://www.show.scot.nhs.uk/sign/home.htm)

(Note: at the time of writing the electronic addresses given are correct, however these are liable to change over time.)

Checklists are available for the critical appraisal of guidelines that have not already been subject to such review. Cluzeau and colleagues designed the most valid and comprehensive appraisal instrument presently available.[22] The following questions, based upon this instrument, help to assess the rigour of guideline development, its content and context, and its application.

Did the guideline development group encompass the right range of skills and experience?

The guideline development group should include professionals with expertise in the clinical topic, literature searching, epidemiology, health services research, facilitating group processes and writing. [23] The clinicians present should represent the range of disciplines who deal with the clinical topic. For example, a guideline group on the investigation of post-menopausal bleeding might include a general gynaecologist, a general practitioner, an oncological gynaecologist, a radiologist and a pathologist.

How was evidence identified and assessed?

The evidence used to formulate recommendations should be based upon a comprehensive search of available and relevant research. An appropriate search strategy might include the Cochrane Library and major literature databases such as Medline and Embase.

The appropriate types of studies to answer questions, such as randomised controlled trials for testing therapy, and cohort studies for assessing prognosis, should be critically appraised according to agreed criteria. Such criteria help to "filter out" or take account of the limitations of studies. Without such explicitly stated methods of quality control it is difficult for the reader to tell whether the guideline developers have inadvertently (or even deliberately) incorporated their own prejudices in the selection of studies.

How was the evidence linked to recommendations?

Guideline users need to know about the nature and strength of evidence informing recommendations, and how the development group arrived at its conclusions. An analysis of guidelines produced by specialty societies over 1988–98 demonstrated that the majority failed to meet certain criteria for good quality, including explicit grading of evidence.[24] Grading systems help discriminate between, recommendations based upon rigorous evidence (for example meta-analyses or randomised controlled trials) and those based upon opinion and clinical experience. Apart from available evidence, other factors can legitimately influence the formulation of recommendations, including the relevance of the evidence to the target population, economic considerations, values of the guideline developers and society, and practical issues concerning implementation.[25]

Has this guideline been externally reviewed?

External review improves the validity and helps pre-test the relevance and acceptability of guidelines. Assessment by clinicians and guideline methodologists, not directly involved in the guideline's development, enables checks on the completeness of the clinical information and rigor of the methods reported.

Is this guideline up to date?

As the evidence base can change over time, all guidelines should carry an expiry date when the recommendations will be reviewed and updated if necessary.

Do the guideline developers have any potential conflicts of interest?

The agency responsible for development of the guideline should be clearly identified and the development process should be editorially independent from the funding body. These criteria help to identify any conflicts of interest. For example, without editorial independence, a guideline sponsored by a pharmaceutical company may implicitly, or otherwise, recommend a course of management favouring a particular drug treatment. Alternatively, a guideline produced by a particular specialty may err towards recommendations requiring the expansion of that specialty.

Where and when can this guideline be applied?

Circumstances when guidelines cannot be applied, such as when appropriate equipment or trained staff are unavailable, should be stated. Similarly, possible management options and subsequent recommendations should be clearly outlined. The role of patient preferences should be considered to help clinical staff to decide when it is appropriate to take these into account, say in deciding between two or more possible treatments. As guidelines usually apply to a group of patients as a whole, individuals may receive inappropriate care if recommendations are poorly worded or interpreted without reference to individual needs and preferences. For example, clinicians following guidelines on the management of hypertension need to be aware of their limitations and take into account pre-existing illnesses and risk factors that might complicate treatment and modify outcomes.[26]

291

What are the potential benefits from following this guideline?

Potential health benefits from following recommendations may include reduced mortality, improved health-related quality of life, reassurance or avoidance of unnecessary procedures. These need to be set out objectively to support clinical decision-making.

What are the potential costs of following this guideline?

Guideline implementation frequently has resource implications, associated both with implementation and from additional costs or savings resulting from following recommendations. Ideally, the evaluation of new healthcare technologies incorporates an assessment of cost-effectiveness. As cost-effectiveness data may not be available, the guideline may need to take account of some approximation of relative costs in presenting its recommendations.[25]

Poorly developed guidelines can not only potentially harm patients. They can add to confusion over best practice and generate hostility to more rigorously developed guidelines. As well as encouraging fairer resource allocation, the adoption of guidelines may also promote the inappropriate provision of healthcare interventions or facilities. Guideline developers should therefore consider the wider implications and possible unknown costs and consequences of their recommendations.[27] For example, recommending routine *H. pylori* testing for patients with dyspepsia with the aim of reducing the workload of diagnostic endoscopy services may paradoxically increase demand because of the high prevalence of this clinical presentation in primary care.[28]

How can we ensure that this guideline is used?

Follow up of ovarian cancer at a multidisciplinary clinic is an independent predictor of survival, reducing the risk of death at five years by 40%.[29] Adherence to locally developed protocols is also associated with better survival.[30] However, major variations in care have persisted, including in or amongst hospitals where guidelines have been developed but not followed.[30] Although they may increase general awareness about clinical issues, traditional methods of disseminating information, such as printed educational materials (for example journals or guidelines) or didactic educational meetings (for example lectures) are unlikely to change clinical behaviour.

Haphazard or indiscriminate distribution of guidelines may alienate professionals. In recent years, clinicians have been overwhelmed by proliferating quantities of guidelines,[31] sometimes of dubious quality and some of which are produced or sponsored by special interest groups, such as the pharmaceutical industry. Dissemination strategies should therefore balance comprehensive coverage against targeting of key groups or professionals.

The content of the recommendations, the receptivity of the target audience and organisational size and culture, availability of resources all pose potential barriers to changing practice. It is important to discriminate between factors that cannot be easily altered (for example resource allocation at a macro level or organisational size and staffing) and those that can be addressed (for example staff knowledge, attitudes and skills). Several theoretical models of change have been described which can be used both to understand the behaviour of health professionals and to guide the development and implementation of interventions to promote change.[32] Inevitably, implementation requires more time and resources and is usually "messier" than originally envisaged.[33] Previous experience highlights the importance of engaging local clinicians, piloting strategies before they are "rolled out" and providing support and training.

Particular problems have been highlighted with the implementation of care pathways. Documentation and information systems for the collection, analysis and feedback of data should be carefully designed and piloted. Many barriers, particularly clinician hostility to structured clinical management, need to be negotiated and overcome over a long time scale.[9,34] Staff should be aware of and practised in using the care pathway for all patients with the chosen condition.

Interventions to overcome specific barriers should ideally be tailored to the nature of anticipated local problems.[35] There is a growing body of evidence to support the prior assessment of barriers and needs.[36] Systematic reviews from the Cochrane Effective Practice and Organisation of Care (EPOC) Review Group provide sound evidence on which to base interventions (see below).[37] Combinations of interventions increase the likelihood of successfully implementing a guideline.

In the context of risk management, effective interventions may reduce inappropriate risk-averting behaviour. For example, a randomised trial has demonstrated the use of local opinion leaders to support the distribution of a clinical guideline resulting in a greater proportion of women with a previous caesarean section undergoing a trial of labour and delivering vaginally.[11] However, the use of audit and feedback had little impact in the same study, illustrating how additional interventions may only work in certain circumstances.

In situations where the probability or consequences of error are high, certain interventions can explicitly reduce clinical risk. For example, in the calculation of drug dosages or in their administration, errors occur which result in patients receiving the right drug but wrong dose, the right drug by the wrong route (e.g. via spinal fluid rather than intravenously), or

---

Interventions to promote professional behavioural change*

Consistently Effective

- *Educational outreach visits (for prescribing in North American settings)* – Use of a trained person who meets with providers in their practice settings to provide information with the intent of changing the provider's performance. The information given may include feedback on the provider's performance
- *Reminders (manual or computerised)* – Any intervention that prompts the healthcare provider to perform a patient specific clinical action
- *Multifaceted interventions* – A combination that includes two or more of the following: audit and feedback, reminders, local consensus process, marketing
- *Interactive educational meetings* – Participation of healthcare providers in workshops that include discussion or practice

Mixed Effects

- *Audit and feedback* – Any summary of clinical performance
- *Local opinion leaders* – Use of providers nominated by their colleagues as "educationally influential"
- *Local consensus process* – Inclusion of participating providers in discussion to ensure that they agreed that the chosen clinical problem was important and the approach to managing the problem was appropriate
- *Patient mediated interventions* – Any intervention aimed at changing the performance of healthcare providers where specific information was sought from or given to patients

Little or No Effect

- *Educational materials* – Distribution of published or printed recommendations for clinical care, including clinical practice guidelines, audio-visual materials and electronic publications
- *Didactic educational meetings* – Lectures

*Adapted from *Cochrane Library Issue 4* [37]

---

wrong drug altogether. These errors occur principally because clinicians' ability to process information accurately and, in urgent situations, rapidly is limited.[38] Therefore, clinical prompts or reminders represent, amongst others, an appropriate intervention to help prevent errors. In hospital settings, computer support systems designed to aid decisions concerning dosage or directly administer drugs (via an infusion) have been shown to be superior at calculating and administering drug dosages compared with doctors acting unaided.[39] Computer support can lead to increased blood concentrations of drugs, reduced time to achieve therapeutic benefits and fewer unwanted effects of treatment.

Although the success of interventions supporting guideline implementation is influenced by the characteristics of healthcare organisations or clinicians, the characteristics of individual guideline recommendations may also have an impact on adoption.[40] A review of published studies reporting compliance with guidelines developed or endorsed by official organisations found compliance was greater for "trialable" recommendations (which could be discarded easily if found ineffective locally) and lower for complex recommendations.[41] Following the dissemination of guidelines in general practice, recommendations which were vaguely worded, incompatible with local norms and values, and which required changes to fixed routines or habits were associated with lower compliance following implementation.[42]

How can we evaluate the impact of this guideline?

Evaluations (or audits) of the impact of guidelines are preferentially planned prior to implementation. Three complementary approaches can be considered.:

- Monitoring one critical aspect of care using a tracer condition, based upon the assumption that it will reflect the overall quality of care. Ideally, a tracer condition should be relatively common, well defined, and responsive to effective healthcare interventions.[43,44]
- Focusing on a small number of critical points in the care process or pathway where greatest scope for error exists or where the consequences of errors are greatest.
- Use of critical incident analysis to explore organisational factors contributing to adverse events (or where a pathway has failed) and assess whether a different course of action would have averted the event.

For example, evaluating the impact of a guideline on the management of major post-partum haemorrhage is potentially problematic. Ideally, relevant and reliable clinical data would be available. However, major post-partum haemorrhage represents a relatively uncommon occurrence within a single maternity unit. Changes in incidence or related mortality over time may occur by chance and may be difficult to attribute to the introduction of a guideline. Furthermore, there should be little need to measure health outcomes if the guideline recommendations are already based upon evidence of effectiveness. An evaluation could therefore begin by testing simple aspects of dissemination, such as receipt by target users and availability. (Guidelines on the management of post-partum haemorrhage are more likely to have an impact on clinical care if they are available in delivery and resuscitation suites rather than on bookshelves.) In evaluating

295

implementation, test runs of emergency protocols or "fire drills" offer opportunities to test and inform further refinement of local protocols.[45] Critical incident analysis can be used following a major haemorrhage to explore possible contributory factors and learn lessons for future clinical management.

Several reasons may explain variance from care pathways, not all of which necessarily indicate failures in care. These include complications in the patient's condition or social circumstances, co-morbidity, changes in the availability of treatments or investigations, clinicians deciding not to use the pathway, and input from staff from other departments or outside the hospital unfamiliar with the pathway.[3] Variances require regular analysis to explore reasons for departure from the pathway before being fed back to staff.

Will the adoption of this guideline make us more or less vulnerable to litigation?

There is confusion as to whether the adoption of guidelines and pathways increases or decreases vulnerability to litigation.[46] On one hand, there is concern that clinicians who fail to follow guidelines or pathways will be accused of falling short of acceptable standards. On the other, the implementation of guidelines may lead to safer and more effective care, thereby reducing clinical risk.

There is no direct evidence that the introduction of guidelines and pathways has directly contributed to increased rates of litigation, particularly from the United States where there is greater experience of pathways. Guidelines have been cited as evidence in 6% of a random sample of cases in claims opening over 1990–91, in roughly equal proportions for the plaintiff and defendant, although more recent data has not yet been published.[47]

In the UK, proof of negligence is based upon proving deviation from accepted and customary patterns of care (the "Bolam test") rather than departure from an "ideal" practice.[48] This "test" recognises that medical opinion may be divided and that the views and practice of a sizeable minority of doctors are legitimate, at least in a legal context.

Guidelines are frequently employed to support changes in clinical behaviour, often beyond customary standards of care. Therefore, it is only once compliance with a guideline recommendation becomes firmly established that it becomes customary care, although a minority opinion may still have legal credibility. There is pressure to supersede the Bolam test with a new definition more related to ideal practice but there is little or no prospect of this happening without reference to a responsible body of medical practitioners.[48]

Attempts to define standards of care often encounter the blurred boundary between appropriate and inappropriate care.[49] By itself, a guideline is too blunt a tool to reliably demonstrate inappropriate care.[50] Clinicians who interpret and follow guidelines in a blanket fashion may fail to take into account uncertainty about the evidence, and patient needs and preferences. Many guidelines pertain to the "usual" case, derived from research findings which average out risks or clinical effects from a range of study subjects. Nevertheless, clinicians who practise outside of accepted guidelines or care pathways should take special care to document their rationale for the variation in practice.[51]

Clinicians following any guideline, even if it is flawed, remain legally responsible for their own actions, as guideline developers cannot be held liable for the actions of individual clinicians. Many guidelines now carry standard disclaimers to this effect. Nevertheless, guideline developers should try to ensure that guidelines are based upon robust evidence and a true consensus. Areas of disagreement or clinical uncertainty should be noted within the guideline.[51] Guidelines also need to be worded cautiously and precisely and avoid incorporating words such as "should" in certain recommendations.

Concerns over litigation also pose a potential barrier to guideline implementation. For example, some guidelines may recommend withholding or withdrawing routinely used treatments or investigations based on evidence of no, or limited, clinical effectiveness. Although such a guideline might be safe to follow from a legal viewpoint, clinicians' fears over a perceived vulnerability to litigation may deter them from adopting it in practice.

Given the potential benefits to be gained from clinical guidelines, it is unfortunate that legitimate but magnified concerns over litigation may hinder their development or implementation. Furthermore, the first and foremost aim of clinical guidelines in the context of risk management is to reduce risk to patients rather than protect clinicians from litigation. But improved standards of care should lead to reduced litigation.

Conclusions

Clinical guidelines and care pathways can help deliver improved healthcare at greater safety margins. However, clinicians and managers should be aware of avoidable pitfalls and the need for carefully planned and executed development, dissemination, and implementation in order to realise potential benefits.

Topics selected locally for guideline development or adoption should be of sufficient clinical and organisational importance. Rather than develop an original guideline, it is usually more efficient to adopt or adapt a guideline from a recognised guideline development programme. Guidelines developed according to a rigorous methodology are more likely to be valid and relevant to clinical practice. Interventions to promote the uptake of a clinical guideline should ideally be tailored to the nature of anticipated barriers. Several active interventions are of proven effectiveness in changing clinical behaviour but multifaceted approaches work most consistently.

Clinical guidelines need to be applied flexibly to a range of clinical and organisational circumstances. The existence of a guideline is insufficient by itself to establish whether compliance, or non-compliance, is negligent. In the longer term, as both patient expectations of care and trends in litigation continue to rise, clinical guidelines should become a cornerstone of risk management.

Acknowledgements

The Health Services Research Unit is supported by the Chief Scientist's Office of the Scottish Executive Health Department (SEHD). Robbie Foy is funded by a health services research training grant from the MRC/SEHD. The views expressed here are those of the authors.

References

1 Smith D. *Delia Smith's Complete Cookery Course*. London: BBC Worldwide Publishing; 1989.
2 Field MJ, Lohr KN, eds. *Clinical practice guidelines: directions for a new program*. Washington DC: National Academy Press, 1990.
3 Campbell H, Hotchkiss R, Bradshaw N, Porteous M. Integrated care pathways. *BMJ* 1998;**316**:133–7.
4 Woods KL, Ketley D, Lowy A, *et al*. Beta-blockers and antithrombotic treatment for secondary prevention after acute myocardial infarction. Towards an understanding of factors influencing clinical practice. *Eur Heart J* 1998;**19**:74–9.
5 Grimshaw J, Russell I. Effect of clinical guidelines on medical practice: a systematic review of rigorous evaluations. *Lancet* 1993;**3421**:317–22.
6 Sackett DL, Richardson WS, Rosenberg W, *et al*. *Evidence-based medicine: how to practice and teach EBM*. London: Churchill-Livingstone, 1997.
7 Muir Gray JA. Where's the chief knowledge officer? *BMJ* 1998;**317**:832–40.
8 McColl A, Smith H, White P, Field J. General practitioners' perceptions of the route to evidence based medicine: a questionnaire survey. *BMJ* 1998;**316**:361–5.
9 Layton A, Moss F, Morgan G. Mapping out the patient's journey: experiences of developing pathways of care. *Qual healthcare* 1998;7 (Suppl)S30–S36.
10 Grimes DA. Evidence-based obstetrics and gynaecology: theory into practice: within a department. *Baillière's Clin Obstet Gynaecol* 1996;**10**(4):697–714.
11 Lomas J, Enkin M, Anderson G, *et al*. Opinion leaders vs audit and feedback to implement practice guidelines: delivery after previous cesarian section. *JAMA* 1991;**265**: 2202–7.
12 Scottish Obstetric Guideline and Audit Project. *The management of mild, non-proteinuric hypertension in pregnancy*. Edinburgh: Scottish Project for Clinical Effectiveness in Reproductive Health, 1997.
13 Reason J. Understanding adverse events: human factors. *Qual healthcare* 1995;4:480–9.
14 Dowsey MM, Kilgour ML, Santamaria NM, Choong FM. Clinical pathways in hip and knee arthroplasty: a prospective randomised controlled study. *Med J Aust* 1999; **170**:59–62.

15 Institute of Medicine. Field MJ, Lohr KN, eds. *Guidelines for clinical practice. From development to use.* Washington: National Academy Press, 1992.

16 NHS Centre for Reviews and Disseminations. Implementing Clinical Practice Guidelines. *Effective healthcare* 1994;(8).

17 Overhage JM, Tierney WM, Zhou X, McDonald CJ. A randomised trial of "corollary orders" to prevent errors of omission. *J Am Med Inform Assoc* 1997;4:364–75.

18 Anderson FA, Wheeler HB, Goldberg RJ, *et al.* Changing clinical practice: prospective study of the impact of continuing medical education and quality assurance programs on the use of prophylaxis for venous thromboembolism. *Arch Intern Med* 1994;154:669–77.

19 Feder G, Eccles M, Grol R, *et al.* Using clinical guidelines. *BMJ* 1999;318:728–30.

20 Russell I, Grimshaw J, Wilson B. Scientific and methodological issues in quality assurance. *Proc R Soc Edinb* 1993;101B:77–103.

21 Littlejohns P, Cluzeau F, Bale R, *et al.* The quantity and quality of clinical practice guidelines for the management of depression in primary care in the UK. *Br J Gen Pract* 1999;49:205–10.

22 Cluzeau F, Littlejohns P, Grimshaw J, *et al. Appraisal Instrument for Clinical Guidelines.* London: St George's Hospital Medical School, 1997.

23 Shekelle PG, Woolf SH, Eccles M, Grimshaw J. Developing guidelines. *BMJ* 1999;318: 593–6.

24 Grilli R, Magrini N, Penna A, *et al.* Practice guidelines developed by specialty societies: the need for a critical appraisal. *Lancet* 2000;355:103–6.

25 Eccles M, Freemantle N, Mason J. North of England evidence based guidelines development project: methods of developing guidelines for efficient drug use in primary care. *BMJ* 1998;316:1232–5.

26 Tudor Hart JT. Hypertension guidelines: other diseases complicate management. *BMJ* 1993;306:1337.

27 Haycox A, Bagust A, Walley T. Clinical guidelines – the hidden costs. *BMJ* 1999;318: 391–3.

28 Foy R, Parry JM, Murray L, Woodman CBJ. Testing for *Helicobacter pylori* in primary care: trouble in store? *J Epidemiol Community Health* 1998;52:305–9.

29 Junor EJ, Hole DJ, Gillis CR. Management of ovarian cancer: referral to a multidisciplinary team matters. *Br J Cancer* 1994;70:363–70.

30 Wolfe CDA, Tilling K, Raju KS. Management and survival of ovarian cancer patients in south east England. *Eur J Cancer* 1997;33:1835–40.

31 Hibble A, Kanka D, Pencheon D, Pooles F. Guidelines in general practice: the new Tower of Babel? *BMJ* 1998;317:862–3.

32 NHS Centre for Reviews and Dissemination. *Effective healthcare: Getting evidence into practice.* University of York, 1999.

33 Dunning M, Abi-Aad G, Gilbert D, *et al. Turning evidence into everyday practice.* London: King's Fund Publishing, 1998.

34 Pearson SD, Goulart-Fisher D, Lee TH. Critical pathways as a strategy for improving care: problems and potential. *Ann Intern Med* 1995;123:941–8.

35 Grol R. Beliefs and evidence in changing clinical practice. *BMJ* 1997;315:418–21.

36 Davis DA, Thomson MA, Oxman AD, Haynes RB. Changing physician performance: a systematic review of the effect of continuing medical education strategies. *JAMA* 1995;274(9):700–5.

37 Cochrane Effective Professional and Organisation of Care Group. *The Cochrane Library.* Issue 4. Oxford: Update Software, 1999.

38 McDonald CJ. Protocol-based computer reminders, the quality of care and the non-perfectability of man. *N Engl J Med* 1976;295:1351–5.

39 Walton R, Dovey S, Harvey E, Freemantle N. Computer support for determining drug dose: systematic review and meta-analysis. *BMJ* 1999;318:984–90.

40 Lomas J, Dunn EV, Norton PG, *et al.,* eds. *Disseminating research/changing practice; teaching old (and not so old) docs new tricks: effective ways to implement research findings.* California: SAGE, 1994.

41 Grilli R, Lomas J. Evaluating the message: the relationship between compliance rate and the subject of a practice guideline. *Med Care* 1994;32(3):202–13.

42 Grol R, Dalhuijsen J, Thomas S. In: Veld C, Rutten G, Mokkink H. Attributes of clinical

guidelines that influence use of guidelines in general practice: observational study. *BMJ* 1998;**317**:858–61.

43 Kessner DM, Kalk CE, Singer J. Assessing health quality – the case for tracers. *N Engl J Med* 1973;**288**:189–93.

44 Irvine D. *Managing for quality in general practice*. London: King's Fund, 1990.

45 Department of Health, Welsh Office, Scottish Office Department of Health *et al. Why mothers die*. Report on Confidential Enquiries into Maternal Deaths in the United Kingdom 1994–1996. London: HMSO, 1998.

46 Carrick SE, Bonevski B, Redman S, *et al.* Surgeons' opinions about the NHMRC clinical practice guidelines for the management of early breast cancer. *Med J Aust* 1998;**169**: 300–5.

47 Hyams AL, Brandenburg JA, Lipsitz SR, *et al.* Practice guidelines and malpractice litigation: a two way street. *Ann Intern Med* 1995;**122**:450–5.

48 Hurwitz B. Legal and political considerations of clinical practice guidelines. *BMJ* 1999;**318**:661–4.

49 Naylor CD. Grey zones of clinical practice: some limits to evidence-based medicine. *Lancet* 1995;**345**:840–2.

50 Jacobsen PD. Legal and policy considerations in using clinical practice pathways. *Am J Cardiol* 1997;**80**(8B):74H-9H.

51 Pelly JE, Newby L, Tito F, *et al.* Clinical practice guidelines before the law: sword or shield? *Med J Aust* 1998;**169**:330–3.

16 The role of human factors engineering in medical device and medical system errors

JOHN GOSBEE, LAURA LIN

Most errors in your hospital cannot be addressed using clinical risk management that focuses on the traditional concerns of litigation, insurance, and personnel discipline. Even systems-oriented thinking is not sufficient. What is also needed is the formal discipline called human factors engineering. Human factors engineering must become part of the vocabulary, consciousness, and recruitment and training strategy of clinicians and risk managers. Much more than an additional set of principles and techniques, human factors engineering provides a tried-and-true framework for building and strengthening that elusive safety culture.

In this chapter we will define and describe human factors engineering. We will discuss its necessary role in medical device, medical software, and healthcare work area design: specifically, how researchers and engineers have proven its need in reducing error-facilitating design. We will highlight the very few publications on how human factors engineering can transform the way clinicians and risk managers approach error in healthcare settings.

Then, we will provide straightforward guidance for you, your facility, and those who develop policy and curriculum. We start with preventive clinical risk management strategies born out of human factors engineering analysis, including the:

- procurement process
- developing software, work areas, and procedures within your own healthcare organisation
- surveillance approaches (for example, audits)
- awareness training for front-line clinical personnel.

Next we outline the "reactive" clinical risk management strategies that are affected by human factors engineering, including:

- structure, techniques, and questioning during analysis of adverse events
- how to improve corrective actions for medical errors and tie them to "preventive" measures.

Finally, clinicians and risk managers would only be equipped to do these new activities with the proper resources, training, and management adjustments. So we give you a checklist that we believe is the least to get started.

Human factors engineering (HFE)

As many as 100 000 deaths or serious injuries occur each year in the USA as a result of medical accidents.[1] It is believed that a significant number are related to the misuse of medical devices.[2,3] While human error is often cited as the cause of medical device mishaps, what is less frequently acknowledged is the notion that a poorly designed human-machine interface can facilitate human error.[4,5] What is also not widely known is that human errors can be significantly reduced by incorporating human factors in the design of medical devices.[6,7] The process of human factors engineering (HFE) can also be applied to other aspects of the workplace setting, ranging from information systems to the layout of workspace (for example, in an ICU), to improve safety. The general idea is not new.[8]

Human factors engineering is a discipline concerned with the design of tools, machines, and systems that take into account human capabilities, limitations, and characteristics. The goals are to design for safe, comfortable, and effective human use.[9] The practice and application of human factors engineering is nicely explained in Nielsen.[10] Ergonomics, usability engineering, and user-centered design are considered synonymous or closely related to human factors engineering, which is based on design-related aspects of several biomedical disciplines. From a systems perspective, the human is receiving input from a machine, processing that input, and creating an output that goes to the machine. Anthropometrics and biomechanics cover most of the physical aspects of input and output. The science of sensation and perception is related to input to the human. Cognitive psychology, which covers models and theories of human performance, memory, and attention, relates to the processing of the input and initiating the output. Understanding how these biomedical sciences can inform an engineer to match humans and systems is the key for human factors engineering.

A human factors engineering process comprises several important elements, all of which revolve around the user of the system, hence, the term "user-centred design". This design process focuses on user needs, user characteristics, and end user testing of the human-machine interface. Another key characteristic of this user-centred design approach is the concept of iterative design and testing. Simply put, the design is repeatedly refined throughout the design cycle based on feedback from user testing (or usability testing) which is also repeatedly conducted, starting from the early stages of the design cycle. This helps to ensure that the system being designed meets its intended purpose and operates in its intended manner. Early testing also helps to ensure that design deficiencies are identified and rectified before the system is fielded. Design deficiencies can cause unnecessary increases in workload, creates greater risks for errors, and reduces productivity. The human factors engineering design process is described in more detail by Wiklund.[11]

In many corners of the world, human factors engineering is already widely practised. In the USA, the Human Factors and Ergonomics Society is the main professional organisation (www.hfes.org). In the United Kingdom and the international community, it is the Ergonomics Society (www.ergo.ac.uk) and International Ergonomics Association (www.iea.org), respectively. The domains of aviation, nuclear power plants, and consumer software have a strong history of implementing human factors engineering to improve usability and safety. This chapter explains how human factors can be implemented within healthcare organisations to do the same.

Human factors engineering and adverse events

There is a diverse set of issues related to human error in medicine. Bogner's book on *Human Error in Medicine*[12] highlights many of the associated human factors issues. One of the primary areas that clinicians and risk managers can directly influence is the reduction of human errors that occur during the operation of medical devices or medical information systems.[13,14]

Human factors engineering and medical device design

The role of human factors in the design of medical devices and medical information systems is the topic of a growing number of published articles.[15] Gosbee[16] talks about the need for user needs analysis in the discovery phase of device design. Aucella *et al*[17] and Brown[18] provide examples of the user-centred design process implemented in the design of a ultrasound machine. Lin *et al*[19] describes the implementation of human factors analytical techniques (for example, cognitive task analysis) in analysing and redesigning an interface for a patient-controlled analgesia pump. Beascart-Zephir *et al*[20] discuss methods for assessing

303

usability of information technology in healthcare. Finally, in a study at the University of Toronto, Lin[6] demonstrates the positive impact of human factors engineering on the design of medical devices, providing evidence of better usability, reduced errors, and reduced mental workload in a system designed using HFE processes.

Ignoring human factors in the design process will more likely lead to a poorly designed human–machine interface, often the culprits in adverse events. Poorly designed systems may originate from external vendors or from internal developers. Both cases present the opportunity for the risk manager or clinician to implement a human factors process. The process to build a better safety culture, methods of error analysis, and preventive measures, starts with an understanding of the effects when human factors engineering is ignored.

More training and more technology may not help

Explanations of errors rarely penetrate the true underlying causes.[16] Therefore the solutions have only a limited effect. For example, some usual solutions are to increase training of personnel or to introduce computers and technology. As you will see, this does not always solve the problem.

Training

In studying errors that occur in medicine, researchers often believe that the source of the problem is the individual committing the error. However, the fact that even highly trained professionals can make errors points to the need for alternative methods to reduce errors. Device related user errors often stem from human–machine interaction rather than from the individual exclusively. Machines that are not designed to accommodate the limitations of human performance or the needs of the task at hand are doomed to promote more human–machine interaction errors, no matter how well trained the individual. Human factors studies of error in medicine provide broader insight into the sources of problems,[12] and as a result, provide a broader set of implications that reach beyond the reprimand of the individual. While the training solution may help to control the problem, the source of the problem will continue to persist.

Technology

Ideally, computers should be used for tasks computational in nature, require flawless and extraordinary memory recall, and perfect vigilance over extended periods. Many in healthcare have identified the role of computers in effectively addressing errors, including medication errors and as reminders for oft forgotten clinical interventions. Examples of effective applications include alerting the provider of allergies and drug–drug interactions,[21] and increasing out-patient preventive measures[22] (for example, cancer screening and immunisation).

When human factors engineering is not considered in the design of computer systems, the user needs and their existing problems are rarely identified and hence not properly addressed. Unfortunately, when this occurs, many computer systems in healthcare solve the wrong problem or do not address the error in a usable manner. At best, the computer does nothing to eliminate errors. At worst, it introduces insidious new problems.[23] A recent empirical study showed that only 4 out of 307 pharmacy computers correctly identified all unsafe medication orders in a field test.[24] The researchers suggested the root causes of the failures were: complex programming, hard-to-use human–computer interfaces, and unrealistic time commitments needed to properly to maintain and use the systems. While there is ample evidence that many pitfalls await the introduction of new technology, some developers of medical information systems have appropriately used human factors methodologies to develop information systems.[25]

A side effect of introducing technology is the change in the nature of the healthcare practitioner's job, thus imposing a new set of cognitive demands on the user of the technology. The net effect is not necessarily a reduction in workload, but rather, an unintentional shift in the type of workload incurred and the type of errors that emerge as a result. It is important to recognise this change in roles and shift of workload in order to understand the systemic causes of user errors appearing with new technology. Furthermore, the increasing number and variety of technologies in the healthcare environment introduces integration challenges. This demands a system-level approach to evaluating the technology. Many of these factors are related to the integration of a new machine or technology into an existing environment. The deficiencies of some technology may not be apparent until you attempt to integrate it into the setting in which it is to be used.

Latent errors

While technology provides increased capabilities, it also introduces increased complexity, making it easy to end up with poorly designed systems if human factors engineering approaches and methods are not used. A poorly designed system (for example, software, devices, and work areas) constitutes a latent error, an error whose effects are not seen until there is a triggering event (for example, nurse misprogramming an infusion pump) that causes the error (pump delivers too much morphine). The natural tendency is to associate the outcome (for example, patient is killed by overdose) with the triggering event (nurse misprogramming the pump), and to designate the triggering event as the cause. However, when the latent error (poorly

Table 16.1 Link between latent errors and their effects in the healthcare setting

HFE Process Ignored	Description	Effects seen in Healthcare Setting
Inadequate Functional Requirement Definition	Not identifying the user need Misunderstanding the user need	Trying to use wrong tool for the job so care delayed or deficient
Inadequate Attention to User Interface Design	Not adopting human factors design methods (user centred design)	Right tool for the job, but does not fit into physical, cognitive, or other human limitations
	Not adhering to design principles	Inefficient, frustrating, error-
	Not designing to meet human performance requirements	prone, and takes too long to train
Inadequate Usability Testing	Not evaluating the usability of product in a representative setting with end users during design	Right tool, but takes too long to use or too error prone Does not fit into flow of work or work area
Inadequate Training Requirements Definition	Not understanding the training level of the end-user or needs for training	Right tool, but make errors while learning on the job, avoiding the tool, or not using all the tool's capabilities

designed programming interface on the infusion pump) is not acknowledged and rectified, the true culprit lies in wait for the next unsuspecting user. Table 16.1 describes the link between latent errors (the neglect of human factors processes) and the effects they have in the healthcare setting.

Example of use of HFE

The role that a poorly designed user interface plays in precipitating user errors during operation of medical devices is not widely recognised. At the University of Toronto, this motivated the study of improving medical device design through the application of human factors engineering.[6,19] Human factors engineers focused on a commonly used device as the testbed, the Abbott Patient Controlled Analgesia (PCA) Infuser. According to Food and Drug Administration (FDA) incident reports reviewed in the study, human error was found to be responsible for a majority (68%) of fatalities and serious injuries associated with the Abbott PCA in a randomly chosen year. This is similar to what was found in other studies.[26] Of the reports where human error was involved, nurse programming errors were found to be the most common type of human error in PCA use. Furthermore, the majority of programming errors involved setting an incorrect drug concentration, all of which led to an over-delivery of medication. Taken together, there was strong evidence that the design of the PCA Infuser had many latent errors and could be improved with human factors engineering.

As the first step towards demonstrating the utility of human factors engineering, the engineers develop a redesigned PCA pump based on human factors analytical techniques and design principles, including cognitive task analysis (field studies, bench tests, and design checklist). In the field studies, for instance, nurses were observed in the recovery room doing many tasks at once and constantly being interrupted while programming the PCA. During bench tests, many difficulties were encountered, even while operating the equipment under ideal conditions with the help of a users' manual. Finally, the design checklist helped the engineers find where design principles were violated. The redesigned PCA pump included such features as logical grouping and labelling of controls, simplified and more natural language in the displayed messages, and improved status display and feedback.

The second step was to evaluate empirically the design with users. Two user groups participated: novice users (nursing students) and experienced PCA users (recovery room nurses). Participants were given a PCA order form (prescription) and their task was to programme the pumps accordingly using each interface (see Lin et al[19] for details on experimental design). The evaluations included performance metrics such as number of errors, time to complete the task of programming, and subjective workload measures (i.e. mental demand, frustration, etc.).

In both groups, there were marked improvements with the redesigned PCA pump. First, there was a reduction in number of errors recorded, 50% and 55% reduction for nursing students and nurses, respectively. Furthermore, there were no errors in setting the drug concentration with the redesigned system, demonstrating a degree of resistance to the most culpable error found in the *Medical Device Reports*.[27]

Accompanying the reduction in programming errors with the redesigned system was a statistically significant improvement in task completion time. Nursing students were able to complete programming tasks with the redesigned system 15% faster. The nurses showed 18% faster completion times despite having no prior experience with the new system, compared to several years of experience with the existing Abbott pump. This improvement can be attributed to, among other things, the fact that significantly fewer programming errors were being made, and thus less time was wasted recovering from errors.

The subjective workload associated with the redesigned interface was found to be lower for both user groups using the redesigned pump compared to the existing Abbott pump: 53% and 14% lower for nursing students and nurses respectively. Finally, post-experiment interviews with the nurses and nursing students showed that an overwhelming majority (100%

of nursing students and 90% of nurses) preferred the redesigned system to the current system.

Collectively, what the findings of this study point to is that quantifiable improvements in equipment safety and efficiency can be achieved by adopting a human factors approach to interface design.

When HFE is ignored during design, these so-called latent errors impact the eventual occurrence of adverse events during patient care. Thus the onus falls upon the risk manager and clinician to recognise the existence and the potency of latent errors and to devise strategies to mitigate them. The challenge is two tiered:

- how to devise strategies that will ensure the purchase of useful and usable products (proactive strategies)
- how to diagnose and devise corrective actions when these products are already in use (reactive strategies).

We will outline proactive and reactive management strategies that incorporate a human factors engineering view.

"Preventive" clinical risk management strategies affected by HFE

There are several "preventive" clinical risk management strategies that incorporate the principles and techniques of human factors engineering.[28] First, risk managers and clinicians need to provide guidance and become involved in procurement of medical devices and software. Secondly, in a similar fashion, they need to work with "in-house" design and development efforts, since many healthcare organisations develop their own software and organise or design complex work areas. Thirdly, clinicians and risk managers should provide systematic surveillance of high risk software, devices, and work areas that are already purchased and in place. Finally, they need to train clinicians and other allies to observe and report human factors issues from the "front lines."

Before you buy . . .

As anyone seeking to improve quality of the final product knows, you need to build them from quality parts that have no hidden flaws. A preventive approach to avoiding troublesome devices and software includes both performing human factors analysis of products before purchase, and demanding human factors data from vendors. The Mayo Clinic in the United States has built usability (i.e. human factors) labs to evaluate many software products before purchase – as well as to use them for their own development projects.[29] During usability testing, many end-users attempt to use the software or device using likely scenarios under conditions that mimic actual operation. Measurements of errors, recovery from errors, and time to complete a task are most often taken. It is not hard to imagine how human factors engineers can also gather "soft" measures like opinion and blend them with observations like counting the number of muttered curse words.

Your hospital may not have resources for extensive usability labs, but other techniques like cognitive walkthrough and heuristic evaluation are also useful.[10] If you applied cognitive walkthrough in a basic manner, you would gather people in a room who would be affected by the use of the device or software. For an intravenous (IV) pump, that might be a nurse, a pharmacist, and a technician. Then you would have each person think through and talk about how they would use the IV pump under consideration. For instance, first an order for IV fluid is sent from pharmacy, then the nurse transcribes the order, then the nurse takes the IV fluid to the bedside, etc. As they "walk through" the usage of the system, questions and issues arise.

Heuristic evaluation is more of a human factors guideline checklist approach. Someone skilled in the area of human factors and medical software and devices is needed. Sometimes more than one expert is used, or the human factors engineering expert does not really know the medical domain. In the case of software, the expert looks at all the computer screens to determine if the design departs from accepted human factors guidelines and principles. Principles include things such as consistency of navigation and logical grouping and organisation of controls (for example, icons).

If your organisation does not have the resources to enact the above methods, you could at least ask a series of questions that considered environmental and stressors issues. For instance, "what effect does the vendor think time pressure will have on performance of basic tasks, and was that measured during development?" For another example, "how are error rates affected by ambient noise and lighting conditions in the areas where the device or system will be used?"

Along the same line of questioning, healthcare organisation should demand human factors engineering data from companies that make devices and software. Questions they should be able to answer include:

- how long does it take to learn operation of the system?
- how long does it take to complete typical set-up tasks?
- what are the types and frequency of errors that could happen and the systems to thwart them?

Some companies will have this human factors engineering data. Some in the medical device and software industry have hired human factors engineers and are following the user-centred design approach. In recent years, more pressure is being brought to bear on industry from governments, standards groups, and professional societies. In the USA, for instance, the FDA requires some validation that the user can operate a device in the manner intended and the environment envisioned.[30] The Association for the Advancement of Medical Instrumentation is working on its third version of human factors design guidelines for devices.[31] International Standards Organization has developed some applicable standards, as well.[32]

Before you build . . .

If your hospital is designing its own software and arranging and integrating devices into a work area (for example, anaesthesia work station), it will need human factors engineering expertise – badly. For example, the internal software development team will need to follow a user centred design philosophy. They will need to learn human factors engineering techniques or contract for people with those skills.[16,33] They should expect to do iterative cycles of creating design concepts, conducting analysis, design activities, testing, etc. Errors should be expected if they do not understand the role and importance of involving end users, performing field studies, and integrating human factors engineering into the design team and design cycle.[34]

The recent United States Institute of Medicine report on addressing error recommends several principles for the design of systems and processes within healthcare organisation.[35] Much like the general discussion of human factors engineering above, they recommend a healthcare organisation should:

- avoid reliance on memory
- use constraints or forcing functions
- avoid reliance on vigilance
- simplify key processes
- standardise work processes.

All of these general recommendations are the underpinnings for human factors engineering principles and methods described and demonstrated through examples cited earlier.

Surveillance strategies

Even before you began to affect procurement or in-house development activities, you can do systematic surveillance of troublesome and risk-related devices and software. This "auditing" occurs in some fashion in most hospitals for other areas such as infection control and fire safety. Armed with an eye to human factors engineering flaws, one does not need to wait for near misses or adverse events.

Where does a person start? As mentioned above, we know that automation and software to aid medication ordering is falling short. The publication, *Institute for Safe Medication Practices Alerts*, contains weekly notices (www.ismp. org). We know that ICUs might be filled with non-standard interfaces. We can guess that look-alike medications or IV bags are stored together in the emergency room or first-response "crash carts" in hospital hallways. Finally, additional targets will arise from more rigorous analysis of errors that is blossoming in places like the United States Veterans Affairs hospitals.[36]

Extend your reach

The final general preventive strategy is to increase human factors engineering awareness by training for front-line clinical personnel. As described, the safety culture change will involve everyone in the healthcare system. A concrete step towards this goal is to help care givers anticipate major errors by "seeing" near misses or troublesome design. This can be tricky since a "Blame and train" mentality will need to be quashed before clinical people will agree to take the time to be trained or change their focus to systems, not the f-word (fault). Some general guidance to helping people whose main job is not risk management per se, is needed before they see that error is not random.

"Reactive" clinical risk management strategies affected by HFE

Almost immediately, clinical risk managers and others could incorporate human factors engineering into existing duties: analysing adverse events and developing corrective actions to prevent similar events. Describing the outcome of the error is usually easy, but without human factors engineering you can often come up short when identifying the root cause. Corrective actions that speak to training and procedure changes need additional human factors engineering-based advice for errors more closely rooted in medical devices and software interface design.

The risk manager and other healthcare personnel will be involved with doing analyses of adverse events – often called root cause analyses. If the general mindset focused on people, not systems, then lack of skill and training are most often considered the culprit. Expanding this mindset and root cause analysis is best described by looking at prompting questions. The checklist of questions offers a concrete path toward systems thinking. Better still, they result in better recommendations.

Considerations include the intended purpose, user population, user's existing skills, user's activities, and the characteristics of the existing

311

environment. Here are some of the questions the people performing root cause analyses should ask:

- Do the systems meet an existing need of the users?
- Is the user given prompts and salient feedback after each action?
- Are the functions of the various controls clear and obvious?
- Are the displayed messages easy to understand?
- What is the load on the user's memory?
- Are there clearly marked exits for the user to leave the system or function or to cancel an action?
- Does existing knowledge or training of the users make it more difficult to learn how to use the system properly?
- Does the system require training that is counter to existing norms or conventions (negative transfer of training)?
- Are there multiple sets of users who will use the machine differently depending on the goals of their job?
- Does the system introduce automation? If so, is the user's primary role to monitor the automation?
- Is there a sense of being aware or in control of the computer-controlled tasks (i.e. automated system)?
- Are there problems associated with the user taking back control when something goes wrong with automation (switching from auto-pilot to manual)?
- Does the system use symbols, alarms, or controls that appear similar to other currently used machines but function differently?
- Does the system create unexpected tasks or procedures (i.e. work-arounds) that need to be performed in conjunction with the operation of the system?
- How does the system affect how current activities are carried out? Does it hinder other activities?
- What environmental conditions (for example, noise, light levels) make the use of the system difficult or impossible?

The investigation team will not get all the answers from their own inspection or experimentation. They can take some simple steps to search for human factors engineering data about the device, software or system under scrutiny. First, you can search medical literature in places like United States' Medline. Whoever searches Medline,[37] needs to be aware of quirks like the key word is "human engineering", and that problems with devices sometimes are "hidden" in articles about training and patient compliance (i.e. adherence). Second, many databases on adverse events with medical devices and pharmaceuticals exist over the World Wide Web. This includes *Medical Device Reports* (*www.fda.gov/cdrh/mdr.html*), Emergency Care Research Institute (*www.ecri.org*), and Institute for Safe Medication Practices (*www.ismp. org*). Finally, literature from human factors and ergonomics societies includes evidence that is specific and helpful. However, it is rarely known or cited in medical circles, and requires you search through databases like *Psych Lit*, *Ergonomics Abstracts*, and *HCIBIB*.

It is not surprising that teams assigned by healthcare organisations to recommend ways of avoiding error often suggest firing or retraining people and redoing standard operating procedures. This incomplete approach is avoided, if the team uses the prompting questions noted above and gets the training described below. In addition, the new focus on device and software design deficiencies provides the justification to move toward the "preventive" risk management strategies described earlier.

What is needed and how much?

The advice to improve the safety culture is nearly useless without an explicit and significant investment in existing and new personnel. The people who lead the new efforts (for example, risk managers, clinical managers) need several human factors engineering (HFE) classes. An ideal curriculum would begin with an introductory class in HFE, followed by HFE methods and techniques, application of HFE to design of equipment and software, and HFE and safety (for example, design of warnings and alarms). Every large hospital or healthcare organisation should have at least one human factors engineering and medicine expert on staff. As combined human factors engineering and medicine programmes and curricula evolve, these cross-disciplinarians will be coveted.[38]

Everyone involved in patient care and management who makes purchasing and operational decisions needs awareness and appreciation of human factors engineering. As an indirect cost, this is the organisation's largest investment. The internal human factors expertise can be combined with nearby universities and professional organisations to help. Professional groups and governing bodies for training medical doctors, nurses, and pharmacists have addressed the need to teach about the nature and reduction of error in medicine. Governing bodies for graduate and undergraduate medical education in the United States have several requirements for teaching quality assurance, continuous quality improvement, and systems thinking. The enumeration of these is beyond the scope of this article. The American Nurses' Credentialing Center, partnered with American Nurses Association, lists human factors engineering (which would include error) as one of seven areas of competency.[39] The American Society of Health-System Pharmacists cites the human factors engineering training of pharmacy directors as one of seven key strategies to reduce adverse drug events in hospitals.[21] The Joint Commission on Accreditation of Healthcare organisations may require the contribution of all these healthcare personnel in root cause analysis of sentinel (significant) events.[40] The

Institute of Medicine's landmark study of error strongly recommends initial and ongoing training of healthcare personnel on human factors engineering and safety.[41]

Closing remarks

There is broad and deep evidence that this relatively new discipline, human factors engineering, can make a big impact on healthcare errors. Better yet, a person could start including human factors engineering into the framework and techniques for error investigation tomorrow. To make the largest reduction in errors and adverse events, it will take application of human factors engineering to procurement, design, audit, and awareness-raising activities. Moreover, it will take an investment in new training, people, and other changes to management activities.

References

1 Van Cott HP. Human error in healthcare delivery: Cases, causes, and correction. In: *Proceedings of the Human Factors and Ergonomics Society 37th Annual Meeting*. Santa Barbara, CA: Human Factors and Ergonomics Society, 1993:430–4.

2 Burlington B. Human factors and the FDA's goals: Improved medical device design. In: *Proceedings of the AAMI/FDA Conference: Human Factors in Medical Devices: Design, Regulation, and Safety*. Arlington, VA: Association for the Advancement of Medical Instrumentation, 1995. [Online]. http: //www.fda.gov/cdrh/humfac/hufacimp. html

3 Carstenson PB. Overview of FDA's new human factors plan: Implications for the medical device industry. In *Proceedings of the AAMI/FDA Conference: Human Factors in Medical Devices: Design, Regulation, and Patient Safety* [Online]. Arlington, VA: Association for the Advancement of Medical Instrumentation, 1995. Available URL: http: //www.fda. gov/ cdrh/humfac/ hufacimp. html

4 Hyman WA. Errors in the use of medical equipment. In: Bogner MS, ed. *Human error in medicine*. Hillsdale, NJ: Lawrence Erlbaum Associates, 1994.

5 Cooper JB, Newbower RS, Long CD, McPeek B. Preventable anesthesia mishaps: a study of human factors. *Anesthesiology* 1978;**49**:399–406.

6 Lin L. Human error in patient-controlled analgesia: Incident reports and experimental evaluation. In: *Proceedings of the Human Factors and Ergonomics Society 42nd Annual Meeting*. Santa Barbara, CA: Human Factors and Ergonomics Society, 1998:1043–7.

7 Welch DL. Human error and human factors engineering in healthcare. *Biomed Instrum Technol* 1997;**31**:627–31.

8 Rappaport M. Human factors applications in medicine. *Human Factors* 1970;**12**:25–35.

9 Sanders MS, McCormick EJ. *Human factors in engineering and design*. 7th edn. New York: McGraw-Hill, 1993.

10 Nielsen J. *Usability engineering*. Cambridge, MA: AP Professional, 1993.

11 Wiklund ME. Medical device and equipment design: Usability engineering and ergonomics. Buffalo Grove, IL: Interpharm Press, 1995.

12 Bogner MS. *Human error in medicine*. Hillsdale, NJ: Lawrence Erlbaum Associates, 1994.

13 Bridger RS, Poluta MA. Ergonomics: Introducing the human factor into the clinical setting. *J Clin Eng* 1998;**23**:180–8.

14 Stanhope N, Vincent CA, Adams S, *et al.* Applying human factors methods to clinical risk management in obstetrics. *Br J Obstet Gynaecol* 1997;**104**:1225–32.

15 Saladow J. Continuum of care and human factors design issues. *J Intraven Nurs* 1996;**19**(3 Suppl):20–4.
16 Gosbee JW. The discovery phase of medical device design: A blend of intuition, creativity, and science. *Med Device Diagn Ind* 1997;**11**:79–82. [Online]. http://www.devicelink.com/mddi/archive/97/11/016.html
17 Aucella A, Kirkham T, Barnhart S, *et al.* Improving ultrasound systems by user-centered design. In: *Proceedings of the Human Factors and Ergonomics Society 38th Annual Meeting*. Santa Barbara, CA: Human Factors and Ergonomics Society, 1994.
18 Brown D. The challenges of user-based design in a medical equipment market. In: Wixon D, Ramey J, eds. *Field methods casebook for software design*. New York: Wiley, 1996: 157–76.
19 Lin L, Isla R, Harkness H, *et al.* Applying human factors to the design of medical equipment: Patient-controlled analgesia. *J Clin Monit Comput* 1998;**14**:253–63.
20 Beascart-Zephir MC, Brender J, Beuscart R, Menager-Depriester I. Cognitive evaluation: How to assess the usability of information technology in healthcare. *Comput Methods Programs Biomed* 1997;**54**:19–28.
21 American Society of Health-System Pharmacists. Top-priority actions for preventing adverse drug events in hospitals: recommendations from an expert panel. *Am J Health-System Pharm* 1996;**53**:747–51.
22 McDonald CJ. Protocol-based computer reminders. The quality of care and the non-perfectibility of man. *New Engl J Med* 1976;**295**:1351–5.
23 Louie C, Luber A. *Automated drug delivery systems and the potential for medication misadventures. A university's experience.* New York. American Association for the Advancement of Science, 1996.
24 Cohen M. Over-reliance on pharmacy computer systems may place patients at great risk. *ISMP Medication Safety Alert!* 1999;**4**:1.
25 Thull B, Janssens U, Rau G, Hanrath P. Approach to computer-based medication planning and co-ordination support in intensive care units. *Technol Health Care* 1997;**5**:219–33.
26 Callan CM. Analysis of complaints and complications with patient-controlled analgesia. In: Ferrante FM, Ostheimer GW, Covino BG, eds. *Patient-controlled analgesia*. Boston: Blackwell Scientific Publications, 1990: 139–50.
27 United States Food and Drug Administration. *Medical Device Reports.* Washington, DC: United States Food and Drug Administration, 1998. [Online]. www.fda.gov/mdr
28 Welch DL. Human factors in the healthcare facility. *Biomed Instrum Technol* 1998;**32**: 311–16.
29 Claus PL, Gibbons PS, Kaihoi BH, Mathiowetz M. Usability lab: A new tool for process analysis at the Mayo Clinic. In: *HIMSS Proceedings*. Chicago: Healthcare Information Management Systems Society, 1997;**2**:149–59.
30 United States Food and Drug Administration. Human factors implications of the new GMP rule: New quality system regulations that apply to human factors. In: *Selections of Center for Devices and Radiologic Health guidance documents*, Washington, DC: United States Food and Drug Administration, 1998. [Online]. www.fda.gov/cdrh/humfac/hufacimp.html
31 American National Standards Institute, Association for the Advancement of Medical Instrumentation. *Human factors engineering guidelines and preferred practices for the design of medical devices* (ANSI/AAMI HE-48). Arlington, VA: Association for the Advancement of Medical Instrumentation, 1993.
32 International Standards Organization. *ISO 9241 Ergonomics requirements for office work with visual display terminals (VDTs)*. Geneva, Switzerland: International Standards Organization, 1998. [Online]. http://www.iso.ch/9000e/9k14ke.htm
33 Gosbee JW, Ritchie EM. *Human–computer interaction and medical software development interactions*. New York: ACM Press, 1997;**4**:13–18.
34 Gosbee, JW. Communication among health professionals: Human factors engineering can help make sense of the chaos. *BMJ* 1998;**316**:642.
35 Kohn LT, Corrigan JM, Donaldson MS. *To err is human: Building a safer health system*. Washington, DC: National Academy Press, 1999: 140–9. [Online] www.nap. edu/readingroom
36 Augustine CH, Weick KE, Bagian JB, Lee CZ. Predispositions toward a culture of safety in a large multi-facility health system. In: *Proceedings of Enhancing Patient Safety and*

Reducing Errors in healthcare. Chicago, IL: National Patient Safety Foundation, 1998, 138–41.

37 United States National Library of Medicine. Medline. [Online]. http://www.ncbi.nlm.nih. gov

38 Marquette University. *Healthcare Technologies Management Program.* Milwaukee, WI, USA. [Online]. www.eng.mu.edu/hctm/index.html

39 Healthcare Information Management Systems Society. *Guide to Nursing Informatics.* Chicago, IL: Healthcare Information Management Systems Society, 1996.

40 Joint Commission on Accreditation of Healthcare Organizations. 1999. Oakbrook Terrace, IL. [Online]. www.jcaho.org.

41 Kohn LT, Corrigan JM, Donaldson MS. *To err is human: Building a safer health system.* Washington, DC: National Academy Press, 1999:116. [Online] www.nap. edu/reading-room

Further reading/websites

Pertinent annotated literature

Bridger RS, Poluta MA. Ergonomics: Introducing the human factor into the clinical setting. *J Clin Eng* 1998;**23**(3):180–8.

These South African investigators cite the direct effect of poor interface design with increased errors. For one example, they cited a failed resuscitation effort caused by inconsistent and misleading graphics on a defibrillator.

Saladow J. Continuum of care and human factors design issues. *J Intraven Nurs* 1996 May-Jun;**19**(3 Suppl):20–4.

Role of human factors engineering in addressing the many design and procedural issues for delivering intravenous medications and fluids.

Stanhope N, Vincent CA, Adams S, O'Connor AM, Beard RW. Applying human factors methods to clinical risk management in obstetrics. *Br J Obstet Gynaecol* 1997;**104**:1225–32.

Role of human factors engineering in addressing the many design and procedural issues in the obstetrics setting.

Welch DL. Human factors in the healthcare facility. *Biomed Instrum Technol* 1998 May–Jun;**32**(3):311–16.

This is one in a series of articles about human factors engineering written for biomedical engineers. This article emphasises the role of human factors engineering in proactive measures, as well as accident/incident investigation. The proactive measures include evaluation of existing systems, evaluation prior to purchase, and design and evaluation of facilities and procedures.

Helpful annotated websites

Emergency Care Research Institute. www.ecri.org

This is one of the premier organisations in the USA that collects, analyses, and reports out recommendations to reduce medical device error. The web site has a very useful search tool to find typical device error reports

Ergonomics Society. www.ergo.ac.uk

The main human factors engineering professional organisation in the United Kingdom.

Human Factors and Ergonomics Society. www.hfes.org

The main professional organisation in the United States.

Institute for Safe Medication Practices. www.ismp. org

Their newsletter is read and used by most clinical risk managers in the USA. This is one of the premier organisations in the USA that collects, analyses, and reports out human factors recommendations to reduce medication error.

Institute of Medicine report/book on error in medicine. www.nap. edu/readingroom

To Err is Human: Building a Safer Health System. This well-referenced text is freely available. Each chapter deals with the highly publicised and controversial recommendations to study and reduce error.

International Ergonomics Association. www.iea.org

The main human factors engineering professional organisation for the international community.

Joint Commission on Accreditation of Healthcare Organizations. www.jcaho. org

Largest US organisation that reviews errors and provide accreditation to most hospitals.

Marquette University's Healthcare Technologies Management Program. www.eng.mu.edu/hctm/ index.html

Unique academic program that blends human factors engineering with medical device design and evaluation – with some focus on error and efficacy.

United States Food and Drug Administration Human Factors Section. www. fda.gov/cdrh/humanfactors.html

The human factors group has created several documents that talk about medical devices, errors, and the design process. "Do it By Design" is especially good.

United States National Library of Medicine. http://www.ncbi.nlm.nih.gov

The Medline search engine to locate references on thousands of biology, medicine, and related journals.

17 Working time, stress and fatigue

LAWRENCE SMITH

Social and organisational changes have contributed to medicine becoming even more of a 24-hour discipline. The admission and treatment of patients at night has added to workloads. However, there has been a change in the nature of the work in a broader sense. In effect, work has become intensified because of a trend towards only admitting patients to hospital with more serious conditions, and their being discharged sooner than was once the case. This concentrates the work of medical staff, who are now dealing with severe and often acute problems but have less opportunity to relax, sleep on-call, and generally take the time to interact with patients and staff. A doctor may experience severe sleep loss during a night on-call and then be expected in theatre the next day for a normal working day shift. Similarly, busy weekends on-call may mean a doctor achieving very little sleep. Doctors themselves are well aware of the potential risks associated with extended work hours, regular night work, and fatigue. Nursing staff can also be subject to the effects of long work hours and regular night duties.[1]

Despite the advent of the "New Deal" on doctors' hours of work, the length and patterning of doctors' work hours remains to be an issue of some concern and debate in both the scientific literature and the media. This is because the working time arrangements experienced, in addition to being stressors in their own right, can also act to exacerbate the stresses and psychological difficulties that have been reported to be prevalent in the medical profession.[2,3] This chapter reviews evidence that "non-standard" working time, including shift and night work, can impact upon the work effectiveness and health of medical professionals. The issues covered range from some fundamental points about the body clock, shiftwork and health, work stress, sleepiness and fatigue, through to doctors work hours and the effects of the New Deal. At the outset, it should be recognised that the implications of working time, stress and fatigue overviewed here are just as pertinent to the lives of nursing staff and other healthcare professionals.[4,5]

Before reading further, ask yourself this question: "If I was in need of emergency, perhaps life saving, medical attention, who would I prefer to be treated by – a fatigued doctor at, or close to the end of a run of busy night duties, or by one who is fresh from a reasonable period of rest and relatively early in a duty period – if given the choice?" Should you have no answer at this point, reconsider it after reading this chapter.

Circadian rhythms

The timing of functions and processes at the individual, organisational, societal, and environmental levels are generally synchronised. Consequently, the desynchronisation of these processes that can stem from regular night work lies at the heart of the potential for disruption to the individual and employing organisation. This potential impairment exists because humans have evolved so that the daily rhythms in their physiology, hormone levels, biochemistry, and behaviour have become entrained to the most reliable and predictable cyclic changes in the physical and social environments.[6] These circadian rhythms, with a periodicity of about 24 hours, are not simply a response to environmental fluctuations. Rather, they are controlled by an endogenous timing mechanism or biological clock and human beings' capacity to both keep and tell the time.

Circadian rhythms confer an advantage because they anticipate changes in the environment. Body systems are primed to be "up and running" for activity early in the day, and to wind down in preparation for rest, recuperation, and sleep at night. A major function of the circadian system is the regulation of sleep and wakefulness. Nevertheless, although rhythms are driven by the biological clock, much of their variation is also a function of exogenous factors such as time cues in the environment (for example, the light and dark cycle) or level of social activity. Therefore, circadian rhythms are, under normal conditions, synchronised to form a dynamic but relatively stable system. Under shift and night working conditions, however, it is a system whose components can be regularly "teased apart" as a result of having to invert the activity-rest cycle and re-aligned when returning to a daytime orientation.

Shiftwork

Shift scheduling is now such a ubiquitous feature of work that it touches the lives of significant numbers of employees in most countries. Clearly, the health service does not shut down at 1700 every day and close at weekends. Rather, it is a major user of shiftwork practices. Shiftwork in this sense refers to the extension of work time beyond "normal" office hours, which requires two or more teams, firms or "shifts", to provide operational cover. It has also come to represent irregular work hours and those on permanent evening or night duty.[7,8] It is a long-established method of organising working time that has been linked to acute and chronic effects in the individual. The potential adverse effects of shiftworking are well-chronicled.[9,10,11,12] Outcomes fall into a number of areas:

- biological disruption to physiological processes, including the sleep–wake cycle[13]
- the impairment of physical health and psychological well-being[7,12]
- alertness, performance and safety may suffer[14,15,16]
- depending on work schedule configuration, there may be consequences in terms of productivity, moonlighting, sickness-absence and turnover[17]
- lastly, there can be interference with social and domestic life.[18,19,20]

Doctors in general, can work longer hours than would be expected or accepted for typical shiftworkers in other sectors of employment. Indeed, it is common to find that many staff work (unpaid) regularly beyond the official hours for which they are contracted. Consequently, difficulties associated with work hours may be increased in doctors regardless of their work schedule. Having said this, the extent to which shiftwork affects the individual depends, largely upon the job being done, characteristics of the individual (personal coping resources, personality), organisational and social environments, and features of the shift system.[21,22] In addition to this, there are models that link shiftwork to health and stress effects.[23,24,25] An important feature of many of these perspectives is the recognition that shiftworkers may engage in more "risky" coping behaviours that contribute to impairment to health, for example increased smoking, caffeine, alcohol, or drug use and changed eating habits.

Summary points

There is concern about the potential impact of work hours, stress and fatigue on clinical performance. Knowledge about the functioning of the body clock and how shift and night work affects our physiology and psychology suggests that the concern is warranted.

Work stress

A number of sources of stress at work have been identified[26]; including:

- factors intrinsic to the job such as work overload/underload, time pressures, work hours and shiftwork, physical work conditions, and repetitive work
- role-based stress such as work role ambiguity, work role conflict, and levels of responsibility (especially responsibility without control)
- conflicting demands between work and home life
- relationships/interactions with subordinates, colleagues and superiors in work, and with partners/family outside work
- career development factors such as lack of job security, under/over-promotion, and thwarted ambition
- organisational structure and culture, including office politics, communications, participation in decision-making, the organisation of work, and organisational trust.

Doctors and nursing staff face many of these issues at work. Medical professionals also face the stresses of dealing with relatives following the death of a loved-one, increasing challenges to medical decision-making, and increased resort to pursuing malpractice claims.[27] Clearly, job conditions can be a major stress factor, and a large part of a health professional's working conditions is, of course, her/his work schedule. The next section considers how stress manifests itself in doctors. Later sections focus on sleep and fatigue effects that are implicated in the genesis of these outcomes.

Stress effects in doctors

Psychiatric disorder among doctors has been suggested to be a relatively unacknowledged problem.[28] Most relevant to this consideration is the incidence of alcohol abuse, drug dependence and affective disorders. A number of studies have reported higher than average levels of alcoholism, drug abuse, and marital breakdown amongst doctors.[29,30] Some of the causes for these psychiatric difficulties reported by doctors included high workload, but a link to inadequacy of sleep and rest in relation to work demands is also possible.[31]

Sleep loss in relation to work scheduling was implicated in a study of the links between stress and clinical care.[32] A large proportion of hospital doctors and general practitioners surveyed, reported stress to have affected patient care detrimentally (this included generally lowered standards, irritability or anger, serious mistakes and some very serious errors resulting in patient death). The deterioration in patient care was attributed to tiredness, pressure of work, depression or anxiety and the effects of alcohol. On this latter point, a relatively stable pattern of drinking over time, and recreational drug use in response to felt stress, was found among junior doctors.[33] It is reasonable to conclude that these behaviours would probably have had some impact upon the work of many of the participants given the high average weekly work hours of the sample (in a follow-up report, doctors' stress levels were more clearly linked to the number of hours worked[34]). Some graphic anecdotes illustrated the way alcohol, used to cope (with stress and long hours), affected work effectiveness. It was also commented that resort to alcohol may have been a successful, if inappropriate, short-term coping strategy to help maintain psychological well being. The "risky-behaviours" noted in Haider *et al*'s model[24] of shiftwork and health is brought to mind here. However, the picture painted isn't always so bleak; for example, McAuliffe and colleagues[35] concluded that doctors were no more vulnerable to alcohol abuse than other professionals. Nevertheless, given the reported extent of substance abuse the problems should not be underestimated.[36]

Firth-Cozens provided a model that usefully summarised the relationships between stress, psychological problems and clinical performance.[2] The model suggests that sustained work and/or reduced sleep contribute to breakdown in medical performance. Individual differences in coping resources moderate the stress effects of long work hours and partial sleep deprivation upon work-related psychological, social, and physical performance. Problems may also arise indirectly when inappropriate palliative coping behaviours are operated. Depression in doctors on work rotations has been noted.[37,38] This may be particularly problematic where sleep deprivation and managing death and distressed relatives are frequent experiences, for example, in intensive care units. It was also reported that, compared to the general population, depression rates are higher in medical practitioners.[39] Although this view has been challenged recently[40] by McManus and colleagues, this is a cause for concern, because depression can result in poorer decision-making, impairment to memory, and concentration, as well as interpersonal problems; all of which may impact upon patient care. In a study that operationalised stress as "caseness" on the General Health Questionnaire, it was found that doctors who were chronically stressed reported a considerably higher levels of error. (However, it should be borne in mind that under-reporting of clinical mistakes is likely[2] compared to those who were never stressed.[41]) It was suggested that a vicious cycle is set in-train, whereby self-blame and guilt concerning mistakes continue to feed the stress and depression that could contribute to errors in performance. This point was re-emphasised more recently by Firth-Cozens who noted that depression was linked to self-critical cognitions during early training, past sibling rivalry and to current levels of sleep loss.[27]

Time pressure and sleep loss have been suggested to be major stresses for junior doctors[42,43] that could interfere with both learning[44] and the provision of medical care[45] but there is evidence that conflicts with the above contentions. Notably, Firth-Cozens found that stress levels were not predicted by work-related stressors such as hours worked, sleep duration or number of beds.[46] This echoed Jex and colleagues' research that found sleep deprivation and excessive work hours to be relatively unimportant predictors of performance (measured as unexplained absences, mistakes, missing deadlines, and conflict with colleagues) compared to abusive patients and changing schedules.[47] The capacity of stress and work conditions to predict work satisfaction in senior house officers has been studied.[48] They used measures such as level of role clarity and work group functioning, stress and workload, all of which significantly predicted levels of job satisfaction. Interestingly, although hours worked was entered into their regression analysis as a predictor variable, in this instance it did not achieve significance. There is, however, support for the view that mood and psychological well being, and by implication attitude and interaction with others, could be significantly impaired by long hours and/or sleep loss.[33,43,49] One reason for the inconsistency in the findings on work-hours and sleep loss effects could be related to the broad individual differences in response to work factors. The shiftwork research literature offers support for this view. For example, Harma reported that people differ considerably in their capacities to tolerate shift and night work.[50]

Lastly, it is noteworthy that the issue of time of day and night-work effects on clinical effectiveness was not a primary focus of many of the studies on doctors cited. However, working time is implicated and these findings not only have important implications for the physiological, psychological, and social well being of doctors, but also the quality of training and patient care.

Summary points

There is substantial evidence that work stress can result in a range of undesirable consequences (such as depressed psychological state, alcohol and drug abuse) that might adversely affect clinical performance. Despite the somewhat inconclusive research reported in relation to the effects of sleep loss and long-hours on doctors, it would be unwise to ignore the extensive literature on shift and night work that suggests that night time performance and well-being can be detrimentally affected, sometimes with catastrophic results.

Effects of fatigue and sleep loss on performance

In an influential report, Mitler and colleagues reviewed scientific and technical reports on the 24-hour distribution of medical health events and performance failures over 24 hours.[51] Their analysis argued that many serious incidents were caused or made worse by human error at times when sleepiness is high and alertness and performance capability are depleted. Available evidence suggests that performance decrements are more likely during the period 0100h to 0600h and to a lesser extent between 1400h to 1800h (the "post-lunch dip"). There appears to be a bimodal potential for reduced safety over the 24-hour period which roughly parallels the physiologically based rhythm in sleep propensity.[52] More recently, Folkard has reiterated these points but has also suggested "non-circadian" time into shift effects on performance.[53]

Problems with sleep are probably the commonest and most serious complaints of shiftworkers. Night (and morning) shift work is typically associated with shorter sleep duration. Complaints include premature awakening, feelings of getting too little sleep and not being rested after sleep. Torsvall et al concluded that not only is the sleep of shiftworkers disturbed but so too is the wakefulness, whereby sleepiness at night often reaches levels at which wakefulness simply cannot be maintained.[54] Obtaining less and sometimes little or no sleep in a 24-hour period results in acute partial sleep deprivation. Although immediately problematic for performance and safety, this deficit can be countered by adequate periods of sleep, and psychological intervention. Interestingly, repeated experience of acute sleep deprivation does not appear to result in the individual becoming "immune" to it.[55] Indeed, the only real solution to loss of sleep is achieving adequate amounts of it! In an ideal world, sleep on rest days and shifts other than the night shift should result in complete recovery from acute sleep loss. The major problem, however, is returning to work duties before recovery is complete (for example, many complain of returning to work still tired and not fully recovered from a block of night duties).

Studies of cognitive performance including vigilance and attention, generally support the view that long work hours contribute to deterioration in performance.[56] Indeed, there are sequelae to sleep loss that are reflected in performance on virtually all cognitive and sustained attention tasks.[57] Sleep loss may contribute to greater fatigue as the length of a task increases, as the difficulty of mental and physical demands increase, as memory load on a task increases, when a task is newly learned, and when a task is externally paced.[58] The increased propensity to fall asleep (that is, the inability to resist falling asleep[52]) at night may be exaggerated if the shiftworker is suffering from partial sleep deprivation. This may manifest itself as increased lapses of attention, or microsleeps of which the nightworker may be completely unaware.[57,59] At greater levels of sleepiness under acute sleep loss, the brain becomes more dependent on the environment to maintain alertness. Consequently, exposure to performance tasks requiring sustained attention may accelerate the sleep deprived

325

brain's tendency to move towards sleep. This could result in a marked deterioration in performance.[60,61,62] It has also been noted that under conditions of extreme sleepiness any type of task performance may be degraded.[7]

If sleepiness and circadian decreases in functioning are as pronounced as those noted in the literature it might be expected that this would be reflected in job performance and safety. Work with flight simulators has shown that flying performance at night can be degraded to a level corresponding to having a 0·05% blood alcohol level such as that following moderate alcohol consumption.[63] Lapses may result in the employee not performing their job appropriately and failing to avoid hazards. People may be unaware of these lapses and associated performance decrements. A field study on nursing staff looked at the incidence of sleep deprivation and sleepiness-related accidents when on rotating shiftwork.[64] The odds of reporting an accident or error were twice as high in rotating shiftworkers compared to day/evening colleagues, and 2·5 times higher for near-miss incidents. Their results were consistent with laboratory research that has shown that sleep deprivation is associated with lapses in attention, increased reaction time and increased error rates on performance tasks.[56] Other studies using EEG recordings have shown evidence of napping or dozing off in work on the night shift.[53]

One of the major justifications for limiting night work is that safety may be compromised at night.[65] Surprisingly, there is little direct evidence to substantiate this.[12] But there are exceptions. For example, analysis of accident data from a weekly rotating three-shift system at a large manufacturing plant indicated that there was a significant increase in the risk of injuries from the morning shift, through the afternoon shift, to the night shift.[66] The results lend some support to the view that night-time accidents may be more serious in nature and suggested that this effect may be limited to self-paced work situations. There was also evidence of a cumulative effect whereby there was a significant increase in night shift accidents from the first to the last two days of the week but no significant differences emerged for the morning and afternoon shifts. The authors suggested that the increased injury rates at night reflected a failure of circadian rhythms in performance capabilities and alertness, to adjust sufficiently to the night shift. The important aspect to this study was that work conditions remained relatively stable across shifts and over time. However, few shiftworking situations meet the criterion of a situation where the *a priori* probability of an accident is, at least on average, constant over the 24-hour period. Determining time of day effects in the healthcare environment could be difficult given constantly changing work conditions.

Summary points

Distinct 24-hour patterns in performance breakdown have been reported. These have been linked to the natural rhythm in the propensity to sleep, and the requirement that shiftworkers have to work in opposition to this natural drive towards sleep as a function of their regular night duties. Sleep loss is likely to contribute to, or combine with, on-shift work fatigue effects and decreases in alertness and performance capabilities at certain times of day to compromise task performance and safety.

Sleep loss and fatigue effects on clinical work

There has been considerable and, often publicly expressed, concern about the potential detrimental effects of long hours and night working on the clinical effectiveness of fatigued and sleepy doctors.[67,68,69,70] The out-of-hours (outside the normal 0800–1700 work period), workload traditionally covered by doctors on call has been highlighted to be particularly onerous.[71] Leslie et al reported that the average hours worked by junior doctors ranged between 83 and 101 hours per week.[72] But, for example, if two doctors were providing cover "out-of-hours", each would work a normal 0800 or 0900 to 1700 or 1800 day and be on-call on alternate days until Friday when one would cover the full weekend. In this case each doctor could work an average of 104 hours per week.

While reported effects of the total hours of work may be rather equivocal in terms of doctors' effectiveness, the requirement to work regular night duties can have a telling impact upon doctors' psychological state and performance.[73,74] A study of Swedish surgeons reported that 8% of doctors felt that their medical performance definitely suffered during on-call night work while another 11% stated that their performance was moderately affected. During the day following the night duty the figures were 17% and 19% respectively.[75] Deterioration in British doctors' job efficiency related to sleep loss has been reported,[76] while in another study, sleep-deprived doctors were reported to have experienced a significant increase in the numbers of errors made in reading ECG output.[77] In a pilot study on sleepiness in doctors on night call duty,[78] sleepiness measured at three-hourly intervals through night duties was at its peak between 0300 and 0600. Doctors used naps as a way of compensating for sleep lost as a result of night duties.

The capacity of on-call duties to interfere with sleep is a major concern because the amount of sleep available on-call is highly variable and the desire for sleep can conflict with responsibilities for patient care.[79] Caffeine may not be used because the work–rest pattern is ill defined, and therefore it may interfere with the ability to sleep when the opportunity arises. There is also the problem of having to perform optimally immediately on waking from sleep. Sleep inertia (a form of "warm-up decrement") experienced immediately after a period of sleep, can affect performance because it can take some time (up to 30 minutes) to dissipate.[60,61,80] In a review of on-call scheduling effects on doctors' sleep, performance, and mood, Bonnett and Arand noted that impaired performance related to sleep loss was more likely for reasoning tasks, for non-stimulating tasks and in less experienced doctors.[81] Sleep loss also results in more negative mood states. In addition, compared to pre-hospital baseline sleep, chronic partial sleep deprivation can result in reductions of sleep durations by one hour. An acute decrement in sleep duration of 2–4 hours in medical settings could be reflected by performance decrements.[82,83,84] The fatigued individual may be disinclined to apply any more effort to a task, resulting in performance decrements. Mental fatigue may involve not only an apparent inability to produce the right quantity of work, but also an inability to do the right kind of work.[85] Unsurprisingly, doctors are aware of the potential risk of deterioration in performance capability and decision-making.[75]

Summary points

Serious treatment errors reported by the media are a manifestation of the concern about the functioning of very tired medical staff working long-hours, often at night, under conditions of high work demands. There is evidence that the psychological state, performance, and attitude of sleep deprived and fatigued doctors can be detrimentally affected. In short, these conditions serve to compound the potential stress of the job.

Motivation and compensatory effort

An all too familiar, and sometimes unsettling, set of anecdotes on the effects of tiredness on medical performance was provided by Firth-Cozens.[2] The accounts bear testimony to both the difficulties experienced in carrying out treatments efficiently, and to the degradation in motivation and attitude in work caused by severe tiredness. Having said this, there has been a tendency to underestimate the ability of individuals to motivate themselves to overcome the effects of sleep loss on performance. For example, the capacity of doctors to "rally in certain circumstances" was noted.[2] Evidently, most night workers do not make mistakes every time they are on duty. It is apparent that we are very resourceful creatures and can exert additional effort for brief periods to reduce performance deficits in adverse conditions.[86] Even extremely tired individuals can demonstrate high levels of performance on complex tasks that stimulate interest.[85]

Dinges and Kribbs[57] noted that sleep loss may affect the "willingness to perform" rather than the capacity to perform. Fatigue has been defined in a similar manner.[85] By using a variety of motivational variables such as incentives, signals, reminders, feedback, and exhortations, performance levels can be raised in sleep deprived individuals. However, this motivated effort cannot be sustained for long if task demands persist, if new tasks compete for significant attention, or if the task is contained within other continuous work. It appears that motivation can be used to sustain performance at near-baseline levels if the amount of sleep achieved has not been reduced below 50% of typical sleep duration and if the period of wakefulness following sleep deprivation does not exceed 24 hours.[87] In a study of cognitive performance that linked night work and workload in house officers, it was reported that some tired doctors performed better than their more alert colleagues.[88] It was also noted that tasks that were more closely related to actual job performance were not detrimentally affected by the more adverse conditions. No significant performance decrements were observed in junior doctors by Ford and Wentz, even when sleep loss increased up to 72 hours.[89] Individual differences in tolerance and coping resourcefulness may have played a part in these results.[2] Compensatory effort may also have been invested in job performance.

In addition, we must not forget that the consequences of making a mistake on a cognitive performance task completed for a research study are insignificant compared to those potential errors committed in the course of treating patients. The stakes are very much higher for real-job failure, therefore, motivational and personal resource factors may well play a part in the maintenance of job performance. This suggests that intervention to increase or improve personal coping strategies is possible and may be a consideration for doctors in training. For example, Jones et al reported the success of a hospital-wide stress-management programme in reducing medication errors.[90] As well as overarching structured policy changes to ensure adequate sleep, appropriate stress coping strategies are possible and treatment for depression is available. The organisational benefits of such an intervention programme have been indicated by reduction in malpractice claims in hospitals that had implemented stress management training.[27] By the same token, there is no reason why the stress of working hours and night working could not be addressed with suitable intervention programmes that included non-pharmacological methods to aid sleep.

Summary points

Professionalism and the high stakes associated with failure mean that compensatory effort is invested in an attempt to maintain satisfactory clinical performance. In general, this can serve to counter the debilitating effects of sleep loss and fatigue. However, there can come a point when tiredness is so great that any task performance, or treatment decision, can be degraded. People do differ in their capacity to tolerate shift and night work rotas. Part of the difference relates to the level and sophistication of personal strategies that can be deployed. In light of this, it is also feasible to provide training in appropriate interventions to help medical staff cope more readily with their work schedules.

Changing work hours

Changing work rotas is the common "catch-all" approach to trying to minimise the sleep loss, fatigue and stress-related outcomes noted above. This was the motivation behind the New Deal on working hours for junior doctors introduced in 1991. The New Deal agreement to reduce hours of work and to improve overall working conditions while maintaining clinical and educational standards has resulted in a number of work scheduling approaches. Recommendations for average hours of duty were advanced for on-call, partial shift and full shift rotas. On-call rotas require doctors to be available (and ready) for work during stipulated rostered work periods. During this time doctors may be able to take some rest or even sleep should there be a lull in work demands. However, such rest periods are unlikely to be relaxing or recuperative as the doctor is always uncertain about when she/he could be "called". For example, when on-call a doctor could work a "normal" day from 0900 but finish their period on-call at 1700 the next day. Being on-call can also entail working a full 48 hours over a weekend and finishing at 1700 on a Monday. Under the New Deal it was recommended that no doctor should be contracted to be on duty for more than 72 hours per week (although under certain circumstances a maximum average of 83 hours could be worked). Partial shift rotas comprise (to a greater or lesser degree) "normal" working days (for example, 0800 to 1700) in combination with a mixture of evening (for example, 0800 to 1900), late (for example, 0800 to 2130 and/or night shifts (for example, 2100 to 0900). Under the New Deal no doctor should be contracted to be on duty for more than 64 hours per week on average. Full shift rotas can be similar in configuration to more typical shift schedules used in other jobs (rotating through early/morning, afternoon/late and night shifts). These rotas can also be very similar in appearance to partial systems. On full shifts doctors should be contracted to work no more than 56 hours per week on average under the New Deal.

The outcome of this initiative, at least in terms of work hours, has tended to be equivocal at best. There still tends to be little evidence of attempts to empirically evaluate this form of work scheduling. Nevertheless, there have been a small number of commentaries and studies on the implications of the New Deal[91,92] in terms of working time. This research helps provide some context to the issue presented thus far. Some have examined on-call systems while others have reported on the applicability of partial shift systems. One investigation looked at the introduction of a partial shift system to a group of pre-registration house surgeons.[93] Although the authors concluded that the partial shift system was generally applicable, the doctors' well-being and performance effectiveness were not systematically studied. An exploration of shiftworking regimes implemented as replacements to on-call rotas noted that the new shift rotas had a negative effect on job satisfaction, psychological well-being and training.[94] Thus, adjustments to work rotas may influence clinical training, and not necessarily in a positive way. Kelty, Duffy and Cooper explored the effects of a reduction in on-call duty over a six–year period (1990–1995) on "relatively uncommon" emergencies in cardiothoracic surgery that occurred out of hours.[95] Under the New Deal arrangement, they suggested that the duration of higher specialist training would be cut by 50%. This was because on a 1:6 rota (equivalent to 56 hours/week) trainees would, on average, experience 2 aortic emergencies only, whereas on a 1:4 rota (trainees available for up to 83 hours a week) the exposure to such emergencies was double. The authors suggested that the New Deal stipulation of 56 hours might require adjustment to include some mechanism to allow trainees to be on-call for specialist training.

Earlier research examined the introduction of a partial shift rota that reduced weekly hours to an average of 64/week. The partial shift system replaced a "one in four" on-call rota on which the working week ranged from 64 to 112 hours (average 88 contracted hours). No detrimental effects on patient care or educational standards were reported. The areas of improvement on the partial system were reported to be: reduced hours, shorter periods of continuous duty, better quality off-duty hours, no chronic fatigue, improved family and social life, and shorter weekend duties. However, there were reservations. These included the timing and nature of the "cover" shift and problems with night duties such as disruption to social life, impairment of firms' "team spirit" and interference with continuity of care. Although the partial shift system was deemed applicable, the house surgeons that participated in the study were equally divided in their preferences between the on-call and partial shift systems.[96]

Work rota preferences were also indicated in a pilot study that compared shift and on-call rotas.(Unpublished study comparing doctors' work rotas by Smith L, Sericki D, Ockford S. 1999.) The study highlighted a number of issues. Perhaps most notably, and in view of the current concern of junior doctors about their work hours, a large number of doctors declined to participate (19% response rate: 87/460). This was disappointing as it ran counter to the very active support of the Yorkshire Task Force on junior doctors' working time. The bulk of returns were from doctors working on-call rotas. The most meaningful comparisons could only be made between those on different kinds of on-call rota (1 in 4; 1 in 5 and 1 in 6 rotas). There was a tendency for variables such as alertness on shift, fatigue after work periods and interference with social and family life to be poorer on the 1 in 4 rota compared to 1 in 5 and 1 in 6 rotas. Doctors were significantly more satisfied with these latter configurations compared to the 1 in 4 or shift-based rotas. After the option of permanent day work, on-call rotas were preferred by doctors, with partial and full-shift systems ranked third and fourth respectively.

Research by Hale and colleagues studied two groups of house surgeons that worked 6 weeks on partial shifts and 6 weeks on a "one in six" on-call rota in a balanced design.[97] They also gained information about work effectiveness from other sources such as consultants, nursing staff and patients. The house surgeons were surveyed for their expectations regarding each form of work time organisation, as well as for their experiences on the schedules. Prior to exposure to each schedule the doctors reported that both partial shifts and on-call duty would result in equal levels of anxiety at work but that the partial shifts would reduce fatigue levels. The partial shifts were also expected to result in poorer communication between medical staff and with patients. The majority of house surgeons would have opted for an on-call rota ahead of a partial shift rota despite the belief that fatigue would be reduced on the latter. The profile of results gained after experiencing the two schedules was somewhat different to expectations. Anxiety levels were greater on the partial shift system. A particular concern was that the house officer "felt isolated" from colleagues during night shifts. Fatigue levels were similar on both schedules. A majority of house surgeons reported impairment to communication with patients and senior colleagues when on the partial shift system. Educational value was considered but the results were equivocal; no clear advantage was afforded by the partial system. In the same study, consultants and registrars indicated their concerns that the partial system impacted negatively on the management of surgical firms (both day and night), and that patient cover was impaired. In addition, a majority of nursing staff felt housemen to be less fatigued on the partial shifts but also that running surgical firms was much smoother with the on-call rota (especially in terms of communications with nurses and the technical skills of the house surgeons). There was low satisfaction with night cover on both systems. Interestingly, patients were also surveyed. They reported no differences between the schedules in terms of the high quality of patient care received. This reflects the professionalism of the staff and their capacity to engage in compensatory investment of personal resources.

Social and psychological well being, doctors' perceptions of sleep quality, levels of fatigue, risk of error, and ratings of patient care were examined in a study that compared the impact of partial shifts with on-call duty.(Unpublished study examining on-call and partial shift rotas by Smith L, Lukman H, Choong Y. 2000.) A standardised working-time related questionnaire battery and follow-up interviews were used in a cross-sectional assessment of work schedule effects. Thirty junior doctors in the general medicine departments at two large teaching hospitals participated (15 worked a partial shift system while the other 15 worked an on-call rota). When compared to doctors working the on-call rota, doctors on the partial shift system did not report experiencing a significantly greater sense of well being, nor improvements in perceived performance effectiveness. The partial shift system did not improve doctors' social life and doctors on both systems reported similar levels of sleep disruption and fatigue. The overall picture was one of little difference between the two schedules for the majority of dependent variables, despite the partial shift system achieving its aim of reducing doctors' working hours. One explanation may lie in the way such systems are configured and implemented in terms of direct participation in decision-making processes about working time.

In Smith *et al*'s study (unpublished study examining on-call and partial shift rotas by Smith L, Lukman, Choong Y. 2000) there was a steep drop in perceived performance effectiveness in the early hours (i.e. the period between 0300 and 0700) on both systems. It was notable that doctors reported feeling most irritated with their patients, nurses, and other medical staff and that levels of concern and empathy for patients were at their lowest at this time. Doctors are well aware of the potential for clinical performance to be debilitated. The perceived probability of making errors was also reported to be greatest during this period. The social consequence of implementing the partial shift system was another important aspect. Although the partial shift system reduced the number of duty hours, it increased the number of nights and weekends on duty. Hence, doctors would have to work more unsociable hours. As social life is an important element for most health service staff, the trade off between reducing the number of doctors' duty hours and their social life may not be as attractive as the New Deal might suggest. It is worth noting that during informal interviews one of the recurrent comments on the disadvantages of the partial shift system was concern about discontinuity of care. This means that, although doctors on the partial shift system clerked their patients on admission, as on-call doctors would, when their shift was over, these patients may be treated by different doctors who may have a different degree of knowledge of the patient's condition. Moreover, doctors who had experience of both systems indicated a preference for working the on-call rota, similar to Hale *et al*'s observation.[97]

Summary points

The existing research evidence suggests that the well-meaning changes to rotas prompted by the New Deal has not necessarily been reflected by improvements to well being and effectiveness in work. It may be the case that new shift rotas are as disruptive to the lives of medical staff as the long on-call hours have been. The overarching issues stemming from the research on working time arrangements concern the potential for sleep disruption and work fatigue. Furthermore, doctors and nursing staff are well aware of the potential reduction in clinical performance as a result of sleep loss and fatigue. Despite this awareness they will sometimes be so tired that, motivationally, they will not be in an optimal state to make appropriate treatment decisions. Mistakes may be made and/or treatment that could or should be completed immediately may be deferred, with treatment decisions passed on to the doctors following on.

Concluding comments

This chapter reviewed the impact of factors such as working time, stress and sleepiness, upon doctors. Non-standard work hours, especially when regular night duty is involved, can harbour the potential for serious consequences. There can be both direct and indirect effects: direct, in terms of disruption to the body clock, sleep, alertness, mood, and performance; indirect, both in terms of the disruption caused to family and social life, and in terms of the way shiftworking can exacerbate already stressful circumstances.[11,98] In the latter case, the pressures of high workload, downturns in psychological state and increase in "risky" coping behaviours may be amplified by the uncompromising work schedule a doctor finds herself/himself working.

In many respects the research suggests that the devil is in the detail. That is, relatively shorter work hours are not necessarily a good or a bad thing *per se*, the crucial issue is how the hours/shifts are configured in relation to operational constraints and demands, and social requirements. Changes to the configuration of on-call and shift rotas, combined with improvements to support staff provision and training in intervention strategies could help doctors cope more effectively with their work hours. The configuration issue is important because even on apparently "better" partial and full shift systems doctors can still be required to work very long hours (blocks of successive work periods) in some weeks. In addition, these blocks of duty periods might comprise a run of night shifts only, for example four 10-hour day shifts followed by three 16-hour night shifts (88 hours), or seven 12-hour night shifts (84 hours). Given the knowledge about the impact of sleep deprivation, it may be the night work requirement that is being reflected in the relatively poor or equivocal outcomes reported in the research literature on the partial shift system. Therefore, the average weekly work hours maximum stipulated under the New Deal arrangement offers little protection on occasions because it depends upon the reference period over which the average is calculated, need for cover for holidays and sickness-absence, and so on.

The message here, then, is that there is relatively little evidence of improvements to conditions in the research literature that has evaluated the relative impact of different work schedules stemming from the New Deal. When compared to doctors working on-call rotas, doctors on partial shift systems do not experience a greater sense of well being, lowered fatigue, and decreases in sleep loss nor improved work effectiveness. In addition, partial shift systems may still have a negative impact upon doctors' social lives. This suggests that junior doctors may still be working too many hours and that their work schedule could be revised to reduce the adverse effect on their social lives. Perhaps the over-riding issue is that of potential high fatigue levels exacerbated by sleep loss and high work demands. The fatigue that appears to be present in both partial shift systems and the on-call rotas should not be ignored. A study of physicians on night call duty showed effects on sleepiness with residual effects (elevated sleepiness) persisting after the on-call duty period.[78] Although doctors will elicit compensatory behaviours and invest extra effort to reduce the negative effects of fatigue on their job, there is a cost involved and a limit to human capabilities, especially at the extreme of tiredness. When doctors are required to work optimally beyond their threshold, their own and patients' well-being and safety may be compromised.

Furthermore, only a few studies have examined the impact of the partial shift rota in general medicine or compared it to full-shift or on-call rotas. It should also be noted that many of the studies cited are cross-sectional, "one-off" situations that do not reflect the complexity of interactions between personal state and work conditions over a career in medicine. So, a further crucial aspect to the issue of long work hours, prolonged night work, workload and stress effects is the potential for interaction effects upon work performance. That is, the end of a run of successive night duties, heavy work demands, fatigue, sleepiness, distractions in the environment, and having to make crucial decisions during the circadian down-turn in alertness and performance could very well combine, irrespective of compensatory effort, to degrade clinical performance. It only takes one such "window of catastrophe" to occur in one working lifetime for the severest consequences to be manifest. Importantly, with regard to strategic issues, it is surprising that no concerted national research effort has been directed at a systematic evaluation of the implementation and effects of New Deal shift rotas. Although a large undertaking, it would be possible to gain a generalised picture of the current status and consequences, for doctors and the Health Service, of the implementation of new rotas. Like Firth-Cozens and Moss[99] we can ask – "have the initiatives to reduce doctors' work hours resulted in lowered stress or is there more to be done?" As noted, the links between stress and depression, and longer work hours can be somewhat equivocal. Based on the evidence from the shiftwork and sleep deprivation literature, there should be concerted action to examine the effects that a lack of adequate sleep and chronic sleep loss (associated with work demands and hours worked) have upon psychological state and clinical performance. So, the answer is "yes!" more can be done, especially in terms of the configuration of working time and the provision of strategies designed to alleviate some of the difficulties commonly experienced.

In conclusion, the interest in possible deterioration in the performance of medical professionals in general, and doctors in particular, as a consequence of the organisation of work hours is not a new phenomenon; there has been research into the topic over the past three or four decades. Despite this research effort, it remains difficult to identify precisely how long a person should work, given the incentives prevalent in the clinical domain and the resourcefulness of human beings. Nevertheless, there may be a point, in terms of work hours, beyond which it is unwise to ask, or require, a medical practitioner to work and expect optimal performance. It is also worrying that despite the extensive scientific literature on the effects of shift and night working, much of it in relation to medical and nursing staff, there remains a lack of current knowledge about the impact of new and persisting work rotas upon doctors, nationwide. Furthermore, there has been little concerted effort in testing, and providing the doctors, nursing staff and other healthcare workers, with a set of tangible interventions targeted at combating the negative impact of shift and night work. Finally, recall the question in the introduction. On balance, and given the choice, how many of us would happily choose to be treated by the sleep deprived and fatigued doctor at the end of a run of busy night shifts?

References
1 Totterdell, Smith L, Folkard S. Nurses as nightworkers. In: McMahon R, ed. *Nursing at night: A professional approach.* London: Scutari Press, 1992.
2 Firth-Cozens J. Stress, psychological problems and clinical performance. In: Vincent C, Ennis M, Audley RJ, eds. *Medical Accidents.* Oxford: Oxford University Press, 1993.
3 Mumford E. Stress in the medical career. *J Med Educ* 1983;**58**:436–7.
4 Hardy GE, Shapiro DA, Borrill, CS. Fatigue in the workforce of National Health Service trusts: Levels of symptomatology and links with minor psychiatric disorder, demographic, occupational and work role factors. *J Psychosomatic Res* 1997;**43**:83–92.
5 Jones G. Stress in psychiatric nursing. In: Payne RL, Firth-Cozens J, eds. *Stress in health professionals.* Chichester: Wiley, 1987.
6 Minors D, Waterhouse J. Circadian rhythms in general. In: Scott AJ, ed. *Occupational Medicine: State of the Art Reviews – Shiftwork.* Philadelphia: Hanley and Belfus, 1990.
7 Akerstedt T. Psychological and psychophysiological effects of shiftwork. *Scand J Work Environ Health* 1990;**16**(1):67–73.
8 Knauth P. Designing better shift systems. *Appl Ergonomics* 1996;**27**(1):39–44.
9 Colquhoun WP, Costa G, Folkard S, Knauth P. *Shiftwork problems and solutions.* Frankfurt am Main, Berlin: Peter Lang, 1996.
10 Folkard S, Monk TH. *Hours of work: Temporal issues in work scheduling.* Chichester: John Wiley, 1985.
11 Scott AJ. *Occupational medicine: State of the art reviews – Shiftwork* (Vol. 5, No. 2). Philadelphia: Hanley and Belfus, 1990.
12 Waterhouse J, Folkard S, Minors D. *Shiftwork, Health and Safety: An overview of the scientific literature 1978–1990.* London: HMSO, 1992.
13 Tepas DI, Mahan RP. The many meanings of sleep. *Work Stress,* 1989;**3**(1):93–102.
14 Akerstedt T. Sleepiness at work: Effects of irregular work hours. In: Monk TH, ed. *Sleep, sleepiness and performance.* Chichester: Wiley, 1991.
15 Folkard S. Circadian performance rhythms: Some practical and theoretical implications. *Phil Trans R Soc Lond,* 1990;**B327**:543–53.
16 Nurminen T. Shiftwork and reproductive health. *Scand J Work Environ Health* 1998;**24**(3):28–34.
17 Smith L, Folkard S, Tucker P, Macdonald I. A comparison of 8-hour versus 12-hour shifts. *Occup Environ Med* 1998;**55**(4):217–29.
18 Barton J, Aldridge J, Smith P. The emotional impact of shiftwork on the children of shiftworkers. *Scand J Work Environ Health* 1998;**24**(3):146–50.
19 Fischer FM, Moreno CR de C, Fernandez R de L. Day and shiftworkers' leisure time. *Ergonomics* 1993;**36**(1–3):43–9.
20 Volger A, Ernst G, Nachreiner F, Hanecke K. Common free time of family members under different shift systems. *App Ergonomics* 1988;**19**(3):213–18.
21 Harma M. Ageing, physical fitness and shiftwork tolerance. *Appl Ergonomics* 1996;**27**(1): 25–9.
22 Knauth P. Innovative working time arrangements. *Scand J Work Environ Health* 1998; **24**(3):13–17.
23 Knutsson A, Akerstedt T, Orth-Gomer K. Increased risk of ischaemic heart disease in shiftworkers. *Lancet* 1986;**2**:89–92.
24 Haider M, Kundi M, Koller M. Methodological issues and problems in shiftwork research. In: Johnson L, Tepas D, Colquhoun P, Colligan M, eds. *Biological rhythms, sleep and shiftwork.* New York: SP Medical and Scientific Books, 1981.
25 Olsson K, Kandolin I, Kauppinin-Toropainen K. Stress and coping strategies of 3-shift workers. *Le Travail Humain* 1990;**53**:175–88.
26 Arnold J, Cooper C, Robertson IT. *Work psychology: understanding human behaviour in the workplace* (2nd edition). London: Pitman Publishing, 1995.
27 Firth-Cozens J. Individual and organisational predictors of depression in general practitioners. *Br J Gen Prac* 1998;**48**:1647–51.
28 Thapar A. Psychiatric disorder in the medical profession. *Br J Hosp Med* 1989;**42**:480–3.
29 Vaillant GE, Sobowale NC, McArthur C. Some psychological vulnerabilities of physicians. *N Engl J Med* 1972;**287**:372–5.

30 Murray RM. Psychiatric illness in male doctors and controls: an analysis of Scottish hospital inpatient data. *Br J Psychiatry* 1977;**131**:1–10.
31 Rubin R, Orris P, Lau SL, *et al*. Neurobehavioural effects of the on call experience in house staff physicians. *J Occup Med* 1991;**33**:13–18.
32 Firth-Cozens J, Greenhalgh J. Doctors' perceptions of the links between stress and lowered clinical care. *Soc Sci Med* 1997;**44**(7):1017–22.
33 Firth-Cozens J. Emotional distress in junior house officers. *BMJ* 1987;**295**:533–6.
34 Firth-Cozens J. Sources of stress in junior doctors and general practitioners. *Yorkshire Med* 1995;**7**(3):10–13.
35 McAuliffe WE, Rohman M, Breer P, *et al*. Alcohol use and abuse in random samples of physicians and medical students. *Am J Publ Health* 1991;**81**:177–81.
36 Brooke D, Edwards G, Taylor C. Addiction as an occupational hazard: 144 doctors with drug and alcohol problems. *Br J Addiction* 1991;**86**:1011–16.
37 Valko RJ, Clayton PJ. Depression in the internship. *Dis Nervous System* 1975;**36**:26–9.
38 Reuben DB. Depressive symptoms in medical house officers: effects of level of training and work rotation. *Arch Internat Med* 1985;**145**:286–8.
39 Hsu K, Marshall V. Prevalence of depression and distress in a large sample of Canadian residents, interns and fellows. *Am J Psychiatry* 1987;**144**:1561–6.
40 McManus IC, Winder BC, Gordon D. Are UK doctors particularly stressed? *Lancet* 1999;**354**(9187):1358–9.
41 Firth-Cozens J, Morrison L. Sources of stress and ways of coping in junior house officers. *Stress Med* 1989;**5**:121–6.
42 Ford GV. Emotional distress in internship and residency: a questionnaire study. *Psychiatric Med* 1983;**1**:143–50.
43 Hurwitz TA, Beiser M, Nichol H, *et al*. Impaired interns and residents. *Can J Psychiatry* 1987;**32**:165–9.
44 Light AI, Sun JH, McCool C, *et al*. The effects of acute sleep deprivation on level of resident training. *Curr Surg* 1989;**46**:29–30.
45 McCue J. The distress of internship: causes and prevention. *N Engl J Med* 1985;**312**:449–52.
46 Firth-Cozens J. The role of early experiences in the perception of organisational stress: fusing clinical and organisational perspectives. *J Organ Occup Psychology* 1992;**65**:61–75.
47 Jex SM, Baldwin JR, Dewitt C, *et al*. Behavioural consequences of job-related stress among resident physicians: the mediating role of psychological strain. *Psychol Rep* 1991;**69**:339–49.
48 Heyworth J, Whitley TW, Allison EJ, Revicki DA. Predictors of work satisfaction among SHOs during accident and emergency medical training. *Arch Emerg Med* 1993;**10**:279–88.
49 McManus IC, Lockwood DNJ, Cruikshank JK. The preregistration year: Chaos by consensus. *Lancet* 1977;**1**:413–17.
50 Harma M. Individual differences in tolerance to shiftwork. *Ergonomics* 1993;**36**(1–3):101–10.
51 Mitler MM, Carskadon MA, Czeisler CA, *et al*. Catastrophes, sleep and public policy. *Sleep* 1988;**11**:100–9.
52 Lavie P. The 24-hour sleep propensity function (SPF): Practical and theoretical implications. In: Monk TH, ed. *Sleep, sleepiness and performance*. Chichester: Wiley, 1991.
53 Folkard S. Black times: Temporal determinants of transport safety. *Accident Analysis Prevent* 1997;**29**(4):417–30.
54 Torsvall L, Akerstedt T, Gillander K, Knutsson A. Sleep on the night shift: 24-hour EEG monitoring of spontaneous sleep/wake behaviour. *Psychophysiology* 1989;**26**(3):352–8.
55 Webb WB, Lewy CM. Effects of spaced and repeated total sleep deprivation. *Ergonomics* 1984;**27**:45–58.
56 Rosa RR Extended workshifts and excessive fatigue. *J Sleep Res* 1995;**4**(2):51–6.
57 Dinges DF, Kribbs NB. Performing while sleepy: Effects of experimentally induced sleepiness. In: Monk TH, ed. *Sleep, sleepiness and performance*. Chichester: Wiley, 1991.
58 Johnson LC, Naitoh P. *The operational consequences of sleep deprivation on sleep deficit*. AGARD monograph No. 190. North Atlantic Treaty Organization, 1974.

59 Johnson LC. Sleep deprivation and performance. In: Webb WB, ed. *Biological rhythms, sleep and performance*. Chichester: Wiley, 1982.
60 Dinges DF Napping patterns and effects in human adults. In: Dinges DF, Broughton RJ, eds. *Sleep and alertness: Chronobiological, behavioural and medical aspects of napping*. New York: Raven Press, 1989.
61 Dinges DF. The nature of sleepiness: Causes, contexts and consequences. In: Stunkard AJ, Baum A, eds. *Eating, sleeping and sex*. Hillsdale, NJ: Erlbaum, 1989.
62 Dinges DF. Probing the limits of functional capability: The effects of sleep loss on short duration tasks. In: Broughton RJ, Ogilvie RD, eds. *Sleep, arousal and performance*. Boston: Birkhauser, 1991.
63 Klein DE, Bruner H, Holtman H. Circadian rhythm of pilot's efficiency and effects of multiple time zone travel. *Aerospace Med* 1970;**41**:125–32.
64 Gold DR, Rogasz S, Bock N, et al. Rotating shiftwork, sleep, and accidents related to sleepiness in hospital nurses. *Am J Publ Health* 1992;**82**(7):1011–14.
65 Commission of the European Communities, Directive on Working Time. *Official Journal of the European Communities* 1993, 93/104/EEC.
66 Smith L, Folkard,S, Poole CJM. Increased injuries on night shift. *Lancet* 1994;**344**: 1137–9
67 Asken MJ, Raham CC. Resident performance and sleep deprivation: a review. *J Med Educ* 1983;**58**:382–8.
68 Beatty J, Ahern SK, Katz R. Sleep deprivation and the vigilance of anaesthesiologists during simulated surgery. In: Mackie RR, ed. *Vigilance: theory, operational performance and physiological correlates*. New York: Plenum Press, 1977.
69 Deaconson TF, O'Hair DP, Levy MF, et al. Sleep deprivation and resident performance. *JAMA* 1988;**260**:1721–2.
70 Leung L, Becker CE. Sleep deprivation and house staff performance: Update 1984–1991. *J Occup Med* 1992;**34**:1153–60.
71 Ferguson C, Shandall A, Griffith G. Out of hours workload of junior and senior house surgeons in a district general hospital. *Ann R Coll Surg Engl* 1994;**76**(2 suppl):53–6.
72 Leslie PJ, Williams JA, McKenna C, et al. Hours, volume and type of work of pre-registration house officers. *BMJ* 1990;**300**:1038–40.
73 Lingenfelser T, Karschel R, Weber A, et al. Young hospital doctors after night duty: Their task-specific cognitive status and emotional condition. *Med Educ* 1994;**28**:566–72.
74 Poulton EC, Hunt GM, Carpenter A, Edward RS. The performance of junior hospital doctors following reduced sleep and long hours of work. *Ergonomics* 1978;**21**:279–95.
75 Arnetz BB, Andreasson D, Strandberg M, et al. Physicians work environment: psychosocial, physical and physiological data from a structured in-depth interview and bio-chemical assessment of general surgeons and general practitioners. *Stress Reports* No. 187; Karolinksa Institute, Stockholm, 1986. (Swedish with English summary)
76 Wilkinson T, Tyler PD, Varey CA. Duty hours of young hospital doctors: effects on the quality of work. *J Occup Psychology* 1975;**48**:219–29.
77 Friedman RC, Bigger JT, Kornfeld DS. The intern and sleep loss. *N Engl J Med Educ* 1971;**285**:201–3.
78 Arnetz BB, Akerstedt T, Anderzen I. Sleepiness in physicians on night call duty. *Work Stress* 1990;**4**(1):71–73.
79 Engel W, Seime R, Powell V, D'Alessandri R. Clinical performance of interns after being on call. *S Med J* 1987;**80**:761–3.
80 Stampi C. Ultrashort sleep/wake patterns and sustained performance. In: Dinges DF, Broughton RJ, eds. *Sleep and alertness: Chronobiological, behavioural and medical aspects of napping*. New York: Raven Press, 1989.
81 Bonnet MH, Arand DL. The use of prophylactic naps and caffeine to maintain performance during a continuous operation. *Ergonomics* 1994;**7**(6):1009–20.
82 Bonnet MH. Sleep deprivation. In: Kryger M, Roth T, Dement WC, eds. *Principles and practice of sleep medicine*. New York: Saunders, 1994.
83 Hartley LR. A comparison of continuous and distributed reduced sleep schedules. *Q J Experim Psychology* 1974;**26**:8–14.
84 Wilkinson RT. Sleep deprivation: performance tests for partial and selective sleep deprivation. *Prog Clin Psychology* 1968;**8**:28–43.

85 Craig A, Cooper R. Symptoms of acute and chronic fatigue. In: *Handbook of Human Performance*, Vol 3. Academic Press, 1992 (Chapter 11, 289–339).

86 Hockey GRJ. Skilled performance and mental workload. In: Warr P, ed. *Psychology at Work*. London: Penguin, 1996.

87 Dinges DF, Orne MT, Whitehouse WG, Orne E. Temporal placement of a nap for alertness: Contributions of circadian phase and prior wakefulness. *Sleep* 1987;**10**:313–29.

88 Deary IJ, Tait R. Effects of sleep disruption on cognitive performance ands mood in medical house officers. *BMJ* 1987;**296**:1513–16.

89 Ford GV, Wentz DK. Internship: what is stressful? *S Med J* 1986;**79**:595–9.

90 Jones JW, Barge BN, Steffy BD, *et al*. Stress and medical malpractice: organisational risk assessment and intervention. *J Appl Psychology* 1988;**4**:727–35.

91 Barrett A. Beat the clock: Junior doctors hours. *Nursing Standard* 1995;**10**(11):18–19.

92 Fisher EW, Moffat DA, Quinn SJ, *et al*. Reduction in junior doctors' hours in an otolaryngology unit: Effects on the out of hours working patterns of all grades. *Ann R Coll Surg Engl* 1994;**76**(2 suppl):232–5.

93 Hartley C, Rothera MP. A new deal for ENT surgeons – The Manchester experience 1992–3. *Ann R Coll Surg Engl* 1994;**76**(2 suppl):228–31.

94 Kapur N, House A. Improving New Deal shifts for junior house officers. *Hosp Med* 1998;**59**(12):960–6.

95 Kelty C, Duffy J, Cooper G. Out-of-hours work in cardiothoracic surgery: implications of the New Deal and Calman for training. *Postgr Med J* 1999;**75**(884):351–2.

96 Vassallo DJ, Chana J, Ingham-Clark CL, *et al*. Introduction of a partial shift system for house officers in a teaching hospital. *BMJ* 1992;**305**(6860):1005–8.

97 Hale PC, Houghton A, Taylor PR, *et al*. Crossover trial of partial shift working and a one in six rota system for house surgeons at two teaching hospitals. *J R Coll Surg Edinb* 1995;**40**:55–8.

98 Smith C, Robie C, Folkard S, *et al*. A process model of shiftwork and health. *J Occup Health Psychology* 1999;**4**(3):207–18.

99 Firth-Cozens J, Moss F. Hours, sleep, teamwork and stress. *BMJ* 1998;**317**:1335–6.

18 Training and supervision

FIONA MOSS, ELISABETH PAICE

Training and education are core activities of the health service. There is an enormous investment in the training and education of healthcare professionals. Lack of doctors trained in understaffed specialities and difficulties in recruitment and retention of nurses can fundamentally limit the effectiveness of a healthcare service. People are central to the delivery of healthcare and over 70% of the NHS budget is on people. Healthcare professionals clearly need to be trained to be competent in the care of individuals. Training is required in many different fields and many different and differing competencies and aptitudes. Some surgeons, for example, must be trained to be technically competent in very complex tasks. Radiotherapists, on the other hand, have to have an understanding of radiobiology that enables them to safely, accurately, and appropriately prescribe radiation. And public health specialists need to be trained to respond appropriately to the discovery of an outbreak of infectious diseases so that risks to public health are minimised. Technical competence is central to the work of many of the healthcare professions. But healthcare professionals need many other skills besides technical competence.

First, healthcare professionals need to know when it is appropriate to perform an intervention; be knowledgeable about other options available, and have the skills to discuss options with patients to enable patients to make informed choice about healthcare interventions. These generic skills are necessary to give good individual care. Secondly, as doctors and nurses, and other healthcare professionals do not work in isolation, and the risks entailed in their work may be lessened by effective and appropriate support, training must include an understanding of the roles of all the others contributing to care and the skills needed to be effective team members. Thirdly, if risks to

341

patients are to be lessened and if the quality of care is to improve, healthcare professionals need to have the skills to recognise and respond to errors, and also the skills and training to enable them to understand and work within and respond to quality improvement and risk management programmes. Training in all three of these areas is an essential component of risk management in the health service.

A significant number of professionals responsible for delivering care within the NHS are working within postgraduate training programmes. They are employed to work, and the employing organisation is paid to train them while they do so. Doctors in training, by definition, lack the knowledge, skills and experience of fully trained specialists. Learning through mistakes is not an option where patient care is concerned. Supervision is the key to safe learning. In this chapter, we will consider how to provide doctors in training with the skills and attitudes to take an active part in risk management. We will consider the risks of training, to the employer, to the trainee, and to the patient, and ways in which these risks can be managed through safe hours, safe supervision, the use of simulators, performance review, and systems designed to allow for human error.

Training in risk management

Risk management and the curriculum

The UK has seen a quiet revolution in medical education, from undergraduate through to higher specialist training.[1] The General Medical Council's report on undergraduate training[2] criticised the burden of facts imposed on students and recommended more emphasis on equipping the new doctor with the essential skills needed at the beginning of the preregistration year. Despite this fresh approach, risk management was not mentioned anywhere in the document. The reforms of higher specialist training included a published curriculum for each specialty. Few of the curricula refer either to risk management or to patient safety or quality improvement. This is despite the fact that the royal colleges (the bodies responsible for developing these curricula) have led the medical profession in developing clinical audit, one of the planks of risk management. In most specialist registrar curricula, there is acknowledgement of the need to be involved in audit, but few provide more. The curriculum for specialist training in geriatric medicine is one of the most explicit and includes the following:

Ability to undertake and contribute to clinical audit requires:

1 Knowledge of the principles of clinical audit and performance indicators
2 Knowledge of different methods of clinical audit, applied to geriatric medicine

3 Trainees must demonstrate participation in clinical audit programmes and provide documentation of at least one audit project which the trainee has carried out during the specialist training.[3]

Training in organisational aspects of care

Many mistakes and errors are attributed to problems in organisational aspects of care.[4] Medical training focuses almost exclusively on the diagnosis and management of illness in individuals and little on the care and clinical management of groups of people with particular conditions. This focus on the individual, whilst central to clinical care, if not balanced by an understanding of the processes of care, limits an individual's ability to be sensitive to the organisational aspects of risk management and quality improvement. The professional focus on individual care may be one of the reasons why it has been difficult for healthcare professionals to be enthusiastic about quality improvement and risk management programmes. It may also explain why it is difficult to develop and implement written care pathways and why healthcare professionals are reluctant to adhere to guidelines. Many practitioners simply do not expect to work closely to protocols and such organisational aspects of care have been described as "cookbook" medicine. Organisational aspects of care are rarely covered in undergraduate education and are not explicit features of most specialist training curricula.

Training in the skills of risk management

Audit is currently the element of risk management that is most commonly covered in training programmes. For many trainees this involves collecting data or presenting data collected by someone else. Very few trainees see the whole audit loop through or have any training in how to implement the changes that will close the loop. In a study of the involvement of junior doctors in audit, Firth-Cozens and Storer found that about one fifth of respondents had not participated in audit at all and that those that had, found the experience of limited educational value.[5] Learning about audit is more than just learning about the process, it should include reflection on the interpretation of data and analysis of the problems, and an opportunity to be involved in the change process. If risk management is to work as an approach to reducing risks in healthcare we need a more open approach to errors, mistakes, and near misses. All training programmes should include an understanding of the inevitability of human error, the factors associated with errors, and the ways in which systems can pick up and alert the practitioner to potential error. Trainees should also be trained in appropriate checking behaviour that will minimise mistakes. They should understand the importance of safe handover. Finally they need to know how to respond effectively to errors and mistakes whether made by themselves or others. The culture of medical teams needs to change considerably before the majority of junior doctors will feel comfortable in admitting to errors, or questioning the decisions of their seniors.[6]

Multiprofessional training

Since error so often occurs in the gaps created by different professionals working together in a complex environment[7] risk management programmes should incorporate all those who are involved in patient care. For the same reason, training in risk management is best delivered in a multiprofessional context. An example of a curriculum designed to cover every aspect of quality is the *Managing Life in the NHS: Education towards Clinical Governance* programme[8] developed in North Thames, in a partnership involving the postgraduate deans, the educational consortia (responsible for commissioning education for nurses and other professions allied to medicine) and local hospitals, where the modular programme is delivered. One of the prerequisites for obtaining financial support is that the programme must be delivered to a multi-professional group, preferably no more than a third of each group being doctors. Early evaluation of the programme showed that the opportunity to train with colleagues from other disciplines was welcomed and recognised as valuable by almost all participants. Formal training in team work, and team and group behaviour is not a routine part of most training programmes, except in general practice. For safe practice all practitioners need to be effective at communication both with patients and with colleagues, and must be able to work effectively within teams and groups. Medical education has for too long been isolated, encouraging doctors to develop competitive, tribal and hierarchical attitudes that are not conducive to successful teamwork, open discussion of errors, or a proper appreciation of the stresses affecting other healthcare workers.[6,9]

Managing the risks of training

Safe supervision

The first postgraduate year is particularly stressful[10,11] and a time when mistakes are likely to occur. Lesar *et al* showed that more prescribing errors occur among those in their first postgraduate year than among other clinicians.[12] and Wu reported that 45% of a large group of medical house officers reported making at least one error, 31% of which resulted in a patient's death.[13] Clearly careful preparation and close supervision are required to protect patients from errors made by recently qualified doctors. Otherwise patient care may be compromised and trainees may be subjected to further stress through errors made while under stress.[14] In the UK, full registration with the GMC requires completion of a year as a preregistration house officer (PRHO). The PRHO can only work in posts that have been approved by the local university's postgraduate dean as falling within guidelines set out by the GMC. Each PRHO must have a named educational supervisor responsible for their development and access at all times to supervision from a more senior doctor. Despite these clear guidelines, the GMC found continuing deficiencies in the education and supervision of PRHOs, and has produced further detailed recommendations in an attempt to improve the experience.[15]

The quality of consultant supervision seems to be one of the most important factors in determining job satisfaction for doctors in training, whatever their level of seniority.[16-18] The reasons for inadequate supervision include poor hospital organisation; lack of training in supervision for consultants who themselves may have experienced inadequate supervision, and lack of time in a hard-pressed service. An audit of colorectal surgery performed in 1990–4 in three parts of the United Kingdom showed that consultants supervised only a fifth of the resections performed by trainees and were present at less than two thirds of the total number of operations.[19] Figures for cholecystectomy were similar. In urology, vascular surgery, ophthalmology, and orthopaedics the data suggested that the figures for trainees operating under supervision might be even less satisfactory.[20] Collins has emphasised the need for dedicated, consultant-supervised operating lists and consultant involvement in all emergency work, including out of hours, so that the service is provided by consultants, trainees are properly supervised, and surgical patients receive the benefit of fully trained expertise in their care at all times.[21]

Safe hours

Traditionally, doctors in training in hospitals have carried responsibility for delivering emergency care, especially at night and at weekends. A long hours culture has developed both in the UK and in the USA, in which doctors learn to deny the effects of fatigue on their performance.[6] As medical advances accelerate, and patient expectations rise, the intensity of work out-of-hours is steadily increasing. Obviously, arrangements must be made to care for patients who genuinely need medical attention at night, but the public's growing expectations of a 24-hour service must be tempered with the realities of affordable staffing and the impact of shiftwork and sleep deprivation on health and on error rate. The report of a confidential enquiry into perioperative deaths (CEPOD) in the United Kingdom[22] has shown that there is increased reluctance by trainees to involve senior

345

members of staff in the night. This results in a lower standard of care, which is reflected by inappropriate preoperative management, inappropriate operation, and deaths related to surgery. It is increasingly realised that sleep deprivation in surgical and anaesthetic junior hospital staff causes significant reduction in performance of mental and physical skills. Stewart and colleagues found an excess of perinatal deaths occurring at night and during months when annual leave is popular and suggested this may indicate an over-reliance on trainees at these times.[23] A study of surgeons' error rate using a simulation showed that surgeons awake all night made 20% more errors and took 14% longer to complete the tasks than those who had had a full night's sleep. They also showed increased stress and decreased arousal, which paralleled the decrease in operative dexterity.[24] The capacity to learn through experience has been shown to be impaired by lack of sleep. [25] It should come as no surprise to learn that doctors work and learn most effectively when they have adequate sleep, and when that sleep takes place at night.[26]

At present there are fewer consultants than trainees in the NHS, and in a health service chronically short of doctors, there are not enough consultants to provide first- or even second-line cover around the clock. The problem of how to cover emergencies out of hours, provide safe supervision for trainees and at the same time ensure rest and a reasonable work/life balance for all doctors has not yet been solved. There are, however, some steps that can and should be taken. Work that could be done by day should not be carried out when people are at their lowest ebb and help is hardest to access if things go wrong. Tasks that need to be done in the middle of the night should be the responsibility of staff trained and competent to do it. The tradition of having doctors in their first year covering the wards at night should be reviewed. Several studies have shown that much of what they are called to do is unnecessary, does not require a doctor or could safely be delayed until morning.[27] The remaining tasks carry the risk of exposing the inexperience and ignorance of such recently qualified doctors, who may be reluctant to ask for help from their supervising senior house officer or specialist registrar, or having asked, may find their seniors reluctant to assist. We carried out a survey of PRHOs, asking for examples of incidents they had found stressful. This revealed that excessive responsibility was the most frequently mentioned theme, especially at night and when medical problems arose on a surgical ward.

The implications for risk management are clear. Similar problems have been reported in New York hospitals. The Bell Regulations, which limited working hours for junior doctors in the state to 80 hours a week, were brought in following the death of a young woman whose care was in the hands of tired and poorly supervised junior doctors. Over two years later, doctors still reported working over 100 hours a week in punishing schedules and feeling poorly supervised. The laws had changed but not the culture.[28]

Stressful incidents in the PRHO year

"On call overnight. Very sick patient in multi-organ failure. Nurses anxious. SHO unhelpful. Rude on phone, would not attend. Totally out of my depth. Nasogastric tube needed, nurses refused, had to pass my first one, patient alert and communicating. I felt I was deceiving patient pretending I knew what I was doing. Long stressful night. Inevitable but harrowing."

"On call at night for general surgery. Two patients becoming very ill at about 3.00am – SHO unsupportive, refusing to come out. Contacting my registrar, medical SHO and medical registrar and having very little support. Having been very distressed, and having put in considerable effort, one patient died."

"Three weeks into my medicine job, I tried to deal with a situation at 4.00am without waking my SHO, as I wanted to do something without asking her and I also thought she may think I was stupid for asking her to get out of bed before I had at least attempted to sort it out. I treated it completely incorrectly and consequently looked really stupid and felt really awful (the patient didn't die)."

"One night on call – three sick patients on three different wards and running between them all night. No clue what was happening with one man who subsequently went to ITU. Unable to interest my registrar at all."

PRHOs in 1997. IC McManus, E Paice (unpublished survey)

Managing the risks of a peripatetic workforce

The UK system of postgraduate training requires trainees to acquire experience in a range of settings and thus they change posts every six or twelve months, moving from hospital to hospital. They have little reason or opportunity to develop loyalty to the organisations they rotate through, or gain a thorough understanding of their processes or philosophy.[29] Despite this they work at the front-line of patient care, under conditions – – such as tiredness, pressure of competing tasks, and unfamiliarity with the environment – associated with increased rates of error. They are at risk of incurring psychological or physical harm from their working environment, and their employers are at risk if they fail in their duty of care for them. It is clearly important that the NHS should take responsibility for training but the risks of depending on trainees for service delivery, particularly when they work in a hospital for short periods, are real and need to be managed.

347

Whilst the NHS is a unified healthcare system, there are many difference in procedures and practice between hospitals and sometimes between departments in a hospital. Lack of understanding of how things work can lead to mistakes or omissions. New trainees joining a unit are a source of increased medication errors.[30] Good induction programmes must be considered essential every time a trainee of whatever seniority, moves into a new post. Induction should be a feature of starting a job, at whatever grade. The programme should include attention to the processes and procedures of the hospital and the department, an introduction to key staff, a copy of relevant protocols and guidelines, a discussion of the duties of the job and the degree of responsibility expected, and clear instructions about whom to call if in doubt, especially out of hours. In surveys of over 6000 doctors in training in North Thames,[18] we found that there was a strong correlation between the quality of induction and not feeling forced to cope beyond their competence or experience, at every level of seniority.

For pre-registration house officers starting their first post within the NHS induction became mandatory in August 1994 The mandatory induction lasts only a day and has to include a wide range of essential employment, and health and safety issues as well as time with the outgoing PRHO for a handover. Several medical schools have co-operated with employing

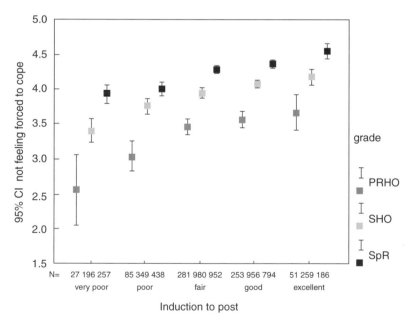

Figure 18.1 Relationship between trainees' ratings of the quality of induction to the post and responses to the question "How often do you feel forced to cope with problems beyond your competence and experience?".(1 = all the time, 2 = daily, 3 = weekly, 4 = monthly, 5 = never.)

hospitals to provide an additional period of "shadowing" for new doctors about to take up their first post. This would appear to be an excellent idea, and does reduce the anxiety of starting,[31] but in the interests of risk management attention should be paid to ensuring that what is passed on is sound and safe practice and is not totally left to the discretion of the outgoing trainee. Otherwise, short-cuts and other bad habits may be passed on. Starting subsequent jobs may be less traumatic for the trainee, but it remains in the interests of the organisation to ensure that time is set aside for a safe induction, to prevent the rise in errors that occurs when new trainees join a unit, especially when it is their first experience of a specialty. In the best run departments, a reduction in clinical work is planned for the whole unit in order to release senior staff to undertake the induction of trainees joining the team. The improved efficiency, confidence, and adherence to local risk management processes of the new recruits amply repays such efforts at the start.

Overseas graduates

Britain has fewer doctors for its population than most developed countries. Although the numbers entering medical school are to be increased by 1000, there is currently a shortfall made up by the employment of doctors from other countries seeking to gain specialist training here. At present nearly a third of doctors in training in the UK graduated abroad. Some, especially those from European Economic Area countries who do not need to pass an English language examination to practise here, may have difficulties in understanding and being understood by patients and colleagues. Others may find difficulty in adjusting to different attitudes to patient autonomy or the role of non-medical members of the team. Doctors coping with living in a foreign country may be particularly keen to demonstrate their competence and reluctant to admit ignorance, ask for help or tolerate questioning, unless given strong encouragement and reassurance. Extra attention should be paid to the induction needs of overseas graduates especially in their first post, and the NHS executive has recently identified special funding for this purpose.

The place of simulators in reducing the risks of training

Comparisons are sometimes made between the extent and effects of errors in the airline industry[32] compared with medical practice and between the process of training doctors and training airline pilots. Training for pilots is based on many hours of work with a simulator that can offer experience of many different conditions and circumstances without risk to themselves, the aircraft or passengers. Simulations also cover interpersonal interactions in the cockpit, because human factors have been

349

shown to be the source of error in accidents.[33] In UK medicine, all but the most basic techniques and procedures are acquired in through working in an "apprenticeship" style, watching, assisting, doing under supervision and finally doing alone. This method has generally served well, but it requires years of apprenticeship to experience the full range of uncommon situations. With shorter working hours and a shortened total training time, there is real anxiety that specialists will complete their training without the breadth of experience of their predecessors. Simulations, although relatively undeveloped in medicine compared with the airline industry, can offer training opportunities without risk to patients. Advanced trauma, life-support training courses simulate a range of emergency scenarios in a lifelike manner, using effectively made up and rehearsed actors. High fidelity anaesthetics simulators use a computerised mannikin and realistic operating theatre equipment to mimic anaesthetic emergencies.[34] Less high-tech but just as valuable for training purposes is the use of role play with actors as simulated patients for training in breaking bad news, handling complaints and dealing with conflict. All of these offer planned exposure to simulated crises and a safe environment in which trainees can gain practice and learn from mistakes without putting patients at risk.

Risks to the trainee

The factors that make trainees prone to perpetrating medical errors also put them at risk of accidental self harm. Needlestick injuries are a good example of this, avoidable in theory, common in practice, especially among students and doctors in training. Needlestick phobia following an injury cost a UK trainee her career and the employing trust £460 000 in compensation.[35] Violence in the workplace is becoming increasingly common, and doctors in training are especially at risk because they are called to deal with difficult situations, often with no training in conflict management or self defence. There have been numerous instances of trainees being physically threatened by angry patients or relatives, or assaulted at night when crossing unlit car parks between the wards and their accommodation. Proper security is the responsibility of the employer, and should be provided for the protection of those bearing the burden of covering the hospital at unsocial hours. Finally, medicine is stressful,[36] and every year about 1% of UK hospital trainees leave the profession, often because they find the workload too heavy and the responsibilities too great.[37] Some become psychologically ill.[38] Failure to address preventable causes of stress such as sleep deprivation, excessive demands, bullying, or harassment in the workplace presents the employer with the risk of incurring significant financial penalty.

Employment issues

Doctors in training – whose responsibility?

Most doctors in training in the UK are employed by NHS trusts, in training posts commissioned by the postgraduate dean. In some regions one trust will act as lead employer, with trainees rotating to other trusts on secondment. At specialist registrar level, recruitment is to 3–6 year rotational programmes that are managed by the postgraduate dean. More junior grades are usually appointed by the employing trust. In all cases, the postgraduate dean is responsible for ensuring continuity of education through rotational programmes, and for ensuring that jobs are not advertised as training posts unless they meet certain standards and have educational approval from the relevant royal college.[39] Consultants undertaking training are expected to provide assessments of competence and progress in the form of trainers' reports, which help determine whether the trainee is ready to move on to the next stage of training. These in-training assessments are reviewed by a panel, under the aegis of the postgraduate dean, that considers both the trainee's progress and the adequacy of the documentation.[40]

Training and disciplinary problems

Problem behaviour of doctors in training can create risks for the employing organisation and compromise patient care.[41] Problems include personal conduct (rudeness, poor punctuality), professional conduct (failing to examine patient, contacting patient at home for reasons unconnected with their care), and professional competence (failing to recognise the significance of signs or symptoms, failing to call for help, isolated but serious errors). Health-related problems have included substance abuse and psychiatric disturbance. In the past, disciplinary procedures have sometimes been dropped, or never commenced, because the trainee was due to leave the trust where the problem occurred soon. Sometimes trainees have been offered the choice between resignation or facing a disciplinary procedure. These approaches are unsatisfactory because they leave the matter unsettled, do nothing to address the problem behaviour, and face the next employer with recognising and tackling the same problems from scratch. In the interests of patient safety, problem behaviour should be tackled when and where it occurs and proper disciplinary procedures followed, as they would be for any other member of staff. Referral to the GMC may be appropriate if educational procedures have been exhausted and the trainee's performance is not considered compatible with good medical practice. It will be also be appropriate where a poorly performing junior doctor is found to be abusing alcohol or drugs, behaving unprofessionally, or impaired by a physical or mental condition affecting fitness to practise.

351

The poorly performing trainee

When a trainee is identified as poorly performing there is usually considerable anxiety and distress on all sides. The trainee will be distressed at the implications for his or her career and the trainer may well feel at risk of counterclaims by the trainee of poor supervision. In our experience, it is usually best to accept that the training relationship has broken down and move the trainee, who will sometimes blossom under a new trainer. It is difficult for a trainee to improve in an environment where other staff have lost respect or confidence in their colleague's competence. Trainees in this situation are usually referred to the postgraduate dean and their deficiencies tackled by a placement that offers remedial training, if necessary in a supernumerary capacity. Where a trainee is moved for such reasons, it is important for the receiving trainer to have information about the areas of practice that gave rise to concern. It is also important that senior management of the receiving organisation know the problems and give consent to the placement. Information is best transferred in writing and in fairness the trainee should be allowed to see what has been said. Poor assessments that result in delay to progress or removal from training have devastating effects on the career and livelihood of trainees and are likely to be the subject of challenge. Assessments should be based on carefully documented objective evidence, should be carried out by several trainers, and should be scrupulously fair. Failure to document and tackle poor performance is also risky, since the trainee may go on to behave in a way that damages patients and raises questions about the adequacy of previous assessments. In balancing lives against livelihoods, there is no choice but to put patient safety first.

Conclusions

Organisations employing doctors in training expose themselves to a number of risks. Less experienced than fully trained doctors, trainees are more prone to active failures through ignorance or misreading a situation. Their working conditions are often rife with factors associated with latent failures: heavy workload, inadequate knowledge or experience, inadequate supervision, a stressful environment, frequent change of working environments, conflict between work and personal life, obstacles to accessing technological support. At the same time, the NHS depends on trainees not only to supply the workforce of tomorrow, but also to make a major contribution to service today. No risk management programme can be effective unless the organisation engages all its staff, and unless training encompasses all the competencies necessary to function safely as part of a team. Medical education, both undergraduate and postgraduate, needs to tackle risk management quite explicitly, and include training in all aspects of quality improvement, teamworking and organisational behaviour. At the same time, attention must be paid to reducing latent error by good induction processes; responsibilities tailored to individual competence and clearly communicated; protocols for managing common problems; easy access to advice from a nominated senior; safe handovers; well-functioning supportive teams; and a rigorous safe hours policy.[42] The tendency of humans to err, and the necessity of developing systems that acknowledge and counteract that tendency, must be instilled early and reinforced at every level for every member of the healthcare team.

References

1 Catto G. Specialist registrar training. *BMJ* 2000;**320**:817–18.
2 General Medical Council. *Tomorrow's Doctors*. London: GMC, 1993.
3 *Curriculum for Higher Specialist Training in Geriatric Medicine*. Joint Committee for Higher Medical Training. London: RCP, 1999.
4 Reason J. Human error: models and management. *BMJ* 2000;**320**:768–70.
5 Firth-Cozens J, Storer D. Registrars' and senior registrars' perceptions of their audit activities. *Qual healthcare* 1992;**1**:161–4.
6 Sexton JB, Thomas EJ. Error, stress, and teamwork in medicine and aviation: cross sectional surveys. *BMJ* 2000;**320**:745–9.
7 Cook RI, Render M, Woods DD. Gaps in the continuity of care and progress on patient safety. *BMJ* 2000;**320**:791–4.
8 Heard S. *Managing life in the NHS: Education towards clinical governance*. London: TPMDE, 1998.
9 Moss F. Junior doctors: waving or drowning? *BMJ* 1999;**318**:1639–40.
10 Hsu K, Marshall V. Prevalence of depression and distress in a large sample of Canadian residents, interns and fellows. *Am J Psych* 1987;**144**:1561–6.
11 Firth-Cozens J. Emotional distress in junior house officers. *BMJ* 1987;**295**:533–6.
12 Lesar TS, Briceland LL, Delcoure K, *et al*. Medication prescribing errors in a teaching hospital. *JAMA* 1990;**263**:2329–34.
13 Wu AW, Folkmann S, McPhee SJ, Lo B. Do house officers learn from their mistakes? *JAMA* 1991;**265**:2089–94.
14 Wu AW. Medical error: the second victim. *BMJ* 2000;**320**:726–7.
15 General Medical Council *The New Doctor*. London: GMC, 1998.
16 Paice E, Moss F, West G, Grant J. Association of use of a log book and experience as a pre-registration house officer: interview survey. *BMJ* 1997;**314**:213.
17 Paice E, Leaver P. Improving the training of SHOs. *BMJ* 1999;**318**:1022–23.
18 Paice E, Aitken M, Cowan G, Heard S. Trainee satisfaction before and after the Calman reforms of specialist training: questionnaire survey. *BMJ* 2000;**320**:832–6.
19 Aitken RJ, Thompson MR, Smith JAE, *et al*. Training in large bowel cancer surgery: observations from three prospective regional United Kingdom audits. *BMJ* 1999;**318**:702–3.
20 Harper, DR. Royal College of Surgeons of Edinburgh gives consultant fellows feedback on their training activity. *BMJ* 1999;**319**:258.
21 Collins C. Surgical training, supervision, and service: Laissez-faire attitudes to surgical training and patient care are unsustainable. *BMJ* 1999;**318**:682–3.
22 Buck N, Devlin HB, Lunn JN. *The report of a confidential enquiry into perioperative deaths*. London: Nuffield Provincial Hospitals Trust and King's Fund Publishing Office, 1987.
23 Stewart JH, Andrews J, Cartlidge P. Numbers of deaths related to intrapartum asphyxia and timing of birth in all Wales perinatal survey, 1993–5. *BMJ* 1998;**316**:657–60.

24 Taffinder NJ, McManus IC, Gul Y, *et al.* Effect of sleep deprivation on surgeons' dexterity on laparoscopy simulator. *Lancet* 1998;**352**:1191.

25 Stickgold R, Whidbee D, Schirmer B, *et al.* Visual discrimination task improvement: a multi-step process occurring during sleep. *J Cognitive Neuroscience* 2000;**12**:246–54.

26 Deary IJ, Tait R. Effects of sleep disruption on cognitive performance and mood in medical house officers. *BMJ* 1987;**295**:1513–16.

27 McKee M, Black N. Junior doctors' work at night: what is done and how much is appropriate? *J Publ Health Med* 1993;**15**:16–24.

28 Green M. Putting patients at risk: How hospitals still violate the "Bell" regulations governing resident working conditions. Office of the Public Advocate for the City of New York, 1997.

29 Dowling S, Barrett S. *Doctors in the making: the experience of the pre-registration house officer year.* Bristol: SAUS Publications, 1993.

30 Wilson DG, McArtney RG, Newcombe RG, *et al.* Medication errors in paediatric practice: insights from a continuous quality improvement approach. *Eur J Pediatr* 1998;**157**: 769–74.

31 Richards C. Shadowing: the Leicester experience. In: Paice E, ed. *Delivering the new doctor.* ASME Educational Booklet, 1998.

32 Berwick DM, Leape LL Reducing errors in medicine. *BMJ* 1999;**318**:136–7.

33 Halamek LP, Howard SK, Smith BE, *et al.* Development of a simulated delivery room for the study of human performance during neonatal resuscitation. *Pediatrics* 1999;**318**: 887–8.

34 Gaba DM. Improving anesthesiologist's performance by simulating reality. *Anesthesiology* 1992;**76**:491–4.

35 Hayes SF. Compensation for needlestick injury is profoundly mistaken. *BMJ* 1999;**318**: 735.

36 Firth-Cozens J, Moss F. Hours, sleep, teamwork and stress. *BMJ* 1998;**317**:1335–6.

37 Paice E. Why do young doctors leave the profession? *J Roy Soc Med* 1997;**90**:41–2.

38 Williams S, Dale J, Glucksman E, Wellesley A. Senior house officers' work related stressors, psychological distress, and confidence in performing clinical tasks in accident and emergency; a questionnaire study. *BMJ* 1997;**314**:713–18.

39 Paice E, Goldberg I. What do postgraduate deans do? *BMJ* 1998;**316**:2.

40 Sim F. Record of in-training assessment (RITA): a look at ethical issues in assessment. *Hosp Med* 1999;**60**:676–8.

41 Paice E, Orton V, Appleyard J. Managing trainee doctors in difficulty. *Hosp Med* 1999;**60**: 130–3.

42 Moss F, Paice E. Getting things right for the doctor in training. In: Firth-Cozens J, Payne RL, eds. *Stress in health professionals.* Chichester: John Wiley, 1999.

19 Teams, culture and managing risk

JENNY FIRTH-COZENS

A fundamental part of risk management is about changing behaviour towards safer care. This change comes about through learning, which takes place at the level of the individual health professional, at the organisational systems level, and at points in between. These levels are captured in the description of organisations as a dynamic balance between the authority and autonomy of the individual, the control that exists in formal structures, and the co-operation that takes place within and between teams.[1] This chapter uses a variety of different literatures and briefly discusses the learning that takes place at the different levels and the cultural change necessary to encourage it. It then focuses on teams and team leaders as potentially powerful forces for bringing about the management of risk and better quality in general.

Individual learning

As we have seen from earlier chapters, risky behaviours are easiest to perceive at the sharp end of care; where the health professional and patient interact. This is the most readily apparent place for allocating responsibility, and many internal reviews of untoward incidents focus at this end, seeing problems in terms of health workers' lack of skills; poor communication with others; or their affective state, such as depression which affected their decision-making, etc.[2] This focus is not surprising since the cause of the mistake is most easily visualised at this level, making it possible to acquire quite detailed knowledge about the professional and the situation concerned. In addition, it creates the smallest possible sense of responsibility for the rest of the organisation.

The learning by the individual health worker seen as responsible may be very long-lasting indeed: certainly early mistakes are a powerful part of memories for doctors.[3,4] However, the learning involved may not always be appropriate in that their clinical care may become more defensive in the future. Janoff-Bulman[5] has described the process of change that takes place for individuals faced with crises:

- first the confrontation with an experience which does not fit their previous assumptions about themselves
- next resistance by means of ignoring or reinterpreting the incident
- followed by validation, where the truth is recognised
- finally integration, which allows the previous and new knowledge about themselves to be synthesised and new learning and behaviours to take place.

These steps, if completed, represent a healthy progression and could equally apply to organisations faced with serious safety problems. Even if the individual responsible for a serious mistake goes through these processes successfully, the learning for the rest of the organisation is likely to be negligible unless it can move forward in similar ways.

Behavioural change after negative events has been shown to be quite narrowly focussed on the person or persons most closely involved and on the behaviours most obviously connected with what happened. For example, the ways that those with the actual experiences can learn, while those just outside the experience do not, is well illustrated by the considerable subsequent precautions taken by the US towns actually hit by Hurricane Hugo compared to those nearby who were fortunate enough to escape its ravages, even narrowly.[6] If we do not personally experience a negative event for ourselves, our sense of control over our future events is almost magical. Based on their lives thus far, those in Pompeii, for example, made a tragic estimate of the chance that Vesuvius might erupt! This optimism may be particularly problematic where confidence is already high; medical students and doctors, for example, are often chosen for their high confidence.

Both individual and organisational learning about risk will also be influenced by the training and education that precedes the taking of formal responsibility. Medical students in particular may need encouragement to see that error and learning are intimately connected, enabling them to help themselves and others learn from their mistakes. Achieving this balance is going to continue throughout training for all healthcare workers; for example, by encouraging the reporting of errors while doing whatever possible to remove the shame and fear that so often follows them.[7]

356

Organisational learning and culture change

The difficulty of bringing about desired changes in organisations is well evidenced by the large number of books that exist on various ways to achieve it. There are certainly numerous examples within management literature of why organisational learning so often fails to occur.[8-10] These include bureaucracy, a lack of clear purpose or feedback mechanisms, poor communication, and cultural issues around a lack of openness, centralised authority, and blame where errors are seen as indicating incompetence.[11] On the other hand, there is a useful body of literature building up around what are termed "high reliability organisations", or HROs – ones which are nearly error free despite operating in highly hazardous fields:[12,13] in particular, these include the ability to react to unexpected sequences of events through constant training, and "redundancy", or having more than you appear to need in terms of staff and equipment – a rare event in healthcare.

The emotional and social contexts of healthcare

In tackling clinical risk by changing culture we need to take note of literature from other sectors, but also to appreciate the special emotional and social context in which this change will take place: this is an arena in which mistakes can actually cause physical harm to others. As Leape[14] and colleagues have said: ". . . patients and physicians . . . live and interact in a culture characterised by anger, blame, guilt, fear, frustration, and distrust regarding healthcare errors. The public has responded by escalating the punishment for error. Clinicians and some healthcare organisations generally have responded by suppression, stonewalling, and cover-up."

This emotional context needs to be worked with rather than ignored or denied. Apart from existing in its own right, it is a contributing factor to the high stress levels that health workers in general experience.[15,16] Stress and error are intimately linked. For example, Houston and Allt[17] found that insomnia and stress increased alongside errors as junior doctors began a new post. Since resistance to change is greater when people are demoralised or under unreasonable pressure, a failure to acknowledge the very real emotional context of healthcare and high stress levels is likely to make any attempts at real cultural change impossible.

The indisputable links between stress, cognitive functioning and error are outlined in detail by Smith (see Chapter 17). The situation of the relationship between stress and error is made more serious because findings consistently show that health professionals – particularly doctors, nurses and managers – are considerably more stressed than other British workers: Wall et al[15] found that 28% of health staff overall were above threshold on the General Health Questionnaire compared to 18% of workers in the British Household Panel Survey of 1993. Nevertheless, there was wide variation between trusts (17–33%) with larger trusts having significantly higher levels than smaller ones. Results indicated that work factors, including management practices, are influential in causing or lowering the stress of staff. Bringing together these findings suggests strongly that one way that management can improve patient care is by lowering the stress levels of staff. A supportive organisational culture which benefits both quality and staff well-being is illustrated by the research into "magnet" hospitals,[18] and from results of the largest patient satisfaction survey ever conducted, which showed the highest correlations were with the cheerfulness, friendliness and sensitivity of staff.[19]

Moreover, so long as management commitment is assured[20] a number of means exist to enable organisations to reduce stress;[21,22] for example:

- increasing participation in decision-making[21]
- improving two-way communication
- providing tangible and intangible reward systems[23]
- improving skill mix through work design[24]
- providing stress management courses[25] and counselling services[26]
- providing a reasonable and supportive approach to doctors facing complaints.[16]

In addition, the development of teams and team leaders is also likely to improve the emotional context of healthcare, as I discuss later in the chapter.

In terms of the social context, humans in all situations make alliances, which can be both productive and disruptive.[27] Wherever possible we tend to forgive those within our alliance for making the mistakes – we don't want to cause them the emotional pain that is associated with blame and criticism.[22,28] So some staff may have their mistakes or their behaviour ignored over time. It may be reinterpreted or forgiven, so long as they are within the alliance (for example, as happened at Bristol), or be scapegoated if they are outside it,[29] as can happen to a junior doctor or a nurse who is cast out through blame, or to patients or other staff groups who were outsiders from the beginning. Whistle-blowers will also be cast out[30] since disloyalty to the alliance is seen as a very serious crime, reflecting our national culture that forbids the "telling of tales". By defending colleagues within the alliance and casting aside those outside it, systemic learning throughout the alliance or the organisation as a whole becomes much more difficult. This makes the structural tying in of clinical teams to management particularly important.

Organisational culture as a target for change

There is no doubt from what has been said above, that organisational culture and the practices that underpin it are essential targets for change towards greater patient safety; in particular, the necessary cultural change towards openness and accountability. This will be a culture where reporting of mistakes, including near-misses, is routine, and where this and demonstrations of learning from mistakes are the behaviours which are most clearly valued and rewarded: a culture which has made air transport safer.[31] It will provide real, rather than ambivalent, support to whistle-blowers and to patients who report that all is not well.[32] Competition between groups is natural and in such an organisation this competition will be used to drive the goal of patient safety, rather than merely those of efficiency or technological advances. Making safety "sexy" rather than dull is essential, and for this reason risk management within the organisation should be given particularly charismatic leadership to help break the mould of its being a split off, tedious and reactive concept.[33]

A systems approach to risk[34] is essential in terms of cultural change in that it has the effect of spreading responsibility throughout all levels of the organisation. So long as the acceptance of responsibility at managerial levels is communicated and seen to be taken seriously, this will help to negate an authoritarian top-down culture. Just as importantly, this sharing of responsibility will reduce the level of emotional response that takes place at the sharp end, which should allow learning to take place more readily and more appropriately.

However, an organisation-wide approach cannot solve everything. Various writers have described how the most successful organisations are small to midsize family businesses of not more than 150 members,[27] very different from most British trusts. Wall *et al*'s[15] work on trust size and stress levels also suggests that "small is beautiful". It may be that the particular size and complexity of healthcare establishments means that they do not lend themselves so well to attempts to intervene directly at the organisational level, other than by creating the appropriate culture and structures to enable smaller groups such as directorates and particularly teams to bring about safer care themselves.

Using teams to tackle patient safety

The benefits of teams in reducing errors and improving the quality of patient care have been recognised in a number of studies.[35–37] For example, Reith[35] looking at lessons from mental health inquiries, found four major themes that recurred throughout:

1 Thoroughness and attention to detail
2 "Real" teamworking including inter-agency co-operation and effective liaison
3 Listening to all members of the clinical team

4 Listening to carers, relatives and patients.

Similarly, Adorian et al[37] demonstrated that using regular team discussions and feedback significantly improves detection, treatment and follow-up of patients with hypertension. Teams clearly play a major role in creating safer patient care.

Outside of healthcare the importance of the team was apparent in a study of flight crews[38] which considered the effects of fatigue on errors. It found that crews in the fatigue condition, where they had flown together for several days, made significantly fewer errors, looking at overall team scores, than the crews who were rested but who had not worked together. It was not that those within the fatigued team made fewer errors – individually they made more, just as expected – but the team was able to compensate for them. This lower rate of errors may be partly due to team attributes such as being able to recognise failures, co-ordinate and compensate better, but may also be through the influence of teams in lowering stress levels.[39] Fatigue does not necessarily lead to stress,[40] and it may be that the increased support which teams are able to give, the greater awareness of each other's ways of working that they allow, and the greater chance of co-ordination, act together to reduce stress levels.

Teams also matter because there is evidence that good teamworking appears associated with lower stress levels. Those in "real" teams – ones with clearly defined roles, whose members work together to achieve them, with different roles for different members, and recognised externally as a functional team – have lower stress levels than those in teams which do not meet these criteria; while these in turn have lower scores than those in no team at all.[39] We are social beings, but also ones who want individual recognition: good supportive teams allow our ideas and participation to gain the essential acceptance and valuing which make up that recognition, from our peers and beyond, and so become an essential part of reducing stress and containing the emotional context of healthcare.

What makes a good team and how can it be measured?

There have been various evaluations of the elements that lead to team effectiveness[36,39,41–44] and the main ones of these[36] are listed below. One of the most important elements, in terms of risk, is that the teams should ensure that they are able to hear the voices of those staff with the most experience of what can go or has gone wrong in patient care, whether or not they are of lower rank than their colleagues.

Morgan's work on naval teams[45] is useful in this context. He found that in effective teams:

- Members monitored each other's performance and stepped in to help out. Trust was an implicit part of this.

Elements leading to team effectiveness

- Clear team goal and objectives
- Clear accountability and authority
- Diversity of skills and personalities
- Clear individual roles for members
- Shared tasks
- Regular internal formal and informal communication
- Full participation by members
- The ability to change and develop
- The confronting of conflict
- Feedback to individuals
- Team rewards
- Monitoring of team objectives
- Outside recognition of a team
- Two way external communication
- Feedback on team performance

- Giving and receiving feedback was the norm for all team members and seen as part of their role. Understanding each other's role is an important part of this and one that does not happen frequently in health services.[46,47]
- Communication was made real: senders checked that messages were received as intended.

However, there is a fundamental problem in assessing the effectiveness of teams, and indeed of organisations, in terms of risk. This is that, at least in the early days of monitoring, a team with a culture of openness and reporting is likely to produce greater numbers of accidents and near misses than one in which errors are linked to incompetence and hidden where possible; for example, those with authoritarian team leaders.[48] Measuring effectiveness, therefore, is not always easy unless you concentrate on the large-scale incidents which are difficult to miss or where you have in place precision monitoring systems, such as in aircraft.[38] One way around this would be to measure as outcomes attitudes about risk and safety, and evidence of change being accomplished. Another useful route would be to develop systems to capture near-misses. This is a relatively rare source of information in the health services, though air travel has used it as a principal route to increasing safety.

Hackman[49] sees three essential ways to capture team performance:

1 Elements of the task itself, which would include accidents and near misses, as well as other indices of care
2 Measures of the team members' ability to work together
3 Measures of team members' well-being and development.

361

Enhancing team effectiveness

There are a number of ways to improve the effectiveness of teams: those listed in the box above, and other broader concepts which underlie them and which are discussed below.

Improving decision-making

I have argued elsewhere,[50] using an analogy from chaos theory, that healthcare behaviours can be divided into those that are habitual and routine; those which are largely routine, but able to be adapted to fit changing circumstances; and those which cannot easily be foreseen and so require a different type of learning activity around anticipation. Although many of the routine procedures come from previous training, guidelines and protocols, there will be other areas within the work which should be tackled through the establishment of habit. The team is an appropriate organisational unit to decide what these are and how they should be tackled, using evidence or guidelines where they exist. Equally, it can periodically horizon-gaze in order to anticipate potential changes and new risks and to share these with the wider organisation. The importance of diversity in teams has been stated frequently[36,50,51] and the broader knowledge this produces increases the team's ability to address its tasks well, so long as all the members feel able to participate in decision-making.[21,52,53]

In order to enhance patient safety, decision-making at both the team and the individual levels can habitually include questions such as those suggested by Snowden[54] in reference to psychiatric care:

- Do we know what the risks are and do we have all the necessary information?
- Are we cutting corners and setting aside enough time for all involved to come to a decision?
- Do we need to take this risk now?
- What is it hoped will be achieved and what might happen?
- Are there discrepancies between the decision and the observation of others?
- Do we have a rigorous formulation of the case?

Listening to patients

To aid decision-making further, clinical teams need to include all those people who can usefully provide information about the patient, but could patients themselves ever be seen team members? This need not involve the same type of membership that health staff have, but it would be a means of listening to their views and their concerns in ways that do not always take place now. Certainly their presence has been found useful within audit groups.[55]

In reality, patients are very much outside any of the alliances within healthcare; in fact, they have been written about as "the enemy".[56] Menzies-Lyth[57] suggests that we keep them outside because we cannot bear to identify with their suffering, disease, humiliation, etc.; worst still in terms of error, that we may play any part in it. This is one of the reasons patients and carers are not listened to properly; another is that they sometimes bear bad news; and a third is that health staff genuinely have less and less time to listen as fewer of them are expected to do so much more.[58,59]

Certainly most mental health enquiries show that staff have not heard or sought the views of carers or other relatives who may have much greater knowledge of patients than they do.[35] Perhaps thinking of them as team members would put an impossible strain on individual healthcare staff; however, providing the means whereby the team itself can listen to, share, and act upon information from patients or carers is essential.

Rewarding teams

Good teams are still not common in healthcare[60] but their importance makes it imperative that we consider how their performance is managed and how good teamworking is rewarded, not just through one individual member but for the team as a whole.[61]

Encouraging innovative solutions

Within healthcare, individual solutions will depend upon local problems and local circumstances. Multidisciplinary teams are often the units best able to identify and tackle such problems; for example, to create work patterns that minimise sleep deprivation by looking at the whole context of patient care.[62] This may involve getting many of the tasks in patient care at night done by staff other than doctors, or organising rotas and on-call commitments in the context of the daily activity of the team, while outpatient clinics and routine surgery can be scheduled to ensure they do not coincide with a team's responsibilities for emergency care.[62,63] Finally, work patterns need to respond to the experience – or inexperience – of team members; for example, consultants may need to adjust clinic lists in order to support the new pre-registration house officers when they begin their first postgraduate job.[62]

Autonomy and accountability

Teams within healthcare correspond well with descriptions of "self-managed teams" regarded in the management literature as reflecting a good organisational structure. Such teams are autonomous in taking operational decisions; responsible for achieving their performance goals; and usually multidisciplinary to allow cross-fertilisation of ideas among members.[64] Despite the benefits perceived in such teams, it is essential that they are tied into the organisation's management structure and goals: as I stated earlier, the strength of an alliance can be a barrier to quality as well as a benefit.

In terms of the accountability of such teams, Brittain and Langill[65] describe how one health organisation is tackling the vagueness of working relationships between clinical teams and senior management, and the lack of clarity around their accountability and authority. Just the process of doing this is likely to be as crucial as whichever framework is finally agreed upon.

Leadership

Finally, none of this will happen without good team leadership and if we want this, then we must hold people accountable to bring it about and ensure that the relevant resources to allow its development are provided.

Teamworking and team leadership

Good teams do not just develop on their own; where the team experience is poor, individual competitiveness is a very real alternative.[44] Good team leadership is essential. Nevertheless, in a recent survey I did to look at development needs of health service staff in terms of clinical governance, I found that almost no consultants, general practitioners or nurses had had any team leadership development.[66] Without such development, teams may experience various phenomena that are peculiar to groups. For example, working in groups is not always as productive as working alone,[36] and teams working in uncertain situations can be subject to the psychological phenomenon of groupthink[67] where members tend to reinforce each other's assumptions rather than test them out or go outside for help. In addition, teams that are not functioning well can be destructive of individuals,[29] just as a good team can support and develop those within it. Organisational studies over the last half of the century have shown that 60–75% of employees in any type of organisation find the most stressful aspect of their job is their immediate boss.[68,69] Much of the credit for a well-functioning team or responsibility for one that distresses its members goes to its leadership.

We humans are hierarchical creatures[26] and the structures we create inevitably and by necessity reflect this, so leadership cannot be avoided. Teams need leaders to pull them together, provide them with a common purpose and develop their skills, expectations and patterns of learning. Leadership skills involve getting things done through others, being adaptable but persistent, breaking down barriers, inspiring and helping their members to succeed. Leadership is not domination, but persuasion, and a large number of studies have shown that certain leadership characteristics are related to enhanced team performance.[68]

Some people may well take to a leadership role much better than others,[26] and we are aware of some of the characteristics which help or hinder leaders in being productive. We know, for example, that a desire for mastery in terms of challenge is important, while strong competitiveness with others is a hindrance.[44] Research with airline crews has shown that error levels are higher where the captains are characterised by arrogance, hostility, boastfulness or being dictatorial. Those with fewest errors had captains who were warm, friendly, self-confident and able to stand up to pressure[70] – what proponents of the Big-Five personality constructs for job selection would label as "Agreeableness" and "Emotional Stability".[68] Hogan[68,69] points out that it is the dark side of the personality that negatively affects their ability to form teams – characteristics such as over-competitiveness, paranoia, or the need to control everything – but these are sadly difficult to recognise at interview. Nevertheless, there is evidence that they can be changed through interventions.[71] The importance in terms of risk is in appreciating that some team leaders, such as consultants or senior nurses, may create not only less productive teams, but also less safe teams than others.

One way that an arrogant or dictatorial team leader will affect care negatively is by refusing to allow juniors to question decisions made by more senior staff;[72] a practice which led to the deaths of hundreds of air passengers and staff[73] until the culture was changed. Of course, if one takes a radical view of the clinical team as one which also includes the patients, then they too might be encouraged to air their views openly in a team that is functioning well. A good leader would be able to contain the anxiety that such feedback could create and so allow the team to truly learn and spread that learning beyond its boundaries.

Conclusions

Although individual learning must take place for healthcare to increase patient safety, the outline above indicates that it is likely to do this best within the context of a well functioning team. Nevertheless, such teams need to be tied into the management structure in ways that allow their accountability to be clearly recognised by everyone. Good teams will be ones which are open to learning from their mistakes as well as their successes, but this is unlikely to take place unless the culture of both the team and the organisation can shift towards welcoming such openness and monitoring the changes that result. Good team leaders will be essential to this process which means that their development across the organisation will be a vital but not inexpensive step in managing risk. Extra resources are essential to do this, but also are needed to provide "redundant" or back-up equipment and personnel to avoid crises, as well as to ensure that sufficient staff are available so that patients and carers can be properly heard.

References

1 Keidel RW. Rethinking organizational design. *Academy Manage Execut* 1994;**8**:12–30.
2 Norman DA. Categorization of action slips. *Psychological Rev* 1981;**88**:1–15.
3 Mizrahi T. Managing medical mistakes: ideology, insularity and accountability among internists-in-training. *Soc Sci Med* 1984;**19**:135–46.
4 Firth-Cozens J, Greenhalgh J. Doctor's perceptions of the links between stress and lowered clinical care. *Soc Sci Med* 1997;**44**(7):1017–22.
5 Janoff-Bulman R. *Shattered assumptions: towards a new psychology of trauma.* New York: Free Press, 1992.
6 Norris FH, Smith T, Kaniasty K. Revisiting the experience behavior hypothesis: the effects of Hurricane Hugo on hazard preparedness and other self-protective acts. *Basic Appl Soc Psychology* 1999;**21**(1):37–47.
7 Casarett D, Helms C. Systems errors versus physicians' errors: finding the balance in medical education. *Acad Med* 1999;**74**(1):19–22.
8 Senge PM. Leading learning organisations. *Training Develop* 1996;**50**(12):36–7.
9 Garvin DA. Building a learning organization. *Harvard Bus Rev* 1993;**71**:78–91.
10 Birleson P. Learning organisations: An unsuitable model for improving mental health services? *Aust N Z J Psychiatry* 1998;**32**(2):214–22.
11 Michael DN. *On learning to plan and planning to learn.* San Francisco, California: Jossey-Bass, 1976.
12 Roberts K. Managing high reliability organizations. *California Manag Rev* 1990;**32**: 101–13.
13 Roberts K, Libuser C. From Bhopal to Banking: organizational design can mitigate risk. *Organisational Dynam* 1993;**21**:15–26.
14 Leape LL, Woods DD, Hatlie MJ, *et al.* Promoting patient safety by preventing medical error. *JAMA* 1998;**280**(16):1444.
15 Wall TD, Bolden RI, Borril CS, *et al.* Minor psychiatric disorder in NHS trust staff: occupational and gender differences. *Br J Psychiatry* 1997;**171**:519–23.
16 Vincent C. Fallibility, uncertainty and the impact of mistakes and litigation. In: Firth-Cozens J, Payne R, eds. *Stress in health professionals: psychological and organisational causes and interventions.* Chichester: John Wiley, 1999:63–78.
17 Houston DM, Allt SK. Psychological distress and error making among junior house officers. *Br J Health Psychology* 1997;**2**:141–51.
18 Aiken LH, Sloane MN. The effects of specialization and client differentiation on the status of nurses: the case of AIDS. *J Health Soc Behav* 1997;**38**:203–10.
19 Regrut B. *One million patients have spoken: Who will listen?* South Bend, Indiana: Press, Ganey Associates, 1991.
20 Jones JW, Barge BN, Steffy BD, *et al.* Stress and medical malpractice: organizational risk assessment and intervention. *J Appl Psychology* 1988;**4**:727–35.
21 Murphy L. Organizational interventions to reduce stress in healthcare professionals. In: Firth-Cozens J, Payne RL, eds. *Stress in health professionals. psychological and organisational causes and interventions.* Chichester: John Wiley, 1999.
22 Firth-Cozens J. Physician well-being and patient care. *Soc Sci Med,* 2000; **52**(2) 215–22.
23 Firth-Cozens J. Healthy promotion: changing behaviour towards evidence-based healthcare. *Qual healthcare* 1997;**6**(4):205–11.
24 Abts D, Hofer M, Leafgreen PK. Redefining care delivery: a modular system. *Nurs Manag* 1994;**25**:40–6.
25 Jones KR, DeBaca V, Yarbrough M. Organizational culture assessment before and after implementing patient-focused care. *Nurs Econ* 1997;**15**:73–80.
26 Firth-Cozens J, Hardy G. Occupational stress, clinical treatment and changes in job perceptions. *J Occup Organiz Psychology* 1992;**65**:81–8.
27 Nicholson N. How hardwired is human behavior? *Harvard Bus Rev* 1998; July–August: 135–47.
28 Blatt SJ, Zuroff DC. Interpersonal relatedness and self-definition: two prototypes for depression. *Clin Psychology Rev* 1992;**12**:527–62.
29 Hirschhorn L. *The workplace within: psychodynamics of organizational life.* Cambridge, Massachusetts: MIT Press, 1988.

30 Wafer A. Lonesome whistle. *BMA News Review* 1999; December:18–21.
31 Berwick DM. You cannot expect people to be heroes. *BMJ* 1998;**316**:1736.
32 Cambridge P. The first hit: a case study of the physical abuse of people with learning disabilities and challenging behaviours in a residential service. *Disability Soc* 1999;**14**(3): 285–308.
33 Hirschhorn L. The psychodynamics of safety: A case study of an oil refinery. In: Hirschhorn L, Barnett C, eds. *The psychodynamics of organizations*. Philadelphia: Temple University Press, 1993:143–64.
34 Reason J. *Managing risks of organisation accidents*. Aldershot: Ashgate, 1997.
35 Reith M. Risk assessment and management: lessons from mental health inquiry reports. *Med Sci Law* 1998;**38**(3):221–6.
36 Firth-Cozens J. Celebrating teamwork. *Qual healthcare* 1998;7:S3–S7.
37 Adorian D, Silverberg DS, Tomer D, Wamosher Z. Group discussions with the healthcare team: A method of improving care of hypertension in general practice. *J Human Hypertension* 1990;**4**:265–8.
38 Fouchee HC, Helmreich RL. Group interaction and flight crew performance. In: Weiner EL, Hagel DC, eds. *Human factors in aviation*. San Diego, California: Academic Press, 1988:189–227.
39 Carter AJ, West MA. Sharing the burden – team work in healthcare setting. In: Firth-Cozens J, Payne RL, eds. *Stress in health professionals*. Chichester: John Wiley, 1999.
40 Firth-Cozens J. Emotional distress in junior house officers. *BMJ* 1987;**295**:533–6.
41 Guzzo RA, Shea GP. Group performance and intergroup relations. In: Dunnette MD, Hough LM, eds. *Handbook of industrial and organisational psychology*. Palo Alto, California: Consulting Psychologists Press, 1992.
42 Belbin RM. *Management realms: why they succeed or fail*. New York: Halsted Press, 1981.
43 West MA. Reflexivity and work group effectiveness: a conceptual integration. In: West MA, ed. *Handbook of work group psychology*. Chichester: John Wiley, 1996.
44 Tjosvold D. *Team organization. An enduring competitive advantage*. Chichester: John Wiley, 1991.
45 Morgan GGJ, Glickman AS, Woodward EA, *et al. Measurement of team behaviors in a navy environment*. Orlando, Florida: Naval Training System Center, 1986.
46 Bond J, Cartilidge AM, Gregson BA, *et al. A study of interprofessional collaboration in primary healthcare organisations*. Newcastle upon Tyne: University of Newcastle upon Tyne, healthcare Research, 1985.
47 Katzman EM, Roberts JI. Nurse–physician conflicts as barriers to the enactment of nursing roles. *W J Nurs Res* 1988;**10**:576–90.
48 Edmondson AC. Learning from mistakes is easier said than done: group and organizational influences on the detection and correction of human error. *J Appl Behav Sci* 1996;**32**(1):5–28.
49 Hackman JR. *Groups that work (and those that don't): Creating conditions for effective teamwork*. San Francisco, California: Jossey Bass, 1990.
50 Firth-Cozens J. Tackling risk by changing behaviour. *Qual healthcare* 1995;**4**:97–101.
51 Ilgen DR. Teams embedded in organizations. Some implications. *Am Psychologist* 1999; **54**(2):129–39.
52 Donnelly P. Decision-making in a community mental health team. *Mental Health Nursing* 1996;**16**:12–15.
53 Collighan G, Macdonald A, Herzberg J, *et al.* An evaluation of the multidisciplinary approach to psychiatric diagnosis in elderly people. *BMJ* 1993;**306**:821–4.
54 Snowden P. Practical aspects of clinical risk assessment and management. *Br J Psychiatry* 1997;**170**:32–4.
55 Kelson M. *Patient-defined outcomes*. London: College of Health, 1999.
56 Aitken S. The patient as enemy. Notes from a fifth columnist. *Changes* 1984;**2**(2):54–5.
57 Menzies-Lyth I. *Containing anxiety in institutions*. London: Free Associations Press, 1988.
58 Senge P. *The fifth discipline: the art and practice of the learning organization*. New York: Doubleday, 1990.
59 Murphy EC, DeJoy S. *Cost-driven downsizing in hospitals: implications for mortality*. New York: Amherst, 1993.

367

60 West M, Field D. Teamwork in primary healthcare. Perspectives from organisational psychology. *J Interprofessional Care* 1995;9:117–22.
61 Bloor K, Maynard A. Rewarding healthcare teams: A way of aligning pay to performance and outcomes. *BMJ* 1998;316:569.
62 Firth-Cozens J, Moss F. Hours, sleep, teamwork and stress. *BMJ* 1998;317:1335–6.
63 Moss F, Paice E. Getting things right for the doctor in training. In: Firth-Cozens J, Payne R, eds. *Stress in health professionals. Psychological and organisational causes and interventions.* Chichester: John Wiley, 1999.
64 Shukla M. *Competing through knowledge.* New Delhi: Response Books, 1997.
65 Brittain B, Langill G. Structuring the design and implementation of leadership and teamwork for program management. *Healthcare Management Forum* 1997;10(2):50–2.
66 Firth-Cozens J. *Clinical governance training needs in health service staff:* NHS Executive Northern & Yorkshire: Durham, 1999.
67 Janis IL. *Groupthink: Psychological studies of policy decisions and fiascos.* Boston: Houghton Mifflen, 1982.
68 Hogan R, Curphy GJ, Hogan J. What we know about leadership. *Am Psychologist* 1994;49(6):493–504.
69 Hogan R, Raskin R, Fazzini D. The dark side of charisma. In: Clark KE, Clark MB, eds. *Measures of leadership.* West Orange: Leadership Library of America, 1990.
70 Chidester TR, Helmreich RL, Gregorich SE, Geis CE. Pilot personality and crew co-ordination. *Int J Aviation Psychology* 1991;1:25–44.
71 Peterson DB, Hicks MD, *How to get people to change.* Eighth Annual Conference of the Society for Industrial and Organizational Psychology, 1993, San Francisco.
72 Moray N. Error reduction as a systems problem. *Human error in medicine.* Hove: Erlbaum, 1994.
73 MacPherson M. *The black box: Cockpit voice recorder accounts of in-flight accidents.* London: Harper Collins, 1998.

20 Creating and maintaining safe systems of medical care: the role of risk management

PETER PRONOVOST, LAURA MORLOCK, CHRISTOPHER CASSIRER

While most efforts to investigate errors in medicine have generally focused on active failures and provider behaviours, greater opportunity for improvement may be found by focusing on the organisational characteristics of health systems. In this chapter we will first present a case that outlines how organisational characteristics can influence the risk for error. Next we discuss recent empirical evidence regarding relationships between organisational characteristics and improved patient safety – first focusing on intensive care units (ICUs) as a high-risk area and next examining the broader influence of hospital risk management programs on organisational safety. Our goal is to demonstrate, with empirical data from Maryland hospitals, that the design of safe systems of medical care directly translates into improved patient safety. While much of the research underlying this association is beyond the scope of this chapter, the interested reader can review the endnotes, as well as several of our recent publications for details on the research methodology.

Case Example

Following an uncomplicated surgical procedure, a 63-year-old man develops an infection in his chest wound. He is readmitted to the operating room for wound treatment, and then transferred to an Intensive Care Unit (ICU) for post-operative care. Although an allergy to penicillin is noted in the medical record, the ICU team chooses to treat his wound infection with a combination of antibiotics, one of which is a derivative of penicillin. Twenty-five minutes after the first dose, the patient experiences a cardiopulmonary arrest. Resuscitation attempts are unsuccessful. Although the results of a subsequent autopsy are inconclusive, the patient's reaction to the antibiotic is regarded as a likely triggering event.

Consistent with hospital policy, an interdisciplinary team is formed to review the case and investigate factors contributing to the adverse outcome. These teams are designed to review care management problems (see Chapter 23) or unsafe acts (see Chapter 1). The team confirms that the patient was prescribed and administered a medication to which he was allergic. Furthermore, the team determines that the providers knew the patient was allergic to the class of antibiotics that was prescribed and knew that the prescribed antibiotic was in the class to which the patient was allergic. However, the patient allergy was not recognised by the physician when the drug was prescribed, or by the nurse when the drug was administered. The pharmacy, which undoubtedly would have detected the problem, never actually received the order. Upon further investigation the team determines that to save time, the first dose of antibiotics administered to the patient had been "borrowed" by the nursing staff from available medication that had been prescribed for another patient who was admitted earlier to the ICU.

The team next decides to investigate what had caused the nursing staff to act in a manner that so obviously violated the hospital's protocol for administering medications. As the team begins to "drill down" into the root causes of the ICU staff's behaviour, failures become apparent in several relevant patient care systems. The team learns that:

System Failure #1:
Borrowing medication is a frequent strategy for reducing time to first administration

It is often important for medications to be started quickly. This is definitely the case for antibiotics in critically ill patients. Indeed, the time to first antibiotic administration for patients with pneumonia is a frequently used indicator for the quality of hospital care. Since antibiotics are not stored in the intensive care units, in order to administer the first dose of antibiotics as quickly as possible to a critically ill patient, antibiotic supplies intended for one patient are frequently borrowed and given to another patient in need. The staff borrow medications from other patients because system factors inhibit them from efficiently sending orders to the pharmacy and quickly obtaining medications. However, when providers borrow medications, they by-pass the pharmacy and its multiple safety checks. Had the order been processed by the pharmacy, the allergy may have been identified and the error prevented. The frequency of medication borrowing, however, is the result of inadequacies in two other systems.

System Failure #2:
The process for ordering medications needed immediately (stat)
is regarded as broken

As the process has been designed, orders for medications needed immediately (stat) are to be faxed to the pharmacy, while routine orders are to be hand carried. Once received by the pharmacy, faxed orders are to be acted upon quickly. However, as the process works in reality, all orders are faxed to the pharmacy and as a result, faxed orders are not necessarily given priority by pharmacy staff. In addition to being faxed, stat orders are sometimes telephoned to the pharmacy, resulting in an interrupted workflow for both pharmacists and nurses. Frequent delays in stat medication delivery cause the nursing staff to lose faith in the timeliness of the stat order delivery system.

System Failure #3:
The process for receiving medications needed immediately also
requires redesign

Once a medication order is processed by the pharmacy, the filled order must be sent to the patient care unit. It should be sent either through a tube system or by a messenger. But the team is told that the tube system is frequently not working, and the limited number of messengers may be elsewhere in the hospital. As a result, nurses doubt that pharmacy orders will be readily available when first needed, leading to the practice of borrowing medications.

In addition to these organisational factors that help shape the reality of daily working conditions for patient care staff, the investigation team learns that on the day of the adverse event the ICU was operating with fewer nurses than usual. Several team members wonder whether the added workload due to short staffing created additional stress and time pressures for the ICU physicians and nurses.

The findings of this investigation are typical in that they illustrate the complexity of the chain of events that often precede an adverse event.[1-4] In this hospital, like many others, the medication ordering and dispensing processes are complex, but partially broken, systems containing many checks that usually prevent error. For example, the physicians prescribing medication orders usually review patient allergies, pharmacists dispensing the medications usually cross check the medications against patient allergies, and nurses administering medications provide a final check against patient allergies. As a result, single mistakes or mishaps generally do not lead to an adverse event.

In this case example, all of these systems failed, enabling the patient to receive a medication to which he was allergic. The systems generally function because they contain many checks (which may appear redundant), and dedicated people adjust their behaviour in recognition or anticipation of system inadequacies. Catastrophe usually requires the convergence of multiple failures, often spurred by production pressures.[3] The team in our case example identified three system failures whose convergence may have allowed this event to occur. Additional factors – including nursing staff absenteeism the day of the event – may also have exacerbated the system problems.

Because catastrophic failures generally require multiple system failures, there may be no single root cause for an incident. Knowledge of the outcome (in this case giving a drug to which the patient was allergic) makes it appear that providers should have seen the events leading up to the mishap. This hindsight bias has often in the past directed our attention to providers rather than systems. But experience during the past decade in healthcare, as well as in other industries, has led to a deeper understanding of accident causation and prevention, with a greater focus on the organisational factors that provide the working conditions in which errors and adverse events occur.[3,5,6] As Vincent has noted,[7] adverse events must be interpreted within a context of systems operating simultaneously at a variety of levels – including the task, team, and work environment, as well as the organisation.

In this chapter we will first briefly review the type of organisational paradigm that is increasingly being utilised in the investigation and analysis of adverse events, as well as in our efforts to create safer systems of patient care. Next we will present results from several recent studies that provide some evidence for the link between organisational factors, working conditions and patient care outcomes. Finally we will discuss some of the implications of these results for the management and reduction of risk in patient care settings.

Understanding and preventing adverse events: Towards an organisational analysis

A decade ago in his analyses of organisational accidents within complex industrial systems, James Reason distinguished between active and latent failures (see Chapter 1).[8] Active failures are further classified into slips or lapses, mistakes, and violations. In this case example a slip may have occurred when the prescribing physician knew of the patient's allergy and knew that one of the antibiotics prescribed was a penicillin derivative, but prescribed it anyway, perhaps due to distraction or preoccupation. "Lapses" may have occurred if one or more members of the nursing staff failed to remember the patient's allergy. A mistake may have occurred if the physician had not identified the specific antibiotic as a derivative of penicillin.

Reason further distinguishes between errors and violations. The latter are usually deliberate deviations from standard operating procedures or practices. Necessary or situational violations may seem to the provider "to offer the only path available to getting the job done".[5,7] Borrowing medicine prescribed for another patient as a way of shortening time to the administration of a first dose deliberately violated the hospital's procedures, but was seen by the staff as a way of delivering better patient care in spite of the "broken" operating systems. Although these distinctions among various kinds of active failures may seem inconsequential, they would require quite different prevention strategies.

According to this perspective, adverse events in complex systems such as medical care usually result from the interaction of active and latent failures.[5,8] Latent failures arise from managerial decisions – or the lack of decisions – that shape working conditions. The decisions often result from economic, political and operational constraints that create production pressures. The damaging consequences of these latent failures may not be evident until the occurrence of a "triggering event".[3,8 10]

Currently there is considerable interest in the creation of a framework that could help guide investigation and analysis of adverse events in medical care by taking into consideration the hierarchy of organisational and other influences on provider behaviour and patient care outcomes.[7,10–16] Vincent,[7] for example, has developed a framework, describing influences on clinical practice, that is based on earlier efforts by Reason[5,8] and others, as well as the healthcare literature on provider errors, adverse events and risk management (see Table 23.1)

Patient characteristics, particularly clinical condition, are undoubtedly the most important direct predictors of patient outcome. Clinical condition has also been shown to be a risk factor for adverse events: seriously ill patients, including those admitted to an ICU, are more likely than other hospitalised patients to experience an adverse event.[17–19] ICU patients may be at higher risk for a number of reasons: the ICU work setting is intense, with many interactions between patients and caregivers. Serious illness reduces both the patient's natural resilience and the ability to rebound from the consequences of human error.[10] In addition, ICU patients receive about twice as many drugs as patients in general care units, which increases their exposure to medical and nursing errors.[10]

Patient care outcomes, including the risk of an adverse event, are also influenced by factors associated with the task, individual providers, the team, and the work environment. A large body of literature, for example, provides evidence that higher volumes of specific services or procedures are associated with better outcomes of care. Explanations for this pattern often reason that higher volumes of selected diagnoses or procedures facilitate the development of specialised task routines, greater provider knowledge and skills and better team communication and co-ordination.

Individual provider and team behaviours are in turn influenced by the immediate work environment, and by policies, procedures and decisions made at higher levels of the organisation which govern the allocation and management of financial resources, people, equipment, space and time.[10] The decisions of hospital leaders and managers are conditioned by opportunities and constraints in the external environment. These include societal and cultural factors, the legal and regulatory framework, and financial pressures. In the USA, for example, in response to cost containment pressures from public and private insurers, hospitals have been downsizing the numbers of registered nurses and using lower paid nursing staff with less training. These hospital-level decisions are likely to have significant influences on the work environment and should be monitored for their effects on team functioning, task performance and patient outcomes.

Influence of ICU organisational factors on patient outcomes

As an example of how we can begin to investigate which hospital organisational characteristics support a culture of patient safety, we will discuss three of our recent studies that have examined associations between ICU organisational characteristics and patient outcomes. Previous studies have revealed wide variation in the organisational characteristics of ICUs and levels of resource use among ICU providers, as well as in risk-adjusted ICU patient mortality and morbidity. The association between ICU organisational characteristics and outcomes, however, has not been well documented. We sought to determine whether the organisational characteristics of ICUs are associated with outcomes for a high-risk population of surgical patients.[21] ICUs are high-risk areas and thus provide an opportunity to evaluate the association between system organisation and patient outcomes.

In the first study, we used hospital discharge data from patients having abdominal aortic surgery and surveyed the medical directors of the ICUs in Maryland that care for these patients. The primary outcomes for this study were in-hospital mortality, hospital length of stay, ICU length of stay and specific medical and surgical complications recorded as discharge diagnoses in the database.

Studies that attempt to isolate the impact of organisational factors on patient outcomes face methodological challenges because patient characteristics may systematically vary among ICUs and these differences must be taken into consideration in order to examine the independent effect of organisational influences. To account for variation in patient characteristics, we adjusted for differences in patient demographics, comorbid disease, and severity of illness. We also adjusted for differences in hospital and surgeon volume.[22,23] The details of this analysis are described below.

374

Details of analysis of study of influence of ICU organisational factors on patient outcomes

- To adjust for patient demographics, we included patient age (in years), gender, and race (white versus non-white).
- We selected the diseases in the Romano Charlson Comorbidity Index (each disease included as a separate variable) to adjust for potentially important comorbid diseases[22].
- To adjust for severity of illness, we classified patients as having a ruptured (ICD-9-CM code 441.3) or unruptured aorta, and used the nature of admission field, which is coded at admission, to identify each case as elective, urgent or emergent.
- We calculated the volume of aortic surgery performed by each hospital and each surgeon in the database, and modelled hospital and surgeon volume as dichotomous variables using a LOWESS smoothing curve.[23] We defined low volume as less than 36 cases per year for hospitals and less than 8 cases per year for surgeons.

ICU physician staffing in Maryland hospitals

After these adjustments, we found that daily rounding by an ICU physician was a particularly powerful predictor of risk-adjusted patient mortality and morbidity. Not having daily rounds by an ICU physician was associated with a three-fold increase in in-hospital mortality, as well as a two- to three-fold increased patient risk for a number of complications including cardiac arrest, acute renal failure, septicaemia, platelet transfusion, and reintubation. In addition, several ICU characteristics were associated with increased ICU length of stay and these included: not having daily rounds by an ICU physician, having an ICU nurse to patient ratio of one nurse caring for more than two patients, not having monthly review of morbidity and mortality, and routinely extubating patients in the operating room.

ICU nurse staffing in Maryland hospitals

In a second study, we wanted to further explore why nurse to patient ratios were associated with average lengths of stay. We began by examining relationships between nurse to patient ratios and rates of complications. We found patients at hospitals that had an ICU nurse to patient ratio of one nurse for three or more patients – versus one nurse for one or two patients – had an increased risk of several specific pulmonary complications including pulmonary insufficiency after a procedure and reintubation of the trachea. These analyses suggest that organisational characteristics of

375

ICUs are related to differences among hospitals in the outcomes of high-risk surgical patients, and that clinicians and managers should consider the potential impact of these organisational influences on the outcomes of patients having high-risk operations.

Synthesis of the literature regarding ICU physician staffing and outcomes

In a third study, we sought to build upon our previous analyses by synthesising the evidence regarding associations between ICU physician staffing and patient outcomes. We conducted a systematic review to identify relevant studies from 1965 through July 1999. We critiqued studies for relevance to our investigation; study design; patient population; comparability of baseline patient characteristics and severity of illness assessment; as well as nature of the ICU intervention. For this analysis, we grouped ICU physician staffing into low intensity (no intensivist or elective intensivist consult) or high intensity (mandatory intensivist consult or closed ICU). An intensivist is defined as a physician with specialised training who provides care to patients in an ICU setting. In a "closed ICU" the intensivist, rather than another attending physician, assumes direct responsibility for the patient's care. The main outcome measures were in-hospital patient mortality, ICU patient mortality, hospital length of stay (LOS) and ICU LOS.

In our literature search, we identified 1560 citations in the literature and 17 studies that met our inclusion criteria. Seven of the studies (41%) were from academic medical centres, six (35%) from community teaching hospitals, three (18%) from nonteaching community hospitals, and one (6%) included all hospitals in Maryland. All studies were observational rather than randomised clinical trials.

Hospital mortality

Ten studies (Figure 20.1) reported the data needed to calculate a hospital mortality rate although one study presented only observed-to-expected mortality ratios. The hospital mortality rate ranged from 6% to 74% in the low intensity ICU staffing group and from 4% to 57% in the high intensity ICU staffing group. Data in Figure 20.1 are presented as the unadjusted hospital mortality rate in the high intensity group divided by the unadjusted hospital mortality rate in the low intensity group together with the 95% confidence interval. The vertical line represents the line of equivalency. Therefore, data points below the line suggest lower unadjusted hospital mortality rates in the high intensity group versus the low intensity group. Data points above the line suggest lower unadjusted hospital mortality rates in the low intensity group. Most studies (7 of 10) reported sig-

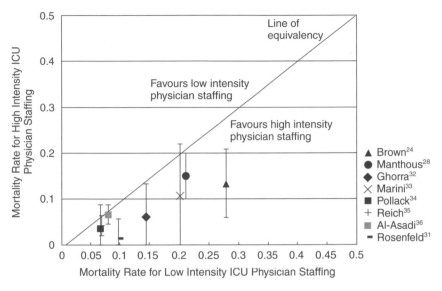

Figure 20.1 Calculation of hospital mortality rates.

nificant reductions in unadjusted hospital mortality with high intensity staffing (ranging from 2% to 17% absolute risk reduction with a median of 10%). These findings persisted when mortality rates were adjusted for baseline patient severity (significant reductions in mortality were reported in 9 of 11 studies). In no studies was there a statistically significant increase in mortality with high intensity staffing.

ICU mortality

Eleven studies evaluated the impact of ICU physician staffing on ICU mortality. Eight of these studies (Figure 20.2) provided data to allow calculation of a mortality rate, two studies reported only risk adjusted mortality rates (observed/expected), and one study provided a mortality rate without denominator data. The ICU mortality ranged from 8% to 51% in the low intensity group and from 6% to 35% in the high intensity group. All nine studies reporting unadjusted ICU mortality rates found a statistically significant reduction in ICU mortality with high intensity staffing. Again, these findings persisted after adjusting for differences in baseline patient severity (10 of 11 studies reported a significant reduction while one found no difference).

Data in Figure 20.2 are presented as the unadjusted ICU mortality rate in the high intensity group divided by the unadjusted ICU mortality rate in the low intensity group along with the 95% confidence interval. The vertical line represents the line of equivalency. As in Figure 20.1, data points

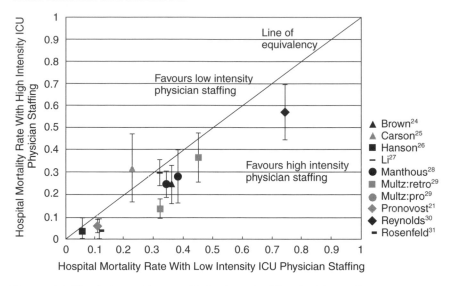

Figure 20.2 Hospital mortality rate with low intensity ICU physician staffing.

below the line suggest lower unadjusted ICU mortality rates in the high intensity group versus the low intensity group. Data points above the line suggest lower unadjusted ICU mortality rates in the low intensity group.

In summary, high intensity versus low intensity ICU physician staffing is associated with reduced hospital and ICU patient mortality (as well as reduced hospital and ICU length of stay). Based on this analysis, and extrapolating to the US hospitalised population, we estimate that providing high intensity ICU physician staffing at all US hospitals could prevent 540 000 deaths per year. Given the magnitude of the effect of staffing by specialists in intensive care, and the variation in ICU physician staffing, we suggest that providing high intensity ICU physician staffing may result in a significant opportunity to improve quality and reduce the resource expenditures involved in prolonged lengths of stay. Moreover, the impact of ICU physician staffing is significantly greater than the majority of therapies often employed in medical care.

Influence of hospital risk management programmes on ICU work environment and patient outcomes

In a fourth analysis we sought to explore how the broader organisational characteristics of hospitals influence ICU work environments and patient outcomes. Creating a culture of safety within a hospital is usually regarded as the specific responsibility of the risk management programme. The objectives of clinical risk management are often defined as reducing the frequency of preventable adverse events, decreasing the number of liability claims, managing those claims that do emerge, and financing risk through the most economical methods. There is relatively little empirical information available, however, regarding how hospitals create and maintain organisational arrangements to facilitate these activities and how effective these efforts are with regard to creating safer work environments, promoting patient safety and reducing patient and organisational risk.

In an effort to examine these issues, a survey was conducted in 1995 of all Maryland hospitals.[37,38] Although this study was independent of the analyses of ICUs in Maryland hospitals discussed in the previous section, the common hospital study population and time frame permitted us to combine the two data sets in order to explore relationships between hospital risk management activities, ICU work environments and patient outcomes.

The risk management study surveyed all Maryland hospitals using a slightly modified version of a questionnaire originally designed by the American Society for Healthcare Risk Management (ASHRM) of the American Hospital Association (AHA). ASHRM was formed in the mid 1980s, following the nation's second medical malpractice insurance crisis, in order to provide an educational and training resource for the growing profession of hospital risk management.

In 1991, the organisation responded to information about the wide variation in hospital approaches to risk management by developing a model approach. ASHRM published its recommendations, based on expert opinion, in a *Hospital Risk Management Program Self-Assessment Manual (1991)* for use by hospital risk managers.[39] Included in this manual is an *Assessment Abstract* designed to represent the key features of a hospital risk management programme that ASHRM believes are appropriate for all hospitals. The model is based on risk management theory, a systems approach to programme development, and a continuous quality improvement model for programme improvement. ASHRM's recommendations were also intended to reflect accepted tenets or "best practices" in hospital risk management as they appeared in the trade and professional literatures.

According to the ASHRM model, every hospital risk management programme should have an organisational structure to support the risk management function that includes governing board support and monitoring, a designated hospital risk manager, and activities in place to motivate physician involvement. Programmes should also include systems to identify and analyse adverse events. Loss prevention activities should be in place that include educational programmes for both clinical and administrative staff, the reviewing of informed consent policies and procedures, and the monitoring of compliance with regulatory and accreditation requirements. Further, loss prevention activities should include an established patient/family relations programme and the analysis of medical liability claims data. The ASHRM model also recommends that hospital risk management programmes include policies and procedures for managing alternative approaches to financing professional liability risk as well as a liability claims management programme to control losses associated with these claims.

In total, the ASHRM Assessment Abstract contains 134 separate risk management programme structure and process components. All hospital risk managers in the State were mailed a questionnaire, and also participated in on-site interviews regarding their responses to the survey. Eighty-nine per cent of acute-care hospitals in the State participated in the study. Analysis results suggested that the level of hospital risk management activity among the not-for-profit, acute care hospitals in Maryland varied widely in 1995. On average, hospitals had adopted approximately two-thirds (66%) of the minimum set of programme components recommended by the American Society for Healthcare Risk Management. There was considerable variation, however, in risk management programme adoption – ranging from 28 to 94 programme components in place. Hospitals were more likely to have high levels of risk management activity if they were self-insured at the primary layer for medical liability (p < 0.06), had residency programmes (p < 0.05), were affiliated with a multihospital system (p < 0.05), and were located in a metropolitan area (p < 0.01). Hospital size was not associated with the level of risk management activity.

In order to explore relationships among hospital risk management activities, ICU work environments and patient outcomes, we combined the data sets from the two Maryland studies. In a series of multivariate analyses, we examined the effect of each risk management programme dimension on the risk-adjusted mortality of ICU patients who had undergone abdominal aortic surgery. The risk adjustment model has been described in the previous section. Analysis results indicate a significant (p < 0.01) relationship after risk adjustment between a strong risk analysis programme activity at the hospital level and better ICU patient outcomes. The risk analysis programme component score measured the extent to which a hospital:

- Had developed a process to analyse and trend risk identification data
- Conducted risk analyses stratified by hospital location, type of occurrence, patient characteristics, and other hospital characteristics
- Had initiated loss prevention activities in response to problems that had been identified.

This programme component was also strongly associated with nurse staffing ratios in the ICU: hospitals with strong risk analysis activities were more likely to have ratios of one nurse to one or two patients than hospitals which paid less attention to risk analysis (Kendall's tau = 0·34; p < 0·001).

These results suggest a significant association between hospital risk management programme efforts with respect to relatively more sophisticated risk analysis activities and lower ICU risk-adjusted patient mortality rates. There could exist a direct causal relationship. It is possible that in-depth analyses of adverse events would target ICUs as high risk locations since there is considerable evidence that ICU patients in general are at high risk for adverse occurrences. But the finding that hospitals with more attention devoted to risk analysis also have higher nurse to patient ratios in the ICU units suggests that each of these indicators may reflect a general awareness and concern with patient safety that is manifest in many aspects of the management of these hospitals.

Managing and reducing clinical risk in patient care settings

The organisational framework used in this and other chapters of the book has a number of applications.[7] First, it can be helpful in stimulating a more comprehensive and systems-oriented approach to adverse event investigation and analysis (see Chapter 23).

It also can be useful in formulating more effective risk reduction strategies. As Vincent has noted, many quality and safety initiatives are limited in their impact because they rely on only one level of intervention – such as staff training or protocol development – and neglect other factors with significant influence on clinical practice. The ICU adverse event investigation team in our case example made a number of recommendations that are interesting in this regard because the strategies target several different organisational levels. The team's first recommendation was to stop the practice of borrowing medications through an educational intervention for staff members that would emphasise the risks inherent in such a practice. A second staff education programme was recommended in order to change staff behaviour regarding the faxing of all – rather than only the immediately required (stat) – pharmacy orders.

Other recommendations targeted the hospital level: in the short run, fixing the tube system would reassure staff that the medication dispensing process can be dependable and efficient. As a longer-term strategy, the team advocated hospital consideration of an electronic physician order entry system that has been shown to reduce medication errors. Finally, the team recommended implementing a practice standard that all stat medications be administered within 30 minutes from the physician's order. The team members recognised that plans would need to be developed for measuring compliance with such a standard at the work setting level. They also suggested the formation of a new multidisciplinary committee at the hospital level who would be charged with monitoring compliance with the new standard and co-ordinating the various efforts to improve patient safety with respect to medication administration.

Using this type of organisational framework to conceptualise the factors affecting clinical practice may also help identify those areas in which empirical studies are needed to better understand significant influences on adverse events and patient outcomes. In this chapter we have discussed results from several studies that have tried to examine the effects of organisational factors – including ICU work setting characteristics and hospital-wide risk management programmes.

Although the risk management field in healthcare has traditionally advocated a systems perspective, the identification, classification and monitoring of adverse events at both the hospital and liability insurer levels have tended to focus on the individual provider. Clearly, a balance must be achieved between the use of a systems approach and the acknowledgement of personal responsibility in managing medical errors.[40] But as Reason has emphasised, at the individual level, the precursors of error (such as inattention, distraction, preoccupation, forgetting, fatigue and stress) are often the last and least manageable links in the chain of events leading to an adverse event.[5,8] As illustrated in the ICU event discussed earlier, the most serious adverse events often involve an individual error coupled with multiple system failures that may include task, team, work environment, and organisational levels.

The results of our studies in Maryland hospitals, for example, suggest that differences in ICU organisational characteristics are significantly related to variation in the risk-adjusted morbidity and mortality experienced by patients following abdominal aortic surgery. Daily rounds by an ICU physician specialist were associated with a three-fold reduction in in-hospital mortality and complications. In addition, an ICU nurse to patient ratio greater than 1:2 was associated with increased ICU days (and thus greater resource expenditures) as well as the greater risk of pulmonary complications.

It is important to note that in many hospital risk management programmes, the patient deaths, and perhaps the instances of "excess" morbidity would have been classified as serious adverse events and possibly linked to specific ICU providers. In many hospitals the almost exclusive focus on the actions of individual physicians and nursing staff, the coding methodologies, and a failure to link events with system factors render invisible the broader organisational influences. Investigations of individual serious adverse events that try to determine the root causes of mishaps will identify some system influences, but will rarely be able to perceive the consequences of factors – like staffing patterns – that form the constant context of care delivery within a particular work setting. These types of influences can only be examined through comparisons over time within a single institution or through multi-institutional comparisons in which it is possible to examine the effects of variation in organisational factors.

Our study of risk management programmes in Maryland hospitals suggests that the more methodologically sophisticated programmes analysed trends in adverse events; examined these events by hospital location, type of occurrence and patient characteristics; and used these analyses to target specific loss prevention activities. Hospitals that had these programme components in place appear to also have ICUs that promote patient safety.

One possible implication of these study results is that hospital risk management programmes must exercise leadership in defining, measuring and monitoring those system factors that may influence adverse events and patient risk. It is important to realise, however, that there are significant challenges for those hospital risk management programmes that select this strategy. Serious adverse events, fortunately, are relatively rare occurrences when viewed as rates whose denominators reflect the numbers of patient days or procedures over a specified time period. Although much can be learned by examining trends within a single institution over time, for the most part, advances in our knowledge about relationships among system influences, adverse events and patient outcomes must come from the collaborative efforts of multiple institutions.

As an analogy, it is interesting to speculate how much would be known today about aviation safety if each individual airport had continued to collect and analyse – according to it's own definitions and methods – each relatively infrequent accident within its own air traffic area. To some degree, that is the current situation in healthcare, and it is reflected in our relative lack of knowledge concerning the full range of factors influencing patient safety. Risk managers must assume a leadership role – both in their own institutions and in the formation of collaborative networks – in examining organisational system factors, as well as the individual provider behaviours, that influence adverse events, patient safety and healthcare quality.

References

1 Vincent C. Risk, safety, and the dark side of quality: improving quality in healthcare should include removing the causes of harm. *BMJ* 1997;**314**:1775–976.
2 Cooper JB, Newbower RS, Kitz RJ. An analysis of major errors and equipment failures in anaesthesia management considerations for prevention and detection. *Anesthesiology* 1984;**60**:34–42.
3 Cook RI, Woods DD. Operating at the sharp end: the complexity of human error. In: Bogner MS, ed. *Human error in medicine*. Hillsdale, New Jersey: Erlbaum, 1994:255–310.
4 Vincent CA, Bark P. Accident investigation: discovering why things go wrong. In: Vincent CA, ed. *Clinical risk management*. London: BMJ Publications, 1995.

5 Reason JT. Understanding adverse events: human factors. In: Vincent CA, ed. *Clinical risk management*. London: BMJ Publications, 1995.
6 Leape LL. Error in medicine. *JAMA* 1994;**272**:1851–7.
7 Vincent C, Taylor-Adams S, Stanhope N. Framework for analysing risk and safety in clinical medicine. *BMJ* 1998;**316**:1154–7.
8 Reason JT. *Human error*. New York: Cambridge University Press, 1990.
9 Leape LL, Brennan TA, Laird N, *et al*. The nature of adverse events in hospitalized patients: results of the Harvard medical practice study II. *N Engl J Med* 1991;**324**:377–84.
10 Joint Commission on Accreditation of Healthcare Organizations. *What every hospital should know about sentinel events*, Oakbrook Terrace, IL: JCAHO, 2000.
11 Vincent C, Taylor-Adams S, Chapman EJ, *et al*. How to investigate and analyse clinical incidents: clinical risk unit and association of litigation and risk management protocol. *BMJ* 2000;**320**:777–81.
12 Moray N. Error reduction as a systems problem. In: Bogner MS, ed. *Human error in medicine*, p. 70. Hillsdale, NJ: Lawrence Erlbaum Associates, 1994.
13 Joint Commission on Accreditation of Healthcare Organizations. *Sentinel events: evaluating cause and planning improvement* (2nd edition). Oakbrook Terrace, IL: JCAHO, 1998.
14 Joint Commission on Accreditation of Healthcare Organizations. *Root cause analysis in healthcare: tools and techniques*. Oakbrook Terrace, IL: JCAHO, 2000.
15 Ammerman M. *The root cause analysis handbook: A simplified approach to identifying, correcting, and reporting workplace errors*. New York: Quality Resources, 1998:66–7.
16 Adapted from Spath PL. *Investigating sentinel events: How to find and resolve root causes*. Forest Grove, OR: Brown-Spath & Associates, 1997:98.
17 Brennan TA, Leape LL, Laird NM, *et al*. Incidence of adverse events and negligence in hospitalized patients. *N Engl J Med* 1991;**324**:370–6.
18 Giraud T, Dhainaut J, Vaxelaire J, *et al*. Iatrogenic complications in adult intensive care units: a prospective two-centre study. *Critical Care Med* 1993;**21**:40–51.
19 Andrews LB, Stocking C, Krizek T, *et al*. An alternative strategy for studying adverse events in medical care. *Lancet* 1997;**349**:309–13.
20 Cullen DJ, Sweitzer BJ, Bates DW, *et al*. Preventable adverse drug events in hospitalized patients: A comparative study of intensive care and general care units. *Crit Care Med* 1997;**25**(8):1289–97.
21 Pronovost PJ, Jencks M, Dorman T, *et al*. Organizational characteristics of intensive care units related to outcomes of abdominal aortic surgery. *JAMA* 1999;**281**:1310–12.
22 Romano PS, Roos LL, Jollis JG. Adapting a clinical comorbidity index for use with ICD-9-CM administrative data: differing perspectives. *J Clin Epidemiol* 1993;**46**:1075–9.
23 Cleveland WS. Robust locally weighted regression and smoothing scatterplots. *J Am Stat Assoc* 1979;**74**:829–36.
24 Brown JJ, Sullivan G. Effect on ICU mortality of a full-time critical care specialist. *Chest* 1989;**96**:127–9.
25 Carson SS, Stocking C, Podsadecki T, *et al*. Effects of organizational change in the medical intensive care unit of a teaching hospital: a comparison of "open" and "closed" formats. *JAMA* 1996;**276**:322–8.
26 Hanson CW, Deutschman CS, Anderson HL, *et al*. Effects of an organized critical care service on outcomes and resource utilization: a cohort study. *Crit Care Med* 1999;**27**:270–4.
27 Li TC, Phillips MC, Shaw L, *et al*. On-site physician staffing in a community hospital intensive care unit. Impact on test and procedure use and on patient outcome. *JAMA* 1984;**252**:2023–7.
28 Manthous CA, Amoateng-Adjepong Y, al-Kharrat T, *et al*. Effects of a medical intensivist on patient care in a community teaching hospital. *Mayo Clin Proc* 1997;**72**:391–9.
29 Multz AS, Chalfin DB, Samson IM, *et al*. A "closed" medical intensive care unit (MICU) improves resource utilization when compared with an "open" MICU. *Am J Respir Crit Care Med* 1998;**157**:T–73.
30 Reynolds HN, Haupt MT, Thill-Baharozian MC, Carlson RW. Impact of critical care physician staffing on patients with septic shock in a university hospital medical intensive care unit. *JAMA* 1988;**260**:3446–50.

31 Rosenfeld B, Dorman T, Pronovost P, *et al.* Remote management improves ICU outcomes. *Crit Care Med* 2000;**27**:A153.

32 Ghorra S, Reinert SE, Cloffi W, *et al.* Analysis of the effect of conversion from open to closed surgical intensive care unit. *Ann Surg* 1999;**229**:163–71.

33 Marini CP, Nathan IM, Ritter G, *et al.* The impact of full-time surgical intensivists on ICU utilization and mortality. *Crit Care Med* 1995;**23**:A235.

34 Pollack MM, Patel KM, Ruttimann E. Pediatric critical care training programs have a positive effect on pediatric intensive care mortality. *Crit Care Med* 1997;**25**:1637–42.

35 Reich HS, Buhler L, David M, Whitmer G. Saving lives in the community. Impact of intensive care leadership. *Crit Care Med* 1998;**25**:A44.

36 Al-Asadi L, Dellinger RP, Deutch J, Nathan SS. Clinical impact of closed versus open provider care in a medical intensive care unit. *AJRCCM* 1996;**153**:A360.

37 Cassirer C. Hospital risk management programs in Maryland (1995). Unpublished Sc.D. dissertation. The Johns Hopkins University, 1997.

38 Morlock LL, Cassirer C, Malitz FE. *Impact of risk management on liability claims experience.* Final report submitted to the Agency for Healthcare Policy and Research, 1997.

39 American Society for healthcare Risk Management. *Hospital risk management self-assessment manual.* Chicago: American Hospital Association, 1991.

40 Casarett D, Helms C. Systems errors versus physicians' errors: Finding the balance in medical education. *Acad Med* 1999;**74**(1):19–22.

PART IV: IMPLEMENTATION OF RISK MANAGEMENT

21 Implementation of risk management

RICHARD W BEARD, ANNE O'CONNOR,
PATRICIA SCOTT

The National Health Service is the main provider of medical care in the UK. However, it is estimated that at least 10% of patients choose the private health sector as a means of obtaining care and treatment. The reasons for this are many and include reduced waiting times, better facilities, receiving better treatment and consultant care. Another major influence is the number of companies that include the provision of healthcare insurance as incentive packages to their staff.

Despite the significant number of hospitals and other specialist units operating within the private sector, there is very little written about risk management and other quality initiatives operating within them, although the authors are aware of a number of schemes working well within these facilities.

In the first edition (1995) of *Clinical Risk Management*,[1] we discussed the implementation of a clinical risk management programme in the maternity services within the NHS. Since then, two of the authors (RWB and AO'C), having gained further experience of working in the private health sector, realised that although provision of care may vary, there are many essential similarities between the private sector and the NHS. These similarities have enabled us to use our previous risk management experiences and to implement programmes tailored to the needs of individual hospitals based on that described in the first edition. Although this chapter focuses mainly on the private sector, the reader will be aware that the principles of risk management can apply to both forms of care.

In this chapter, we will look at the main areas of clinical claims within the private healthcare sector, how risk management can affect insurance

389

premiums and we will give examples of good clinical risk management systems that are likely to reduce premium rates. We will discuss differences between the NHS and private healthcare sector and how this may affect the quality of care and the system of risk management that is appropriate. We will also provide a practical example of how such a system has been implemented successfully in a private obstetric hospital.

The main clinical claims within the private healthcare sector

Looking at the increasing number of claims originating from the private sector and the resulting cost implications, it is advisable that robust, safe systems should be in place since many of the existing systems do not appear to be working satisfactorily. The claims from the private sector reflect much of the NHS experience and include:

- Slips, trips and falls
- Incorrect drug administration and transfusion accidents
- Suspicious deaths after operations or other treatments
- Failures of communication
- Failure to obtain informed consent for invasive procedures
- Inappropriate decisions by individuals with insufficient experience to make them.
- General lack of nursing or medical care
- Failure to transfer a patient to a more appropriate medical environment or to obtain a second opinion
- Plastic surgery, in vitro fertilisation, and sterilisation
- Post-operative infection
- Performing the wrong operation
- Damage to teeth during operation

It should be noted that the number of successful claims represent only a small proportion of the total claims made. Claims are frequently indefensible due to poor or missing documentation.

It needs to be recognised that there is already quite a strong incentive to provide safe practice in the private sector. While private hospitals have to take out insurance against accidents, which will cover the cost of medico-legal action, insurance companies are likely to reduce their premiums if private hospitals can provide evidence of safe practice. Examples of such practice are shown on page 391.

Examples of good clinical practice and attention to risk management that are likely to reduce insurance premiums

- Attention to good clinical standards, particularly in high risk areas
- Good operating theatre procedures
- Pre-operative assessments
- Attention to technology, e.g. double checking to calibrate equipment for laser surgery
- Establishing standards and procedures, e.g. use of evidence-based protocols to guide obstetric practice
- A robust accident and incident reporting system
- An active clinical governance committee
- A high standard of documentation
- An effective complaints procedure
- Evidence that all staff are applying the above in their daily practice

---

National initiatives to improve the quality of healthcare

To date initiatives to improve the quality of healthcare in the UK have focussed on the NHS, but recent government proposals, discussed later in this chapter, indicate that the private health sector will be expected to conform to quality standards required of the NHS. Some of these issues are laid out and discussed in detail in Chapter 4 by Secker-Walker and Donaldson of this book.

It is clear from publications emanating from the Department of Health and the NHS Executive, that quality of care has to go hand in hand with economic restructuring of the NHS if the ultimate goal of improved efficiency is to be achieved. In the last 10 years, recommendations on medical and clinical audit,[2,3,4,5] have been followed by guidance on complaints procedures.[6]

Then, in 1996, the importance of professional education and training in this development was highlighted in the circular *Clinical Effectiveness; a framework for action.*[7] Thus, having planned the basis for improvement in the publications already referred to, practical proposals on how to implement these plans, generally referred to as clinical governance, were made in a series of publications.[8,9,10] Clinical governance is defined as "a framework through which the NHS organisations are accountable for continuously improving the quality of their services and safeguarding a high standard of care by creating an environment in which excellence of care will flourish". How this is to be achieved has been laid down in a number of papers which place on NHS Trusts the responsibility of establishing clinical leadership,[2,3]

391

creating a development plan to improve quality of care,[4] accepting account-ability through annual reports with patient involvement, leading, in time, to independent scrutiny. Initially, these directives were interpreted as meaning that clinicians, aided by managers, should develop evidence-based clinical guidelines, establish appropriate education and training programmes and set up audit programmes to monitor clinical practice.[5] However, recent additional directives specifically require the development of clinical risk management, combined with continued professional development, leading to regular revalidation of specialists.[11,12] If these proposals are to be become a reality, we believe that it is clinical risk management which will drive the others. Equally, if risk management is to succeed, the drive must come from a bottom-up as well as a top-down approach. Finally, it should be under-stood that establishing risk management in the private sector is equally as important for hospital managers as it is for clinicians.

Summary of differences between the NHS and private healthcare providers

Contrary to common public belief, the private health sector is not regu-lated in the same way as the NHS. This leads to a lack of uniformity between the two sectors, which can be confusing and lead to gaps in regulatory con-trol. There is little doubt that the government intends that standards laid down in the NHS will be applied to the private care sector. In a recent con-sultation document from the NHS Executive, *Regulating private and volun-tary healthcare*,[13] the shortcomings of the present regulatory system in the private sector are recognised. It states "Private hospitals are inspected under the Registered Homes Act (1984). These regulatory arrangements are . . . out of date, unsatisfactory and not sufficiently independent. They do not reflect the growth in the scale and complexity of treatments provided by the private and voluntary healthcare sectors, nor do they provide the protection to which the public is entitled". The consultation paper goes on to state ". . . healthcare is not a service which should be bought or sold in an unregu-lated market with individual patients being required to satisfy themselves about the safety of services being provided. Regulation is essential to provide public protection . . ." Finally, it states, "it is also important that new arrange-ments are robust for the future, and clearly independent of the NHS".

It is proposed in the above document, that a new national statutory reg-ulatory body should be set up that is responsible for overseeing the quality of the service provided by the private healthcare sector. It recommends that attention should be paid to specific activities to determine whether or not a hospital may be registered. These are:

- management
- staff recruitment

- financial activity
- operational policies
- complaints procedures
- quality assurance
- information provided to patients
- clinical professional standards
- clinical activities.

It proposes that risk management should be used by the new statutory regulatory body to determine the effectiveness of these activities in individual private institutions. While such an approach would avoid any tendency for a private institution to hide its defects, the generation of valid data presents major logistical problems. An alternative, which we describe in this chapter, is to require management and professional staff at a local level to establish their own risk management process, details of which could be made available to the national statutory regulatory body. Despite recent media reports to the contrary, there is a long history, in Britain, of effective and safe regulation of practice by both the medical and nursing professions that should be utilised.

Specific problems to be considered when setting up risk management in the private sector

To be effective, risk management, whether it is in the NHS or private sector, requires healthcare personnel to collaborate with each other by agreeing to accept the process and the recommendations resulting from it. Before making recommendations on how this can be achieved in the private sector, it is important to recognise that practice in the private sector differs in a number of important details from that of the NHS.

- Most consultants working in a private hospital have a maximum part-time contract with the NHS. This means that their allegiance is mainly to their NHS hospital and, in consequence, their style of practice is likely to be heavily influenced by this. This may make it more difficult to establish a protocol to regulate clinical practice in a private hospital, particularly in London, with consultants coming from several NHS hospitals. It also means that most of these consultants are so busy that they have little time for committee activity in their private hospital(s).
- There is much competition between private hospital managers to encourage consultants to work within their institutions. In consequence, there is little incentive to impose regulations or apply sanctions if those regulations are disregarded.
- Heavy responsibilities are placed on resident medical officers (RMOs) who provide night cover in private hospitals. This cover involves the care

393

of patients of consultants from a wide variety of specialties, for most of which the RMOs have received little or no training. In addition, many private institutions are small and consequently may not be able to afford the expensive, high-tech facilities such as those required in adult or neonatal intensive care units.

- Clinical records may be incomplete because there are often two sets of notes for a patient – one in the hospital and the other with the consultant.
- At present, medical staff who are suspended from an NHS post may continue to practice in the private sector.

While it is important to recognise that these problems exist, it does not follow that some of them cannot be overcome or circumvented, to make clinical practice safe.

Principles guiding implementation of a risk management programme in the private sector

Many of the existing risk management principles have been successfully re-modelled and implemented within some private institutions. To this end, we will revisit the model discussed in the first edition of *Clinical Risk Management*,[1] and show how it can be altered to suit the needs of practice in the private sector. Risk management systems cannot be set up in isolation but must be accepted as part of a total quality improvement programme. Local, national and international requirements in practice must also be built into that programme. Examples of such requirements include clinical governance guidelines, the clinical negligence scheme (CNST),[14] and the recent changes to our legal system which specifically outlines timetables and pre-action protocols for the management of clinical negligence.

Clinical negligence pre-action protocols[14]

Healthcare providers must:
- Ensure key staff know some healthcare law
- Implement clinical risk management and clinical governance
- Monitor and audit clinical practice
- Set up adverse outcome reporting systems
- Use audit of selected outcome to improve the quality of the service
- Ensure patients know how to raise concerns or complaints
- Establish sound systems for managing records of all patients treated in the hospital
- Give advice and explanations early after an adverse outcome

---

Setting up the system

It is essential that the risk management system is supported from the top. Without the backing of the hospital administration and particularly of the hospital manager and the hospital medical committee, it will not succeed. The other ingredient necessary for success is that all staff feel supported and secure that they will not be victimised for reporting their concerns. It is hoped that this last issue will be dealt with in a paper, soon to be produced by the government which will include the protection of those who voice their concerns ("whistle blowers").

Managing risk within a hospital that has many specialties, is not an easy task. It is advisable to set up risk management systems in small manageable steps, taking one specialty at a time. Where to start? Initially, you need to concentrate on complaints and claims data that give cause for concern.

The hospital risk management group

Composition

The composition of such a group will depend on the size and mixture of specialties in a hospital but a working example could include the following:

- a chairman who should have a position of authority, such as being one of the clinical directors
- a clinical director from each specialty
- a financial representative
- the hospital claims handler or risk manager
- the director of nursing
- a non-executive director, particularly if he/she has some legal or insurance experience.

Responsibilities of the group

Following identification and evaluation of clinical risk, decisions must be made by the hospital as to whether risk can be eliminated, controlled or accepted. If a risk is identified as being unavoidable because of its particular nature, then action must be taken by the relevant departments to minimise that risk.

Local specialty group

The composition and responsibilities of a risk management group representing a particular hospital speciality, will depend on the nature of that specialty. This is well illustrated in the description of an obstetrics risk management committee that follows.

Actions taken to minimise clinical risk

These may include:

- Examination of staffing levels, grades, skill mix and supervision
- Developing patient management protocols and guidelines
- Job and risk management training
- Medical equipment review, e.g. fitness for use, obsolescence issues, user training, maintenance schedules, etc.
- Monitoring risk controls and modifying as appropriate
- Infrequently, where there is a serious concern regarding the practice of an individual practitioner, admitting privileges may have to be suspended

---

The process

Figure 21.1 is a flow diagram showing how the findings of local groups of any specialty can be communicated to the hospital risk management or clinical governance board on a regular basis. Reports should include recommendations that are made by the group to eliminate or minimise clinical risk.

The forging of links between the local clinical risk management committees, the clinical audit group, quality assurance bodies and hospital clinical governance group is essential if the system is to be effective.

Rationale for selecting obstetrics as an example of risk management in the private sector

Obstetrics provides a good model for illustrating the development of risk management in the private healthcare sector. It is a relatively compact specialty in which there is general agreement as to what constitutes good practice. The Royal College of Obstetricians and Gynaecologists (RCOG) provides general guidance on good practice, most recently in a report entitled *Towards Safer Childbirth – minimum standards for the organisation of labour wards*.[15]

In addition, the use of evidence based practice protocols and audit is generally accepted by the profession as being a part of routine practice. In the private sector 24-hour cover is provided by midwives who are independent practitioners used to looking after women with normal pregnancies but are also proficient at recognising complications which require referral to a doctor.

Considerable experience already exists in the NHS in the development and practice of maternity risk management.[1,16] Probably the most compelling

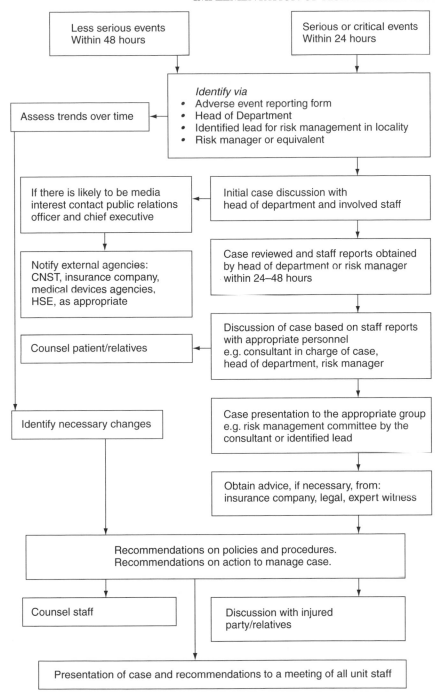

Figure 21.1 General risk management process.

argument of the need for risk management in a private maternity service is the existing high rate of litigation in the UK in the specialty. The 1998 National Confidential Enquiry into Stillbirths and Deaths in Infancy (CESDI)[17] reported that 77% of intrapartum stillbirths studied had received suboptimal care, which underlines the continuing risk of litigation. Most recently, the NHS Litigation Authority[14] reported that between 1995 and 1998, the cost of settling claims in obstetrics was £242 782 343. Managers of hospitals with a private maternity unit know only too well the implications of this figure, even though it is taken from the NHS.

The description that follows is of the experience from five years ago of setting up a risk management group in a private maternity unit, the staff of which had had no previous experience of the process.

Description of the Birth Unit

The Birth Unit is a part of the private Hospital of St John and St Elizabeth in North London. It currently delivers approximately 300 women a year with defined "low risk pregnancies". It offers two choices of care, midwife-led and consultant-led, which will be described later in this chapter. The philosophy of the Unit is to offer women a freedom of choice during pregnancy and delivery which includes the use of a birthing pool, and the appropriate application of complementary therapies, combined with conventional medical facilities and obstetric management. Much of what *Changing Childbirth*[18] recommends, has been achieved by the Unit. Obstetricians, anaesthetists, paediatricians, ultrasonographers, and pathologists and operating theatres provide round the clock cover. In addition, neonatal intensive care back-up is provided by the nearby Neonatal Unit at St Mary's Hospital, Paddington. The paediatric and midwifery staff of the Birth Unit are all highly experienced practitioners trained in neonatal life support. Midwives achieve maximum continuity of care by working 12-hour shifts.

How risk management began in the Birth Unit

In 1994, the hospital manager instigated an independent confidential enquiry to investigate a series of worrying, untoward events that had occurred in the Birth Unit over a period of four months. The enquiry was carried out by a panel of independent experts and co-ordinated by the North Thames Regional Health Authority. They reviewed all case notes, Birth Unit statistic protocols, etc. and interviewed members of the medical and midwifery staff. The following recommendations were made.

- The concept of "low risk" needs to be defined, and applied when women are being booked for care in early pregnancy.

- Existing practice protocols need to be reviewed and made more evidence based.

- Patients need to be given clear information about the service provided and facilities made available to them by the Birth Unit.

- It was noted that the Birth Unit was at risk of being isolated from mainstream maternity care, and recommended that a system for auditing practice and outcomes should be established.

- Midwives and medical staff should obtain updating experience in an NHS maternity unit.

The recommendation which was to have the most profound impact on future care and the working of the Birth Unit, was that an external adviser in obstetrics should be appointed, to guide the Unit, leading ultimately to the establishment of the risk management process.

What was to be done?

The introduction of risk management on to the Birth Unit was aided by the high level of enthusiasm and commitment of the staff to ensure that a quality service was provided. Before risk management was established, adverse events were always privately discussed at Unit meetings, often agonised over but rarely acted upon. There was general agreement that if risk management was to be effective, everyone had to accept the proposed procedures. On the positive side, it was recognised that as the Birth Unit was relatively small compared with larger maternity units, communication was less of a problem. The need for locums and agency cover was less common than in a larger maternity unit. However, it was also recognised that the philosophy of the Birth Unit of freedom of choice and the high expectations of the women who came to the Unit, brought problems that, although not unique to the private sector, are probably more prevalent than in the NHS.

In 1995, the Maternity Risk Management Committee (MRMC) was set up and a senior midwife (PS) from the Birth Unit, with a particular interest in this subject, was appointed the risk manager. She was to be responsible for co-ordinating the risk management process and understanding the natural anxieties of staff about the outcome of the whole process. A detailed list of her duties is provided in the chapter by Beard and O'Connor in the first edition of this book.[1] She attended a risk management training course and spent some time at St Mary's Hospital, Paddington where risk management had been effectively applied for the previous two years.

To initiate risk management, a series of in-house study sessions were held to explain the purpose and benefits, and what it involved. These were attended by all midwifery staff, including bank staff, who are midwives experienced in the practice of the Birth Unit, although no longer working there. The sessions were designed to gain their co-operation and to help dispel fears or misunderstandings. This approach served the purpose of raising the profile of risk management and of allaying fears that risk management was a punitive tool. All newly appointed midwifery staff are now required to attend these sessions as a part of their orientation programme and this proved to be vital for the future success of risk management. A folder was created by the risk manager, containing information for staff to learn about risk management, record keeping and advice on how to write reports. Specimen signatures of all medical and midwifery staff were kept by the risk manager so that she could determine who was responsible for writing the notes of patients whose case histories were to be discussed at the MRMC meeting. A list of Adverse Events (shown in Box below) identical to those used by Beard and O'Connor,[1] was used by the risk manager and midwives to alert them to cases that might need to be discussed by the MRMC. A flow diagram in Figure 21.2, illustrates the process that was implemented once a case requiring discussion at the MRMC had been identified by the risk manager.

Adverse events

1 Birth Injury

- Shoulder dystocia

- Fracture clavicle

- Paralysis such as Erb's palsy

- Fractured skull

- Fracture of any long bone

- Tear of falx cerebrum or subdural haematoma

- Any serious soft tissue injury to mother or baby, e.g. third degree tear, ruptured uterus or bladder injury

- Iatrogenic injury following birth

2 Condition of Baby at Birth

- Seizures within the first 24 hours

- Apgar score of 4 or less at 5 mins

- Iatrogenic respiratory distress syndrome after elective induction or caesarean section

---

- Stillbirths and neonatal deaths in infants of 24 weeks gestation and over, unassociated with lethal congenital anomaly
- Any major congenital anomaly first detected at birth
- Unanticipated admission to SCBU

3 *Maternal Complications*

- Need for blood transfusion
- Postpartum haemorrhage >1000 ml
- Transfer to high dependency unit
- Convulsions
- Extended length of stay in hospital after vaginal delivery for medical reasons greater than five days or greater than 7 days following a caesarean section
- General or epidural anaesthetic problems
- Drug errors
- Injury due to equipment failure

4 *"Near Miss" cases as judged by risk manager*

An incident report form was designed to be kept on the Birth Unit for staff to complete after the occurrence of an adverse incident. It was recognised as important that these forms should be user-friendly. They were collected by the risk manager as possible cases for discussion by the MRMC. She would ensure that all the information, such as fetal heart rate traces, case notes, and staff reports were available and complete. A photocopy of all records used for this purpose was made and kept separately by the risk manager. One great strength of adverse incident reporting, which was soon apparent, was that the information collected soon after the event, was fuller and more accurate than that previously obtained for perinatal mortality meetings. The risk manager would then inform the consultant or midwife, under whom the patient to be discussed had been booked, of the date when the MRMC would be discussing the case, giving at least two weeks' notice.

In creating the above system, the support of all staff was an essential part of the successful development of risk management in the Birth Unit. Obtaining reports from the medical and/or midwifery staff continued to

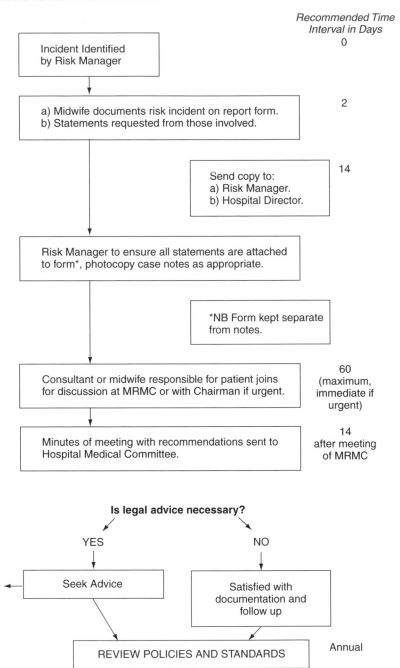

Figure 21.2 Maternity risk management process.

present an occasional problem. The main reasons for this usually proved to be a busy workload or often, a need for some advice and support on how to write the report.

Composition of the Maternity Risk Management Committee

The selection of members of the committee was made, recognising that maternity care is a multidisciplinary activity and that it was necessary to have a representative from each of the disciplines involved. Individuals with specialist expertise, relevant to a case under discussion, are invited to the meeting as required.

The established members of the MRMC are as follows:

- Senior consultant obstetrician from outside the Birth Unit (chairman)
- Consultant obstetrician ⎫
- Consultant anaesthetist ⎬ representing their specialist colleagues
- Consultant neonatologist ⎭
- Midwifery manager of the Birth Unit
- Risk manager (a midwife from the Birth Unit with aptitude for the job)
- Hospital manager
- The possibility that a lay member of the public who has had a baby in the Birth Unit should become a member of the Committee, is currently under discussion. Other desirable credentials for such a person are legal and/or risk management experience.

The inclusion of a lay person on the MRMC may be a matter of concern to some professional members and hospital management because of the issue of confidentiality. However, there is no reason to believe that a layman or woman is less likely to respect the confidentiality of the proceedings of the Committee than professional colleagues. In addition, all members of the MRMC are asked to sign the Terms of Reference which include a clause on confidentiality. On the positive side, the availability of a balanced opinion from a knowledgeable member of the public adds greatly to the decision-making and credibility of a hospital risk management committee.

Setting up risk management

Preliminary decisions to be made by the MRMC are shown in the box on page 404. Before starting risk management, these decisions must be agreed with all consultants and midwifery staff on the Unit and by the Hospital Medical Committee.

Initial check list for the MRMC to implement before starting risk management

Organisation of the committee
- Terms of reference*, objectives, method of working and protocols agreed by MRMC
- Frequency of meetings sufficient for needs of the Unit
- Agreed list of low-risk admission criteria (box, see page 405) and adverse events (box, see page 400)
- Definition of appropriate sanctions
- Support for the MRMC agreed with all Unit staff and Hospital management

Communication with patients
- Full information should be made available to all patients before booking for care, about the philosophy and activities of the Birth Unit and the Hospital
- Consent should be obtained from patients before any invasive procedure
- Patients/partners should be informed at the earliest opportunity, of details of clinical disasters/near misses
- Effective system available for dealing with complaints

Requirements from attending consultants and midwives
- Knowledge of practice and adherence to protocols
- Maintain CME requirements
- Clear understanding of professional relationship with and importance of good communication with midwives as a part of team building
- Minimal use of agency staff

Requirements from hospital management
- Availability of advice from hospital solicitors and insurance company
- Agreement that the MRMC will review all applications from consultants applying for admitting rights to work on the Birth Unit
- Availability of appropriate support service at all times, such as pathology, imaging, etc.
- Provision of appropriate equipment on the Birth Unit and its effective maintenance, for example fetal heart rate monitors, infusion pumps, etc.
- Support for the whole risk management process.

* See Appendix 21.1

Organisation and principles

- Terms of reference (see Appendix 21.1) must be agreed which include the objectives and responsibilities of the MRMC. In addition, its composition, duration of membership and the method of replacing members and of working should be agreed.
- In a low risk maternity unit, it is essential to have a list of criteria to exclude women at the time of booking if they have risk factors. A list of these factors used by the Birth Unit is shown below.

Protocol of exclusions at booking for low-risk maternity care

1 Maternal medical disorders:
- Chronic heart disease
- Chronic renal disease
- Chronic hepatic disease

- Diabetes
- Gross obesity: use body mass index to assess
- Cerebro-vascular accident or previous brain surgery
- Psychosis or previous serious psychiatric disorder

- Hypertensive disease
- Coagulation disorder
- Multiple sclerosis
- Epilepsy
- Any major medical complications

2 Obstetric history:
- Primigravida over 39 years of age
- Grand multiparae (5 or more viable pregnancies)
- Multiple pregnancy
- Recurrent miscarriage (3 or more clinical miscarriages)

- Previous injury or operation on the uterus, vagina or bony pelvis

- Infertility over 3 years
- Assisted conception (IUI, IVF, or GIFT)
- Previous perinatal death
- Premature delivery (<37 weeks gestation)
- Previous postpartum haemorrhage (>1000 ml)

- Previous caesarean section
- Previous difficult forceps delivery

Communication between staff and patients

- Informing patients of facilities provided by the Birth Unit, in an honest manner, before they decide to book for care, is an essential component of an open approach, which inspires confidence.
- Most women seeking maternity care in a private hospital understand that neonatal intensive care, at the highest level, is rarely available but they do wish to know what arrangements are in place should their baby require this type of care. They will also wish to know how available their consultant obstetrician will be during labour, particularly when choosing midwife-led care, if complications arise which may require transfer from a midwife to a consultant obstetrician.
- The mother and her partner should be kept fully informed as soon as possible of any complications affecting her or their baby. This principle is also relevant if the baby is stillborn or dies in the neonatal period, when a full explanation from the consultant obstetrician, and if relevant, a consultant paediatrician or anaesthetist, is required. An open approach from the outset of such cases is good practice and also reduces the possibility of litigation at a later date.

Requirement from consultant and midwife

- Evidence-based practice protocols should be regarded as guidelines to practice and never as a dictat. Consultants and midwives should follow guidelines unless one of them decides that the clinical circumstances are such that an alternative approach is justified. Deviation from protocol should always be accompanied by a written explanation in the case notes by the individual responsible for it.
- Maintenance of in-service, regular education for both consultants and midwives is particularly important. Consultants are required to maintain continuing medical education (CME) of their Royal Colleges, and midwives to conform to their statutory educational requirements.
- All staff working on the Birth Unit need to recognise when complications of pregnancy are developing that may necessitate transfer of a patient to a high risk unit.
- Midwives working in a small private maternity unit, need to be more experienced than those on a larger unit because of the responsibility they carry in making decisions in the absence of on-site medical cover. If possible "bank" rather than agency midwives should be employed when locum cover is required.
- Availability of midwife-led care in a maternity unit implies that midwives are accepted as independent practitioners there. However, the possibility that medical advice may be required at any stage in a pregnancy is

given substance by assigning the name of a consultant to every patient at the time of booking. This implies that a consultant is only responsible for a patient, booked for midwife-led care, when she is transferred to the care of her nominated consultant.

- Ease of communication between consultant and midwives is an important component of successful practice in any maternity unit. This is particularly so in a unit with midwife- and consultant-led care working alongside each other. If good relations exist between midwives and consultants, then the handover of care of a patient will be easier when a complication of pregnancy develops.

Proposal on how sanctions may be used by the MRMC

Sanctions of some kind are necessary once substandard care is identified by the MRMC if risk management is to be effective. For the Birth Unit, these range from:

- Most commonly – a discussion with the staff involved in the case about where practice was considered to be at fault, and what might have been done to avoid the adverse event(s).
- Occasionally, when care is considered to be seriously at fault or after a member of staff has been involved in two or more cases of suboptimal care, a warning will be issued that this individual may be suspended from practice if this recurs.
- Very rarely – a recommendation may be made that a member of staff (consultant or midwife) who has been previously warned about suboptimal care, should be suspended from active practice. A national procedure already exists with appropriate sanctions for investigating midwives involved in such cases. However, for a consultant, a procedure for suspension with sanctions, which is based on Department of Health recommendations, is proposed in the box on page 408.

It can be seen that a number of safeguards are proposed that recognise the negative impact of the enquiry process on the consultant. The adverse effect of suspension on the morale and reputation of a consultant is recognised, so that emphasis is placed on the importance of limiting the duration of an independent enquiry to determine whether the recommendation by the MRMC is upheld.

Requirements from hospital management

- The MRMC should have an agreed line of communication with the medical committee of the hospital of which it is a sub-committee, and with the hospital manager. Matters relating to disciplining of a member

---

**Proposed process to be adopted following recommendation
that an attending consultant should be suspended** (based on
DOH Circular *Disciplinary procedures for hospital staff* 1990 HC (90/9)).

- Recommendation and reasons for the suspension agreed by MRMC,
  the chairman of the hospital board and the hospital manager.
- Consultant to be suspended is informed of decision and reasons
  for it.
- Hospital board ratifies the recommendation.
- The Independent Enquiry – two senior clinicians, an obstetrician,
  a paediatrician or an anaesthetist depending on the case, and a layman who may be the preferred person to chair the Enquiry) who
  are not involved with the hospital, are invited to investigate the case
  and report to the MRMC on whether suspension is justified. The
  legal advisors of the consultant and the hospital may attend the
  hearing of the enquiry.
- MRMC considers the report of the Independent Enquiry. If suspension is upheld a recommendation on the sanction to be applied
  will be made. In general, this will range from:

  (i) a warning
  (ii) an agreed period of retraining and definition of objectives to
  be achieved. A consultant colleague is selected to act as a
  mentor to the suspended consultant during the period of
  retraining
  (iii) termination of the admitting rights of the consultant

- The recommendation must be ratified by the Hospital Board.
- Every effort should be made to complete the above procedure
  wthin 3 months. During this time, the consultant who has been
  suspended should be kept fully informed of progress and may raise
  an objection if he/she considers any part of the process is unfair.

---

of staff, dealing with complaints from patients, and advising on consultant appointments to the Birth Unit are examples of the need for such
links.
- Safety of patients should be safeguarded by a check being made by the
  MRMC on the suitability of medical staff applying for admitting rights
  to work on the maternity unit.
- Hospital management should agree to remedy any deficiency and availability of support services that are essential to the Birth Unit such as
  pathology, imaging, and the use of theatres, and the availability of up-
  to-date functioning technology.

- The management may also occasionally, be asked by the MRMC to provide expert legal or insurance advice.

Regular proceedings of the Maternity Risk Management Committee

The Committee regularly audits the clinical practice of the Unit, considering cases with serious adverse events (see box, page 401–2) and is required to decide whether care was substandard. Particular attention is paid to how things could have been handled better so that recommendations can be made to prevent a recurrence. Often these cases highlight lack of judgement, of communication, of planning or of seeking advice from others too late. A major role of the MRMC is to feed back information to staff, patients and management about what happened and proposals for improving care in the future. Good practice as well as bad are included. At all times, proceedings of the MRMC are strictly confidential. Consultants on the Birth Unit and midwives are invited to attend one meeting so as to become familiar with the functions of the MRMC. This not only helps to give risk management a higher profile but allays anxiety amongst the staff that risk management is a "witch hunt" rather than the positive activity it is designed to be.

Example of a case history which might be brought to the MRMC by the risk manager

The case history shown in the box (see page 410) would normally be discussed by the MRMC, with the consultant concerned present. The following conclusions would probably have been drawn by the Committee.

- Insufficent attention was paid antenatally and during labour to the clear evidence that the baby was large for dates.
- The clinical management of a large for dates baby should have been discussed with the patient and her partner at 41 weeks gestational age. Two choices existed at that time, either induction and trial of labour, or elective caesarean section.
- Inappropriately high doses of both Prostin and Syntocinon were used resulting in uterine hyperstimulation. Delivery by caesarean section should have been done as soon as there was evidence of failure of the labour to progress. Attempting vaginal delivery was contra-indicated because of the clear evidence that existed at the time of cephalo-pelvic disproportion.
- The consultant should have come to see the patient earlier during the labour.

409

Example of the case history that would be brought to the MRMC by the risk manager

- A healthy 30-year-old, obese primigravida was booked at 11 weeks gestation for consultant-led care.
- Antenatal care was uneventful until 38 weeks gestation.
- 38 weeks' gestation. The fetus was noted to be large for dates with an estimated fetal weight on ultrasound scan of 3.8 kg.
- 41 weeks. Concern was expressed by the midwife to the consultant at the continued growth of a large baby and failure of the head to engage. The midwife suggested induction of labour.
- At 42 weeks, labour was induced with vaginal Prostin 2 mg at 0800. Fetal head not engaged 3/5.

    at 1600. Labour was established with the cervix 3 cm dilated but poor contractions, and fetal head still not engaged. The consultant was contacted who recommended that intravenous Syntocinon should be started.

    at 2400. The cervix had been fully dilated for one hour with the fetal head engaged 2/5 but poor uterine contractions. The consultant was contacted who recommended increasing the Syntocinon infusion from 30–40 milliunits per minute.

    Uterine hypertonus developed, accompanied by fetal bradycardia. Again the consultant was contacted who asked the midwife to prepare for a ventouse delivery by calling the anaesthetist.

    at 0100. Attempted delivery by ventouse failed.

    at 0120. Limp baby delivered by caesarean section (Apgar scores 2 at 1 minute and 6 at 5 minutes). Baby weighing 4.5 kg.

    Irritable with large cephalo-haematoma transferred to Special Care Baby Unit.

The baby remained in the Special Care Baby Unit for five days, irritable and feeding poorly. The consultant obstetrician did not discuss the case history, in any detail, with the parents.

- The consultant should have discussed the case with the parents as soon as possible after the delivery.

In a case such as this, it is likely that the MRMC would decide that care had been suboptimal and a warning would have been issued to the consultant by the chairman.

Achievements of risk management

Since risk management has been functioning at the Hospital of St John and Elizabeth, the MRMC has faced many debates and challenges but there is no doubt that it has helped to influence change. Broadly, the following changes have come about as a consequence of its activities:

- There is now a more established practice of maternity care on the Birth Unit, which is adhered to by consultants and midwives.
- Early recognition that a complication may develop in a pregnancy has been improved by a more concise and detailed collection of the information at the time of booking, such as the use of a high body mass index as a maternal risk factor. Risk factors are now highlighted in the case notes and future management laid down in care plans.
- Clear lines of responsibility for the type of case that can be accepted for midwife-led and consultant-led care are now laid down. Midwives also have clear guidelines as to when to call for medical assistance or to refer patients for a medical opinion.
- Information given to patients has improved. The Birth Unit brochure outlines the type of care available and what is included in a package. Information on the full range of services available and not available is clearer as is information on clinical procedures such as blood tests, external versions, induction of labour, amniocentesis, and epidurals.
- Informed consent is now obtained for all invasive procedures such as amniocentesis, induction of labour and operative delivery.
- There is a successful, in-house programme of education of midwives and medical staff. It is compulsory for all staff, working on the Birth Unit to attend record keeping, epidural updates, and advanced neonatal resuscitation. Guest speakers are invited throughout the year to lecture on subjects designed to keep knowledge of the staff up-to-date.
- Emergency call training sessions are held regularly to cover such conditions as acute haemorrhage, crash caesarean section, cord prolapse, and neonatal resuscitation.
- A protocol committee has been established which reviews existing protocols using evidence based research with feed-back to the whole team at Unit meetings.
- Record keeping has improved and writing of "care plans" is now an accepted practice.
- Communication has improved between all staff. For example, after a case has been discussed by the MRMC, the Risk Manager will feed back the conclusions and recommendations to staff and to the patients concerned with an invitation to discuss the matter further with her.
- Cord pH values are now obtained on all babies with low Apgar scores at birth.

- Management of sick newborn babies has been improved by creating formal links and clear guidelines between the Birth Unit and St Mary's Hospital Neonatal Unit for the transfer of babies and for their crash team to come to the Birth Unit in emergency situations.
- Auditing of Birth Unit statistics is an annual event that started in 1994. Changes in practice such as a rise in the caesarean section rate has resulted in a detailed enquiry requested by the MRMC which will lead to appropriate action being recommended.
- Criteria for booking low risk women and criteria for transfer of care from midwife-led to consultant-led care. These criteria have been repeatedly refined and conditions considered unacceptable for a low risk Birth Unit such as multiple pregnancy and women wishing to have a vaginal delivery with a breech presentation, have been introduced. The criteria for the transfer of care from a midwife to a consultant and when to refer a patient to another maternity unit with facilities for high risk care are clearer and more generally accepted.
- The curriculum vitae of all consultants requesting admission rights to work on the Birth Unit are now submitted to the MRMC by the hospital manager for consideration.
- An agreed policy has been formulated for the rare occasions when a midwife may find herself differing from a consultant over the management of a patient, particularly if it conflicts with the Unit protocol. On such occasions, the midwife may discuss the problem with the senior midwife and if the matter still cannot be resolved, the final opinion of the on-call consultant for the Unit will be obtained.

Comment

Clinical risk management, whether done in a private hospital or in the NHS, is about ensuring that the risk of clinical care provided by any specialty is as low as possible. Before starting the risk management process, it is necessary for the RMC to do some essential groundwork to ensure that the facilities and practice guidelines on the Unit are acceptable to all who work on that Unit and to review current practice on the Unit.

In the private sector, this is a particularly important preliminary activity as these hospitals are often small with consequent limitations on their clinical activity in certain areas. Examples are: limited medical cover at night, the ready availability of the consultants under whom the patients are admitted, and the lack of an intensive care unit. Agreement about how the risk management process will be carried out by an RMC or its equivalent and the sanctions available to that committee, must be agreed with the hospital management and the medical and senior nursing staff.

These are early days for the risk management process to be applied in the private sector but we believe that over the next two to three years it will be an essential part of clinical activity that these hospitals must undertake.

References

1 Beard RW, O'Connor A. Implementation of audit and risk management: a protocol. Vincent C, ed. *Clinical risk management*. London: BMJ Publishing Group, 1995:350–74.
2 Department of Health. *Working for patients. Medical audit (1989)*. London: HMSO, 1989.
3 *Clinical audit. Meeting and improving standards in healthcare*. NHS Management Executive 1993.
4 *Clinical audit in the NHS. Using clinical audit in the NHS – a position statement*. NHS Executive 1996.
5 Burnett AC, Winyard G. Clinical audit at the heart of clinical effectiveness. *J Qual Clin Pract* 1998;**18**:3–19.
6 *Guidance on implementation of the NHS complaints procedure*. NHS Executive, 1996.
7 *Clinical effectiveness: a framework for action in and through the NHS*. NHS Executive, 1996.
8 Baker R, Fraser RC. Development of review criteria: linking guidelines and assessment of quality. *BMJ* 1995;**311**:370–3.
9 Donaldson LJ, Muir Gray JA. Clinical governance: a quality duty for health organisations (1998). *Qual healthcare* 1998;**7**: (suppl.) S37–44.
10 *Clinical governance: quality in the NHS*. NHS Executive, 1999.
11 Department of Health. *Supporting doctors, protecting patients*. Consultation Paper (1999). London: HMSO, 1999.
12 Department of Health. *A first class service: quality in the new NHS*. London: HMSO, 1998.
13 *Regulating private and voluntary healthcare: A consultation document*. NHS Executive, 1999.
14 The NHS litigation authority. *Clinical negligence scheme for Trusts' Hospital Doctors*. 26th Feb (1998):64–5.
15 Royal College of Obstetrics and Gynaecology. *Towards safer childbirth – minimum standards for the organisation of labour wards*. London: RCOG Publication, 1999.
16 Department of Health. *Why do mothers die? Report on confidential enquiries into maternal deaths in the United Kingdom (1994 –1996)*. London: DoH, HMSO, 1999.
17 Department of Health. *Confidential enquiry into Stillbirths and Deaths in Infancy (CESDI)*. Fifth Annual Report. London: Maternal and Child Health Consortium, 1998.
18 *Changing childbirth: Report of the Expert Maternity Group*. London: HMSO, 1993.

Appendix 21.1

Terms of Reference

The Maternity Risk Management Committee (MRMC), established in 1992, is a sub-committee of the Hospital Medical Advisory Committee, to which it reports.

1 *Objectives of the Committee*

   a   To carry out a continuous review of the practice of the Birth Unit so as to ensure that at all time, every effort is made by the staff and management to promote and maintain practice.

   b   To advise the Medical Advisory Committee on all matters affecting the practice of the Birth Unit.

2   *Membership of the MRMC*

Chairman	a senior obstetrician who is not personally involved in the clinical practice of the Birth Unit

Medical members

A consultant obstetrician*.
A consultant paediatrician } who are working on the Birth Unit and will
A consultant anaesthetist represent their colleagues

A lay representative
Risk Manager   –   Usually a senior midwife on the Birth Unit.
Ex-officio members   –   Midwifery Manager of the Birth Unit.
                         Hospital Manager.

* The obstetric representative of the MRMC will also sit as a member of the Hospital Medical Advisory Committee representing his/her colleagues (obstetricians, paediatricians, anaesthetists, and midwives) who work on the Birth Unit.

3   *Confidentiality and adherence of consultants and midwives wishing to work on the Birth Unit to the Terms of Reference*

Any consultant or any midwife who has applied to work on the Birth Unit, must sign before they are appointed that they have read and accept the Guidelines of the Birth Unit and the Terms of Reference of the MRMC, and that they will agree to keep all matters discussed or circulated by the MRMC as confidential.

4   *Meetings of the MRMC*

a   Any member of staff who has been responsible for the care of a patient whose case history is to be discussed by the MRMC will be expected to attend that meeting. In the event of the patient having had midwife-led care, both the midwife involved in the care at the time of the "adverse event", and the consultant under whom she was nominally booked, will be invited to attend the meeting.

b   All members of the MRMC, and those to be invited to the next meeting, will be informed by the Risk Manager of that meeting at least 3 weeks before it is due.

c   In the event of a member being unable to attend a meeting of the MRMC, he/she may nominate a suitable locum with the consent of the Chairman.

d   In the event of a member of staff, who is responsible for the care of a patient with a history which is to be considered by the MRMC, being unable to attend the appointed meeting, the case will be deferred until the next meeting when it *must* be discussed, unless in exceptional circumstances the Chairman decides otherwise.

e   Any individual with specialist expertise relevant to a case to be discussed, can be invited by the Chairman to attend that item of business at a meeting of the MRMC.

f   All medical and midwifery staff who work on the Birth Unit are invited to attend one meeting of the MRMC of their choice in order to understand the workings of the Committee. They should give the Risk Manager notice, of at least one week, of their intention to attend. At his/her discretion the Chairman may refuse the request of any member of staff for a particular meeting.

g   All staff who are not members of the MRMC, but who are attending a meeting of the Committee, are entitled to see the papers of that meeting that are relevant.

5   *Functions of the Risk Manager*

a   She is responsible for bringing cases containing defined "adverse events" to the attention of the MRMC. She is entitled to request any members of staff involved in such a case to prepare a report on the events surrounding that case. This report must be returned to her at least 2 weeks before the meeting.

b   She will regularly present to the MRMC, audit data on the activities of the Birth Unit.

c   She will give at least 3 weeks' notice to all those being invited to attend the next meeting of the MRMC.

d   She will be responsible for creating the agenda, in consultation with the Chairman, keeping the minutes of all meetings, and for distributing the relevant papers to members and invited visitors.

e   She will be responsible for reminding members of the Committee who have agreed to take on a task(s) at the preceding meeting, that they should complete that task by the next meeting.

f   She will alert the Chairman to any possibly serious clinical incidents* or near misses** that may require urgent discussion. The reasons for either of these descriptions being applied to any case report discussed by the MRMC will be minuted.

* A clinical incident is any occurrence which is not consistent with professional standards of care of the patient or the routine operational policies of the organisation (CESDI Report – see item 7.2).

** A "near miss" has a case history with no defined adverse event but contains evidence that but for luck or skilful management, could have led to a major adverse event(s) (CESDI Report – see item 7.2).

6   *Functions of the Committee*

a   The MRMC will meet regularly every two months. The Chairman may decide to hold additional meetings or to defer a meeting with the agreement of the Committee.

b   In general, the MRMC will consider any item of business that the Risk Manager considers may have increased the risk to a mother(s) or baby(ies) whilst under the care of the Birth Unit. All cases of perinatal or maternal deaths and possible near misses will be on the agenda.

c   If a member of staff is considered by the MRMC to have been responsible for a clinical incident, the procedure outlined in item 7 will be implemented.

d   The MRMC may establish working groups for activities such as the creation or revision of protocols or the audit of particular clinical practice or any other subject which members consider relevant to the objectives of the Committee.

e   The Medical Advisory Committee have agreed that the MRMC will give their opinion of any doctor applying to work on the Birth Unit, before he/she is given Admitting Rights.

f   The Medical Advisory Committee may, at any time, ask the MRMC for advice on any matter relevant to maternity care, including complaints from patients.

7   *Procedures that will follow designation by the MRMC of care having resulted in a clinical incident*

a   The MRMC will only consider a clinical incident to have occurred if the following conditions are fulfilled:
i   a majority of the members of the MRMC after a vote have agreed this to be so.
ii   The individual responsible for providing care (a consultant if care has been consultant-led, and a midwife if it has been midwife-led) is present when the case is being discussed by the MRMC. (See item 4.4d.)

b   When a clinical incident has occurred, the MRMC will use the CESDI* system for grading suboptimal care which is as follows:
i   Grade 1 – Suboptimal care, but different management would not have altered the outcome.
ii   Grade 2 – Suboptimal care – different management might have made a difference to the outcome.
iii Grade 3 – Suboptimal care would reasonably have been expected to have made a difference to the outcome.

* *Confidential Enquiry into Still Births and Deaths in Infancy* (CESDI 1999) p. 11, *6th Annual Report of the Maternal and Child Health Consortium*, 188 Baker Street, London NW1 5SI.

c   The following action will be taken when a clinical incident is designated by the MRMC as being associated with any degree of suboptimal care: -
i   The Medical Advisory Committee will decide whether any recommendation(s)

should be made and appropriate action taken concerning the facilities available for the management of the case and whether procedures or protocols were available and adhered to which covered the case.

ii The Chairman will convey the views of the MRMC as soon as possible to those individuals who are considered to have contributed in any way to the suboptimal care.

d Action to be taken when suboptimal care (grade 3) is identified:

When the individual responsible is a consultant

i On the first occasion when care has been found to be suboptimal (grade 3) a verbal and written "warning" will be given by the Chairman to the individual concerned. This will include the reasons given by the MRMC for the designation.

ii On the second occasion, the individual will be given a "severe warning" by the Chairman. Issuing a "severe warning" implies that if a further case of suboptimal care occurs, there will be an automatic recommendation that the admitting rights of the consultant should be suspended by the Hospital (see item 7.4 for procedures to be adopted following this recommendation).

iii The MRMC may recommend suspension of Admitting Rights of a consultant, even if no previous "warnings" have been issued to him/her, if the circumstances are considered to be sufficiently serious to warrant such action being taken.

When the responsible individual is a midwife

i If, at any time, a midwife is involved in the delivery of suboptimal care, he/she should work closely with a named supervisor of midwives to address any identified deficiencies in practice (as laid down in the statutory framework for midwifery supervision.

ii Reference will also be made to the Local Supervising Authority (LSA) when appropriate. The LSA midwifery officer will decide whether suspension from practice is necessary.

e Suspension of Admitting Rights of a Consultant

This can occur after a recommendation by the MRMC and with the concurrence of the Chairman of the Medical Advisory Committee and the Hospital Manager.

When a consultant is suspended:

i He/she will be informed of the decision.

ii An Independent Board of Enquiry will be set up.

f The Composition of the Independent Enquiry Board will be:

i Two consultants not involved in any way with the Hospital, with expertise relevant to the case (usually two obstetricians, but alternatively, an obstetrician and a consultant paediatrician or anaesthetist, depending on the case history).

ii A lay member not involved with the MRMC and selected by the Chairman of the MRMC after discussion with the consultant involved in the case.

g The Board will function as follows:

i The Board may take evidence from any individual.

ii Full documentation of the case and any documents requested will be provided to the Board by the Risk Manager.

iii The consultant who is under investigation and/or the Board may have a legal representative(s) present at the Hearings of the Board.

h After the deliberations of the Board have been completed, the Board will decide if they agree that suspension of Admitting Rights was justified.

i If the Board agrees, they will be asked to recommend one of the following:
   – a period of retraining with withdrawal of admitting rights for a specified period of time of at least 3 months.
   – permanent withdrawal of admitting rights.

ii If the Board does not agree with the MRMC that suspension of Admitting Rights is justified, the suspended consultant will be reinstated with full Admitting Rights. However, the MRMC may still issue a "severe warning" to him/her.

i In the event of Admitting Rights being withdrawn from a consultant, the MRMC will appoint a consultant colleague to act as a mentor and friend to that consultant.

He/she will be responsible for ensuring that the period of retraining is properly supervised and carried out and will report back to the MRMC.

8 *Appointing the Chairman and Members of the MRMC*

a   The Chairman will hold office for three years, renewable for a further three years. He/she will be appointed after full discussion, with the consultants and midwives on the Birth Unit, and with the Chairman of the Medical Committee and the Hospital Manager. Only if consultation fails to produce any individual acceptable to the majority, may the outgoing Chairman hold an election. The Chairman elect may be invited to attend one or more meetings of the MRMC before taking up his/her appointment.

b   The three representatives of the consultants will serve n the MRMC for two years, renewable for a further two years. The appointments will be staggered to avoid all representatives standing down from the MRMC at the same time. Their appointment will follow full consultation with staff working on the Birth Unit. Only if this fails, may the Chairman call an election.

c   The lay member of the MRMC will serve for two years renewable for a further two. His/her appointment will be the result of consultation between the consultants and midwives working on the Birth Unit.

22 Clinical incident reporting

JONATHAN SECKER-WALKER,
SALLY TAYLOR-ADAMS

Human error is one of the major contributory causes of accidents. Joschek suggests that between 80 and 90% of the chemical industry's incidents involve human error, ranging from design faults to maintenance errors.[1] The fatality rate due to errors in medicine in the United States has been estimated to be the equivalent of three jumbo jets crashing every two days.[2] The aviation, nuclear power, transport, and chemical industries share many parallels with healthcare. They too operate in a complex socio-technical system, where serious incidents such as the Trident "Papa India" Air Crash (1972), Three Mile Island (1979), Bhopal (1985), Chernobyl (1986), the Herald of Free Enterprise (1987), and the Paddington rail accident (1999) have led to loss of life, negative media attention, large costs, and the introduction of more rigorous retrospective and prospective safety measures. Trusts will only be able to accurately identify their risk issues by full notification, recording, analysis and feedback of information, in relation to these adverse incidents. Continuous monitoring of incidents relies on staff reporting organisational process deficits as well as individual errors.

Learning the right lessons from past events

Incident reporting: the experience from other industries

Critical incident reporting was originally described by Flannagan in 1954 as a technique to improve safety and performance.[3] The concept arose from studies in the Aviation Psychology Program of the United

419

States Air Force during and after the Second World War.[4] The introduction of incident reporting systems assist organisations in understanding the size of the safety problem, for example lost-time accidents, staff/patient injuries, prioritisation of investment resources, desire to avoid repeat incidents, and a need to aid organisational learning.

Aviation accidents are always public, whereas many accidents in medicine go unreported. Yet both industries can be conceptualised as sociotechnical and the problems associated with blame, lack of motivation to report incidents, etc. are similar across industries and organisations. It is therefore vital that medicine learns from the mistakes of other industries and utilises the "best practices" in incident reporting. In both aviation and the nuclear power industry, successful incident reporting systems have the following attributes.

1 There is a balance of incident-reporting activities, whereas in healthcare, though a huge resource is placed on data collection, only limited resources are in place to rigorously analyse data and rectify faults based on this analysis.
2 Incident reporting is complemented by methods to understand why people sometimes succeed/fail, such as prospective safety assessment. The tools and techniques used by safety professionals in other industries may also be of help in medicine, for example task analysis, human reliability assessment, failure modes and effects analysis.[5,6]
3 Positive outcome incidents are investigated, so organisations can learn which factors lead to successful outcomes.
4 A corpus of similar cases is investigated and analysed, so as to avoid idiosyncratic case features.

Woods (see Table 22.1), has identified four basic activities relevant to an iterative loop incident reporting system, which allow organisations the opportunity to learn effectively from their organisational accidents.[7] Each phase of the iterative loop will be explained in more detail.

a. Input

The data acquisition or input phase suggests that the system needs to be independent and non-punitive to enhance a safety learning culture. An incident reporting system lacking these attributes is doomed to fail.

b. Data

To facilitate learning at the data phase of the iterative loop, a reliance on the primacy of narratives must be emphasised. It is therefore vital that the staff and patient involved in the incident are given the opportunity to provide their version of events. Obviously secondary data sources such as medical records, protocols and other pertinent material must be reviewed where appropriate, but these should complement the information received

Table 22.1 Sample Issues in the Iterative Loops in Incident Reporting, Woods (1998)

Activity	Issues
a. Input	• Non-punitive • Independent
b. Data	• Primacy of narratives • Indexing
c. Analysis	• Expertise • Effort after learning • Sets of contrasting cases • Targeted issues/themes • Proactive learning/reactive studies • Linking what happens with why
d. Feedback	• Multiple feedback and organisational learning • Demonstrate learning to practitioners • Co-ordinate with other methods • Separate learning from interventions

from staff and patient. Learning about human performance requires capturing the multitude of factors that link in the evolution of an incident, for example, context, psychological demands of the task, etc.[8] Data on these factors can be used to build up patterns and trends across incidents. Healthcare, like many other industries, has developed classification schemes to organise and categorise data meaningfully. However, these classification systems can obscure, simplify or discard cases, thus preventing organisational learning from system failure.

Due to the problems associated with classification, the Aviation Safety Reporting System (ASRS) utilise an indexing system to collect related subsets of narrative cases from a database that pertains to a theme or question.[9] Therefore a detailed textual chronology of the event is obtained and stored electronically. This allows the database to be interrogated more thoroughly by key-word searches, which is less restrictive.

c. Analysis

The third phase is concerned with case analysis. (See Chapter 23 for a review of an investigative and analysis tool developed for medical accident analysis.) Woods suggests this phase requires the use of experts; system, speciality, and human performance (or safety) experts who can interrogate the data and generate meaningful learning recommendations.[7] The use of safety experts outside medicine can offer a useful dimension to understanding accident causation. Often these individuals will question the system standards and set-up and will be less accepting of organisational culture inhibitors. These practitioners are also trained in disciplines such as ergonomics, human factors, and proactive safety methodologies, thus

421

making them an ideal member of the accident analysis team. It is probable that the analysis phase will be the lengthiest and will require experts to link system failures (what happened) with reasons why. Where possible it is also important for experts to review similar cases to identify any trends and to facilitate further organisational learning. Obviously, within a healthcare setting, it is often only the various serious incidents that are investigated fully. Therefore it seems sensible that if a standardised investigation and analysis methodology was adopted within medicine, cases could be stored on a database which other trusts could access to help facilitate organisational learning and adopt a more proactive safety culture.

d. Feedback

Finally, the goal of feedback is to learn from mistakes and to ensure that the system performs better in the future. This requires all parties involved in the change to share ideas, abandon defensiveness and put blame and recriminations aside. Therefore lessons learnt from accidents must be fed down through all members of an organisation. Where staff can see something positive has been achieved through incident reporting, it is more likely to facilitate continued participation in the process. System changes that follow accident analysis are not the end of the process; it is vital that these changes are monitored either through audit or other proactive safety mechanisms to ensure the changes are having the required positive effect and that they are not negatively impacting other sub-systems or processes. Safety is an on-going proactive and reactive process, which requires the assistance and co-operation of all staff.

Incident reporting: in healthcare

In the United States in the 1950s, and before the overwhelming increase in litigation that was to occur in the 1970s, most litigation concerning medical injury was directed against hospitals and their nursing staff as opposed to their medical staff. Most early risk management using the reporting of problems was directed at reducing patient falls, medication errors, mis-identification of patients, and retained swabs at operation. As an example of success, review of reports led to the recommendation of a third swab count at skin closure, which in turn led to a precipitous drop in retained swabs and resultant claims.[10]

Dentistry was the first medical speciality to introduce this approach into their medical speciality.[11] Thereafter it was introduced into nursing and pharmacy.[12] Anderson et al confirmed the validity and reliability of the critical incident technique in 1964.[13] The technique was then introduced as a mechanism to study patient care by surgeons, physicians, paediatricians, and obstetricians in the early 1970s. It was not until 1978 that Cooper et al used this approach to improve patient safety.[14] This work has stimulated ongoing research throughout the world.[15,16,17,18] All of these early efforts tended to focus exclusively on "critical incidents", with their innate implication of both "error" and preventability.[17] This approach was applicable in these early studies to emphasise the fact that errors are normal.[19] Morgan has suggested that any positive (potentially good for the patient) or negative (potentially harmful to the patient) constitutes valid data for incident reporting and safety improvement.[20]

An untoward incident is an event which gives rise to, or has the potential to produce, unexpected or unwanted effects involving the safety of patients, users or other persons. Incident reporting is a process whereby a hospital worker is required to fill in a form when a patient has been harmed, or there has been the potential for harm.[21] In some jurisdictions and according to the American Hospital Association, an incident is whenever there has been a significant departure from the routine care of a patient.[22] It is up to individual trusts to define and agree their incident definition, a simple wide-ranging definition, derived from the Hospital for Sick Children in Toronto and used by many UK trusts is

> *any occurrence which is not consistent with the routine care of the patient or the routine operation of the institution, whilst a near-miss can be defined as an occurrence which but for luck or skilful management would in all probability have become an incident.*

The Clinical Negligence Scheme for Trusts (CNST) was set up in 1995 "to protect Trusts against the effects of the higher and relatively infrequent clinical negligence claims . . ." The CNST has established a comprehensive set of 14 clinical risk management standards, one of which is the introduction of a clinical incident reporting system. In Wales, the Welsh Risk Pool has set up similar – but not identical – standards and one of these requires a clinical incident reporting system and database.

Purpose of incident reporting

The primary purpose of incident reporting in clinical risk management is to reduce injuries to patients and staff. Incident reporting permits the collection of trust wide incident data and this allows the analysis of trends that may identify organisational, system and environmental problems. These problems may increase the likelihood of human error.

In addition, early warning of specific incidents allows the Trust to investigate the problem rapidly, collect witness statements whilst recollection is fresh, and secure the relevant medical records, pathology, CTGs, and imaging reports. This allows the trust to investigate the incident and recommend an early position on probable liability, which is likely to reduce legal costs. An empirical study by Lindgren *et al* in 1989–90 was undertaken to confirm or deny the contention that incident reporting could improve claims management and legal outcomes.[23]

423

The results suggested that early warning by incident reporting could identify claims worthy of early indemnity payments, facilitate the opening and closing of claims more quickly and produce substantial savings in legal costs. Early warning of an accident from an incident report also allows the organisation to manage any subsequent media coverage in a proactive manner instead of being caught on the back foot. Finally and perhaps most important, the structured analysis of specific incidents allows lessons to be learnt to improve future practice.

Why current clinical incident reporting systems do not work

The reporting and analysis of adverse incidents seems at face value a worthwhile undertaking. However, little is known about the effectiveness of the systems in detecting cases that lead to complaints or claims, or about their broader use in enhancing the quality and safety of care provided. Examination of trends in databases that record incidents will be unreliable unless all incidents are reported. Certain types of events might be reported more often than others and so give a misleading impression of their true nature and frequency. It is crucial, therefore, to establish the reliability of incident reporting schemes if they are to be relied upon as an accurate data source within hospitals.

Research from the United States, where risk management programmes have a considerably longer history and development time than the UK, would suggest that the degree to which incident reporting provides early warning of a claim varied greatly across 30 hospitals. It also varies within hospitals by specialty with obstetrics, gynaecology and paediatrics having pre-warning of claims 68% of the time whilst other specialties are under 50%.[24] Few studies have tested the efficacy of clinical incident reporting systems. O'Neil et al found that although physicians reported 89 adverse medical events compared with the 85 uncovered by retrospective case note review, only 41 of these related to the same patients.[25] Other studies have shown that about 30% of anaesthetic incidents and just 6% of adverse drug events were reported.[26,27] A study of errors made in an intensive care unit showed that 48 were reported by the clinical staff but that 78 errors were noted by trained observers over the 24-hour period investigated.[28] To examine the reliability of adverse incident-reporting systems in the UK, Stanhope et al examined the reliability of adverse incident reporting systems by retrospectively reviewing obstetric notes at two London teaching hospitals.[29] From 500 deliveries, 196 adverse incidents were identified. Staff reported 23% of these and the risk managers identified a further 22%. The remaining 55% of incidents were identified only by retrospective case note review and not known to the risk manager. Staff reported 48% of serious incidents (incidents likely to result in complaints and/or litigation) 24% of moderately serious and 15% of minor incidents. The risk managers identified an additional 16% of serious incidents that staff did not report. We can therefore conclude that current adverse incident reporting does not reveal the true number of incidents that occur.

If adverse incident reporting is to become a reliable tool for detecting problems and monitoring changes to systems and procedures, it is clearly important that incident reporting rates are improved. However, to understand why less that a quarter of incidents are reported via incident reporting systems we need to understand why reporting is so low. Vincent *et al* suggest that the main reasons why clinicians do not report incidents centre on junior staff feeling they will be blamed, high workload, and the belief (even though the incident was designated as reportable) that the circumstances or outcome of a particular case did not warrant a report.[30] It was also found that 30% of clinical staff did not know how to find a list of reportable incidents.

Prerequisites for a successful clinical incident reporting system

Establishing and maintaining a successful clinical incident reporting system is not an easy task. Success of a system is dependent on a change of culture within the organisation, where staff must be convinced of the importance of safety. This is probably best achieved by staff being the catalysts for change and seeing organisational safety developments. Experience from America, Australia and of introducing risk management programmes into UK hospitals, suggests that there are important steps to take at the beginning of the process that are usually common to all institutions.

1 The Trust Board and the Risk Management Committee

The board must make clear its position on disciplinary policy and incident reporting. Staff are unlikely to report mistakes and accidents if they fear for their job. Once the board has agreed a "no-blame" culture the committee should ensure that staff reporting incidents or near-misses are not subject to discipline unless the behaviour deviates from the board's published policy.

The role of the Risk Management Committee should be to provide a systematic and strategic approach to the management of all clinical, and health and safety risks within the trust.[31] The committee should establish and maintain a timetable for an ongoing programme of risk assessment throughout the trust and receive reports from areas that have been surveyed. The committee should monitor the level of compliance with the insurer's risk management standards. Regular reports of trust-wide incident trends and receipt of recommendations after specific incident investigations are a significant part of the committee's business.

The development of clinical directorates in many trusts has often clarified the vertical chain of command from trust board to clinical area but at the expense of managing the horizontal forces working in the organisation. These horizontal forces may relate to the resident pathogens that Reason describes with latent human failure.[8] For example, infection surveillance and control crosses most directorate boundaries as does pathology requests, reporting, and medical records. The Risk Management Committee will act as a means of horizontal scanning for fault lines in the trust where an incident occurrence is too infrequent for one directorate to take much note of but may be significant trust-wide. It should therefore receive regular reports from committees that monitor horizontal or cross-directorate factors in the organisation, such as the Control of Infection Committee, the Clinical Audit Committee, the Drug and Therapeutics Committee, the Resuscitation Committee, the Blood Transfusion Committee and other monitors of clinical performance.

The Risk Management Committee should be composed of senior staff who have the ability to effect change within the organisation and ideally should have the medical director, the director of nursing and the risk manager as members.

2 Incident and Claims Review Committee (see also Chapter 28)

Formation of an Incident and Claims Review Committee (ICRC) provides an excellent and instructive mechanism for learning lessons from patient incidents – often the precursor to a claim or complaint – and for taking an early view of the standard of care and the degree by which it was, or was not, below that which should be expected.[32]

Experience suggests that about a quarter of incidents are definitely defensible, a quarter indefensible and half are less easy to determine. Trusts usually have senior medical staff with considerable medico-legal experience who are more than capable of deciding such matters. There will be a few occasions when outside expert opinion should be sought.

The Committee's role is to:

- review clinical incidents where risk management considers litigation possible
- review relevant clinical complaints or claims
- monitor the progress of litigation already underway
- recommend improvements in practice arising from consideration of the cases
- advise the chief executive whether care provided met, fell below, or, exceeded the established standard of care together with the issue of causation.

Analysis of the incident into its component parts as described by Reason should allow the committee to recommend to the clinical directors changes and modifications in the rendering of care that is likely to reduce risk and lead to improved practice in the future.[8] Vincent has described a structure for the investigation of incidents.[33] However, a simple mnemonic DIME (Defences, Individual, Management, Environment) should help the committee remember to consider the four major stages of accident progression. Discussion of cases can be either in the presence of the clinician involved or in their absence. There are advantages and disadvantages to both methods, although overall the former probably facilitates a more open style of discussion and subsequent recommendation.

A decision to settle may be taken on economic grounds despite the ICRC having assessed the case as showing a good standard of care, and in these cases it will be of significant comfort to the individual clinician concerned that they have had the support of their peers. The committee should also make clear any specific recommendations for improving clinical process or practice in the light of discussions about the case. These recommendations should be discussed and agreed with clinical directors, implemented and then tested for compliance by audit after an appropriate interval of time.

3 Which indicators should be reported?

There are some events that occur within medicine and surgery that indicate that something in the disease process or the treatment has caused damage to the patient that was not expected, such as cardiac arrest or the development of paraplegia after surgery. These events are usually not related to negligence but maybe so viewed by the patient or their relatives. To keep track of these events or indicators, it is important that clinical staff recognise the need for themselves, their junior staff, or nursing colleagues to report them to the risk manager. An important component of a successful incident reporting system centres on an agreed system for the reporting of clinically related patient incidents and near misses. It is therefore essential for a trust to develop an agreed set of terms to describe incidents across specialties. Many core sets of indicators have been developed, for example by the JCAHO, the Maryland Hospital Association in the USA, the UK Quality Indicator Project; the medico-legal claims administrators LADD in South Australia. MMI Companies Inc., after research into its claims, has developed speciality-specific indicators in perinatal care, anaesthesia, surgery, emergency medicine, and other specialities.

The company has demonstrated a reduction in the number and value of claims if its simple guidelines are followed, for example, the use of fetal monitoring whenever oxytocin is used.[31]

The California medical insurance feasibility study in the mid-1970s discovered that out of 20 criteria looked for in the review of 20 864 casenotes, 11 identified virtually all the injuries and adverse outcomes discovered; see box below.[34] However, it is important to point out that only a small proportion of these events – 8.8% – were judged to be due to clinically caused injuries or adverse outcomes. These today, with the exception of admission in the previous 6 months and with the addition of unplanned admission to ITU from within the hospital, can be considered useful as general indicators to be reported as clinical incidents.

Generic adverse event indicators[34]

- Admission in the previous 6 months
- Admission for conditions suggesting prior failure or adverse result of treatment
- Trauma incurred in hospital
- Unplanned return to surgery
- Unplanned removal of an organ during surgery
- Acute MI during the admission
- Wound infection
- Neurological deficit occurring during the admission
- Death (unexpected) in hospital
- LOS exceeding 90th percentile for the region
- Unlisted complication of clinical management

It is, however, the authors' opinion that UK Trusts should develop their own speciality-specific clinical indicators relevant to national practice to aid analysis. One of the duties of the Risk Management Committee should be to review a list of "indicators". Most are self evidently the possible precursors of claims and whilst the core sets may apply to most specialties, individual specialties such as theatres, obstetrics and paediatrics may wish to develop their own. Involvement of junior and senior staff in the development of indicators is vital to their acceptance and use within a department.[35] The box on page 429 provides an example of a list of indicators developed by specialist clinical staff; see Appendix 22.1 for further examples of indicator lists.

4 How to report clinical incidents

All trust staff need to be educated about the purpose and benefits of risk management, including the incident reporting system, on a regular and continuous basis. Risk management also needs to form a part of the induc-

---

**Example clinical indicator lists from mental health and
paediatrics mental health indicators**
(Courtesy of North Herts NHS Trust)

- Overdose taken by in-patient on unit or while on leave
- Deliberate self-harm by patient
- Discovery of an object in patient's possession that could be used for self-harm
- Discharge against medical advice by a patient not detoxing from alcohol or drugs
- Absconding from unit
- Fire-setting in unit
- Unexpected/sudden death in unit or outside of a patient known to mental health services
- Patient requesting to see their medical notes
- Serious physical assault or aggression
- Discovery of illicit drugs/alcohol on unit
- Correspondence from solicitor suggesting litigation
- Injury of unknown origin
- Drug error

---

tion programme. Staff specifically need information on what to report, how, when and why it is relevant, see the box on page 430 for an example.

To encourage early reporting of incidents, it is essential that the reporting system is simple. The reporting form should be concise and contain as many aids as possible to ease completion, for example, tick boxes. Many trusts have introduced a single incident form covering clinical, health and safety, and security risks. It is sensible to route the forms to a single destination so that staff do not have to worry about where to send them. It is then essential to ensure that the forms reach the appropriate managers (occupational health for example) in good time, by use of fax, for example. Forms should be completed by the person who notices the incident, irrespective of whether this person was involved in the incident or not.

The incident reporting system should operate outside the disciplinary procedure (unless the incident is malicious or criminal). Completed incident reporting forms are disclosable in the event of litigation. It is therefore important that details are accurate and factual and do not contain opinions or apportion blame. Completed incident reporting forms should be assessed by the relevant personnel (clinician, risk manager, etc.) within 24 hours and appropriate remedial action taken. As an aid to indicating the priority for action, incidents may be graded for severity, see Tables 22.2 and 22.3.

A sample clinical incident, indicators and reporting strategy

A 44-year-old man attended the day surgery unit for a diagnostic laparoscopy at 1130 on Friday. The consultant was on holiday and a locum specialist registrar undertook the procedure. Postoperatively the patient felt too unwell to go home and was admitted to the surgical ward overnight. The surgical on-call team of SHO and Sp Reg for Saturday felt the patient might have signs of some intra-abdominal bleeding and adopted a wait and see policy. The (different) on-call team on Sunday felt that some peritonism was present and when the consultant returned from leave to do rounds on the Monday morning, frank peritonitis was present. The patient was taken to theatre at 1400 and needed admission to ITU post-operatively. He died two weeks later after suffering septicaemia and adult respiratory distress syndrome.

Incident Reported by: ICU Ward Manager

Date Reported: Monday pm, after admission to ITU

Indicators: admission after day-surgery, unscheduled return to theatre, unscheduled admission to ITU, perioperative death.

Reporting System Instituted: telephoned risk manager and completed clinical incident reporting form, which was then sent to risk manager

Resulting change in practice: After a full investigation and review of this case the trust discovered it had no formal policy covering consultant staff directly deputising for colleagues on holiday – hence no direct supervision of contents of operating lists or regular consultant led ward rounds – they only had rotas that ensured "on-call" cover for the unit.

---

5 Rating the level of risk

Risk can be considered in terms of the likelihood of it occurring and the severity of the consequences if it does. To allow trains to continue to run at speed in the absence of functioning signals is an example of high likelihood and great severity. It is possible therefore to allocate some sort of score to a reported incident. The greater the score, the more individuals or

Table 22.2 Incident Risk Level Estimator Risk Rating Chart

Frequency *Severity*	V Likely 4	Likely 3	Less Likely 2	Unlikely 1
V Severe 4	16	12	8	4
Serious 3	12	9	6	3
Less Serious 2	8	6	4	2
Not Serious 1	4	3	2	1

Table 22.3 Risk Rating Calculation

Potential Frequency □ × Potential Severity □ = □ Risk Rating Number (RRN)

Using the Incident Risk Level Estimator in Table 22.2 consider what the frequency of the risk is and what the potential outcome may be based on the information on the incident form. Use the RRN number to decide action required.

RRN	Situation	Action
16–12	Intolerable, Unacceptable,	Stop Activity
6–9	Substantial, Very High Risk	
3–4	Moderate, Significant Risk	
1–2	Tolerable, Low Risk	

the organisation are at risk. The grid below (see Tables 22.2 and 22.3) has been adapted by the Clinical Risk Management Department at the University Hospital of Wales from that used and published by the Health and Safety Department at the University of Wales College of Medicine.

Categorisation of incidents can be made a complicated procedure. It is likely that the more complicated it becomes, the less compliance is achieved. Using the very simple scoring system illustrated in Table 22.3 allows a Risk Rating Number (RRN) to be assigned to the incident. This will never be an exact science but it does allow a rough and ready guide to the level at which various risks should be considered – perhaps very high scores should always be reported to the medical director; general managers should review all scores above 8 etc.

Other rating systems have been reported, for example that of Roberts and that used at Worcester Royal Infirmary.[35,36]

6 Data management

Incident forms should be sent to a central point for collation and placement on a database. The database needs to be compatible with the incident form. The stark choice is to use a relatively unstructured simple form, which promotes improved compliance from staff, or a longer, rigid tick-box form that staff generally dislike. The problem with the former is that the data-inputter needs to be able to interpret the data on the form into consistent coded format. This requires considerable training and intelligence to do a job that is intrinsically seriously boring. The structured form can be handled by any data-inputter as no interpretation is required.

Much time is expended by risk managers and their support staff in the data input of incidents to software systems, leaving minimal time to interrogate the data. Most incident reporting systems become overwhelmed by slips and falls in the elderly or violence in mental health. Future development should consider the introduction of scanner read incident reporting forms to speed up this process. To do this would require a simple one-sided form to allow the report to be completed on screen on site. In the long run the solution must be to have the system networked to clinical work areas and this would allow hospital staff to record incidents directly via a networked incident reporting system. This solution creates problems about data access and data management – which are soluble. The decision then needs to be made as to which data items are essential to collect – the minimal dataset. It is probable that too much data is currently collected, much of which will never be recalled or be of any use.

The use of relational databases or other semi-intelligent computer software allows risk managers to examine the data for trends and assess areas of concern. There are several suitable incident-reporting databases on the market. The most important requirement is that the system can manage incidents, complaints and claims as separate modules and yet have common databases relating to patients, staff, locations, directorates and so on, thus ensuring that patterns occurring can be recognised. Simple clear screens without too many fields, simple to use look-up tables in alphabetical order, and ease of producing reports, both written and graphical, are some of the features that make it likely that the data-inputter will stay in post.

The adverse incident reporting system must produce reports that are timely and informative for the risk management committee. The system should identify areas where certain adverse incidents are occurring with a frequency that suggests some abnormality in process. A true example of this was increasing numbers of reports that day-surgery patients were not being adequately assessed pre-operatively. Analysis of the data indicated which surgical specialities were most involved and the clinical director and directorate manager were informed and provided with the data. Organisational changes were instituted to provide a dedicated patient assessment clinic and the problem was largely resolved.

The risk manager needs to be trained on how to identify significant adverse clinical incidents, that is, events likely to lead to a complaint, claim or adverse media attention. Further to this, risk managers require training on how to investigate and analyse adverse clinical incidents systematically (for further information, see Chapter 23).

7 Ensure organisational learning by providing regular feedback to staff

The experience of most hospital staff is that clinical incident forms depart for a black box, never to be seen again. The risk manager should endeavour to provide regular feedback to staff following incident reporting, with the provision of incident trends by type and frequency. The motivation of staff to report adverse clinical incidents is enhanced if they see that risk management has positively improved the system. For example: following a continued trend of third degree tears in obstetrics, staff were provided with training; an elderly and unreliable operating table in a delivery room was replaced after pressure from the risk management committee placed it first in the annual capital equipment programme; incident reports about bed shortages and inappropriate trauma patients as outliers in medical beds prompted a review of bed allocation across the trust. Following adverse incident reporting which has led to an event being investigated and analysed, it is vital that staff feel supported and are provided with feedback. This will lead to positive reinforcement for the programme as staff notice that action follows their use of the form.

A trust can establish an adverse clinical incident reporting system, which is working well, within a short time to produce the following advantages:

- early identification of risks
- early communication with injured patients (and with staff to reduce the likelihood of subsequent injuries)
- improved handling of clinical complaints
- reduction of solicitor's bills
- potential for reduced premiums if subscribing to the central fund or other insurance
- using a concurrent claims database, more accurate projections of future likely liability
- identifiable improvements in the quality of clinical care.

8 How to make adverse incident reporting work

It has been suggested that the following should be implemented within trusts to improve staff reporting of clinical adverse incidents.

Making adverse incident reporting work

1   Induction training for all clinical and nursing staff (permanent, locum and agency) on risk management and incident reporting
2   Continuing education on the aims and importance of risk management and incident reporting
3   A clear statement that all members of staff, regardless of profession and grade are responsible for reporting
4   A clearly defined list of reportable incidents/indicators drawn up in consultation with medical and nursing staff and a clear definition of incidents to be reported
5   User friendly incident reporting forms (one side of A4, tick box, minimal writing, etc.)
6   Clarity on how to report
7   Encouragement for staff to report an incident even if they are unsure whether it is necessary to do so
8   A designated person on shift who is responsible for checking that any incident occurring during that shift is reported
9   A trust/hospital policy of no blame and no disciplinary action except in cases of gross misconduct, repeated errors despite retraining, or criminal negligence
10   Regular feedback to staff regarding the action taken as a result of their reports[33]
11   Design of corrective strategies to reduce undesirable incidents in the future
12   Introduction into clinical practice of these specific corrective strategies by general consensus
13   Re-evaluation of the efficacy of introduced corrective strategies by continued accident reporting.[17]

Conclusion

Clinical risk management needs to be introduced in a fairly structured manner into a trust for the first time. Reporting of incidents in hospitals that involve staff and patients – as opposed to adverse events involving patients – has been required in both North American and European hospitals for many years and is part of health and safety legislation. NHS trusts therefore have the basic mechanisms for incident reporting already in position and this process needs to be extended to include incidents occurring to patients. It is helpful if the medical staff are persuaded that it is a supportive process and they understand the human factors science that lies behind the various components of risk management. In time, the organisational culture should allow for clinical incident reporting to be an accepted and natural part of the work of the directorate and seen as a quality measure that allows improvement in clinical care by learning lessons from particular incidents.

It is easy to become obsessed by the need to fill in a form in order to report an incident; however any means of communication, telephone, e-mail or corridor conversation with the risk manager should be welcomed – provided the latter makes a note of it. Whilst it is the responsibility of the directorate managers to receive incident reports and act on them, the analysis of trends across the trust or in individual directorates will generally be carried out by the risk manager. This task needs to be combined with a good working knowledge of the trust, since staff will often use incident reporting to make particular points when management is perceived to be failing to listen or to improve situations.

A typical example will be reporting of staff shortages in a particular ward when the nurses become frustrated by lack of any improvement. This does not undermine the use of the reporting system, since it should send clear signals to the manager or clinical director that the staff is expressing anxiety about safety, which is likely to be genuine. The problem with biased reporting is that it misrepresents trends of incidents, thus altering the risk profile and care needs to be taken when interpreting this data.

References

1 Joschek HI. Risk assessment in the chemical industry. In: *Proceedings of the ANS/ENS Topical Meeting on Probabilistic Risk Assessment*. Port Chester, New York: American Nuclear Society, Sept, 1981.
2 Leape L. Error in medicine. *JAMA* 1994;**272**(23):1851–7.
3 Flannagan JC. The critical incident technique. *Psychological Bull* 1954;**51**:327–58.
4 Banks IC, Tackley RM. A standard set of terms for critical incident recording. *Br J Anaesth* 1994;**73**:703–8.
5 Kirwan B. *Human reliability assessment: an integrated approach*. London: Taylor and Francis, 1995.
6 Kirwan B, Ainsworth LK. *A guide to task analysis*. London: Taylor and Francis, 1993.
7 Woods D. Learning from incidents. In: *Proceedings of Conference on Enhancing Patient Safety and Reducing Errors in Health Care*. Nov 8–9, 1998.
8 Reason JT. The human factor in medical accidents. In: Vincent C, Ennis M, Audley RJ, eds. *Medical accidents*. Oxford: OUP, 1993.
9 Billings CE. Some hopes, and concerns, regarding medical event reporting systems: lessons from the NASA Aviation Safety Reporting System (ASRS) 1998. *Arch Pathol Lab Med*; 122:3:214–15.
10 Mills DH, von Bolschwing GE. Clinical risk management: experiences from the United States. In: Vincent C, ed. *Clinical risk management*. London: BMJ Publications, 1995.
11 O'Donnell RJ. The development and evaluation of a test for predicting dental student performance. *University Pittsburgh Bulletin* 1953;**49**:240–3.
12 Safren MA, Chapanis A. A critical incident study of hospital medication errors. Part 2. *Hospitals* 1960;**34**;53.
13 Anderson B, Nilsson S. Studies in the reliability and validity of the critical incident technique. *J Appl Psychology* 1964;**48**:398–403.

14 Cooper JB, Newbower RS, Kitz RJ. An analysis of major errors and equipment failures in anaesthesia management considerations for prevention and detection. *Anaesthesiology* 1984;**60**:34–42.

15 Derrington MC, Smith G. A review of studies of anaesthetic risk, morbidity and mortality. *Br J Anaesth* 1987;**59**:815–33.

16 Cooper JB, Newbower RS, Long CD, McPeek B. Preventable anaesthesia mishaps: a study of human factors. *Anesthesiology* 1978;**49**:399–406.

17 Williamson JA, Webb RK, Pryor GL. Anaesthesia safety and the "critical incident" technique. *Aust J Clin Rev* 1985;**5**:57–61.

18 Tirat L, Desmonta JM, Hatton F, Vourc'h G. Complications associated with anaesthesia – a prospective survey in France. *Can Anaesth Soc J* 1986;**33**:336–44.

19 Reason JT. *Human error.* New York: Cambridge University Press, 1990.

20 Morgan C. Incident reporting in anaesthesia. *Anaesth Intensive Care* 1988;**16**:98–100.

21 Capstick B. Incident analysis and claims analysis. *Clinical Risk* 1995;**1**:165–7.

22 Robbins D. Incident report analysis: the experience of one large labour and delivery unit. *J Perinatal Neonatal Nurs* 1987;**1**:9–18.

23 Lindgren OH, Christensen R, Mills DH. Medical malpractice risk management early warning systems, *Law & Contemporary Problems* 1991;**54**:22–41.

24 Lindgren OH, Secker-Walker J. Incident reporting systems: early warnings for the prevention and control of clinical negligence. In: Vincent C, ed. *Clinical risk management.* London: BMJ Publications, 1995.

25 O'Neil AC, Petersen MD, Cook EF, *et al.* Physician reporting compared with medical-record review to identify adverse medical events. *Ann Intern Med* 1993;**119**:370–6.

26 Cullen DJ, Bates D, Small SD, *et al.* The incident reporting system does not detect adverse drug events: a problem for quality improvement. *Jt Communications J Qual Improvement* 1995;**21**:541–8.

27 Jayasuriya JP, Anandaciva S. Compliance with an incident reporting scheme in anaesthesia. *Anaesthesia* 1995;**50**:846–9.

28 Donchin Y, Gopher D, Olin M, *et al.* A look into the nature and causes of human errors in the intensive care unit. *Crit Care Med* 1995;**23**:294–300.

29 Stanhope N, Crowley-Murphy M, Vincent C, *et al.* An evaluation of adverse incident reporting. *J Eval Clin Pract* 1999;**5**:1,5–12.

30 Vincent C, Stanhope N, Crowley-Murphy M. Reasons for not reporting adverse incidents: an empirical study. *J Eval Clin Pract* 1999;**5**:(1)13–21.

31 Secker-Walker J. Clinical Risk Management. In: Lugon M, Secker-Walker J, eds. *Clinical governance: making it happen.* London: RSM Press, 1999.

32 Lugon M. Claims management. In: Lugon M, Secker-Walker J, eds. *Clinical governance: making it happen.* London: RSM Press, 1999.

33 Vincent C, Taylor-Adams SE, Chapman J, *et al. Protocol for the investigation and analysis of clinical incidents.* London: RSM Press, 1999.

34 Mills DH, ed. California Medical Association and California Hospital Association. *Report on the medical insurance feasibility study.* San Francisco: Sutter Publications, 1977.

35 Roberts G. Untoward incident reporting: quality improvement and control. *Clin Risk* 1995;**1**:168–70.

36 Dineen M. Worcester Royal Infirmary. Personal communication, 2000.

Appendix 22.1 – taken from Lugon and Secker Walker (1999)

Non-specific indicators that have been shown to be associated with claims of negligence

- Unexpected or trauma related deaths
- Brain damage or neurological deficit not present on admission
- Unexpected amputation due to poor outcome of any procedure or treatment

- Unplanned removal of an organ during surgery
- More extensive surgery than planned preoperatively
- Any unplanned return to the operating theatre
- Operations to repair damage due to an invasive or endoscopic procedure
- Failure to act upon an imaging or pathology result
- Pathology / image report to wrong patient
- Medication error, including infusion pump problems
- Hospital incurred trauma
- Equipment failure leading to patient injury
- Wrong patient or wrong side – surgery or radiology
- Self-harm or suicide
- Complication for which patient was not prepared
- Misdiagnosis
- Unplanned admission to ICU/HDU
- Swab/instrument count incorrect at end of procedure
- Absent medical notes
- Unplanned readmission within 5 days

Indicators in obstetrics may include:

Infant

- neonatal deaths
- stillbirths
- Apgar <4 at 5 minutes
- any paralysis
- subdural haematoma or tear of falx cerebri
- unanticipated admission to SCBU
- major congenital abnormality first detected at birth
- any fracture
- shoulder dystocia
- meconium aspiration
- fits in nursery within first 48 hours
- iatrogenic injury up to one week after birth
- drug errors
- very low birthweight (?<900 gm)

Mother

- maternal deaths
- transfer to ITU
- convulsions
- major anaesthetic problems, either GA or epidural
- PPH >1 litre or need for transfusion
- 30 minutes' delay in caesarean section
- soft tissue injury, 3rd degree tear, ruptured uterus, bladder injury
- injury caused by equipment
- drug errors

Care of the elderly (Courtesy of North Herts NHS Trust)

- Threatening behaviour
- Damage/loss of property
- Significant equipment failure
- Drug errors
- Failure of follow-up arrangements
- Failure to act on a clinically significantly abnormal result

- Falls leading to severe injury or bone fracture
- Injury due to equipment
- Lack of adequate equipment
- Missing patient
- Missing medical records
- Misfiled investigations
- Pressure sores grade 3 & 4 developing on ward
- Unable to contact doctor for ill patient
- Unprofessional behaviour by staff.

Paediatric Indicators (Courtesy of North Herts NHS Trust)

- Extravasation of iv fluid leading to tissue necrosis
- Drug dose or fluid prescription error or administration error
- Failure to recognise the severity of a baby or child's condition or recognise a serious diagnosis
- Child protection procedures not followed
- Problems during transportation to a tertiary referral centre
- Major organisational problems during resuscitation
- Failure to act on a pathology or imaging result
- Equipment failure impeding medical provision
- Unexpected death
- Delayed diagnosis of severe neonatal hyperbilirubinaemia
- Sustained hyperoxia grade 3 plus r.o.p. (neonates)
- Delayed diagnosis of important malformations
- Neonatal icu – accidental extubation > once in 24 hours

23 The investigation and analysis of clinical incidents

CHARLES VINCENT, SALLY TAYLOR-ADAMS

Why do things go wrong? Human error is routinely blamed for disasters in the air, on the railways, in complex surgery, and in healthcare generally. However quick judgements and routine assignment of blame obscure a more complex truth. The identification of an obvious departure from good practice is usually only the very first step of an investigation. While a particular action or omission may be the immediate cause of an incident, closer analysis usually reveals a series of events and departures from safe practice, each influenced by the working environment and the wider organisational context. While this more complex picture is gaining acceptance in healthcare,[1-3] it is seldom put into practice in the investigation of actual incidents.

In a series of papers[4-8] the Clinical Risk Unit, University College London, has developed a process of investigation and analysis of adverse events for use by researchers. Two years ago a collaborative research group was formed, between the Clinical Risk Unit and members of the Association of Litigation and Risk Management (ALARM). This group has adapted the research methods to produce a protocol for the investigation and analysis of serious incidents, for use by risk managers and others trained in incident analysis. The protocol gives a detailed account of the theoretical background, process of investigation and analysis, with detailed case examples and standard forms for use in the investigation process.[9] In this chapter we introduce the main ideas and present sections of two case analyses to illustrate the methods in practice.

The protocol is restricted to the process of analysis and investigation. In the case of a serious incident inquiry there will no doubt be many additional procedures to follow, explanations to many of the parties involved,

439

together with legal and perhaps media involvement. These are clearly all important matters, but beyond the scope of this chapter. However, we would suggest that subsequent decisions and actions would be more effective if grounded in a thorough and systematic investigation and analysis of the initial circumstance, irrespective of the nature of the incident and the complexity of the issues stemming from it.

Research foundations

The theory underlying the protocol and its application derives from research in settings outside healthcare. In the aviation, oil and nuclear industries for instance, the formal investigation of incidents is a well-established procedure.[10,11] Studies in these areas and in medicine have led to a much broader understanding of accident causation, with less focus on the individual who makes the error and more on pre-existing organisational factors. Such studies have also illustrated the complexity of the chain of events that may lead to an adverse outcome.[1,2,5,6] The root causes of adverse clinical events may lie in factors such as the use of locum doctors and agency nurses, communication and supervision problems, excessive workload, educational and training deficiencies.

In healthcare the development of prevention strategies from such analyses has not yet been fully exploited. However the potential for these approaches is apparent in other domains. For instance, the enquiry into the Piper Alpha oil disaster led to a host of recommendations and the implementation of a number of risk reduction strategies, which covered the whole industry and addressed a wide range of issues. These included the setting up of a single regulatory body for offshore safety, relocation of pipeline emergency shutdown valves, the provision of temporary safe refuges for oil workers, new evacuation procedures, and requirements for emergency safety training. Most interestingly oil companies had henceforth to actively demonstrate that hazards had been minimised and were as low as could reasonably be expected.[12-14]

In considering the general goals of incident analysis in any industry Hale[15] has distinguished between the traditional approach, strongly associated with judicial proceedings, and the standpoint of "organisational learning". The objectives of organisational learning are not to apportion blame, but to profit from the events that have taken place. Interestingly, among many other points, he suggests that it is not the exact sequence of events that is ultimately important, because that may be of such low probability that it can never recur. Rather, the accident is an opportunity to learn what the gaps and shortcomings were in the way the organisation managed the process or technology in which the accident occurred. This learning paradigm therefore has a completely different feel to it compared to the judicial. It is a mutual search for opportunities for improvement.

Reason's organisational accident model

The protocol and the methods described below are based on Reason's[3,11] organisational accident model. Reason's model was originally developed for use in complex industrial systems as a means of understanding the relationships between the various factors involved in the genesis of accidents, and to identify methods of accident prevention. The model is described in Chapter 1. We are only concerned in this chapter with practical methods of application.

The method of investigation implied by the model is first to examine the chain of events that leads to an accident or adverse outcome and consider the actions of those involved. The investigator then, crucially, looks further back at the conditions in which staff were working and the organisational context in which the incident occurred.

The first step in any analysis is to identify active failures – unsafe acts or omissions committed by those at the "sharp end" of the system (pilots, air-traffic controllers, anaesthetists, surgeons, nurses, etc.) whose actions can have immediate adverse consequences. These may be slips, such as picking up the wrong syringe, lapses of judgement, forgetting to carry out a procedure or, rarely, deliberate departures from safe operating practices, procedures or standards. In our work we have substituted the term "care management problems" (CMPs) for active failures. In practice, care management problems may encompass a series of active failures, such as failure to monitor over a period of time. Having identified the CMPs, however, the investigator then considers the conditions in which errors occur and the wider organisational context. These are the factors which influence staff performance, and which may precipitate errors and affect patient outcomes.

A framework for the analysis of risk and safety in medicine

We have extended Reason's model and adapted it for use in a healthcare setting, classifying the error producing conditions and organisational factors in a single broad framework of factors affecting clinical practice.[7]

At the bottom of the framework are "patient factors". In any clinical situation the patient's condition will have the most direct influence on practice and outcome. Other patient factors, such as personality, language and any disability may also be important as they can influence communication with staff, and hence the probability of an incident.

Higher up in the framework are individual (staff) and team factors. Individual factors include the knowledge, skills and experience of each

441

member of staff, which will obviously affect their clinical practice. Each staff member is part of a team within the inpatient or community unit, and part of the wider organisation of the hospital or mental health service. The way an individual practises, and their impact on the patient, is constrained and influenced by other members of the team and the way they communicate, support, and supervise each other. The team is influenced in turn by management actions and by decisions made at a higher level in the organisation. These include policies regarding the use of locum or agency staff, continuing education, training and supervision, and the availability of equipment and supplies. Management decisions also affect the conditions in which the team work, including staffing levels, workload, and the physical conditions of the building and the environment. The organisation itself is affected by the institutional context, including financial constraints, external regulatory bodies, and the broader economic and political climate. Each level of analysis can be expanded to provide a more detailed specification of the components of the major factors. For example, "Team factors" includes items on verbal communication between junior and senior staff and between professions, the quality of written communication such as the completeness and legibility of notes, and the availability of supervision and support (see Protocol for full framework).

Table 23.1 Framework of factors influencing clinical practice

Factor types	Influencing contributory factors
Institutional context	Economic and regulatory context
	National health service executive
	Clinical negligence scheme for trusts
Organisational and management factors	Financial resources & constraints
	Organisational structure
	Policy standards and goals
	Safety culture and priorities
Work environment factors	Staffing levels and skills mix
	Workload and shift patterns
	Design, availability and maintenance of equipment
	Administrative and managerial support
Team factors	Verbal communication
	Written communication
	Supervision and seeking help
	Team structure (congruence, consistency, leadership, etc.)
Individual (staff) factors	Knowledge and skills
	Competence
	Physical and mental health
Task factors	Task design and clarity of structure
	Availability and use of protocols
	Availability and accuracy of test results
Patient factors	Condition (complexity & seriousness)
	Language and communication
	Personality and social factors

Definitions and essential concepts

Reason's model and our framework provide the conceptual foundations of the investigation process. Before describing the actual procedural steps of the investigation we will be define some basic terms. These are all explained in greater detail below and examples are given in the two case analyses.

The incident

This is essentially something that happened to a patient, a clinical outcome probably with harmful or potentially harmful effects. The criteria for selection of an incident for investigation are discussed further below.

Care Management Problems (CMPs)

The CMPs are actions or omissions by staff in the process of care. They have two essential features, both of which are necessary for a CMP to be listed:

- Care deviated beyond safe limits of practice and
- The deviation had a direct or indirect effect on the eventual adverse outcome for the patient. (In cases where you cannot be sure of the impact on the patient it is sufficient that the CMP had a potentially adverse effect.)

Note that each CMP is to be identified individually and each will be analysed separately to examine the reasons for its occurrence. Examples of CMPs are given in the box below.

Examples of care management problems

Failure to monitor, observe or act
Delay in diagnosis
Incorrect risk assessment (e.g. of suicide or self harm)
Inadequate handover
Failure to note faulty equipment
Failure to carry out pre-operative checks
Not following an agreed protocol (without clinical justification)
Not seeking help when necessary
Failure to adequately supervise a junior member of staff
Incorrect protocol applied
Treatment given to incorrect body site
Wrong treatment given

Clinical context and patient factors

For each CMP identified, the investigator records the salient clinical events or condition of the patient at that time (for example, bleeding heavily, blood pressure falling) and other patient factors affecting the process of care (for example, patient very distressed, patient unable to understand instructions).

Specific contributory factors

For each CMP the investigator uses the framework (Table 23.1), both during the interview and afterwards, to identify the factors that led to that particular CMP. For example:

- Individual factors may include lack of knowledge or experience of particular staff
- Task factors might include the non-availability of test results or protocols
- Team factors might include poor communication between staff
- Work environment might include high workload or inadequate staffing.

All of these might contribute to the occurrence of a single CMP.

General contributory factors

A further distinction needs to be drawn between specific contributory factors and general conditions in the unit. The investigator should differentiate between those contributory factors that are only relevant on that particular occasion and those which are longstanding or permanent features of the unit or, in some cases, of a member of staff. For instance there may be a failure of communication between two midwives contributing to a care management problem. If this is unusual, and seldom occurs, then it is a specific contributory factor but not a general factor with wider implications. If, on the other hand, this problem is quite frequent then the investigator would also want to note a general contributory factor of "poor communication" which would have clear implications for the safe and effective running of that unit.

Similarly the investigator might ask:

- Does the lack of knowledge shown on this occasion imply that this member of staff requires additional training?
- Does this particular problem with this guideline mean that the whole guideline needs to be revised?
- Is the high workload due to a temporary and unusual set of circumstances, or is it a more general problem affecting patient safety?

Starting the investigation

Which incidents should be investigated?

Broadly speaking, an incident will either be investigated because of its seriousness for the patient, and perhaps for the organisation, or because of its potential for learning about the functioning of the clinical department or organisation. What marks out a serious incident as requiring detailed investigation is the nature, scale and consequences (see Chapter 22). Some incidents require immediate initial investigation, whilst others can wait a few hours (for example until the following morning).

For serious clinical incidents the protocol facilitates rapid, yet comprehensive and effective investigation. It will of course always be necessary to investigate serious incidents but this may not always be the most productive clinical risk management activity from the point of view of "organisational learning". There is much to be said for investigating a "near miss" or a well-handled incident, as these are less emotive and are not generally open to external scrutiny. Such "lesser" incidents may be just as fruitful in terms of revealing the strengths and weaknesses of the unit and the care process.

The investigation process

Reviewing the case records

Accounts of the incident may be taken from written reports of staff members, case notes or interviews with staff. The analysis may be limited if only written reports are considered, in that it may not be possible to explore the full range of conditions that allowed the event to occur. The first task, from the information immediately available, is to record the initial summary of the event and identify the most obvious CMPs. In some instances there may only be one, but nearly always several problems conspire to create the event. Make an initial summary of the principal events (an outline chronology), as recorded in the notes, before starting the interviews. Next list the key staff involved and decide who should be interviewed, and in what order to see them.

Framing the problem

The next task is to decide which section of the process of care to examine. This is not always straightforward. It depends less on the condition of the patient at any particular time and more on when and where problems first arose, which may only become apparent during the investigation.

For instance, a haemorrhage may have been badly managed leading ulti-mately to the patient's death two weeks later. The chronology may sum-marise three weeks of care, most of which may be of high standard. However the analysis will concentrate on those aspects where problems were apparent, for example, in the preparation for surgery, conduct of the surgery and postoperative monitoring, in order that appropriate lessons may be learnt.

Undertaking the interviews

Interviews should be undertaken in private and, if at all possible, away from the immediate place of work in a relaxed setting. The purpose of the interview is simply to find out what happened and this should be explained at the outset. The style adopted should be supportive and understanding, not judgmental or confrontational. Where it becomes clear that a profes-sional shortcoming has occurred, this should be allowed to emerge natu-rally from the conversation, and should not be extracted by cross examination. Most staff are genuinely disturbed when it becomes clear that something they have done has contributed to an incident. The staff mem-ber will normally require additional support at this point and should be allowed, through supportive discussion, to start to come to terms with what has happened.

The investigators and the person in charge of the unit must also decide early in their investigation, if events have been sufficiently traumatic, whether to send any member of staff off duty. This should not normally be considered as a suspension from duty, simply a compassionate mea-sure to enable recovery. The member of staff may also not be able to work safely and effectively in the immediate aftermath of an incident (see Chapter 25).

There are several distinct phases to the interview and it will generally be more effective to move through these phases in order. Each interview should take between twenty and thirty minutes depending on the degree of involvement. Ideally two interviewers are used, one leading the interview and the other taking notes and asking supplementary questions.

What happened? – Establishing the chronology and outcome

First the investigator should establish the role of the member of staff in relation to the incident as a whole and record the limits of their involvement. They then establish the chronology of events as the staff member saw them.

How did it happen? – Identifying the Care Management Problems (CMPs)

In the second phase, the investigator should first explain the concept of a care management problem. They then ask the member of staff to identify the main care management problems as they see them, without concerning themselves about whether or not anyone is or is not to blame for any of them. The task is to identify all important acts or omissions made by staff, or other breakdowns in the clinical process, that were (with hindsight) important points in the chain of events leading to the adverse outcome. Subsequent questions may elicit the reasons behind their actions (for example, Why did you not call for help at that stage?) and explore references to strong emotions, such as anxiety and anger, which sometimes highlight crucial points in the management of the patient.

Why did it happen? – Identifying the contributory factors

In the third phase, the investigator goes back and asks separately about each of the care management problems that the staff member may have information about or experience of. Questions should cover contributory factors at all levels of the framework (Table 23.1). Each care management problem may be associated with several factors at different levels of the framework that were implicated in its occurrence. These might include, for example, poor motivation (*Individual*), lack of supervision (*Team*) and inadequate training policy (*Organisation and Management*). Although the framework has higher level, organisational factors at the top, it may be more natural in clinical terms to begin by enquiring about patient factors, then moving up the table through task factors, individual, team and so on. The full protocol contains a much more detailed framework of factors, which may be helpful at this stage when formulating questions.

Distinguishing specific and general contributory factors

Where a member of staff identifies a clearly important contributory factor the investigator should be sure to ask a follow-up question. Was this factor specific to this occasion or would you regard this as a more general problem on the unit? The prevention of future incidents relies on identifying general, systemic problems, rather than isolated difficulties that are unlikely to recur.

Closing the interview

In previous analyses a contributory factors questionnaire (see Protocol) has performed well as a tool to get clinicians to think about the non-clinical factors that they felt affected their performance. It also acted as an effective prompt, jogging a person's memory about factors not mentioned in their account and as an encouragement to provide details about other issues they might otherwise have considered trivial and not worth mentioning. Finally the investigator should ask the staff member if they have any other comments to make or questions to ask.

447

Analysis of the case

The core of the process is to ask: What happened? How did it happen? Why did it happen? What can we learn from this and what changes should we make, if any? In the analysis the same basic format is followed, this time drawing together the material from the case records, interviews and the investigator's own observations.

The first step in the analysis is simply to produce an agreed chronology of events, identifying any important areas of disagreement between accounts or between the case notes and the memories of the staff. The starting point for the chronology will generally be the point at which the patient entered hospital, though relevant events before their arrival (for example, previous treatment, a misleading referral letter) may also need to be recorded. However it is then important to identify and focus on the most important part of the chronology (see "Framing the problem" above).

The next stage is to identify the key care management problems. These may be provided by the staff themselves or from the investigators' own clinical knowledge and expertise. The investigator should look back over the list and ensure that all the care management problems are specific actions or omissions on the part of staff, rather than more general observations on the quality of care, which should be recorded elsewhere. It is easy to note down "poor teamwork" as a care management problem, which may be a correct description of the team but should properly be recorded elsewhere as a contributory factor.

The next step is to attempt to specify the conditions associated with each of the care management problems, using the framework as a guide and as a way of reflecting on the many factors that may affect the clinical process. Interviews with staff will already have provided lists of both specific and general contributory factors. Where these conflict it may be necessary to make a judgement as to the most important causes of the events.

A separate analysis should be carried out for each care management problem though the depth and detail of the contributory factors identified may vary for each one. It is particularly important to distinguish Specific Contributory Factors, which describe the reasons for the care management problem on that particular occasion, from General Contributory Factors which the investigator judges to be more longstanding features of the individual, team or working conditions. Factors that are specific to that occasion, and which do not reflect more general problems, probably have no long term implications for the quality and safety of practice and therefore probably do not require action or changes of any kind. The final list of general contributory factors for each care management problem is examined and those that have implications for action are identified. The protocol contains blank forms with appropriate headings, to facilitate both the interview and analysis.

Preparation of the report

Once the interviews and analysis are completed, make a composite of all of them, detailing the whole incident from start to finish. If the protocol is followed systematically and the interview and analysis conducted thoroughly, the report and implications of the incident should emerge from the analysis in a relatively straightforward fashion. When the composite is complete, there should be a clear view of the problem, the circumstances which led up to it, and the flaws in the care process should be readily apparent. The final report will:

- Summarise the chronology
- Identify the care management problems and their contributory causes, giving most emphasis to general contributory factors
- Emphasise positive features of the process of care
- Recommend action and time-scales for each one of the general factors requiring attention.

The report will then consider what implications this incident has for the department or organisation. This section will summarise the general contributory factors and the implications for action. The lessons learnt can be drawn out and action plans to deal with the problems which occurred can be formulated. A summary outlining the main components of the investigation and analysis process can be found in the box below.

A summary of the investigation process

All investigations contain a series of steps, which should be followed, as a matter of routine, when an incident is investigated.

1 Ascertain that a serious clinical incident has occurred and ensure it is reported formally. Alternatively identify an incident as being fruitful in terms of organisational learning.
2 Trigger the investigation procedure. Notify two of the senior members of staff who have been trained to carry out investigations.
3 Investigators will establish the circumstances as they initially appear and complete an initial summary. Decide which part of the process of care requires investigation and prepare an outline chronology of events. Identify any obvious care management problems (CMPs) and record them.
4 Interview staff using the structured approach

  - Establish the chronology of events.
  - Revisit the sequence of events and ask questions about each of the clinical management problems identified at the initial stage.

- Use the framework to ask supplementary questions about the reasons for the occurrence of each clinical management problem. Record each CMP and its contributory factors.
- Give staff the post interview checklist to complete and comment on.

5 If new CMPs have emerged during the interviews add them to the initial list. Re-interview if necessary.
6 Collate the interviews and assemble a composite analysis under each of the CMPs identified at the start. For each CMP identify both specific and, where appropriate, general contributory factors.
7 Compile the report of the events, listing the causes of the CMPs and make recommendations to prevent recurrence.

Submit report to senior clinicians and management according to local arrangements. Implement the action arising from the report and monitor progress.

Case examples

The case examples are based on real clinical events, but have been altered in various respects to preserve the anonymity of those involved.

Death of a baby following a difficult delivery

The history of this tragic event was taken from case records and interviews with obstetricians and midwives involved. The case (in box opposite) is described and fully analysed in the protocol. Only some aspects are presented here. The main care management problems identified were as follows:

- Care plan formulated but not communicated
- Inadequate fetal monitoring in first and second stage of labour
- Inadequate pain control in first stage of labour
- Delay in management in second stage of labour.

Each of these care management problems was analysed separately. Only the second, inadequate fetal monitoring, is shown here with the contributory factors in Figure 23.1. A number of contributory factors influenced the care given in this stage of labour, operating at several different levels of the framework. Staff faced a very distressed patient who did not easily accept their recommendations. Scalp electrode removal was not covered by a unit policy, the midwives were distracted because of the mother's distress, the consultant's care plan was not seen because the notes were not retrieved, and the maternity unit was disrupted because of building works.

Death of baby following a difficult delivery

Mrs B was booked for shared care. Her last child was born weighing 4.4 kg and slight shoulder dystocia was noted at delivery. Mrs B was referred to the consultant by the community midwife at 38 weeks as the baby felt large for dates. The ultrasound scan estimated the weight of the baby as 4.5 kg. A graded response to the findings on palpation and ultrasound was made bearing in mind the patient's previous obstetric history. First, the pregnancy should not progress more than 6 days beyond its due date before induction of labour, rather than the usual 12–14 days. Second, it was recorded that no attempt should be made at a difficult mid cavity instrumental delivery. Third, the possibility of shoulder dystocia was anticipated and recorded explicitly to forewarn the labour ward staff.

Chronology:

05.55 Mrs B was admitted with a history of ruptured membranes. Labour commenced shortly afterwards.

06.50 Vaginal examination showed her cervix to be 3 cm dilated. The fetal heart was monitored using external Doppler. At this stage Mrs B requested an epidural, but the anaesthetist was not immediately available as he was finishing handing over on the intensive care unit. Mrs B's labour proceeded rapidly and therefore an epidural was not carried out.

07.15 A scalp electrode was placed on the baby's head as the midwives were unable to monitor the foetal heart easily in view of maternal size and maternal distress. The trace showed the fetal heart rate to be normal.

07.50 A further vaginal examination was carried out. Mrs B's cervix was 6 cm dilated, the fetal heart rate was normal with good variability. Pethidine was administered.

08.05 Mrs B's cervix was fully dilated. Pushing commenced. Mother unable to co-operate with staff as she was in pain and very distressed.

08.14 Scalp electrode was removed as the head was crowning. The final readings of the foetal heart before the scalp electrode was removed showed marked decelerations with a decreasing trend. The delivery did not proceed, the head remained stationary and the external Doppler was re-attached showing foetal heart rate at 160–170 beats.

> *08.33* Medical assistance was sought. The Obstetric registrar and the duty consultant came immediately and quickly diagnosed shoulder dystocia. They carried out a McRoberts manoeuvre, and then supra pubic pressure was applied and the baby was delivered at 08.39.
>
> The infant was severely compromised with no heart beat. He was resuscitated and ventilated and then transferred to SCBU, but died the following day.

Only some of these factors had more general implications for the running of the unit, specifically concerning the retrieval of notes, cardiotocograph training, and policies on the removal of scalp electrodes.

The final report of this case concluded that "with the benefit of hindsight, the outcome of this delivery might, on a balance of probabilities, have been different". Subsequent to the analysis of this case and discussion of the implications a number of changes were made to the organisation and policies of the unit. These included:

- a new protocol stipulating that where there was a conflict between information provided by different types of monitoring equipment, best practice would be to assume the worst case and seek medical advice
- individual training programme for specific members of staff
- programme of further education for all midwives in the assessment and management of shoulder dystocia
- review and eventual replacement of all outdated fetal monitoring equipment.

Attempted suicide in an inpatient psychiatric unit

Eight members of staff were interviewed, six nurses and two senior house officers (SHOs). Three of these people were closely involved in the incident reported. The other five staff members had been peripherally involved but had also been disturbed by the incident and approached the interviewer directly because they wanted to discuss it. The case summary is shown in box on page 454 and an analysis of the second care management problem in Figure 23.2.

The main care management problems identified were as follows:

- There was no formal risk assessment in the ward round, confirmed by the medical notes that are very sketchy in this respect. The SHO (MR) stated that B was not specifically asked about urges to self harm or suicidal ideation.

Care Management Problem
Fetal monitoring of first stage and second stage of labour

Clinical Context and Patient Factors
Painful and relatively short first stage of labour. Fetal heart rate difficult to monitor. CTG scalp electrodes placed on head at 7.15. Cervix fully dilated at 8.05. Patient very distressed and unable to cooperate. Episiotomy recommended but resisted. Argument involving husband for several minutes. Episiotomy done. Scalp electrode removed as head crowning at 8.15. CTG prior to removal shows marked decelerations of heart rate and a slowing trend.

Contributory Factors

Specific	General
Work & Environment Maternity building undergoing extensive building works whilst still in use. Normal geography disturbed.	None
Team Factors Notes not retrieved from library promptly. Care plan set out by Consultant not seen. Unit normally staffed & workload average.	Shift change procedures, need to ensure records recovered fast
Individual Factors Midwives failed to heed slowing heart rate on the CTG as they were distracted by the mother's distress and resistance to advice.	CTG awareness and training
Task Factors Midwives not aware of possible dystocia. Delay between crowning and complete delivery. Scalp electrode not covered by policy.	Lack of clear policy guidelines

Organisational, Management and Institutional Context Factors
Unit has been without a Head of Midwifery Service for 2 years. Function carried out by G grade Supervisors.

Figure 23.1 Contributory factors to case of neonatal death.

453

An attempted suicide

Events preceding the incident

Thursday B admitted to ward. Her medical notes recorded a recent overdose, but no other attempts at self harm.

Sunday B's father telephoned to tell staff that he thought B might harm herself and that she was unlikely to be honest about her mental state. The notes recorded that B was depressed but had no thoughts of self-harm.

Monday The ward round was conducted by a locum consultant and a new senior house officer (SHO). The notes contain no evidence of a risk assessment, but an entry stated that she was not feeling depressed or suicidal. Later that day B asked if she could go on home leave. The nurses felt she was very depressed and were concerned that she was expressing ideas of self-harm and hopelessness. They advised her to stay in hospital.

The incident

Wednesday B was very subdued throughout the day. The nurses were just coming out of the shift handover when the alarm sounded, having been activated from B's room. Two nurses found B with her wrist and neck lacerated. A broken bottle was on the bed and there was blood all over the floor. A nurse wrapped a towel round B's wrist and another round her neck. The nurses walked with B to the clinical room on the ward. Once the towels had been removed, it appeared the cuts were not very recent (although deep and jagged). The blood had clotted and they estimated the cuts had been made 20–30 minutes earlier.

Nursing supplies had to be found to clean B's wrist and neck. B became faint and said she had passed out in her room before pressing the alarm. When the duty doctor (another SHO) arrived a few minutes later, he found B slumped in a chair. She was lifted onto the treatment couch. Her pulse and blood pressure were taken – her BP was slightly low – and she was given oxygen. The doctor tried several times to insert a cannula for an IV infusion, but found it impossible as B's veins had shut down because of the blood loss. Fluid was unavailable for the infusion because all supplies had been used previously by another patient on the ward.

An ambulance was called and arrived quickly. B was transferred to Accident and Emergency (A&E) for intravenous infusion and suturing under anaesthetic. On the ward a nurse called A&E to tell them B was coming. She also rang the nursing agency to arrange for an extra nurse because it was felt B should be put on total observation. CL completed an incident form and informed B's father and the consultant on call. A&E later reported that B's blood tests, blood pressure and pulse were normal.

Care Management Problem

When the SHO (MR) saw B the day before the incident he recorded that B was not depressed and not suicidal.

Clinical Context and Patient Factors

Nurses commented that B was "not one of their regulars" and that they therefore did not know her well enough to interpret her mood or behaviour. Sufficient weight may not have been given to her father's concern about B. Although relatives and friends are sometimes more worried about a person's condition than warranted, the fact that B was not well known to staff suggests that perhaps she should have been monitored more closely.

Contributory Factors

Specific	General
Work & Environment	
None relevant to this care management problem	None
Team Factors	
Supervision: The SHO did the first on-call shifts without help/supervision. After first meeting, consultant went on extended leave. Three different consultants covered in successive weeks. In effect, for his first few weeks in post, MR got no real support or supervision.	Lack of co-ordination of consultant cover Inadequate supervision of junior staff
Individual Factors	
SHO did not feel that he had sufficient experience to assess patients such as B	Training needed in risk assessment
Task Factors	
No guidance given on assessing suicide risk	Consideration should be given to formal risk assessment instruments

Organisational, Management and Institutional Context Factors

Organisational factors: education and training policy
SHO had no clinical induction training to the ward/unit. SHOs are meant to have one formal training/supervision session a week. In his first seven weeks in post, SHO had only one. His current consultant had no time to supervise him and was also having to get to grips with his new job.

Organisational factors: safety culture and priorities
SHO discussed the situation regarding (lack of) supervision with his clinical tutor who said nothing could be done. There appear to be no formal channels through which problems like these can be resolved.

Figure 23.2 Contributory factors to case of attempted suicide.

455

- When the SHO saw B the day before the incident he recorded that B was not depressed and not suicidal.
- To avoid the risk of fainting, B should have been taken to the clinical room in a wheelchair. In addition, she should have been put on oxygen and had her pulse and BP taken before the duty doctor reached the ward. B's wrist had not been bandaged properly.
- When B was first taken to the clinical room, the nurses did not lie her down as a precaution against fainting. When the doctor arrived, B was sitting with her arms hanging down. The nurses should have had her hold her arms up above her head to prevent further bleeding.
- The second SHO could not insert a cannula for an IV infusion.
- Staff had to look for supplies to clean B's neck and wrist. Although this did not take long, any delay could have severe consequences with more serious cases.
- There was no formal, structured and supportive discussion of the incident focusing on how staff felt and whether the incident could have been dealt with better or even prevented. Some staff talked about it briefly with one or two colleagues when they had time, while others went home still disturbed and discussed it with friends.

Whether or not this incident is regarded as preventable, lessons can certainly be learnt from it. B was seen by several doctors at different times, many of whom were inexperienced and/or unsupervised, and/or getting to grips with a new job. Actions of some of the staff could have been questioned but when the broader picture is considered and the contributory causes are examined, more general, and perhaps more worrying, problems can be identified. The SHOs, through no fault of their own, were acting beyond their competence on several occasions. Clear training needs are apparent in regard to the induction of new staff and the medical abilities of psychiatric nurses. Equipment and supplies were poorly maintained and no one appeared to have had overall responsibility for this important task. The poor design of the ward also appears to have been a contributing factor in that B was able to harm herself without fear of being observed and without much chance of being discovered quickly.

The lack of support and supervision is perhaps the most glaring problem, at least in the view of the SHO. On his first day, another patient had a medical problem that MR had never encountered before. He had not been told how to contact the consultant for help and the consultant's secretary did not know how to contact him either. MR eventually managed to get help from another junior doctor. He tried subsequently to discuss the issue with the consultant, who was very dismissive. MR was quite disturbed by his unhelpful and unsupportive attitude. MR felt very strongly that he did not have enough experience to deal with a patient like B, and was keen to discuss the difficulties he had encountered as he considered that they had profound implications for the safe functioning of the unit.

Positive features

It is sometimes too easy to concentrate only on what went wrong, or what could have been done better in relation to a case. This analysis also revealed several positive features in the management of the incident. Pointing these out explicitly is important for staff morale, and helps present a more balanced picture of the functioning of the team and the system in general. For instance, staff had correctly advised B to stay in hospital when she had wanted to return home; there were no delays or difficulties in summoning and getting help, either from other nurses on the ward, the SHO, or the emergency services; once B had been discovered the staff worked efficiently, calmly and effectively as a team; staff recognised the seriousness of the incident and subsequently put B on total observation.

Discussion

The method described above has been tested on over forty incidents, initially in a research context and later by clinicians and risk managers. Incidents have been investigated in obstetrics, anaesthetics, accident and emergency, orthopaedics, general medicine and psychiatry. The structured and systematic approach means that the ground to be covered in any investigation is, to a significant extent, already mapped out. While the process may initially appear complicated and time consuming, our experience is that using the protocol actually speeds up complex investigations by focusing the investigators on the key issues and bringing out the systemic factors that must ultimately be the target of the investigation. These systemic features are those that are addressed when long term risk reduction strategies are implemented. Members of the research team have found that once the general contributory factors are identified, these lead automatically to the implications and action points. The final report "almost writes itself".

We have noted that even very experienced clinicians find following a systematic protocol brings additional benefits in terms of comprehensiveness and investigation expertise. Clinicians are accustomed to identifying the problematic features in the management of a case, and so can easily identify the care management problems. However, the identification of contributory factors and the realisation that each care management problem may have a different constellation of contributory factors are less familiar tasks. A systematic approach pays dividends when exploring these. The protocol does not attempt to supplant clinical expertise. Rather the aim is to utilise clinical experience and expertise to the fullest extent.

A formal, systematic approach also brings benefit to the staff involved. The methods used are designed to promote a greater climate of openness and to move away from finger pointing and the routine assignation of blame. This is quite different from the quasi-judicial approach that can be brought to bear in formal enquiries. If a consistent approach to investigation is used, members of staff who are interviewed tend to find the process less threatening than traditional unstructured approaches, especially when the same procedure is being followed with everyone involved.

Early experience with the protocol has suggested that some formal training and practice is needed before it can be used to its full effectiveness. Presentations and training sessions have suggested that the basic ideas can be grasped relatively quickly, but that the full method takes time to absorb. Guided practice on the investigation of incidents, preferably in a local context, is essential to become familiar with the methods. Initially this protocol is likely to be used by the risk manager, with additional clinical input. However, we suggest that the next step is to designate and train investigators in each clinical area who can carry out an investigation to agreed guidelines. For instance in obstetrics the investigators might be the head of midwifery and specialty director.

While the first case had a tragic outcome, the second demonstrates the benefits of investigating an incident that did not result in lasting harm. Serious incidents can be extremely distressing to staff, accompanied by guilt, self-recrimination, and loss of confidence. Investigation of a serious incident, however sensitively conducted, is bound to be difficult for all concerned. In contrast, with incidents that are less serious or even "routine", staff are not distressed and usually quite willing to discuss the incident quite openly. There is no reason to suppose that the background conditions and precursors to less serious incidents differ fundamentally from those with a more serious outcome. An in-depth analysis of less serious incidents will still reveal any basic problems in the functioning of the service and the management of risk and will bring much greater dividends than the cursory examination of a large number. If several minor incidents are investigated, patterns, trends and common factors will emerge. Recognition of the contributory factors in minor incidents can assist the development of more proactive methods of managing risk and implementing preventative strategies to reduce the number of serious incidents in the future.

Organisational changes should only be implemented after investigation of a series of incidents rather than after just one, which might be unusual or untypical. This is far preferable to making hasty ad hoc changes in response to a single serious incident, which may have idiosyncratic features. If similar problems are found to emerge regardless of the type of incident (for example, both self-harm and violence), there will be a much stronger basis from which to implement change. In the longer term a database of adverse and potentially dangerous incidents that have been subjected to detailed analysis might be established, in which clinical management failures, conditions of work and organisational factors are separately indexed.

While we believe that the protocol is an effective and valuable tool, we consider that it is still at a relatively early stage of development, both conceptually and practically. Formal evaluation is needed and a great deal more practical testing is required. We plan to revise and develop the protocol in the light of experience and formal evaluation. We also believe that the protocol has potential as a research instrument in that analyses of a series of incidents will be considerably more powerful if a common method is applied to all. In the meantime however it is already proving a powerful means of investigating and analysing clinical incidents, and drawing out the lessons these incidents have for enhancing patient safety.

Acknowledgements

We wish to acknowledge several people who have been closely involved in the work described here, in a collaborative enterprise over several years. Pippa Bark co-authored the chapter in the previous edition and carried out early research on the analysis of incidents. Nicola Stanhope collected data in mental health settings and collaborated in the development of the framework and methods of analysis. Members of the ALARM research group, who developed the protocol with the two authors are Jane Chapman, David Hewett, Sue Prior, Pam Strange and Ann Tizzard.

Further Information

Copies of the full protocol are available from the Association of Litigation and Risk Management, Royal Society of Medicine, 1 Wimpole Street, London W1.

References

1　Eagle CJ, Davies JM, Reason JT. Accident analysis of large scale technological disasters: applied to anaesthetic complications. *Can J Anaesth* 1992;**39**:118–22.
2　Cook RI, Woods DD. Operating at the sharp end: the complexity of human error. In: Bognor MS, ed. *Human error in medicine.* Hillsdale, New Jersey: Lawrence Erlbaum Associates Publishers, 1994.
3　Reason JT. Human error: models and management. *BMJ* 2000;**320**:768–70.
4　Vincent CA, Bark P. Accident analysis. In: Vincent CA, ed. *Clinical risk management.* London: BMJ Publications, 1995.
5　Stanhope N, Vincent CA, Taylor-Adams S, *et al.* Applying human factors methods to clinical risk management in obstetrics. *Br J Obstet Gynaecol* 1997;**104**:1225–32.
6　Taylor-Adams SE, Vincent C, Stanhope N. Applying human factors methods to the investigation and analysis of clinical adverse events. *Safety Sci* 1999;**31**:143–59.
7　Vincent CA, Adams S, Stanhope N. A framework for the analysis of risk and safety in medicine. *BMJ* 1998;**316**:1154–7.
8　Vincent CA, Taylor-Adams S, Chapman EJ, *et al.* How to investigate and analyse clinical

incidents: Clinical Risk Unit and Association of Litigation and Risk Management protocol. *BMJ* 2000;**320**:777–81.

9 Vincent CA, Taylor-Adams S, Chapman EJ, *et al. The investigation and analysis of clinical incidents: a protocol.* London, Royal Society of Medicine Press, 1999.

10 Reason JT. *Human error.* New York: Cambridge University Press, 1990.

11 Reason JT. *Managing the risk of organisational accidents.* Aldershot: Ashgate, 1997.

12 Cullen, The Hon Lord. *The Public Inquiry into the Piper Alpha Disaster.* Department of Energy. London: HMSO, 1990.

13 Hughes, H. The offshore industry's response to Lord Cullen's recommendations. *Petroleum Rev* 1991;Jan:5–8.

14 Ferrow M. Offshore safety – formal safety assessments. *Petroleum Rev* 1991;Jan:9–11.

15 Hale AR, Wilpert B, Freitag M, eds. 1997. *After the event: from accident to organisational learning.* Pergamon. London.

24 Caring for patients harmed by treatment

CHARLES VINCENT

Patients and relatives may suffer in two ways from injuries due to treatment; first from the injury itself and secondly from the way the incident is handled afterwards. Many people harmed by their treatment suffer further trauma through the incident being insensitively and inadequately handled. Conversely when staff come forward, acknowledge the damage, and take the necessary action the overall impact can be greatly reduced. Injured patients need an explanation, an apology, to know that changes have been made to prevent future incidents, and often, also need practical and financial help. The absence of any of these factors can be a powerful stimulus to complaint or litigation.[1]

The impact of a medical injury differs from most other accidents in two important respects. First, patients have been harmed, unintentionally, by people in whom they placed considerable trust, and so their reaction may be especially powerful and hard to cope with. Secondly, and even more important, they are often cared for by the same professions, and perhaps the same people, as those involved in the original injury. As they may have been very frightened by what has happened to them, and have a range of conflicting feelings about those involved, this too can be very difficult, even when staff are sympathetic and supportive.

Many of the people dealing with injured patients are not directly involved in clinical work. It is not easy to appreciate in say, the quiet of a barrister's chambers, just what a lifetime of chronic pain means. Those acting for hospitals may never even meet the patients involved, except in court. Staff involved in the original incident may not be those involved in rehabilitation and later treatment. The experience of injured patients therefore tends not to be fully appreciated, especially when they become tarred as litigants. Their psychological and social problems, and some-times their medical problems, are complex, fluctuating and not well under-stood. Appreciating the impact of such injuries is a prerequisite of providing useful and effective help, and the first part of the chapter con-centrates on describing some of the main forms of trauma. The second half of the chapter then addresses the principles and practicalities of helping such people, first by identifying some key principles, and then with exam-ples of good practice which show that even very serious incidents can be resolved and their traumatic impact greatly reduced.

Stress and medical procedures

People who are seriously ill are obviously worried about their poor health and its impact on their work and family. In addition to the stresses associated with the illness itself, there are a number of additional stresses associated with treatment. These include difficulties in understanding diagnosis and treatment, coping with a hospital environment, adverse effects of diagnostic or therapeutic procedures, forced life-style changes, and difficulties in relationships with staff.[2] Reports are also appearing sug-gesting that even routine procedures may produce post-traumatic symp-toms. For instance Clark and colleagues[3] found that a quarter of patients in a general surgical unit developed high levels of acute post-traumatic stress symptoms, which were associated with depression on admission and intra-hospital stress. Normal childbirth can also lead to post-traumatic symptoms of varying degree. In a recent study[4] about a quarter of women giving birth showed some traumatic responses, such as intrusive memories of the event, and a small number (3%) showed clinically significant levels of symptoms. Higher levels of symptoms were associated with perceptions of low levels of support from the partner and staff, patterns of blame, low perceived control in labour, and personal factors, such as previous mental health problems.

These studies are only illustrative and it is not possible to review the nature and extent of psychological problems in hospitalised patients here. However it is clear that patients are often in a vulnerable psychological state, even when diagnosis is clear and treatment goes according to plan. When they experience harm or misadventure therefore, their reaction is likely to be particularly severe.

Psychological reactions to injury

The speed and extent of recovery from any injury depends on many dif-ferent factors; the nature and extent of the injury, the level of pain, and the degree of subsequent disability are crucial. The personality of the patient involved, the history of previous trauma and loss in their life, their financial security, and employment prospects may also influence subsequent adjustment. While reactions vary greatly, certain constellations of symptoms recur.

Traumatic and life-threatening events produce a variety of symptoms, over and above any physical injury. Anxiety, intrusive memories, emotional numbing, flashbacks are all common sequelae and are important components of post-traumatic stress disorder.[5,6] Sudden, intense, dangerous or uncontrollable events are particularly likely lead to such problems, especially if accompanied by illness, fatigue or mood disturbances.[7,8] Awareness under anaesthesia is an example of such an event.

Most medical adverse events do not produce post-traumatic stress disorder in its pure form. The long-term consequences of the event, in terms of pain, disability and effect on family relationships, and ability to work will be much more important than the initial incident and depression is a more usual response. Whether people actually become depressed and to what degree, will depend on the severity of their injury, the support they have from family, friends and health professionals, and a variety of other factors.[9,10]

Studies of people involved in serious accidents (for example, road accidents) suggest that 20–30% of patients suffer long-term psychological impairment.[5,11] Accidental injury during treatment, although little researched, also appears to produce serious psychological symptoms. Vincent et al[12] reported a study of patients injured during surgery and involved in or considering litigation. Damage to organs and nerves, perforations and wound infections accounted for the majority of the injuries. The consequences of these injuries were both sustained and severe. The overall effect on the patients' lives, as judged by them, was considerable including increased pain, disability, psychological trauma, effects on their work and social lives. They frequently suffered from disturbing memories, depression and anxiety. Three quarters of them considered that the incident had had a severely detrimental effect on their life.

When a patient dies

Any bereavement involves multiple losses: the widow or widower loses companionship, a confidant, their sexual relationship, and may experience a loss of identity. Many bereaved people describe the loss in almost physical terms – as having part of them torn away.[13] Bereavement may be particularly severe if the loss is untimely or unexpected[14] or when the bereaved has had little forewarning about the loss.[15,16] A bereavement that follows a sudden, accidental death may be exceptionally severe. Lehman et al[17] studied people four to seven years after they had lost a spouse or child in an accident. Many continued to ruminate about the accident and what could have been done to prevent it, and they appeared unable to accept, resolve, or find any meaning in the loss.

Relatives of patients whose death was sudden or unexpected may therefore find the loss particularly difficult to bear. If the loss was avoidable in the sense that poor treatment played a part in the death, their relatives may face an unusually traumatic and prolonged bereavement. They may ruminate endlessly on the death and find it hard to accept the loss.

The experiences of injured patients and their relatives

Reports of studies help us understand the main effects of injury to patients, but it is still difficult to grasp the full extent of the trauma that patients sometimes face. Appreciating and understanding their experiences is essential if one is going to provide individually appropriate and practical help. The cases described below illustrate the principal forms of trauma, encompassing chronic pain, bereavement and loss, depression, anxiety, and post-traumatic stress disorder. The focus of each case description is therefore on the effects of the incidents described, rather than the clinical events that preceded them. The stories described below were all gathered in the course of interviews for reports. All the patients were involved in legal action, though not necessarily for large sums of money. There was evidence of sub-standard treatment in all cases although in some the most disturbing aspects of their care were not, strictly speaking, negligent. None of the people involved had any prior history of psychological problems of any significance or of serious physical illness. The trauma they describe was attributable to their treatment, or that of their relative. The quotations are the patients' or relatives' own words taken from the interviews. Names and other details have been changed to protect the identity of those involved.

(i) Perforation of the colon: chronic pain and depression

Mrs Long underwent a ventrosuspension – the fixation of a displaced uterus to the abdominal wall. After the operation she awoke with a terrible pain in her lower abdomen, which became steadily worse over the next four days. She was very frightened and repeatedly told both doctors and nurses but they dismissed it as "wind".

On the fifth day the pain reached a crescendo and she felt a "ripping sensation" inside her abdomen. That evening the wound opened and the contents of her bowel began to seep through the dressings. Even then no one seemed concerned. Finally the surgeon realised that the bowel had been perforated and a temporary colostomy was carried out.

The next operation, to reverse the colostomy, was "another fiasco". After a few days there was a discharge of faecal matter from the scar, the wound became infected and the pain was excruciating, especially after eating. She persistently asked if she could be fed with a drip, but the nursing staff insisted she kept eating. For two weeks she was "crying with the pain, really panicking – I just couldn't take any more". She was finally transferred to another hospital – where she was immediately put on a drip and a liquid diet.

A final operation to repair the bowel was successful but left her exhausted and depressed. She only began to recover her strength after a year of convalescence. Three years later she was still constantly tired, irritable, low in spirits and "I don't enjoy anything any more". She no longer welcomes affection or comfort and feels that she is going downhill, becoming more gloomy and pre-occupied.

Mrs Long's scars are still uncomfortable and painful at the time of her periods. Her stomach is "deformed" and she feels much less confident and attractive as a result. As her depression has deepened, she has become less interested in sex and more self-conscious about the scar. Three years later the trauma of her time in hospital is still very much alive. She still has nightmares about her time in hospital and is unable to talk about it without breaking into tears. She feels very angry and bitter that no one ever apologised to her, or admitted that a mistake has been made.

Traumatic experiences, chronic pain and physical weakness combined to produce a serious depression which lasted several years. The depression was marked by classical symptoms of low mood, tiredness, fatigue, low self esteem, and sleep disturbance (see below) – but nevertheless went unnoticed by any of the health professionals involved in her care. Although the term "post-traumatic stress disorder" is frequently used as a "catch all" for reactions to injury, this is in fact seriously inaccurate and misleading. Depression is a far more common response, particularly where chronic pain is involved, although other post-traumatic symptoms may be present to some degree in the early stages.

Principal symptoms of depression

Continual depressed mood
Loss of interest or pleasure in daily activities
Significant weight loss (when not dieting), or loss of appetite
Insomnia or excessive sleeping
Fatigue and loss of energy nearly every day
Strong and frequent feelings of worthlessness or guilt
Diminished ability to think, concentrate or make decisions
Recurrent thoughts of death, suicidal ideas or suicide attempts

---

(ii) Asphyxia during labour: caring for a handicapped child

Mrs Farr's daughter Polly, now six, suffers from severe cerebral palsy following a birth injury. Polly's intellectual abilities do not seem to be seriously impaired, but she is severely physically handicapped.

After the birth Mrs Farr was told that Polly had sustained an injury to her brain, but at first could not really take in this information or comprehend the full implications – "we were just in total shock". Polly had been taken to Intensive Care and, when she came back to the ward, it took a long time to convince Mrs Farr that Polly was actually her child. After she returned home with Polly, she hid herself away and pretended everything was alright. It was some weeks before she telephoned a friend and told her "Polly's brain-damaged". She said that this was one of the worst things that she had to do.

For the first eight months of Polly's life Mr and Mrs Farr had very little professional help. They had the usual paediatric check-ups, seeing registrars who "didn't want to know about Polly" and an "absolutely hopeless" health visitor. They desperately wanted more information and to talk to other people who had children with similar disabilities. They had no idea what to expect or what kind of future Polly might have. After eight months Mrs Farr joined a small support group of mothers and children with similar problems run by a physiotherapist who "became my lifeline". Otherwise she was extremely isolated, apart from nightly phone calls to her mother.

In the first years of Polly's life Mrs Farr cried constantly and blamed herself for everything. She felt that "they'd taken away the baby I should have had and I'd been given Polly". It seemed to her that her real baby had died and she was grieving for the child she never had. She felt that Polly would be better off dead and on many occasions threatened to kill both herself and Polly. Mr Farr would leave the house each morning knowing that they both might be dead when he returned. The physical demands of caring for Polly coupled with the anguish and threats of suicide all but destroyed the marriage. There was no improvement in her mood for three years until she became pregnant again and Polly started school. Until then Polly needed 24-hour attention and she felt "totally trapped".

Mrs Farr copes remarkably well with the enormous physical and emotional demands of caring for Polly. However she is constantly on edge, and finds it almost impossible to relax – "Always in the back of my mind there's something I have to do. I dream about this – I'm always in a panic, always disorganised and out of control". She does everything possible to make Polly's life as good as it can be, but "even now I don't really feel bonded to Polly – I just care for her".

Most of Mrs Farr's problems face all mothers of seriously handicapped children. The grief at the loss of the child that was expected combined with the grinding responsibility of 24-hour care can break the strongest person. It is remarkable then that almost none of the various professionals involved with Polly thought to ask how Mrs Farr was; a few brief questions would have quickly elicited the fact that she was actively suicidal and profoundly depressed.

Mrs Farr's problems were compounded by the attitudes of the hospital and their lawyers, who took five years to admit liability. Even then no help was offered. The solicitors then entered another battle for interim payments to provide some basic facilities for Polly. The hospital's duty of care to Mrs Farr appears to have ended, as far as they were concerned, once litigation began. An early offer of compensation, probably in the form of a structured settlement, would have been comparatively cheap for the trust concerned to institute. Polly's needs could then have been reviewed and payments adjusted accordingly, to the benefit of everyone concerned.[18]

(iii) Neonatal death: bereavement and post-traumatic stress disorder

Mr Carter's son, Jamie, sustained injuries at birth, due to inadequate obstetric care, causing irreparable spinal cord injury. He died when he was two months old without regaining consciousness.

Three days after the birth a paediatrician confirmed that their son was, as they suspected, severely handicapped. He suffered from fits and was partially sighted. He never cried or made any sounds because his vocal cords had been damaged. In spite of these injuries he continued to grow and put on weight. Two weeks after Jamie's birth they were told that he would not live. They then spent a terrible two months, mostly at the hospital, waiting for him to die.

Mr and Mrs Carter had a number of meetings with hospital staff but Mr Carter never felt he had received a full explanation. He remembers being told that "it was just one of those things – that really sent me sky-rocketing. No one said it was a mistake, that's what wound me up. Till this day I've got many questions. No one acted quickly enough. No doctor came at all until the paediatrician arrived".

Mr Carter's reaction to Jamie's death was intense, violent and prolonged. For a year he suffered from disturbing memories and horrific dreams. He became quiet, withdrawn and remote even from his wife, feeling "empty and hopeless". He was tormented by disturbing images and memories of Jamie, of the birth, his slow death, and particularly of his small, shrunken skull toward the end. Images of Jamie's birth still "popped into my head at the most unexpected times. Very vivid, just like looking in on it. It just grabs you round the throat . . . ". He suffered from a persistent stress-related stomach disorder. His sleep was interrupted by violent nightmares of a kind he had never previously experienced. "There was all this blood and gore, fantasy-like stuff". During the day violent images, sometimes of killing people, would come into his head, which absolutely horrified him.

Before Jamie's death, Mr Carter had always been relaxed and easy-going person. Now he was easily irritated and there were many arguments between him and his wife. At work his irritability would often turn to anger, leading to confrontations and sometimes to fights. "I was really angry all the time, so aggressive – I wanted to hurt people, and I'm not like that at all. I felt I had to blame someone all the time for everything".

About a year later Mrs Carter became pregnant again. Mr Carter was very anxious during the pregnancy but his symptoms began to subside after their daughter was born. Two years on he still breaks down and cries occasionally, and is generally a sadder and quieter person. When he passes the cemetery where his son is buried he still becomes angry, but now the feelings subside.

Many of the symptoms and experiences reported by Mr Carter are common in any bereavement. Depression, distressing memories, feelings of anger, and dreams of the person who has died are not unusual. However the intensity, character and duration of Mr Carter's reaction indicates that this was far from an ordinary bereavement. Anger of that intensity and violent day-dreams are not usual, and show that he was suffering from post-traumatic stress disorder (see below). The staff of the paediatric unit clearly tried to help Mr and Mrs Carter, although they did not seem to appreciate what he was suffering and did not ask about traumatic reactions. Even if Jamie's death had been unavoidable it would probably still have been very difficult for Mr Carter to accept an explanation given the severity of his emotional reaction. The necessary explanation would have to have been given gradually, over several meetings, and combined with some attempts to support him and ease the intensity of his reaction.

Principal symptoms of post-traumatic stress disorder

1 The person has been exposed to a traumatic event in which there was actual or threatened death or serious injury, to themselves or someone close to them
- The person's response involved intense fear, helplessness or horror

2 The traumatic event is persistently re-experienced in one or more of the following ways:
- recurrent and intrusive distressing recollections of the event
- recurrent distressing dreams
- acting or feeling as if the event was re-occurring
- intense distress at thoughts or reminders of the event

3 Persistent avoidance of reminders of the event
- avoiding thoughts and feelings associated with the event
- avoiding activities and places associated with the event
- inability to recall important aspects of the trauma
- feelings of detachment from others
- restricted range of feelings

4 Persistent symptoms of increased arousal
- difficulty falling or staying asleep
- irritability or outbursts of anger
- difficulty concentrating
- hypervigilance
- exaggerated startle response

(iv) Suffering and loss associated with childlessness

Ms Pine experienced a series of problems with cervical smears which led to a long delay in diagnosis of cervical cancer. By the time it was diagnosed, the cancer was well advanced. Conservative treatment was no longer possible and a hysterectomy and oophorectomy were carried out in a 30-year-old woman with no children.

The operation itself was terrifying to her and disturbing, in spite of the kindness of the staff. The full implications only gradually sank in. "For a long, long time I just felt numb". She felt different physically, irrevocably altered. "I couldn't have children, I'd lost my femininity, no one would think I was attractive. Relationships would be impossible – there seemed no point if I couldn't have children". In spite of being tormented by these thoughts, she resolutely maintained that she was fine whenever she was asked. The effect of this was that very few people knew how she felt and she took care not to become too close to anyone. "I never felt womanly. I never gave anyone the opportunity. I never went anywhere where I might meet anyone new. I was incredibly lonely for years".

It was ten years before Ms Pine felt able to trust someone enough to begin a relationship. Twelve years on, with a close relationship now established, Ms Pine was generally cheerful and in reasonably good physical health, though still vulnerable to depression. She was working full time, had a full social life and feels herself very lucky to be in a close and enduring relationship. However the loss of her womb and her chance to have children remains a constant sad theme in her life. Her relationship, while marvellous in itself, has intensified the feeling of loss as she and her partner would like to have children. His brother's wife has just had a child which "cuts me up terribly". Ms Pine still had deeply disturbing dreams, from which she wakes tearful and sad. For instance in one recurring dream "a doctor puts a baby inside me, makes me have it, then takes it away".

This sad story illustrates a number of important themes: first, that a deep sense of loss does not only arise from a death; second, and particularly important in a medico-legal context, that suffering does not equate with psychiatric disorder. Ms Pine was at no time sufficiently depressed to be diagnosed as suffering a psychiatric disorder, yet her suffering was intense and prolonged. Third, it is useful to note that Ms Pine was very successful in maintaining her cheerfulness and sociability. While this was in many ways admirable and protective, it also served to mask her feelings from those around her. It is also easy for clinicians and risk managers to assume that someone has "got over it" simply because they are able to be bright and cheerful when the occasion demands. Finally, it is worth noting that Ms Pine's suffering was both prolonged and intensified by allegations of instability made by defence solicitors that bordered on the malicious – which appalled Ms Pine's partner, a solicitor himself.

Principles for helping patients and families

Every injured patient has their own particular problems and needs. Some will require a great deal of additional help, others will prefer to rely on their family and friends. Some will primarily require remedial medical treatment, while in others the psychological effects will be to the fore. There are nevertheless a number of basic considerations that will help in dealing with anyone who has been injured or seriously distressed by their treatment, whether or not negligence or litigation are involved. These suggestions are derived from patients, their relatives, research in this area and from other writers on this topic.[18,19] There is valuable material in other complementary chapters in this volume. James Pichert and Gerald Hickson's chapter contains an important section on communication after a serious incident. Chapters on mediation (Simanowitz and Brown) and handling claims (Chapman) also show how trauma can be minimised with flexible, efficient and sensitive approaches to resolving disputes.

(i) Commitment to openness by the organisation

Successful handling relies on the sensitivity and courage of individual clinicians and risk managers, but also requires a commitment to certain basic principles at the highest level of the organisation. It is quite unrealistic, indeed quite unfair, to expect openness and honesty from individuals without the backing of a policy of honesty and openness approved by the trust board.

(ii) Believe people who say their treatment has harmed them

Patients who consider that they have been injured during their treatment should in the first instance be believed. In many cases it may turn out that they had unrealistic expectations of their treatment, or had not fully understood the risks involved. In a few cases they may be malingering or hypochondriacal. However, given the frequency of adverse events (see Chapter 2), a report of such an injury should at least be seen as credible. It should certainly not be automatically seen as evidence of personality problems, or of being "difficult". Being believed is extremely important for accident victims and, conversely, not being believed is always frustrating and can be intensely disturbing.

(iii) The Continuing Duty of Care

Injured patients may receive support, comfort, and practical help from many sources. It may come from their spouse, family, friends, colleagues, doctors or community organisations. An especially important source of support will be the doctors and other health professionals who are involved in their treatment. It is vital that the duty of care is paramount.

An honest explanation and a promise to continue treatment may enhance the patient's trust and strengthen the relationship. After an initial mistake it

470

is extremely reassuring for a patient to be overseen by a single senior doctor who undertakes to monitor all aspects of their treatment, even if it involves a number of different specialties. Where care has been sub-standard the patient must be offered a referral elsewhere if that is what they wish but:

> Our experience is that, even under such circumstances, the patient will often choose to continue under the care of the same doctor. Paradoxically her faith in that doctor may well have been enhanced.[18]

(iv) Honesty and Openness

> The awful sinking feeling that comes with the realisation of a clinical error, particularly one whose consequences for the patient may be serious, must be familiar to all experienced practitioners . . . . Sharing with the patient the realisation of that error, admitting that it has occurred and facing squarely the responsibility for it requires courage. Nevertheless such an approach is appreciated by the patient . . .[18]

A patient harmed by treatment poses acute and painful dilemmas for the staff involved. It is natural to avoid that pain by avoiding the patient, yet the staff's response is crucial to the patient's recovery. When patients think that information is being concealed from them, or that they are being dismissed as troublemakers, it is much more difficult for them to cope with the injury. A poor explanation fuels their anger, may affect the course of a bereavement, and may lead patients to distrust the staff caring for them. They may then avoid having further treatment – which in most cases they very much need.

When something has gone wrong a senior doctor needs to give a thorough and clear account of what exactly happened. At the first interview, junior staff involved with the patient may also be present. The patient and their relatives need to have time to reflect on what was said and to be able to return and ask further questions. Remember that people may be numb with shock after an incident and be unable to cope with very much information. Several meetings may be needed over the course of weeks or months. Similar considerations of course apply when doctors are breaking bad news of any kind.[20]

(v) Ask specific questions about emotional trauma

A common theme of interviews with injured patients is that none of the professionals involved in their care appreciated the depth of their distress. In many cases outright psychiatric disorders were missed. Risk managers, clinicians, and others involved with these patients can ask basic questions without fear of "making things worse". The case histories illustrate some of the most common reactions and experiences of people suffering from depression and post-traumatic stress disorder. Other crucial areas of enquiry are feelings of anger, humiliation, betrayal, and loss of trust – all frequently experienced by injured patients.

471

When something truly awful has happened, staff are naturally also affected. In most clinical situations the need to think clearly and act decisively mean that emotions must be kept under control. Conversely it is of no help whatever to patients, and may be quite damaging, if staff are obviously unable to cope with the tragedy that has occurred. However, many patients have derived comfort from the empathy and sadness of staff involved in tragic incidents describing, for instance, the warmth and support they found in the staff's own sadness at the event.

(vi) Consider counselling or psychotherapy

A proportion of patients is likely to be sufficiently anxious or depressed to warrant formal psychological or psychiatric treatment. While it is important that a consultant is involved in giving explanations and monitoring remedial treatment, it is unrealistic to expect the staff of say, a surgical unit, to shoulder the burden of formal counselling. They have neither the time nor the necessary training to deal with the more serious reactions.

A referral to a psychologist or psychiatrist may be clearly indicated, but must be carefully handled. Injured patients are understandably very wary of their problems being seen as "psychological" or "all in the mind". This may be especially true of referrals to a psychiatrist who may (however unfairly) be seen as dealing with mental illness rather than simply offering support and treatment. In a large trust a specialist counsellor may be warranted. This would be of benefit both to injured and traumatised patients and to the staff who care for them. Whoever the therapist is, it is fundamental that they accept the reality of the patient's injury and do not attempt to explain the patient's reaction away on the basis of past pathology. Some patients report that their therapist found it extremely difficult to talk straightforwardly about injuries caused by treatment.

Even the best and most sympathetic care can lead to unexpected difficulties. After one avoidable stillbirth a full explanation was offered and the parents were given extensive support. In a final interview the parents expressed their gratitude to the staff. However the mother was left with a sense of emptiness and frustration:

> *I sometimes think it would have been better if I had had somebody to hate. As it was everybody said how sorry they were and I couldn't even get angry even though my baby had died.*

This example illustrates that in some circumstances it may be better if the therapist or counsellor is not connected with the trust or practice concerned. Clearly this is necessary if the patient no longer trusts the staff who cared for them but it may be helpful even where the staff are continuing to care for the patient. One of the great values of an outside therapist, not involved with the incident, is that the patient can safely rage, break down and admit to violent and irrational feelings in safety and without fear – provided the therapist has the necessary qualities of equanimity and acceptance.

(vii) Inform patients of changes

Patients' and relatives' wish to prevent future incidents can be seen both as a genuine desire to safeguard others and as an attempt to find some way of coping with their own pain or loss. The pain may be ameliorated if they feel that, because changes were made, then at least some good came of their experiences. Relatives of patients who have died may express their motives for litigation in terms of an obligation to the dead person to make sure that a similar accident never happens again, so that some good comes of their death.

The implication of this is that if changes have been made as a result of the error, it is very important to inform the patients concerned. While some may regret that the changes were made too late for them, most will appreciate the fact that their experience was understood and acted upon. It is however clear that letters from administrators not involved in clinical work stating simply that "the necessary steps have been taken to prevent a recurrence" do not convince, and may fuel people's anger.[21]

(viii) Financial assistance and practical help

Injured patients need help immediately. They need medical treatment, counselling, explanations but they often need money as well. They may need to support their family while they are recovering, pay for specialist treatment, facilities to cope with disability, and so on.

Mrs Farr's life would have been immeasurably improved with an early, properly structured, settlement providing her with facilities to care for her daughter and respite care. In less serious cases a few thousand pounds early on to provide private therapy, alterations to the home, or additional nursing may make an enormous difference to the patient both practically and in their attitude to the hospital. Clearly there are ethical reasons for offering compensation where a patient has been injured; it should be seen as part of continuing care. There are also sound financial ones, help someone at an early stage and the trust or general practitioner will face lower legal bills and much smaller claims for pain and suffering.

The way forward

In contrast to the earlier descriptions, the emphasis here is on the intervention, rather than a detailed description of the incident and its effects.

Note that not all of them are strict cases of "negligence" – but all involve patients whose care has been problematic and who certainly need help. Most of the principles described above are applicable to each case, but usually one or two are highlighted as being of particular importance. As before they have been made anonymous to protect those involved.

(i) Explanations and apology after iatrogenic cardiac arrhythmia

Mrs A was admitted for minor day case surgery, expecting to return home later that day. A surgeon requested a weak solution of adrenaline to induce a blood free field, but was given a stronger solution than requested. As soon as the liquid was applied the patient developed a serious cardiac arrhythmia, the operation was terminated and she was transferred to the intensive therapy unit, where she gradually recovered.

The clinical risk manager was alerted immediately and assessed the likely consequences for the patient and her family. The first task was clearly to apologise and provide a full explanation. However, with both the patient and family in a state of shock, this had to be carried out in stages. The consultant and risk manager had a series of short meetings over a few days, to explain what had happened and keep the family informed about ongoing remedial treatment. Each time the family was given the opportunity to reflect on what they had been told and come back with further questions.

In the longer term the patient was put in touch with an expert claimant lawyer, one who could offer independent advice but who was also committed to early resolution of disputes. A package of compensation was arranged, primarily aimed at providing the necessary clinical and psychological support. The whole incident was resolved within six months and the patient expressed her thanks to the hospital for the way in which the incident had been handled, particularly the openness about the causes of the incident.

(ii) Emotional trauma after respiratory arrest

A young mother was having a mole removed. She was given a muscle relaxant in an unlabelled syringe, in place of local anaesthetic. This led to a respiratory arrest and paralysis. She was intubated and it was three hours before she was able to breathe again herself. She was conscious for much of this period.

The patient had been terrified throughout this incident. It was clear early on that there was the potential for long term traumatic reactions. However the immediate concern of the patient was the care of her children, for her a greater worry than her own condition. This was therefore clearly the priority for intervention. An immediate payment was made to enable her to pay for part time child care, which was of enormous help in allowing the mother to recover and in assuring her of the hospital's determination to help.

In the longer term the risk manager maintained regular contact with her and remains on good terms with her, continuing to support and assess her need for assistance. The hospital also arranged for her to receive psychotherapy to ameliorate the long term effects of the trauma. Compensation was paid, but in a negotiated settlement with no litigation.

(iii) Anaesthetic awareness: reducing the fear of future operations

A woman was admitted for an elbow replacement. During the operation she awoke, paralysed and able to hear the discussions amongst the surgical team. She was terrified, in great pain and absolutely helpless. The lack of anaesthetic was fortunately noticed, and she was next aware of waking in recovery screaming.

The risk manager visited the patient on the ward as soon as practicable, maintained contact, offered psychological treatment for trauma, and advised her on procedures for compensation, including an offer to pay for an independent legal assessment of the eventual offer of compensation. As in the above example, emotional trauma was the principal long term concern. In this case a fear of future operations was one of the major factors, very important in a woman suffering chronic conditions requiring further treatment. This problem required some additional, imaginative measures.

Some months later, when the patient she felt ready, she was given a tour of the operating theatre and the anaesthetic failure was explained in great detail, as were the procedural changes that had been made subsequent to the incident. This was clearly immensely important in reducing her understandable fear of future operations and minimising the long term impact of the incident.

(iv) Working with a family after the death of the mother following a failure of care

A very active working woman died suddenly, following a delay in diagnosing coeliac disease. There had undoubtedly been a failure of care, but it was in fact unlikely that the delay had worsened her prognosis. The family however, not unnaturally, suspected that their mother might have been saved with prompt treatment.

In this case there was no clear negligence and no real chance of a claim. However, the hospital's emphasis on the duty of care, their concern to learn from errors and care for the patients underpinned a very active intervention strategy – greatly aided by a thoughtful consultant. Everyone involved understood the depth of the family's feeling, and the potential impact of the failure of care on the subsequent bereavement.

The consultant and the team concerned, genuinely saddened by the failure of care, invited the entire family to an evening meeting. In this he outlined the nature, causes and progressions of coeliac disease, and explored the familial factors that were potentially involved. With both the complexity and seriousness of the disease clearly understood, the delay seemed less important. The openness of the doctors and their willingness to discuss the family's doubts allayed fears of a "cover-up".

(v) Learning from experience, encouraged by a parent

A baby's major heart defect was not diagnosed, although clearly visible, on ultrasound scan. The child's mother was therefore not referred to the paediatric centre at a teaching hospital. The mother was discharged home after the birth with no diagnosis of the child's condition having been made. The baby had a cardiac arrest at 10 days old, was resuscitated and transferred to the paediatric centre and thereafter given appropriate treatment. The eventual outcome was positive, but the mother suffered dreadfully, and unnecessarily, in the first weeks of the child's life.

Investigations revealed that a number of staff had missed important signs, both during the ante-natal period and after the birth, and that the mother's anxieties about the baby's condition had been dismissed. Explanations were given and the long term implications for mother and baby considered. In the event the mother recovered quickly, did not want any form of compensation or to make a formal complaint. However she was calmly insistent on knowing that changes were made to prevent future similar missed diagnoses.

A number of changes to training and procedures were made in response to this incident. The task for the risk manager was to keep the mother involved and informed, and maintain good relations with her. Meetings were arranged with the assistance of the community health council to explain the changes in training and procedures that had been introduced and followed up with written accounts.

(vi) Interim solutions when the long term outcome is unclear

There are many occasions, particularly with the very young or the seriously ill, when the long term impact of deficient care is not clear. The usual solution, if a claim is involved, has been to wait until the outcome is clear, which may be years later. In the meantime the patient receives no help.

There was a delay in diagnosis of prostate cancer, of four months in a man in his sixties. The patient was referred to a consultant, who was ill at the time of the appointment. He eventually saw a junior doctor who ignored his complaints of pain and haematuria and marked him for three-month review. There were further delays then due to equipment failure. During this time the man's health deteriorated seriously. Opinion in the hospital was divided as to how much delay had affected prognosis, but all were agreed that care had been well below standard and had certainly affected the patient's quality of life.

The whole of the patient's family used the hospital, and his wife was a frequent attender. Neither the family or the hospital wanted to jeopardise this relationship or the future treatment of other members of the family. A small amount of financial help was given immediately to provide some additional aids and comfort to the patient, in the full knowledge that it was possible that a larger claim might later result if he died suddenly. The risk manager delivered the cheque in person, which was particularly appreciated by the family – who continue to use the hospital.

Problems and difficulties facing the pro-active risk manager

Advocates of open and proactive approaches are frequently questioned by more cautious colleagues about the potential adverse consequences of such policies. Generally there is a wish to be more open, but a fear of being overwhelmed by complaints and litigation, the mindless assaults of the media or by the anger and bitterness of patients and relatives. Problems certainly do arise, but rather less than those that arise from defensiveness and covering up. In fact, even after serious incidents and considerable trauma, patients and relatives can be grateful and appreciative of efforts made to help them. The risk managers who provided these cases were however emphatic that a more proactive policy emphasising the continuing duty of care had not led to unreasonable demands. Their impression was, if anything, that providing support and behaving in a decent manner reduced the stress of all concerned, maintained good relationships, and was very much welcomed by staff who were generally very keen to find ways of making amends. Certainly openness can be abused by a minority of grasping individuals who take the opportunity to make a claim. However, a proactive policy does not mean simply giving in to any demands, and should always be coupled with a robust defence of unreasonable claims and complaints

The principal problems for proactive risk managers and clinicians do not appear to come from the patients, but from other agencies involved in these incidents, who may be working to different timetables and different agendas. One medical director, for instance, had been asked by the coroner not to explain an incident to a family until after the coroner's own investigation. This would have meant a four-month wait for the family to find out how their father had died, which was clearly inhumane and untenable. There also can be difficulties with a trust board or trust solicitors who see the risk manager's task simply as protecting the trust and saving money. Clearly these are important responsibilities, but the duty of care to patients demands that cost-cutting is not the over-riding objective.

With large claims the Clinical Negligence Scheme for Trusts must be involved at an early stage. The involvement of lawyers and the administrative procedures inevitably involve delays and make it more difficult to implement creative solutions or to offer interim payments. All this takes time, which makes continuing contact with the family more difficult, and increases the anger and stress of the patient and family, in turn making an early resolution less likely. The separation of complaints and claims, and the difficulty in offering compensation to settle a justified complaint add to these problems. There would seem to be an urgent need to allow risk managers to take action on an interim basis, with no liability admitted, while major claims are resolved.

Concluding remarks

The aim of this chapter has been to draw attention to the impact of adverse events on patients and offer some suggestions for methods of intervening to minimise the trauma. The risk managers who operate such policies all consider that they are still exploring the best ways to help injured patients, and that there is still much to learn, particularly about how best to provide long term support where needed. Nevertheless, there have been major changes in the care of injured patients in the last five years, in at least a small number of hospitals and this provides much encouragement for the future

Acknowledgements

I thank the people who gave permission for their stories to be used. I am also grateful to Jane Chapman, Allen Cole and Gillian Jacomb who generously shared their experiences of assisting injured patients and their families and provided the later case studies.

References

1 Vincent C, Young M, Phillips A. Why do people sue doctors? A study of patients and relatives taking legal action. *Lancet* 1994;**343**:1609–13.

2 Koenig HG, George LK, Stangl D, Tweed DL. Hospital stressors experienced by elderly medical inpatients: developing a Hospital Stress Index. *Int J Psychiatry Med* 1995;**25**: 103-22.

3 Clarke DM, Russell PA, Polglase AL, McKenzie DP. Psychiatric disturbance and acute stress responses in surgical patients. *Aust NZ J Surg* 1997;**67**:115–18.

4 Czarnocka J, Slade P. Prevalence and predictors of post-traumatic stress symptoms following childbirth. *Br J Clin Psychol* 2000;**39**:35–52.

5 Landsman IS, Baum CG, Arnkoff DB, *et al.* The psychological consequences of traumatic injury. *J Behav Med* 1990;December **13**(6):561–81.

6 Davidson JRT, Foa EB. Diagnostic issues in post-traumatic stress disorder: considerations for DSM-IV. *J Abnormal Psychology* 1991;**100**:346–55.

7 Rachman S. Emotional processing. *Behav Res Therapy* 1980;**18**:51–60.

8 Brewin CR, Dalgleish T, Joseph S. A dual representation theory of post traumatic stress disorder. *Psychol Rev* 1996;**103**:670–86.

9 Brown GW, Harris T. *Social origins of depression.* London: Tavistock Publications, 1978.

10 Kessler RC. The effects of stressful life events on depression. *Annual Rev Psychol* 1997;**48**:191–214.
11 Malt U. The long-term consequences of accidental injury. A longitudinal study of 107 adults. *Br J Psychiat* 1988;**153**:810–18.
12 Vincent CA, Pincus T, Scurr JH. Patients' experience of surgical accidents. *Qual Healthcare* 1993;**2**:77–82.
13 Parkes CM, ed. *Bereavement: studies of grief in adult life*. London: Penguin, 1988.
14 Vachon MLS, Rogers J, Lyall A, *et al.* Predictors and correlates of adaptation to conjugal bereavement. *Am J Psychiatry* 1982;**139**(8):998–1002.
15 Lundin T. Morbidity following sudden and unexpected bereavement. *Br J Psychiatry* 1984;**144**:84–8.
16 Lehman DR, Lang EL, Wortman CB, Sorenson SB. Long-term effects of sudden bereavement: Marital and parent–child relationships and children's reactions. *J Fam Psychol* 1989;**2**(3):344–67.
17 Lehman DR, Wortman CB, Williams AF. Long-term effects of losing a spouse or child in a motor vehicle crash. *J Personality Soc Psychol* 1987;Jan **52**(1):218–31.
18 Clements R. The continuing care of the injured patient. In: Clements R, Huntingford P, eds. *Safe practice in obstetrics and gynaecology*. London: Churchill Livingstone, 1994.
19 Bennet G. After an accident around childbirth. In: Clements R, Huntingford P, eds. *Safe practice in obstetrics and gynaecology*. London: Churchill Livingstone, 1994.
20 Finlay I, Dallimore D. Your child is dead. *BMJ* 1991;**302**:1524–5.
21 Bark P, Vincent CA, Jones A, Savory J. Clinical complaints: a means of improving quality of care. *Qual Health Care* 1994;**3**:123–32.

25 Supporting staff involved in serious incidents and during litigation

DAVID HEWETT

This chapter explores the reactions which clinical staff may experience when there is a serious mishap in their practice that may then lead on to the instigation of civil proceedings on the part of the patient. Based upon that understanding, some practical responses are proposed which directly relate both to the formal investigation protocol which has been described in Chapter 23, and the often protracted legal process.

Although much of the discussion primarily relates to doctors, it is equally applicable to other clinical professions such as nurses, therapists, and technical staff. As the complexity and diversity of clinical practice grows it is inevitable that these groups will become increasingly exposed to the possibilities of mishap, complaint, and litigation.

An existential paradox for clinicians

People who work with patients normally exhibit a very highly developed sense of vocation, something that dominates their attitudes and values in life. The personal rewards of working in a clinical setting are often very great and usually sustained, but the inherent stresses are also considerable.

Delivering clinical care to sick patients contains within the process deep seated and potentially disturbing contradictions.[1] Some (such as increased patient expectations, continual erosion of professional autonomy, constrained resources, a rigid and exclusive model of training etc.) are discussed below. Understanding them is the key to both anticipating and dealing with the psychological trauma which clinical professionals may experience, not only when a mishap occurs, but also recurrently during the conduct of any subsequent litigation.

In recent decades social change has been rapid. Individuality has been emphasised at the expense of group identity. Within these major changes, public expectations of medical care have risen greatly, with the result that certainty is often expected when the state of knowledge can at best only offer probabilities.[2] In the past, tensions between aspiration and reality in medical care were suppressed by a great disparity of power, both charismatic and knowledge based, between the health professional (usually the doctor), and a largely uninformed patient. Now, the public is both more informed and assertive, demanding explanation and justification for life altering decisions that would, hitherto, have been accepted unquestioningly. In turn, this has greatly increased the collective insecurity of professionals who find their actions, and particularly their errors, called to account.

As if this erosion of traditional autonomy was not threatening enough, there is an almost unspoken paradox in simply being a clinician. Clinical care is delivered in settings that are often problematic and sometimes border on the chaotic. Successive governments have exercised unrelenting pressure for efficiency. Hospitals have been required to reduce lengths of stay, as well as increasing the throughput of elective surgical work to satisfy performance targets and reduce waiting lists. This has occurred against a continuing background of limited resources, increasing numbers of emergency admissions, and greater complexity in the treatments being given. Under such conditions, mistakes are very easy to make.

Pre-qualification training in both medicine and nursing imparts a deep seated ethic of obligation as well as perfection in most clinical staff. Medical undergraduates are exposed over a long period to a curriculum which is overburdened in factual content and which remains stubbornly didactic in its delivery. The selection process for entry is heavily weighted in favour of examination success, and does not necessarily select those personalities most able to cope with the uncertainties and contradictions of professional life.

Many currently practising doctors have been trained under a system of ritual humiliation on the teaching ward round, which, although now perhaps less severe than in the past, unfortunately appears to remain alive and kicking. Competition for hospital training and ultimate career posts also serves to keep young doctors (particularly surgeons) constantly aware not only of their current performance, but also their route upwards through a highly structured and innately conservative system.

Such an extremely stylised and rigidly controlled regime tends to be almost completely unforgiving of error, and is behaviourally self-perpetuating. Long hours of work, frequent disturbance of rest, and poor working conditions also combine to create a fertile ground in which errors can occur.

Error and self perception

Error in medical care is different. In many situations encountered in daily life, error may be remedied simply by an apology, a smile, and a cheque or free gift.[1] The consequences of mistakes are transient, mildly uncomfortable, and usually quickly resolved. In others, of which healthcare is one, transport of passengers for reward is another, the price of error can be truly catastrophic. Thus an ethic in which error is believed not to be permissible tends to characterise these service organisations.

When error is believed to be impossible, there are serious consequences for the way individuals, organisations, commentators, and the media respond when accidents do happen. Traditional responses have been based on authority, blame, and quasi-judicial approaches to determining what went wrong. Individual reactions to mistakes are often profound because falling below the accepted standard of perfect practice is perceived as personal failure. It may be helpful to explore how concepts connected with error interact with notions of the self in health professionals.

To begin, Reason (see Chapter 1) describes a general theory of how accidents may be passively facilitated by the environment in which they take place, coupled with failure of preventive mechanisms when challenged by an error. Errors may be those derived from the faulty execution of a plan (lapses, slips etc.), and those inherent in its formulation (mistakes, departures from accepted practice).[3] This thinking, by emphasising multiple causation, runs counter to more traditional naming and shaming organisational cultures.

However, in a healthcare context these rather neat categories may not be entirely distinct because decision making takes place against a constantly changing clinical picture. Thus, what at one point is justified, can later become erroneous. Some situations are so difficult to interpret, the facts so uncertain, that error is almost inevitable. This has been termed "necessary fallibility",[4] a concept based upon viewing medicine almost as an engineering process; the unique application of science to individual situations.

However they are defined, research shows that errors in clinical care are very common. This too runs contrary to the received ethic of perfection. Errors may be ignored or overlooked especially if they do not produce adverse outcomes. In the NHS, it has been estimated that there may be as many as 90 000 adverse events a year leading to as many as 13 500 deaths. From these events about 9000 claims are generated, leading to payment in 2000 cases.[5] From what little is known about the claims epidemiology in the United Kingdom, obstetric practice accounts for the largest proportion of payments measured by value (64%, 1995–98), with gynaecology and orthopaedics being the largest represented numerically.

Based upon litigation in the United States it has been shown that male medical practitioners are on average about three times as likely to be

483

involved in litigation as females.[6] This study also found that the likelihood of being sued varies with age, peaking at around 40. This latter finding is perhaps more difficult to apply in the United Kingdom where training tends to be more intensive and extends over a longer period. The study hypothesised that the lower rate amongst females might be due to their better interaction with patients, although no evidence was adduced to support this particular view. It is perhaps dangerous to assume that litigation correlates with adverse events. Studies show that a decision to litigate is related to the severity of the remaining disability for the patient.[7] Furthermore, doctors who are litigated against more often than others are not less competent. Competence is a function of both knowledge and performance, and those who are most knowledgeable are sued more frequently.[8]

In summary then, errors are common, the risks are greatest if one is a male gynaecologist or orthopaedic surgeon, and in the early stages of unsupervised practice. Errors in medicine may be catastrophic and the prevailing work ethic means that mistakes are unacceptable. Therein lies the root of great personal and professional conflict.

The unacceptability of medical error

The implications for those who are involved in serious adverse events are therefore profound, and operate at several different levels. The most important of these is self-perception. Because error is unacceptable, the fact of its existence is often perceived initially as personal failure. This is well described by Leape:[9]

Physicians are socialised in medical school and by residency to strive for error free practice. There is a powerful emphasis on perfection, both in diagnosis and treatment. In everyday hospital practice the message is clear: mistakes are unacceptable. Physicians are expected to function without error, an interpretation that many of them translate into the need to be infallible. One result is that physicians, not unlike test pilots, come to view error as a failure of character – you weren't careful, you didn't try hard enough. This kind of thinking lies behind a common reaction in physicians: "how can there be an error without negligence?"

Leape has gone further in arguing that role models in medical education constantly reinforce the notion of infallibility, leading to pressure for intellectual dishonesty, with the result that errors are rarely discussed.[9] At a practical level, all clinicians accept that errors are inevitable, but this seldom spills over in to accepting the frequency with which they occur, and there is little research into errors or how to investigate them. Thus, rather like speed limits, their existence is universally accepted, but they are often ignored.

Rosenthal has made a special study of the problems doctors face in the USA, UK and Sweden. She has, through ethnographic studies, identified how doctors practise in a state of "permanent uncertainty" and must accept (against their training) that "fallibility is an intrinsic part of the practice of medicine".[10] All doctors have made mistakes, often serious ones, and their experiences "create a powerful tool of mutual empathy and an unforgettable sense of shared personal vulnerability". Living this way doctors are unsurprisingly "quick to forgive" and "non criticism" is the norm. "Where uncertainty surrounds all members of the profession daily and all see themselves as vulnerable to accidents, it is not difficult to understand a tacit norm of non-criticism, a conspiracy of tolerance."[11]

When an adverse incident occurs the result is an often painful clash between reality and deeply embedded belief systems. Such conflict has been meticulously recorded in a small study which also highlighted some important themes which are generally applicable:[12]

- The ubiquity of mistakes in medical practice
- The lack of self-disclosure about mistakes to colleagues, friends and family
- The often unexpected degree of emotional impact on the physician
- The durability of memories so that events can be recalled in detail years later
- The influence of personal beliefs about personal responsibility and medical practice.

Research in the USA suggests that doctors who are the subject of litigation frequently feel that the claim is quite unjustified, and that settling them is tantamount to an admission of guilt.[13,14] This perception is perhaps reinforced by the traditional advice from medical defence institutions, namely that following an adverse event, apology and explanation should be given to patients without any admission of liability.

Whilst this is clearly a counsel of perfection in a strictly legal sense, adhering to it in practice may be extremely difficult. Patients may think the doctor is being evasive as he or she avoids saying anything that could be construed as an admission of liability. Doctors may feel that being careful in what is said militates against displaying the necessary candour that preserving the professional relationship with the patient may require. This conflict often crops up when doctors help frame written responses to formal complaints. Inability to resolve it then leads to further dissatisfaction, manifest by subsequent requests for Independent Reviews.[13] The whole process then increases the anger, alienation, and sense of outrage experienced by the clinician. Thus the period after an incident, when attempts to deal with the consequences are experienced can be as problematic for the clinician as the incident itself.

Doctors report strong feelings of anger and guilt following adverse incidents and particularly when legal action is taken. Because of the prevailing culture, loneliness is very common in this situation. Silence and suppression are the prevailing coping strategies in medicine. The aftermath, either

485

in terms of investigation or litigation threatens individual standing, and may even extend to uncertainty about future livelihood.

Research in the UK[16] by Genn shows that doctors do not generally take litigation in their stride. Whilst the initial incident may be dealt with effectively, subsequent litigation serves to administer further stress intermittently in a random and highly damaging way. An example of what may happen was described in detail in Genn's paper. The case involved a consultant who caused a spinal injury at operation. Despite great care in undertaking a risky procedure paralysis had been caused.

I didn't think I had been negligent. I think it was just one of those things. I knew it was a dangerous area . . . I felt at the time and I still feel very sorry for the woman who was injured . . . The Medical Defence Union had to ask some rather unpleasant, pretty straight questions about the incident which was fairly painful at the time . . . you would have an interview or two and then the thing would go fallow for several months at a time, then it would rear up again, and that in itself was unsettling.

I didn't feel at the time that it was an attack on my professional competence, but the trial went on for four days, and I obviously didn't like the judgement . . . it is very painful to the person at the time, because someone is casting a slur on your professional capabilities.

I still feel desperately sorry that I caused damage to someone, most of us don't go into medicine with that intention. I don't know how much it really did get to me, because I used to bottle up emotions, but not long after the case I had a depression . . .

I don't think it was the cause of my depression but I would not like to say that it wasn't one of the factors. I think that if I thought that I was negligent I would have found it incredibly difficult. I suppose that because you are a perfectionist, I would have found it very difficult to live with the fact that I had actually done someone some harm by something I should have avoided.

This narrative shows clearly the conflicts and personal struggle experienced by the consultant at the centre of this case, and how difficult coming to terms with it all was over a long period of time.

In the United Kingdom, centralised pooling of liabilities managed by the National Health Service Litigation Authority (NHSLA) has meant that hospital doctors are no longer named as defendants in legal actions. The element of being sued personally may have been removed in practice, but the effects will inevitably linger on as an individual perception, so long as doctors (rightly) see themselves as being primarily accountable to their patients. The process of centralisation may serve to increase the feelings of isolation and powerlessness in the ensuing legal process.

Other reactions to adverse events and litigation

So far the impact of an adverse event and ensuing litigation has been considered at the personal psychological level. This of course may only be part of the overall response. Individual reactions may be characterised by more florid, sometimes morbid features. These are partly conditioned by the pre-existing personality, by past experience, and a multitude of other co-existing factors including latent physical and mental illness.

In some specialties (and obstetrics is probably the best example) the risk of litigation is high and situations in which the outcome is not perfect, despite the best of care, are more regularly encountered. Clinicians working in such areas become used to reviewing carefully what took place, and in time come to view regular legal enquiries philosophically. For others though, the experience is both rare and distressing.

Pre-existing personality traits may become exaggerated.[17] A person, hitherto a natural worrier, may become totally consumed with concern, exhibiting sleeplessness, poor appetite, and thoughts which constantly return to the incident. In severe manifestations, panic attacks coupled with feelings of impending doom may appear. Such a post-traumatic stress disorder can be extremely disabling and call into question the person's ability to work. Someone hitherto rather shy and introverted, may avoid social contact, and possibly experience uncontrollable anxiety in certain places such as the operating theatre or street. Others may turn to stress waking, very low mood, profound feelings of guilt, unreasonably exaggerated notions of personal responsibility and blame may appear. In these situations the possibility of suicide has to be seriously considered.

Responses in the aftermath of clinical accidents

There is much that a well organised trust can do to alleviate the stress encountered by staff faced with a serious incident or who become involved in litigation. Essentially these interventions can be classified into two principal groups, those operating at the organisational level, and action directed towards supporting individuals.

Organisational responses

At the organisational level, key values and principles should be clearly and explicitly set out to help create a climate within which both management and staff become aware of the way in which adverse incidents will be handled. This is an important aspect of the total organisational culture, and can be articulated through policies, procedures and training. Public reference to these ideas by the trust board, backed up by reiteration from the executive team members when they meet staff groups goes a long way in setting the tone. Within the Clinical Negligence Scheme for Trusts (CNST) standards, particularly at level 2 of the assessment hierarchy, the main policy issues are clearly set out by the NHSLA. These provide a solid foundation for the pan organisational response.

487

1 Openness

From the foregoing analysis it is clear that in clinical care beliefs are often not aligned with reality. This conflict can be attacked at an organisational level, and the response starts with developing a culture of greater openness both with patients as well as within and between professional groups. Newly revised standards for CNST level 2 assessment are aimed at fostering this change. Standard 4.2.7 states:

> *In the interests of patient safety, openness and constructive criticism of clinical care is actively encouraged.*[18]

In practice this means that clinical audit, or whatever that activity becomes as clinical governance is established, is a powerful tool which can be used to stimulate debate through regular observation and the application of evidence. The activity provides a forum within which debate can take place. The regular reporting of the outcomes and lessons learned from investigating significant incidents will, in time, break down defensive barriers and help to de-sensitise the subject. Within trust policy statements, specific reference to these will signify top level support and encouragement.

Openness at a professional level goes hand in hand with openness towards patients. Again, the CNST standards call for a clear policy on consent to treatment.

> *Appropriate information is provided to patients on the risks and benefits of the proposed treatment or investigation, and the alternatives available, before a signature on a consent form is sought.*[19]

This particular standard goes on to specify the general content of information leaflets, refers to guidance on the structure of consent forms and the level of competence expected of those who seek consent from patients. Beyond that, the need to inform patients of any mishap, and make a suitable apology, must be reinforced. Apologies do not imply an admission of liability, and it should be accepted that giving information takes precedence over whatever administrative or legal considerations might be thought to apply.

2 Consistency and Objectivity

Trusts need to demonstrate consistency and fairness in investigating adverse incidents. This starts with CNST standard 5.

> *There is a policy for the rapid follow up of all serious clinical events.*[20]

Implementing this standard provides a major opportunity to confront the issues outlined at the beginning of this chapter. The policy statement should set out when and how such incidents will be handled. It will acknowledge that error exists, and that it must be openly acknowledged. Furthermore, not all serious clinical events represent errors.

For example, a maternity unit may decide to review every case where a baby is born in a shocked condition. In many of these situations it will be found that everything had been done properly. In only a small proportion of these, avoidable errors may be detected, but it is necessary to look at them all in order to detect what is avoidable. Establishing a routine process may in itself change the way in which the process is viewed.

Having acknowledged error exists, the next step is recognise that in most situations staff do not make intentional errors. Moreover, errors arise in complex ways the causes of which extend beyond the individuals concerned. In such circumstances it is pointless to apportion blame and make accusations. Rather a systems approach must be adopted which examines why adverse events occur.[21] This approach should be explicitly acknowledged within policy statements, guidelines, and training associated with a formalised incident investigation (see Chapter 23).

We have described elsewhere the use of a formalised method of investigation. This is essential, not only to ensure that a comprehensive investigation is carried out, but also to demonstrate objectivity and fairness in its execution. From such a process, reliable conclusions may be drawn and the requisite preventive action taken. By involving staff in the investigation, sharing the emerging conclusions, and seeking commitment to remedial action, much of the anxiety associated with the process can be avoided.

3 Discipline

Inherent in the use of any formal investigation process is the question of its relationship with disciplinary action. Clearly the latter cannot be entirely ruled out, as standards of practice may be discovered which breach the minima required by professional regulatory bodies. Personal conduct may transgress the boundaries set out in personnel policies and very rarely, the criminal law may have been transgressed. All these situations require managers to take specific action.

Thus it is not possible to assure staff participating in enquiries that disciplinary action can be entirely ruled out. On the other hand, taking a systematic approach and examining all the factors at work will often avoid unnecessary and premature disciplinary action. Premature disciplinary action may prejudice the investigation process and obscure the real determinants of failure because once this is invoked all involved naturally adopt defensive attitudes.

Disciplinary action is more likely to be associated with persistent and habitual problems with a member of staff or a group of staff. It rarely arises completely unannounced, and is often an indicator of previous failures of the organisation to deal with well recognised problems.

In general the benefits of objective and consistent investigation of serious clinical events should outweigh the potential disadvantages, which may be perceived by those whose actions undergo detailed scrutiny. The process, when carried out regularly and predictably, will convey important messages about the way mistakes and their prevention are perceived by top managers and board members.

4 Education and Training

Professional education in many spheres concentrates mainly on developing core knowledge and its application in practice. Other, important, but perhaps peripheral subjects, tend to be either squeezed out or poorly covered in busy curricula. This is certainly true of risk awareness, assessment, and management in the medical curriculum.

The process of investigation and subsequent litigation is often a completely new experience for clinical staff. Coupled with the psychological conflicts described earlier this added uncertainty compounds the problems staff face. It is important therefore to provide specific education to different staff groups, designed to familiarise them with these problems. The content of such education should cover the notion of risk itself, how the trade off between risk reduction, costs, and practicability is achieved. Also it provides an important opportunity to state explicitly the key organisational values contained in the relevant policy statements and procedures.

For those in the front line, particularly doctors, a knowledge of the elementary principles of medical law, namely the concepts of negligence, liability, and causation will help them navigate between the rocks when explaining a mistake to a patient. A simple outline of the procedures followed in managing a case can take away some of the apparent randomness of the periodic stresses involved. Advantage can be taken of local induction programmes for newly recruited staff, postgraduate seminars, and other training opportunities.

Supporting the individual

At the individual level there is also much that trusts can do to minimise the adverse impact of investigations and litigation. This starts with the immediate care of individuals involved in incidents and then periodic and sometimes sustained support through the legal process that may follow.

First of all not everyone will require support. For less serious errors, junior doctors may be counselled and supported by their seniors as a normal part of their training. This will also apply to nurses and others working under the general supervision of more senior colleagues. In more serious situations, familiarity, because such events are inherent in that particular field, may mean that clinicians are well able to cope.

In many other situations a proper support mechanism is needed. This starts by considering whether immediate practice should continue. This matter was recently considered during a fatal accident inquiry in Scotland.

An endoscopic surgeon continued to operate after the first patient on his list unexpectedly died. However, the eighth patient and last patient on his list that day also died. The surgeon was cleared of any blame for the deaths.

A leading specialist in endoscopic surgery said to the inquiry "My own view is that a death on the table is a harrowing experience for a surgeon . . . the surgeon is emotionally and mentally not in the frame of mind to continue to operate that day".

The president of the Edinburgh Royal College of Surgeons said "We can understand the pressure that single handed surgeons are under but I think there would be a very strong feeling that when a surgeon loses a patient, he should not continue to operate that day."[22]

Subsequent commentary on this case pointed out that the anaesthetist was often in a similar position and that he or she too should not continue on that day.[23] It is important not to confuse stopping work in this way with suspension, especially if the individual concerned leaves work and goes home. This is not a form of suspension rather it is a compassionate response to a traumatic experience. There is unfortunately a bad history of prolonged suspension of senior medical staff in the NHS which may lead some senior doctors to reject this advice.[24]

During the investigation phase, familiarity with the process to be followed will be of some limited help to those undergoing it. The style of interviews is important. Investigators should be specifically trained. Interviewees should be offered the opportunity to be accompanied. It is perfectly proper for investigators to ask leading questions, to approach difficult areas with tact and sensitivity, and to make supportive comments. Such interviews should not be confrontational, and cross examination of witnesses is to be avoided. Senior clinicians should be actively discouraged from behaving as though they were examining for a higher professional examination. Judgmental comments are always unhelpful.

After the investigation is complete the findings must be shared with those involved whose comments must be seriously considered. This will foster confidence in objectivity and fairness as well as reducing the understandable paranoia associated with it. Continuing support mechanisms may be needed after the initial phase, especially if litigation is contemplated. The claims manager inevitably provides some of this assistance as the conduit through which the trust communicates with its legal advisers. In difficult cases meetings with the solicitor handling the case are often helpful.

It is essential that clinicians feel confident in what is being done on their behalf. This has been made more difficult to achieve by the central handling of larger claims by the NHSLA and the fact that it is the trust and not the clinician who is being pursued. Research in the USA suggests that being involved with the claim helps considerably to reduce the stress

491

involved.[25] In the UK we appear to have made that well nigh impossible to achieve.

Whilst claims managers can provide factual and procedural assistance to staff, purely professional support may also be needed. Medical directors and clinical directors are well placed to offer professional support, and with the development of appraisal systems for senior clinicians their relative isolation in the system may be ending.[26]

In the formal phases of litigation the claims manager has a very important role to play in supporting clinicians. This runs throughout the life of the case. The initial writing of the statement may require help. It is surprising how many senior medical staff have no experience of this and require help in producing a properly structured and systematic account. Tact and diplomacy is required in helping otherwise highly trained individuals.

Presence at, and preparation of, case conferences is essential as these can prove very stressful as the potential negligence comes to be defined. The formal setting, the eminence of experts, and the seniority of the legal advisers involved can all combine to make a conference a very uncomfortable experience. Debriefing on the journey home is often needed.

Similarly with the Coroner's Court, the purpose of an inquest may be poorly understood, and the relative informality of open proceedings can be deceptive. Staff who have no experience of this find the experience traumatic. They need to be prepared beforehand, accompanied and supported throughout. A trust policy for appearances in court is a good way of codifying the support available to staff, and helps them to deal with direct approaches either from claimants' solicitors, from the Coroner's Officer and others. Even in the best managed hospitals these will occur from time to time. Below is an illustration of the need to support a junior member of staff in the Coroner's court.

Illustrative case: an inappropriate discharge from A&E

A senior house officer (SHO), with some three years post-registration experience in two other A&E departments discharged a young female student who had been brought in as an emergency, following an acute episode of vomiting during which blood was produced.

The doctor was, at that time, unaware that the patient had low oxygen saturations and a tachycardia on admission. Another A&E doctor who was fully engaged with other patients, had been concerned about the patient earlier when he was consulted by the triage nurse. Responding to the nurse he told her to administer oxygen and immediately place the patient in a cubicle The A&E department was full at the time, and the first one available was used. When the patient

---

began to feel better during her wait for assessment, she removed the oxygen mask and moved to a chair chatting and laughing with the friends who had accompanied her

After an hour, the SHO arrived. She sent the patient's friends out whilst she interviewed and examined her. She made a diagnosis of viral gastro-enteritis, noting that the blood might have been due to trauma during vomiting. The patient was anxious to leave, wanting to go out with her boyfriend that evening as he was leaving the area for a while to fulfil a contract.

Next day the patient returned by ambulance at the insistence of her college nurse. Again she had low oxygen saturations and a pronounced tachycardia. This time a chest radiograph was undertaken which showed a dense consolidation of one lung. She was immediately given antibiotics and admitted to a medical ward where unfortunately she died a few hours later following a cardiac arrest in the face of a fulminating pneumonia.

The SHO later wrote a statement for the coroner's officer in which it was clear that she had not read the casualty records properly on the previous afternoon, failing to note the tachycardia and oxygen saturation at 89%, observations which were clearly recorded by the triage nurse. The oxygen administration had not been recorded. Thus in ignorance of these facts the SHO had not appreciated how ill she really was.

The incident was investigated systematically using a protocol, and highlighted not only this error, but also:

- Design faults in the department which meant that ill patients were out of sight of the nursing station.
- A medical staffing structure that had only one senior member, a single handed consultant, which meant that supervision was inevitably poor and "experienced" SHOs were required to make decisions for which in other settings they would seek approval.
- The standard of record keeping and communication within the department was less than satisfactory especially when the department was busy.
- Current procedures meant that patients could be "lost" within the department if cubicles were used that were not clearly visible from the central nurses' station.

The SHO was supported in her statement writing, by talking about what had happened and exploring how she felt about it. She was covered in the department during her court appearance, but also enabled to take several hours out before returning to her shift.

> The Coroner's questioning, although sensitively handled, had nevertheless, in a very formal setting with the patient's relatives present, allowed the facts of the matter to speak in a way that was very clear and direct. This had a considerable personal impact and rendered the doctor unable to carry on in her work without further time for reflection and recuperation. She needed considerable subsequent support from her consultant.

Finally, most clinicians who have to go to Court in those rare cases that are defended fully find the process baffling and potentially humiliating. The loss of control, exposure to public criticism in a highly ritualised and coercive procedure, and the protracted nature of it all combines to assault the esteem of even the most self-confident. By being there, understanding what is happening, and keeping contact with the legal team and the NHSLA, the claims manager is able to support the clinician who will still feel that, whatever the administrative niceties, he or she is the real defendant.

Conclusion

The effects of error in clinical care are often underestimated or ignored. Professional and cultural factors mean that staff who are involved in major clinical accidents are often isolated and may experience deep psychological trauma. Almost all will experience a crisis of confidence, and a sense of frustration and anger.

To alleviate this, there is much that can be done by trusts. As employers they can foster a more appropriate culture by demonstrating that accidents lead to learning, and adjustment to prevent recurrence. Also by ensuring that investigations are fair open and thorough, and by providing support to those involved in adverse events, it can be demonstrated that there is commitment to learning from mistakes.

All this is worthwhile simply because it can lead to higher quality services and better care for patients.

References

1 Vincent C. Fallibility uncertainty and the impact of mistakes and litigation. In: Firth-Cozens J, Payne RL, eds. *Stress in health professionals*. London: John Wiley, 1999.
2 McCue JD. The effects of stress on physicians and their medical practice. *N Engl J Med* 1982;30(8):458–63.
3 Reason JT. *Human error*. New York: Cambridge University Press, 1990.
4 Gorowitz S, MacIntye A. Towards a theory of medical fallibility. In: Egelhardt HT,

Callahan D, eds. *Science ethics and medicine*. Hastings-on-Hudson, New York: Hastings Centre, 1976.

5 Towse A, Danzon P. Medical negligence and the NHS: an economic analysis. *Health Econ* 1999;**8**(2):93–101.

6 Taragin MI, Wilczek AP, Karns, ME, *et al.* Physician demographics and the risk of medical malpractice. *Am Med J* (1992);**93**(5):537–42.

7 Brennan TA, Sox CM, Burstin HR. Relationship between negligent adverse events and the outcomes of medical-malpractice litigation. *N Engl J Med* 1996;**335**(26):1963–7.

8 Ely JW, Dawson JD, Young PR, *et al.* Claims against family physicians are the best doctors sued more? *J Fam Pract* 1999;**48**(1):23–30.

9 Leape LL. Error in medicine. *JAMA* 199;**272**(23):1851–7.

10 Lens P, Wal G van der. *Problem doctors: a conspiracy of silence.* Amsterdam: JOS Press, 1997.

11 Smith R. All doctors are problem doctors. *BMJ* 1997;**314**:841.

12 Christensen JF, Levinson W, Dunn, PM. The heart of darkness: the impact of perceived mistakes on physicians. *J Gen Intern Med* 1992;**7**:424–31.

13 Vincent C, Ennis M. The effects of medical accidents and litigation on doctors and patients. *Law and Policy* 1994;**16**(2):97.

14 Charles SC, Wilbert JR, Kennedy EC. Physicians' self reports of reactions to malpractice litigation. *Am J Psychiatr* 1984;**14**:4.

15 Yamey G. Report condemns NHS complaints procedure. *BMJ* 1999;**319**:804.

16 Genn H. Effects of claims on doctors. *Clin Risk* 1996;**2**:181–5.

17 Hirst DA. Supporting staff during litigation – managerial aspects. *Clinical Risk* 1996;**2**: 189–94.

18 CNST, The Standard 4.2.7. *Clinical Risk Management Standards*, NHSLA, 1999.

19 CNST, The Standard 7. *Clinical Risk Management Standards*, NHSLA, 1997.

20 CNST, The Standard 5. *Clinical Risk Management Standards*, NHSLA, 1997.

21 Leape LL. A systems approach to medical error. *J Eval Clin Pract* 1997;**3**(3):213–22.

22 Christie B. Inquiry says surgeons should stop operating if patient dies. *BMJ* 1999;**318**: 349.

23 Adams AP. The anaesthetist has been forgotten again. *BMJ* 1999;**318** (response to reference 22).

24 Medico-political digest. Suspension unfair to doctors say peers. *BMJ* 1999;**318**:267.

25 Horan DW. How to select counsel and participate in your own defence. *Clin Plast Surg* 1999;**26**(1):79–80, vii.

26 Noble BA. Network of "medical buddies" is needed. *BMJ* 1997;**314**:190.

26 Dealing with clinical complaints

JUDITH ALLSOP, LINDA MULCAHY

Complaints present a challenge to healthcare providers in a number of ways. First, in having to respond, professionals or managers are put in a position where they must investigate and explain the matters that led to the complaint. This may cut across the tasks and routines of day-to-day work. Records must be examined, past events pieced together to establish what happened and, possibly, information obtained from other agencies. A complaint may also be a challenge to the clinical work of a professional. He or she may have to explain what particular decision was made and why it was made. Moreover, it is the patient or relative who determines the agenda. A complaint may begin a process the end point of which cannot be predicted, and over which the service provider has little control. Complaints can lead to the allocation of blame, disciplinary action or litigation. In short, they can be seen as an irritating intrusion, as time consuming and stressful and there appears to be little reward for good complaint handling.

Complaints can also be viewed in a more positive light. They present an opportunity for engagement with the service user. In order to be sure they are providing good care, health providers need to know what patients and their relatives think of services and particularly, what causes dissatisfaction and can lead to complaints. Patients and their relatives have a unique view of their medical care. For example, only patients can know the intensity of their pain or the discontinuities and contradictions in the treatment process. The sympathetic consideration of a complaint can be seen as part of building a partnership with the patient by addressing their concerns. If things are shown to have gone wrong, there is an opportunity to put them right and to maintain a relationship. Even if this has broken down, the intervention of a third party can present the possibility of a repair. Complaints

497

can also provide a valuable insight into how a service is experienced by the people who use it. It is a perspective not open to healthcare providers, particularly if they are senior managers, unless there is specifically commissioned research. Complaints can also identify practices which, if repeated, could be a danger to other patients. They may therefore act as an early warning system – particularly if they are categorised, analysed, and reviewed as part of a wider system of quality and risk management.

A final more instrumental reason for taking complaints seriously is the costs of not doing so. In 1995 the Cabinet Office Complaints Task Force, on the basis of data they collected, estimated that the costs of dealing with a complaint were £3 £45 for informal handling by front-line staff; £370 for a review by senior staff; £770 for external review by a National Health Service (NHS) trust and £11 200 for a full investigation by the Health Service Commissioner.[1] In 1999, the National Audit Office estimated that the potential liabilities of the NHS through litigation were £1·8 billion for 1997–8.[2]

In this chapter, we begin by looking at the shift in government policies for dealing with complaints, which we see as part of a new regulatory regime concerned with standards and safety. In the second section we describe the NHS complaints system introduced in 1996 and what research has shown are some of the barriers to effective complaint handling in healthcare settings. A final section looks at some key aspects of effective complaint handling at the local level.

The changing emphasis in national policy

The 1991 *Citizen's Charter*[3] introduced a programme for the reform of public services. Each sector or department was required to produce a charter which listed entitlements, set performance targets, and outlined mechanisms for the redress of grievances. A further examination of complaints procedures was promised. Subsequently, a review of public sector complaint systems was undertaken by the Cabinet Office Complaints Task Force.[4] In 1994, complaint systems in the NHS were reviewed by the Wilson Committee.[5] Three common themes ran through all these documents. First, there was a concern to improve management within public services to make them more responsive to patient's needs. Second, there was a view that in monopoly services, where the opportunity for exit and using alternative services was limited, consumers should be encouraged to voice their concerns. Third, there was a belief that private sector business offered an appropriate model for learning from complaints. The effective company aimed to satisfy the customer and complaints data were reviewed at board level.

Since coming to power in 1997, the Labour government has laid stress on achieving higher standards in health care; better and more equal outcomes from healthcare interventions; greater partnership with patients and greater accountability within health authorities, trusts and primary care groups. Complaints also remain on the agenda. For example, in 1999, the Cabinet Office published new guidance on how to deal with public sector complaints[6] and the new complaints system is being evaluated. However, policy objectives will be achieved within the context of a stricter regulatory regime designed for early identification of poor practice by professionals or managers. Furthermore, in the wake of recent public investigations and inquiries, concerns about the safety of patients have come to the fore.[7,8,9]

There is a commitment to "modernising" the NHS[10] and proposals to improve quality are set out in *A First Class Service*.[11] They are described more fully in Chapter 3. The monitoring of complaints, both content and handling, is likely to play a part in reviews carried out as part of clinical audit and clinical governance within health authorities, trusts and primary care groups, as well as in the reviews undertaken by the Commission for Health Improvement.

Professional bodies have also introduced changes which increase the amount and extent of regulation. The General Medical Council (GMC) has brought in measures to improve the performance of doctors who have been identified as performing poorly. There is also a scheme for regular revalidation of practising doctors.[12] The Royal Colleges are currently discussing ways of working with the GMC to ensure good quality specialist care. One proposal is that the GMC should keep personal portfolios on all consultants, which would include evidence of participation in audit, continuing professional development and details of any complaints received. Portfolios would be reviewed by doctors and a lay person.[13] Changes are also underway in the regulation of nursing that have a similar purpose.[14] There are signs that the various regulatory bodies are more willing to pool and exchange information.[9,15]

Handling complaints: The current system

The new complaints procedure

In the 1990s, pressures from consumer groups, managers, and doctors led to the introduction of new NHS complaints procedures from April 1996. All trusts, health authorities, and primary care practitioners are now required to establish a complaints procedure and to publicise it. There are two main stages. Complaints are initially handled through the process of "local resolution" but where a complainant remains dissatisfied they may ask for their complaint to be referred to an Independent Review Panel

(IRP). Service providers must appoint a designated officer to administer the procedure and ensure that complaints are dealt with. In addition, health authorities are required to provide conciliators to facilitate the resolution of primary care complaints where either the complainant or staff request conciliation.

NHS Executive guidance is not prescriptive about how health organisations should conduct the process of local resolution. Instead, emphasis is placed on the principles which should guide good practice, such as openness, flexibility, fairness, and understanding what complainants want. The rationale behind local resolution is that it enables complaints to be dealt with promptly and at the point of service delivery, whilst also encouraging accountability by requiring providers to investigate, explain and reflect on their activity.

Complainants who are dissatisfied with the outcome of local resolution may request that an IRP look at the complaint again. Requests for a panel are made to a convener who is usually a non-executive director of the health authority or trust and has responsibility for deciding whether a case should be referred. In reaching their decision conveners are not permitted to investigate the complaint nor should they attempt to resolve it. Their options are to:

- Refer the complaint back for further action at local resolution, if they think that more could be done at that stage to satisfy the complainant
- Refuse a panel if they think that all practicable action has been taken and a panel would not add to the process
- Convene a panel if nothing short of independent review will achieve resolution

When considering a request, conveners must seek advice from an independent lay chairperson. Where the complaint involves clinical judgement, a convener must also seek advice from clinicians. However, it is for the convener to decide whether a panel should be set up.

IRPs are normally made up of three people: the lay chair, the convener and a third panel member from a regional list. Where the complaint relates to clinical judgement, panels must also be advised by at least two clinical assessors. The function of the panel is to investigate the complainant's grievance, as outlined in the convener's terms of reference, and to write a report setting out its conclusions. If appropriate, the panel's report should make suggestions for remedying any failings.[16] The convener's decision about whether to refer a case and the conduct of a panel may also be the subject of an investigation by the Health Service Commissioner. In 1996, the Commissioner acquired the right to consider complaints about clinical care as well as those about administrative matters.

Complaints: context and substance

A complaint shows that the complainant is hurting in some way. It reflects their subjective feelings about a perceived failure in the provision of care. This failure may relate to something which a doctor or nurse has done or not done. It may be a criticism of professional behaviour or an expression of concern about the process of delivering a service or outcomes. Typically, complaint letters take the form of a narrative that catalogues events, and make justifications for complaining. Most complainants are distressed or angry.

Most complaints contain a number of allegations, some of which are expressed and others implied. These can vary considerably in severity from allegations of poor care leading to death to concerns about the standard of bedlinen. Many complainants have suffered some form of loss, even if it is only to their dignity. A common complaint by patients is that their concerns have not been listened to. Others may feel that they have paid out good money for poor workmanship, as in the case of dental work or that there have been side effects of medication. In yet other complaints, the clinician or the care given is seen to have been incompetent. Some will believe that a disaster has been avoided by their own efforts. This is the case in general practice when a decision by a doctor not to visit, or a diagnosis with which the carer does not agree, leads to a hospital attendance where a more serious condition is diagnosed. Many people who complain have been bereaved and attribute the death or the care of the dying to poor clinical care.[17] How their dissatisfaction has been handled is also a frequently cited additional reason for complaint. Figure 26.1 presents recent data on the main allegation made by complainants as categorised by officials and researchers. These isolate a single category of allegation and are unlikely to be presented so clearly in a letter of complaint.

The first act of a complaints manager when receiving a letter of complaint may well be to pose the question: what issues are of concern to this person? The act of complaining should be seen as a social activity outside the norms of everyday behaviour. For most people making a complaint, either verbally or in writing, requires an act of will and an investment of time, and draws on emotional, social and other resources. This means that the issue is important to them and to others within their social network. Furthermore, when people complain, their identity as competent social actors is at stake. Typically, many letters of complaint give accounts which demonstrate that the patient or carer is a competent and reliable person. Qualitative research on complaints has shown that the way in which a complaint is presented is likely to reflect a person's social position, cultural background, skills and knowledge and that certain groups are disadvantaged. A complaints manager will need to take this into account when responding to a letter of complaint.

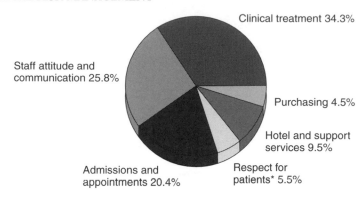

* This includes complaints about privacy, dignity, confidentiality, consent and complaint handling.
Source: Department of Health. *Handling complaints: Monitioring the NHS complaints procedures, England 1997-8.* 1998, Table 5, p5.

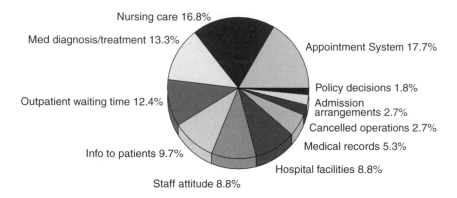

Source: Kyffin, R., Cook, G. and Jones, M. *Complainants' satisfaction with NHS Trust complaints procedures.* Liverpool: University of Liverpool, 1999, Table 3.3, p32.

Figure 26.1 The substance of complaints and the nature of clinical complaints.

The incidence of complaints

The incidence of complaints, and particularly clinical complaints, has been rising over the last decade (see Table 26.1). The subject matter of complaints varies according to the service being complained about. Figure 26.1 shows the type of allegations made in written complaints in hospital and community services across England. The category of clinical care is very broad. Allegations relating to communication, information. and staff attitude may also involve clinical staff.

Table 26.1 The rise in complaints 1991–8

	1991/2	1997/8
Clinical complaints in hospitals[18]	17 991	28 473
Complaints to the General Medical Council[9]	1087	3066
Grievances received by the Health Service Commissioner[19]	972	2660

Barriers to making complaints in the existing system

Despite the rise in complaints, there are still barriers to people expressing their concerns: first, they must be aware that something has gone wrong; and second, they must know where and how to make their views known. Even if they make a complaint, they may not receive the response they would wish for.

The relationship between voicing concerns, adverse events and legal claims is not straightforward. Adverse events can occur which do not become the basis of a complaint because neither the patient nor carer is aware that anything has gone wrong. The Harvard study of medical records showed that there were more adverse events occurring than were ever reported through complaints or claims. Conversely, claims were made where no adverse event had occurred.[20]

Research suggests that much dissatisfaction does not mature into a complaint because the level of knowledge of how to complain continues to remain low[21,22] and people find the various systems confusing.[9] A household survey by Mulcahy and Tritter found that 18% of householders who claimed to be dissatisfied with NHS care said they had failed to complain because they lacked knowledge of how to do so.[23] The box on page 504 provides some typical comments made by people who don't complain.

Research by MORI has also suggested that dissatisfied service users are most likely to fear recrimination in relation to complaints about healthcare and about the police. The same study demonstrated that ethnic minority women and elderly people were the groups least likely to complain.[21]

Complainants' views of the complaint process

If people do decide to raise their concerns, research suggests that staff are not always willing or able to help them. This can happen at any stage of the process. Recent research by the Public Law Project[24] shows that whilst local resolution can work well, complainants and their representatives were concerned about the lack of impartiality and visibility. Particular problems were identified in the primary care sector where complainants felt daunted by the prospect of having to complain directly to the practitioner they were

---

Why people don't complain

My mother did not want me to complain because she felt that she would be victimised and it would affect her treatment.

If you take them on, you may suddenly find you cannot get a doctor locally.

I don't see any point. You'll never prove anything against doctors. They just club together. I just moan.

When I came out [of hospital] I was glad to be alive. It seemed trivial. It was just a relief I hadn't got cancer, I thought that was enough.

I just thought I'd try to keep clear of NHS people – I dreaded the fact I may get old and may have to use them more frequently.

I'm afraid of making a fool of myself.

And you're not going to complain about the nurses because you know they're under pressure.

> *Source*: May A, Allsop J, Coyle, J. *High Hopes: Charters and Complaints, an Account of People's Experiences in NHS Complaints Systems*, 1993. Social Sciences Research Centre, London: South Bank University and Mulcahy L, Tritter J. *Dissatisfaction, grievances and complaints in the NHS: A report for the Department of Health*, 1993.

---

criticising. Some were sceptical about whether they would receive an open and impartial explanation and many feared that they might suffer some form of retribution (see box above). The Health Service Commissioner has deplored the fact that some GPs have asked patients, and sometimes their families as well, to leave their practice following a complaint. It has been recommended that changes be made to the GP contract so that GPs must give reasons for removing a patient.[19]

The Public Law Project research has also shown that there are weaknesses in how local resolution is being conducted. Conveners in the survey sent back nearly half (47%) the cases referred to them for further local resolution. Figure 26.2 shows the reasons for cases being sent back.

The same research revealed that the ways in which independent review panels are established and conducted did not give complainants confidence in their independence or effectiveness in holding the NHS to account. There was a lack of transparency in the ways in which the panels were conducted. For example, the parties to the complaint typically were seen separately and consequently there was no opportunity for them to question each other about their accounts and explanations. Panel hearings were rarely held on neutral premises and they were sometimes administered by the same staff who were involved in local resolution.

What is wrong with local resolution?

Inadequate responses

Local resolution means nothing to the defensive practitioners who merely "play the game" in order to pacify the complainant. This does not result in either a change of practice or attitude.

Much of the formal language used in communications with the complainant makes it appear that they have entered into a structured and fundamentally indifferent system.

Too complicated and time consuming

[The process] is far too complicated. It's taken so much out of us to go through it – I wonder how many other families have the strength to follow it through.

Defensiveness

[T]here was no question of accepting responsibility. It was just instant non-acceptance of blame.

They washed all hands of responsibility. The response was defensive and condescending, it was collective back covering. All the allegations were denied, they twisted everything, made out as if I was telling lies.

> *Source*: Wallace H, Mulcahy L. *Cause for Complaint? An evaluation of the effectiveness of the NHS complaints procedure.* London: The Public Law Project, 1999.

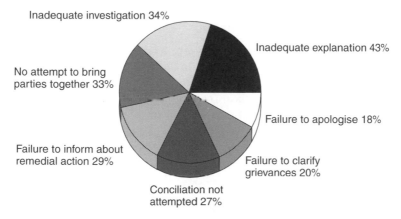

Figure 26.2 Conveners' reasons for sending complaints back for local resolution.

Finally, research has suggested that complainants are doubtful about whether their complaint would help to raise the quality of services, although one of the main reasons for complaining may be to prevent the same thing happening to someone else. Whilst many health organisations endeavour to use complaints for quality management this is often hampered by fragmentary co-ordination of data from these and other sources of information, such as audit, adverse clinical incidents and other sources of information on quality. The box below shows what complainants have said they want to happen as a result of their complaint.

What do people want to happen as a result of complaining?

- Prevent a recurrence
- Make their dissatisfaction known
- Get an explanation
- Get an apology
- Admission of responsibility
- Better treatment
- Have disciplinary action taken

Source: Kyffin R, Cook G, Jones M. *Complaints handling and monitoring in the NHS: a study of 12 trusts in the North West Region.* Liverpool: University of Liverpool, 1997.

Research conducted on the former hospital complaints procedure suggested that claims for retribution through compensation or disciplinary action are relatively rare.

The response of complaint handlers: attitudinal and organisational barriers to learning

Research shows that when people voice a complaint, they tend to do so to the person they hold to be responsible for their care – that is doctors and nurses.[25] This suggests that clinicians' responses are critical in the process of establishing the nature of, and responding to, the grievance.

If complaints about clinical care are taken as an attack on the professional judgement and the personal integrity of a clinician then it is not surprising that strong feelings are aroused. As a consequence, defensive strategies such as denial, or even a counter attack, may be adopted rather than a detached attempt to discover the complainant's problem.[26,27] Another reason for defensiveness is the cost to the person concerned if the complaint escalates. This may lead to enquiries by senior colleagues and the possibility of disciplinary action, both of which threaten reputation, promotion and livelihood. However, although it is important to understand the reasons for these responses, they cannot justify overtly defensive reactions to complaints. For example, a recent report from the Health Service Commissioner has criticised some GPs for refusing to offer an apology when one was clearly due. He has also found that some doctors do not know what the new complaint procedure is and therefore fail not only to inform their patients, but may also pass on misinformation.[28]

In a study of complainants' views undertaken in three NHS acute trusts in a northern region, Kyffin and colleagues found that three quarters of the respondents stated that they were partially or wholly dissatisfied with responses to their complaint.[29] The principal source of dissatisfaction was with the formal letters received. Fifty-nine per cent felt that the response had failed to address all their concerns. Other research has found that negative responses tend to exacerbate complaints. One study of GPs showed that if after a complaint a GP removed a patient from the practice list, showed a lack of sympathy, was hostile or failed to address the issues raised, these could then become issues in the dispute.[30] Similarly, an analysis of letters of response to hospital complaints showed that incomplete explanations, dismissive letters, "pseudo-apologies", technical language and defensive responses played a part in hardening the complainants' attitudes. The length of time taken to deal with the complaint, the lack of openness, not informing the complainant of progress, and an unwillingness to take action when incompetence has been disclosed can also produce disillusionment and a determination to pursue the complaint.[31]

Manager's response to complaints

The response of managers to complaints can also be unsatisfactory. Mulcahy and Lloyd-Bostock[32] found that in some trusts managers tended to act merely as clinicians' agents and in others they failed to involve clinicians at all. Sometimes, although they began an inquiry process, managers did not undertake a systematic investigation but simply copied the complainant's letter to the people concerned and asked for a response. In other instances, little attempt was made to translate technical and derogatory material taken from medical statements into simpler language. Significantly, investigating officers did not always ask the complainant for additional details of their criticisms, despite the fact that many accounts were insufficiently detailed to be useful for either investigation or risk management.

The Public Law Project research also highlighted concerns about the convening role and the ability of conveners to establish an impartial stance.[24] Almost half (46%) of the 169 conveners in this survey felt that their independence was compromised by existing links to the healthcare provider and a number were also concerned that they did not have a sufficient case load to have gained enough experience of the role. The research also drew attention to conveners' and IPR chairs' concerns that they were stepping beyond their formal remit and trying to resolve complaints. Such activity can appear confusing to complainants who may have been led to expect a greater element of impartiality at this stage of the procedure.

Complaints recording and monitoring

Despite the recommendations of the Wilson Committee that complaints should be recorded and used for quality and risk management, little guidance has been given and a national classification system for complaints has not been developed. The data required by the Department of Health does not break down the largest single category, clinical complaints, into further sub-sets. GPs are not required to give information on complaints made to them. Furthermore, in their study of 12 trusts, Kyffin and colleagues argue that oral complaints are often not recorded at all and that complainants' letters which contain a number of allegations are in practice reduced to a single category.[33] This therefore under-records the sources of dissatisfaction.

Key aspects of effective complaint handling

We have drawn attention to the attitudinal barriers to effective complaint handling and to the weaknesses in the new complaints system. These findings must be set against the undoubted shift towards a more open and flexible system and the valiant, and often successful, attempts by under-resourced complaint managers to satisfy complainants. In this section, we concentrate on issues which research, good practice guides,[6,34] and our knowledge of practice have indicated are key issues. We have not attempted to be comprehensive.

The attitude and commitment of senior management

The most critical factor in any complaints system is the attitude and commitment of senior management. Every health service organisation should have a clear and comprehensive written policy for complaints. This should reflect an explicit commitment to particular values. The guidance introduced in 1996 refers to accessibility, simplicity, speed, fairness, confidentiality and effectiveness. To these we would add openness, impartiality, thoroughness and equity. The lead must come from the top and permeate through the organisation, as all staff at some time will be at the receiving end of a complaint. Because complaints can range from very minor matters to the extremely serious in terms of their impact on future patients or the liability of the organisation, staff need to be aware of when to deal with issues themselves and when to pass matters on, and to whom. A corporate approach to complaints is illustrated in the box below.

A corporate approach to complaints

- An ethos of taking complaints seriously
- Senior level commitment to reviewing complaints and outcomes
- A clear delineation of staff responsibilities
- An assessment of the complaints system against evaluation criteria such as:
- Does the organisation learn from complaints?
- Do the procedures encourage good practice and deter poor practice?
- Are complainants and staff satisfied with the procedures?

Understanding the complainant's perspective

It is important for the person responding to the complaint to try to see matters from the complainant's perspective. The British Standards Institute guidance on complaints says:

> From the customer's point of view, only three things matter if something goes wrong. They need to know where to complain, they need to know how to complain and they need to feel confident that their complaint will be dealt with seriously.[34]

Those to whom the complaint is made need to treat the complainant with courtesy and respect. If a complaint is made face-to-face, then the aim should be to listen and to accept that what the complainant says as valid until the matter can be investigated. If a complaint is made in writing, then the initial response should express sympathy for the complainant's predicament and tell them what the enquiry process will be and how long it is likely to take.

Making a complaint is a process in which complainants are faced with a series of choices about what to do next. Initially, they may not be clear about what they want and they probably do not know the details of the system. How a complaint is responded to will affect how the complainant proceeds and this is the case for each subsequent interaction. As we have already pointed out, responses that are dismissive and do not address all the complainant's concerns can lead to a hardening of attitudes. This very contingency presents both opportunities and threats. Informal methods of identifying what the complainant's issues are and what they want from the process may well be more effective in the first instance than written replies.

However, all complaints and the action taken will need to be recorded as fully as possible.

Openness

A complaint system should allow the service user or relative to access it at any point using the medium that they prefer, whether this is by letter, telephone, fax, email or face-to-face contact. All publicity material, whether in the form of notices or leaflets, should give guidance on who to contact for further information both inside the organisation and outside it, if complainants want additional help. Information about the trust or general practice, including their complaints system, could also be made more widely available through the CHC, the GP surgery and other local organisations. Some hospitals use the local press and radio. Others have a freephone number. Community organisations can also be useful in providing feedback on the appropriateness of publicity and its visibility.

Equity is also important – that is, treating complainants in the same way no matter who made the complaint and by whatever route it was made. Some people will need help to express themselves and to identify their concerns, or help with writing their complaint. There will be those with particular difficulties with literacy or language. Such help may be provided within the organisation. For example, trusts in Brighton and Newham have appointed patient or health advocates. In the latter trust, where ethnic minority patients make up nearly half the population, post holders work specifically with these groups. External help should also be available from the local CHC as well as other voluntary organisations. These organisations can be used to clarify the issues for the complainant and help manage expectations.

Openness also means that the complaints policy should be well known throughout the organisation and responsibility should be delegated to front line staff to take action themselves. If a complaints policy is seen as part of caring for patients, then it is more likely that priority will be given to dealing with investigations related to complaints. Candour is important. Patients and relatives should be given full, accurate and honest explanations. If, during the course of a complaint or claim, people find that they have not been told the truth, it may be impossible to reach a resolution of the complaint. At the stage of independent review, the principle of openness requires that, unless there are good reasons, a case should be investigated and conducted in front of the parties involved. Failure to do this will seriously undermine the credibility of the procedure and could serve to enforce the complainant's view that there is a "closed shop".

Confidentiality

The principle of confidentiality requires that the identity of those who complain needs to be protected. The investigation of a complaint means that letters and notes related to the case may be circulated more widely than usual. A policy may need to be developed on the issue of confidentiality and papers circulated on a "need to know" basis. The same principle applies to staff. Allegations against staff should only be known to those investigating the complaint and those investigations generally should not be carried out by the staff member's line manager or someone who can affect their career. Reports to the management board cannot be made anonymous as action may need to be taken. The box below gives some guidelines for staff undertaking an investigation.

Principles of investigation

The person investigating should:

- Not have a direct interest in the complaint
- Keep notes on the information collected and from whom
- Identify conflicts in accounts and attempt to resolve them

and where this is not possible:

- Be open about the information collected and what has been said
- Report the findings to a senior person
- Reach a view and have reasons for that view

Thoroughness and impartiality

The principle of thoroughness relates to the investigation of issues and is critical. Complaints should be investigated by a person with sufficient authority to challenge senior staff and clinicians if necessary. All information relevant to the case should be collected and this may mean going back to the complainant or to their friends or relatives for additional information. It is important to establish areas of agreement and, where people disagree, to seek verification wherever possible.

Impartiality is vital in investigating complaints and establishing the legitimacy of the process. Those investigating should distance themselves from those being complained about. They should not privilege the accounts of colleagues over those of complainants. This is not only important in written responses to the complainant but also in any meeting that may take place or if third parties become involved.

If the complainant asks for an independent review, they will need to have access to a summary of the issues and all the relevant documents. It has been noted above that many complaints are sent back for local resolution and some more than once. This is usually because there was an insufficient investigation of the issues in the first place. If there is a panel hearing, an investigation by the Health Service Commissioner, or a claim is made, again the initial investigation will be crucial in clarifying what the issues are.

Support for staff

We have also shown that staff often react defensively to complaints whether they think they have made a mistake or not. Both research and accounts given by doctors and nurses show that sometimes lives can be blighted by a long drawn out complaints and disciplinary process. There should be ready access to advice and support and information about where to go for help included in the complaints policy documentation. If something untoward occurs, accident analysis suggests that adverse events are rarely due to a single error by a single individual and it is important for senior managers to assume responsibility for what has happened.[35] They should undertake an investigation and work to maintain staff morale. Thereafter, there is a tension between supporting staff where there has been an honest error, and dealing with poor performance, which presents a challenge for organisational leaders. Usually, poor performance is marked by a history of previous events. Although the separation of disciplinary systems and complaint handling supports a less defensive approach and should encourage the free flow of information, there will be occasions when the Chinese walls need to be breached in the interests of patients.

Responses to complaints

All the above principles should be reflected in how staff respond to complaints. Written complaints should be dealt with through specialist, trained staff. In the interests of visibility, the initial response could be a reply telling the person what the process of investigation will be. It has been noted in good practice guides that not enough use is made of the telephone to make direct contact with the complainant initially or at particular stages in the process.[6] This may be quicker, cheaper and more effective. However, the content of telephone calls needs to be recorded.

Those who respond to complaints should try to put themselves in the position of the complainant. After an investigation has been carried out, the letter written to the complainant should answer all the points of concern, be factually correct, clear and easy to understand. Too often response letters simply copy text from doctors' accounts or fail to address the issues.

This is not reporting the findings of an investigation and the action to be taken but rather a co-ordination of defences.

A letter should offer a sincere apology if mistakes have been made. It should also tell the complainant of any action taken to avoid the same thing happening again. It should contain a contact name and telephone number, and tell the person what to do next if they are not satisfied. Depending on the nature of the complaint, this may mean directing the complainant to other avenues for complaint within the NHS. Because more patients within the NHS are receiving a combination of private and public care and because services may be contracted out to other agencies, response letters must be clear about who is responsible for what and why. This is too complicated an issue for complainants to sort out on their own. As far as they are concerned, the NHS is responsible. Remedies should also be offered if this is appropriate. As a general principle, people should not be disadvantaged because something has gone wrong. If possible, they should be put in the position that they were in before the events giving rise to the complaint. A summary of the key issues in complaint responses is given in the box below.

Principles of complaint handling

- Understand what the complaint is about
- Find out what the complainant wants
- Acknowledge the complainant's feelings
- Address all the complainant's concerns
- Keep the complainant informed about progress
- Offer a sincere apology if appropriate
- Act on issues raised and tell the complainant about the action taken

---

Arranging meetings with complainants

If the complainant agrees, it is often useful to arrange a face-to-face meeting between complainant, clinicians, and managers. Kyffin and colleagues' research into complainant satisfaction found that trust policy varied in whether a meeting was offered or not.[32] Where a meeting was taken up by the complainant, over three quarters found them helpful or partially helpful. Meetings can be arranged by the complaint manager and should be at a venue agreed with the complainant. These may well be intimidating for the complainant so their purpose, the process, and who will be present should be clarified for all parties. It is important that all parties come to meetings with the relevant information and there is agreement to the process. It may be useful to have someone neutral to chair the meeting and the complainant should be offered the opportunity to bring a friend if they wish. If it is clear that there are strong differences of opinion about what happened, or complainants have views about what they want in terms of redress which differ from what the organisation concerned is prepared to offer, a trained conciliator could also be asked to help resolve the issue. The conciliation process should be geared to achieving what the complainant wants in a fair way. If the complainant is not satisfied with the initial responses, then the final stage of the local resolution process should be an internal review involving senior staff to ensure that the process has been carried out correctly and that nothing more can be done.

"Difficult complaints"

Two types of complaint may pose particular difficulties for complaint handlers. First, some complaints have a high emotional content because of the outcome of the illness episode to which they relate. For example, we referred above to research that showed that a substantial proportion of complaints related to the medical care of patients who had died during or soon after treatment. Relatives often need support at the time of the bereavement and throughout the grieving process and this is particularly the case where something has gone wrong. The Health Committee, in its enquiry into clinical incidents, recommended that healthcare providers should provide support for the bereaved either within their organisation or in liaison with community groups.[9] It is important if there is subsequently a complaint, that senior managers investigating the complaint or claim are separate from those concerned with bereavement support.

Second, every system has complainants who appear unsatisfiable. Their complaint should not be dismissed without investigation just because it appears "trivial" or "vexatious". It is easy to stereotype people in order to avoid addressing their concerns. Research has shown that among some clinicians there is a tendency to pathologise complainants and see a complaint as a manifestation of an illness.[26] This has the effect of disenfranchising the complainant. However, it is also the case that, for a few people, complaining becomes an end in itself. If one issue is dealt with, another arises. Some complainants avoid meetings but continue to write letters. In such cases, an endpoint may have to be reached as nothing more can be achieved. It is important in such cases to give a clear account of what has been done and the reasons why no further action can be taken. If a request is made for an independent review, or an appeal is made to the Health Service Commissioner, decision takers at this level will need a full account to guide their own decision making. A complaint manager in this position should provide paperwork that explains the issues within the complaint and, in chronological order, what action was taken when and why.

The responsibilities of senior management: resources and training

Senior management must take responsibility for linking complaint management to quality management. This obligation has been underlined by the new arrangements for clinical governance. In practical terms this is likely to lead to senior clinicians and managers meeting to review the results of audit, adverse incidents and complaints on a regular basis. To achieve feedback, action plans and follow-up should be part of the process. At some of these meetings, there is an argument for including community or patient representatives to incorporate a range of views. As well as publicising the policy, this means devoting resources to dedicated staff, to training, and to monitoring process and outcomes. Organisations should know what resources they are devoting to complaints and be able to assess whether these are sufficient for the job. It is particularly important that dedicated complaint staff are well trained and that they work alongside other staff undertaking quality management tasks. There should be ready access to senior management, and there should also be a regular exchange of staff between complaints and other departments so that expertise is spread.

The importance of training in how to deal with complaints, whether these are verbal or written, cannot be over-estimated. All staff employed, whether temporary or not, should have some training in handling complaints as part of their induction. This should include role play in dealing with distressed, anxious or angry people. It is only when people feel what it is like to be a complainant or someone who has to respond, that they become aware of the emotions which are aroused. Training should also cover issues of confidentiality. Again, it is the responsibility of senior management to set aside the resources to undertake this activity.

Responsibilities of senior management: achieving satisfactory outcomes

Complaints' systems should achieve two aims. First, research and accounts from practitioners suggest that all the parties to complaints want an opportunity to present "the facts" as they see them and resent any suggestion of a cover-up. Even though it may not be possible to please everyone in terms of outcomes, managers could see the complaint process as offering the possibility of restorative rather than retributive justice. An open process that allows accounts to be voiced can help to quiet the demons of anger and revenge. Second, lessons can be learnt for the future. If complaints are properly categorised, they can provide a user's view of the service – if things have gone wrong why they have gone wrong, what improvements people would like, and whether action has been taken as a consequence of the complaint. If the feedback loop is to be accomplished, then all complaints, and not just those that are made in writing, need to be carefully and consistently recorded. In a larger organisation, this may mean issuing simple carbon copy pro formas for front line staff to return. The organisation itself needs to reflect on the lessons to be learnt from each complaint and how the same situation can be avoided in the future through, for example, an "outcome" meeting. There may be evidence of resource shortages or indications of poor practice which contributed to the complaint. These may require further investigation and action after the complaint itself has been resolved. Complaint information should be published and circulated regularly. This may mean identifying patterns of poor performance by individuals as well as patterns of complaint in relation to particular services. Reports should include numbers and categories of complaint received, speed in processing against target times, user satisfaction with the process and the action taken to improve services.

Networks with organisations in the community can be an important way of obtaining feedback on the way a complaints system is operating. CHCs, other voluntary organisations or lay people can be included in outcome meetings or in discussing ways to improve the complaints system. Other local health organisations can also be sources of advice and expertise. This exchange of views between providers is likely to become increasingly important as joint arrangements between health and social services for the provision of community services will require the harmonisation of different complaint systems.

Conclusion

For some years, it has been clear from Health Service Commissioner reports and other research sources that the new complaints system, introduced in 1996, has a number of design flaws and there are also problems in its implementation. In particular, there has been a lack of investment in training and a lack of drive within the Department of Health to introduce common systems to learn from complaints. There are also problems in the primary care sector due to a lack of visibility of what practices are doing and problems which derive from the dependence of patients on a particular GP or practice. Given the current level of criticism, it is likely that there will be further changes to the complaints system. Changes in who is the lead authority in community care services will present further challenges in integrating the two complaint systems.

We have argued that complaints provide an opportunity for greater partnership with patients and relatives. Complaint handling should be considered part of patient care – an opportunity to provide information and explanations about what occurred. There is strong evidence that many complainants still receive evasive or inadequate accounts and that this increases their dissatisfaction. Patients and relatives should be given honest reports of why certain decisions were made and why certain incidents occurred, even if these were adverse. We have also suggested that greater partnership can also be achieved by involving lay people and community groups in evaluating the efficacy of the complaints system. This can be a potent way of ensuring that action is taken if weaknesses are identified following an investigation and that the system remains open to those who wish to use it.

References

1 Cabinet Office, Complaints Task Force. *Putting things right.* London: HMSO, 1995.
2 NHS (England) Summarised Accounts 1997–8. HC 382 1998/99, para 5.6.
3 *The Citizen's Charter.* Cm 1599, London: HMSO, 1991.
4 Cabinet Office, Complaints Task Force. *Putting things right.* London: HMSO, 1995; Cabinet Office, Complaints Task Force *The Good Practice Guide.* London: HMSO, 1995.
5 National Health Service Executive. *Being Heard: Report of the Review Committee on NHS Complaint Procedures.* Leeds: NHSE, 1994.
6 Cabinet Office, Service First Unit. *How to deal with complaints.* London: HMSO, 1999.
7 Anon. Children undergoing heart surgery at the Bristol Royal Infirmary. *BMJ* 1998;**316**: 1924.
8 Problems with examinations of cervical smears at Kent and Canterbury Hospital. *Daily Telegraph* 31 January 1998.
9 Health Committee. *Procedures relating to adverse clinical incidents and outcomes in medical care, Sixth Report 1998–9* (HC 549–1). London: HMSO, 1999.
10 Department of Health. *The New NHS: Modern, Dependable.* Cm 387. London: HMSO, 1997, para 1.1.
11 Department of Health. *A first class service: Quality in the new NHS.* London: HMSO, 1998, paras 3.6, 3.7.
12 General Medical Council. *Good Medical Practice.* London: GMC, 1998.
13 Dunne R, Finlayson B. Colleges' revalidation programmes come together. *Hospital Doctor* 1999;1st October:18.
14 JM Consulting Ltd. *Report on a review of the Nurses, Midwives and Health Visitors Act 1997,* report to the Health Departments, 1998.
15 Department of Health. *Supporting doctors, protecting patients. A consultation paper on preventing, recognising and dealing with poor clinical performance of doctors in the NHS in England. A consultative document.* London: DoH, 1999.
16 NHS Executive. *Complaints: Listening . . . acting . . . improving. Guidance on the implementation of the NHS complaints procedure.* Leeds: NHS Executive, 1996.
17 A recent study shows that in almost half of the complaints to a medical service committee ($n = 110$) there had been a death. Allsop J. A form of haunting: complaints where the patient has died. In: Mitchell M, ed. *Remember me: the socio-psychological aspects of dying and death.* Routledge (forthcoming).
18 Department of Health. *Handling complaints: monitoring the NHS complaints procedures, England 1997–8.* London: DOH, 1998.
19 Select Committee on Public Administration. *Annual Report of the Health Service Ombudsman for 1997–98,* HC 54 p xxv.
20 Brennan T, Leape L, Laird N, *et al.* Incidence of adverse events and negligence in hospitalised patients: the results of the Harvard medical practice study 1. *N Engl J Med* 1991;**324**:370–6.

21 MORI. *Attitudes towards and experiences of complaints systems.* Cabinet Office, HMSO, 1994.

22 MORI. *Attitudes towards and experiences of complaints systems.* London: MORI, 1997.

23 Mulcahy L, Tritter J. Pathways, pyramids and icebergs: Mapping the links between dissatisfaction and complaints. *Soc Health Illness* 1998;20,6:825–47.

24 Wallace H, Mulcahy L. *Cause for complaint? An evaluation of the effectiveness of the NHS complaints procedure.* London: The Public Law Project, 1999.

25 Mulcahy L, Tritter T. Hidden depths. *Health Services J* 1994;24 July:26–7.

26 Allsop J, Mulcahy L. Maintaining professional identity: doctors' responses to complaints. *Soc Health Illness* 1998;20(6):847–69.

27 Mulcahy L. From fear to fraternity: doctors' construction of rational identities in response to complaints. *J Soc Welfare Fam Law* 1996;18(4):397–412.

28 Health Service Commissioner for England, Scotland and Wales. *Annual Report 1997–98.* HC (1997/8) 811.

29 Kyffin R, Cook G, Jones M. *Complainant satisfaction with NHS Trust complaints procedures.* Institute of Medicine, Law and Bioethics, University of Liverpool, 1999.

30 Allsop J. Two sides to every story: The perspectives of complainants and doctors. *Law and Policy* 1994;16(2):148–83.

31 Lloyd-Bostock S, Mulcahy L. The social psychology of making and responding to hospital complaints: An account model of complaint processes. *Law and Policy* 1994;16(2): 123–47.

32 Mulcahy L, Lloyd-Bostock S. Managers as third-party dispute handlers in complaints about hospitals. *Law and Policy* 1994;16(2):185–208.

33 Kyffin R, Cook G, Jones M. *Complaints handling and monitoring in the NHS: a study of 12 trusts in the North West Region.* Liverpool: University of Liverpool, 1997.

34 British Standards Institute. *Complaints management systems – Guide to design and implementation.* BS 8600, 1999.

35 Vincent C, Reason J. Human factors: approaches to medicine. In: Rosenthal M, Mulcahy L, Lloyd-Bostock S, eds. *Medical mishaps: pieces of the puzzle.* Buckingham: Open University, 1999.

Further reading: Good practice guides

Cabinet Office, Service First Unit. *How to deal with complaints.* London: HMSO, 1999.

British Standards Institute. *Complaints management systems – Guide to design and implementation,* BS 8600, 1999.

The Public Law Project. *Making a complaint about the NHS: a guide for patients* 2000. Address: The Public Law Project, Birkbeck College, University of London, Malet Street, London WC1E 7HX.

27 Resolving disputes about clinical accidents

ARNOLD SIMANOWITZ, HENRY BROWN

Barely five years have passed since the first edition of this book was published. As the former Lord Chief Justice, Lord Bingham, has observed elsewhere,[1] that is not by historical or legal standards, a long period. But during that period, there have been extraordinary changes in the nature and scope of dispute resolution processes, both generally and in the specific area of clinical negligence.

- Radical procedural reforms of litigation introduced by Lord Woolf have transformed the legal landscape.
- A multi-disciplinary Clinical Disputes Forum has been established, comprising representatives of all stakeholders, which has developed less adversarial dispute resolution procedures including a clinical negligence pre-action protocol.
- The NHS has established a Litigation Authority to manage litigation, develop a risk management programme and minimise the overall cost of clinical negligence.
- A government-backed mediation pilot scheme has reported on mediation as an option for clinical negligence disputes.[2] The government's Chief Medical Officer has also published a detailed consultation paper on preventing, recognising and dealing with poor clinical performance.[3]
- Public funding of litigation funding is undergoing significant change.
- An innovative Arbitration Act has been enacted, signalling new ways of thinking about dispute resolution.
- First steps have been taken towards the establishment of a Community Legal Service.

- As observed by Lord Bingham, there has been "governmental recognition that ADR offers an economical and socially desirable way of resolving some civil disputes . . . " and that there is "evidence of increased resort to ADR, with (very often) startlingly successful results".[4]

These changes cannot be before time for health sector disputes. A House of Commons Select Committee ("the Committee") undertook a significant enquiry into "the adequacy and effectiveness of the procedures, including investigative procedures, undertaken following adverse clinical incidents and outcomes in medical care". It reported in November 1999, expressing concern and observing the criticism of the current systems "voiced not only by patients and their carers but also by health professionals and managers." The Secretary of State told the Committee that "the present system really is a bit of a shambles . . . and at the end of it all none of the people concerned, neither the person complained about, nor the patient, nor the patient's relatives, is satisfied, and if you have got a long, protracted and expensive process that satisfies nobody, there is clearly something seriously wrong with it".[5]

Dispute resolution review

This chapter will review the approaches that risk managers can take towards the management of disputed claims. While this necessitates considering some aspects on a conceptual basis, the intention is to provide practical guidance as to the range of possibilities and available resources.

In addition to considering processes and resources currently available, the chapter will also consider possible further reforms and procedures that can build on the extensive work that has been done in this field.

Complaints, claims, disputes and discipline

The efficacy of the 1996 NHS complaints procedure[‡1] has been questioned. The Committee, noted that "when people did complain, it appeared they often became even more dissatisfied with the process and the outcome of the complaint and confused by a regulatory system which gave them a number of options for taking action".[5] The Health Service Ombudsman has referred to patients' "complaint fatigue".[6] A Report by the Public Law Project also disclosed serious procedural deficiencies.[7]

Furthermore, a serious defect in the procedures for addressing clinical complaints and claims is that these are corralled into rigidly separate compartments. The Ombudsman will not deal with a complaint "where the complainant can seek a remedy in the courts" unless "he is satisfied that in the particular circumstances it is not reasonable to expect the complainant to resort to a legal remedy".[8]

The Legal Services Commission (LSC) on the other hand would prefer to create a connection between complaints and litigation by requiring the would-be litigant to make a complaint before public funding will be granted in certain circumstances.

Notwithstanding any reasons for separating processes, putting a compensation award within the remit of the complaints procedure would have a dramatic effect on the whole complaints/compensation scene. Delay and cost would be reduced and patient satisfaction would be immeasurably improved. It could, at a stroke, eliminate with relatively low cost many cases that might otherwise proceed to litigation.

To compound the problem, disciplinary procedures are dealt with separately from complaints or claims, with each trust having its own disciplinary procedure, based on guidance from the NHS. This differs from primary care disciplinary processes, because the NHS does not directly employ GPs. An attempt is made to address these and related issues in *Supporting doctors, protecting patients*.[3]

The Committee was concerned about the lack of linkage between these systems.[9] It recommended that links be clarified and complexities reduced.[10] It further recommended that the initial investigation of a complaint should be:

> much more thorough and should be carried out by well-trained, dedicated staff . . . the report from investigations relating to adverse clinical incidents or potential adverse clinical incidents must contain a detailed account of events and be robust enough to be used by other bodies, such as the GMC and UKCC, NHS disciplinary committees, or the courts.[11]

The pre-action protocol

The Clinical Disputes Forum has created a pre-action protocol, forming part of the Woolf reforms. It encourages a climate of openness, provides guidance and recommends a timed sequence of steps for patients, healthcare providers, and their advisers to follow. It sets out a code of good practice that parties should follow when litigation is a possibility. Particulars of the protocol are contained in Chapter 28.

Overview of dispute resolution processes

Dispute resolution processes should be viewed against the background described above. There are three basic methods of dispute resolution.

1 Adjudication involves a neutral hearing for the parties and making a binding determination. This can be divided into litigation through the courts and adjudicatory ADR (alternative dispute resolution) which does not use the courts.
2 Negotiation is usually bilateral between the parties themselves, perhaps through representatives.
3 The third dispute resolution method comprises various forms of non-adjudicatory ADR, in which a neutral third party is appointed, who has no authority to make any binding decision but instead helps the parties to arrive at their own binding settlement agreement.

Some non-adjudicatory ADR processes involve evaluating the merits of the dispute or proposed settlement terms on a non-binding basis. Others do not consider merits, but leave this to the parties and their professional advisers. Parties reserve the right, if they cannot resolve the issues by agreement, to have them resolved by adjudication, usually litigation.

Forms of adjudication

Litigation

Litigation is the main adjudicatory process used in clinical negligence cases. However, it is costly, lengthy, and its adversarial nature inherently leads to mutual suspicion and antagonism. It

damages the relationship between patient and clinician or hospital

and

channels money into the hands of the professional resolving the dispute rather than into compensation or patient care . . . The rise in litigation has encouraged a defensive attitude amongst trusts, who may be wary of communicating with patients . . . Unfortunately it is this very defensiveness which may persuade a patient or relative to pursue legal action.[12]

In litigation, everything has to be reduced to claims for financial compensation. Although this may be important to claimants, that is by no means universally the case. The financial claim may often have little more than symbolic value for people seeking accountability.

The Woolf court reforms should help disputes to be resolved fairly, expeditiously, and at a proportionate cost. Following a "multi-track" approach, the court has flexible powers to deal appropriately with claims of over £15 000. These reforms also provide for parties to make early attempts to settle their disputes, for example by making written settlement offers and payments or through ADR.

Other forms of adjudication

Arbitration

This is a private process in which a third party neutral, selected by the parties, makes a binding determination of the issues. The Arbitration Act 1996 recognises and reinforces the principle of party autonomy. The process must be fair, impartial and expeditious. The arbitrator must adopt suitable procedures, avoiding unnecessary delay or expense.

The Department of Health's 1991 consultation paper on proposals for the arbitration of medical negligence claims by a lawyer and two doctors encountered little enthusiasm. However, the new arbitration law with its procedural flexibility and focus on party autonomy may offer new possibilities for clinical negligence cases.

Expert determination[12]

This differs from arbitration in that the expert's functions and authority arise contractually. The expert's determination is binding on the parties. There is no statutory framework. Provided that there is no fraud or collusion and the expert makes a decision within the terms of his or her brief, which may not necessarily involve hearing oral or written submissions, there is not usually any basis for reviewing or appealing the decision.

An expert determination may be appropriate in some circumstances, but disputants seeking adjudication may prefer the benefit of court procedures and appeal or review possibilities.

Ombudsman[13]

Health service commissioners (ombudsmen) may investigate complaints against health authorities or trusts of alleged failures to provide services or of injustice or hardship suffered by their actions. However, the ombudsmen's investigative powers have limitations in relation to clinical negligence claims. For example, they may not investigate complaints about clinical judgment arising from events before 1 April 1996. Nor will the ombudsman deal with complaints where the person has a right of appeal or review to a tribunal or a remedy by way of court proceedings.

The Health Service ombudsman has the power to make non-binding recommendations based on his investigation of complaints. This may include recommending financial compensation, but usually only for losses or costs arising from maladministration.

Negotiation

An important distinction lies between problem-solving and competitive approaches to negotiation. The competitive or "positional" approach considers that there are limited resources for distribution and the more that one party achieves, the less there will be for the other. The problem-solving approach aims to increase the joint gains for both or all parties. This often involves a more principled approach, although the ultimate aim may also be to achieve the best outcome for each party.

Bilateral dispute negotiation inherently tends to be competitive. Non-adjudicatory ADR processes, however, tend to encourage parties to seek a more problem-solving approach. There is, though, a middle view that seeks to find a balance between the competitive and problem-solving approaches.[14] This view considers that both kinds of process may be present in negotiation, and that there is an "essential tension" between them.

Mediation and other ADR forms introduce a new dynamic into negotiations, with established procedures and skilled mediators to help in those cases that cannot easily settle by way of ordinary bilateral negotiations.

Mediation and other non-adjudicatory processes

Shared attributes

Non-adjudicatory ADR processes including mediation share many characteristics. They are confidential and evidentially privileged, with the right reserved to seek adjudication if agreement cannot be reached. They are generally relatively low-risk, low cost, and expeditious. They tend to heal rather than exacerbate differences; and their success rate is relatively high. On the other hand, they do not constitute a panacea; there are situations in which their use would be inappropriate and where third party adjudication is necessary and proper; and they need to be handled with care and skill.

In risk management terms, consensual processes are more effective than adjudication. This is because in adjudication significant decisions are taken out of the hands of the parties, who become dependent on lawyers, expert witnesses, and an adjudicator. However, in non-adjudicatory ADR such as mediation, decision-making remains in the hands of the parties (or managers of health authorities or trusts) and no outcome can be unacceptable to them (apart from reverting to adjudication). Inevitably, this is the most effective way to manage the risk of a dispute.

These processes offer a forum in which parties can communicate more freely, express concerns and offer explanations and apologies if appropriate. They afford the opportunity for patients to understand the considerations that may have made a clinical decision more problematical, and for practitioners to understand the feelings and concerns of the patient.

Mediation (Conciliation)[1,15,16]

Mediation is the most widely used form of non-adjudicatory ADR. In it, disputing parties engage the assistance of an impartial mediator, who has no authority to decide their issues, but who facilitates the resolution of their dispute by helping them to negotiate an agreement without adjudication.

The term "mediation" is sometimes understood to be more pro-active than "conciliation"; but sometimes the reverse usage is employed. There is no consistency of usage, and in this chapter these terms are treated as interchangeable. This is not, however, to be confused with conciliation under the general practitioner complaints procedures. While that form of conciliation can be helpful, it does not address all the issues worrying the patient and specifically does not deal with compensation.

Mediation has considerable potential for resolving clinical negligence disputes out of court. The dynamic offered by a skilled third party facilitator, the opportunities to discuss the issues off the record, and the possibilities to explore settlement options and terms creatively within a controlled procedural framework, combine to provide a constructive and effective forum. The doctor–patient relationship was a caring and trusting one that is likely to have been damaged by the negligence claim. Mediation allows an opportunity for care to be demonstrated and trust (at least in the healthcare system) to be restored. Specific attention will accordingly be given to mediation below.

The mini-trial (Executive Tribunal)[‡3]

The mini-trial is not a "trial", but an assisted negotiation. Respective lawyers, following an agreed procedure and timetable, present the case to the parties on an abbreviated non-binding basis, to enable them to assess its strengths, weaknesses and prospects. Ordinarily no witnesses are called, but expert witnesses might explain technical aspects. In effect, the parties become an informal tribunal, gaining insights that enable them and their lawyers to discuss settlement on a realistic basis.

A key figure is an authoritative neutral adviser, who chairs and manages the process, asking questions and clarifying aspects. The neutral adviser may help the parties to form a view on the case, or may give a non-binding opinion. The adviser may also adopt a mediatory role in any subsequent settlement discussions.

Non-binding neutral evaluation

Under this process, a non-binding evaluation of the medical and/or legal merits of a case can be obtained from a third party neutral. It might range between a formal opinion to both parties, to giving a brief informal indication to either or both separately.

Evaluation may have different purposes. Parties may wish to achieve settlement terms that broadly accord with their respective rights. Or they may have had different advice from their respective lawyers and may not be able to agree what those rights are. Or one party may be unrealistically refusing to accept reasonable terms because of a mistaken perception as to the strength of his rights.

The main form of evaluation is case evaluation, in which a neutral third party or panel makes a reasoned evaluation of the dispute. It is not a judicial or arbitral process, but written and oral submissions can be made, and in some models witnesses can be heard. The evaluation is off-the-record and non-binding and may be used as a basis for settlement discussions, through mediation if required.[44]

In another form, early neutral evaluation (ENE), in addition to the non-binding evaluation, the neutral considers how to conduct the litigation rapidly and economically. The neutral will also consider effective and expeditious case disposal by means other than litigation and may help the parties to explore the possibility of settlement.

In some models of mediation, while the primary focus is on facilitation, evaluation may also be introduced. If the parties can resolve the matter based on their interests, concerns, and their own evaluations of the issues, neutral evaluation is unnecessary.[45]

Other non-adjudicatory ADR processes

Another relevant ADR process is the neutral fact-finding expert in which the parties jointly appoint a neutral expert to investigate facts, form a legal or technical view either about certain specified issues, or on all issues generally, and make a non-binding report to the parties. This helps to inform any settlement discussions that may then take place.

Under the pre-action protocol and the Woolf reforms, experts appointed by both parties may meet to see if they can agree on any of the clinical issues. If lawyers or the parties are not present, there is a risk that one expert may prevail on the other inappropriately, with profound implications for the case. The absence of transparency may make any agreement between experts, suspect in the eyes of the party whose expert makes concessions in this private meeting. Similarly, there is a risk that a single independent expert expressing a neutral view might be viewed as inappropriate and potentially biased.

"Med-arb" is a process in which the neutral attempts to assist the parties to settle their dispute through mediation; but if this is unsuccessful, he or she then makes a binding determination as arbitrator. "Med-arb" has dangers as well as advantages and needs to be selectively and carefully chosen and applied.[16]

The "Multi-Door Courthouse" helps parties to choose an appropriate process. The concept envisages " . . . a flexible and diverse panoply of dispute resolution processes, with particular types of cases being assigned to different processes . . . according to . . . rational criteria for (allocation)."[17] Although not used in the UK in its original court-attached form, it could be adapted to local requirements within a context of case management.

Using the mediation process

Facilitative and evaluative mediation has been differentiated, including by the authors of this chapter in the first edition of this book. While it is essential to appreciate these two ways of working, a clear perspective is needed. All mediation is facilitative, with parties helped to explore their mutual interests. In some cases, it may also contain an evaluative element, in which event the mediator, personally or with other professionals, may evaluate the merits of the issues. While some mediators will only work in a facilitative mode, others will do both. Care and skill are needed in evaluating, because of the responsibility in doing so and because once a mediator evaluates, his or her impartiality may be regarded as suspect. Some practitioners fear that an evaluative process may perpetuate some of the problems and attitudes inherent in litigation. However, provided that the facilitative approach remains dominant, it can sometimes be helpful for a mediator to offer some evaluation, but only if the parties want this, it is appropriate, and he or she is suitably qualified to do so.

Risk managers should enquire whether a mediator offers an evaluative element in addition to the facilitative process. If both parties might perhaps want this (provided always that the mediator thinks that it would be useful at the time), it should be specified as a possible part of the process. The period required for mediation depends on the complexity of the matter. It might range between a few hours and a few days. In most cases, one or two days would ordinarily suffice. If the parties needed more time, this could then be arranged.

Mediation procedure is straightforward. The parties or their lawyers ordinarily provide preliminary information about the dispute to the mediator and to one another, through written submissions and documents. In clinical disputes, these might include medical reports and other relevant documents available to both parties, including those relevant to quantum.

527

If legal proceedings have commenced, copy statements of case would generally also be furnished.

Where the issues are complex, the mediator may initially meet the parties or their lawyers to agree the timetable and ground rules. In the substantive mediation meeting, the mediator is likely to start with a joint meeting of the parties and their lawyers. Each party or their lawyer will make an oral presentation of their case. Witnesses are not usually called, though the broad nature of their evidence might be outlined. The mediator then facilitates negotiations. These may be in joint session or more usually in a series of private meetings ("caucuses") with each party. The mediator will maintain the confidentiality of matters discussed in the caucuses, except as each participant may agree to disclose. By gaining an overview, shuttling from one side to another, and employing various skills and techniques, the mediator helps the parties to narrow and resolve their differences and to arrive at mutually acceptable settlement terms.

The mediator may use other strategies, such as seeing parties without their lawyers, or vice versa. Or the mediator may allow an opportunity for explanations, discussion or apology, or may liaise with respective experts, separately or, if so agreed, together, or seek additional information; or adjourn the mediation to enable the experts to consider certain aspects or for any other reason. The mediator is responsible for managing the process, but the parties remain responsible for agreeing the outcome.[47] If a settlement is reached, it will usually be recorded immediately as a binding agreement or, where court proceedings are pending, as a consent order.

Defence organisations, insurers, indemnifying authorities or the NHSLA will need to authorise the mediation and any binding settlement. They may privately stipulate parameters for acceptable levels of settlement. Their representative may attend the mediation meeting, or may arrange for the settlement terms to be confirmed at its conclusion. It is not usually acceptable to conduct mediation, with its preparation and perhaps some days of meetings, if either side does not have the authority to record a binding settlement if it is reached.

Mediator's role, attributes, skills and qualifications

Role and functions

Mediators combine a number of roles and functions. These include managing the process; gathering and providing information; developing and narrowing options and facilitating settlement discussions; helping parties to appreciate whether their ideas, perceptions or proposals are realistic; and if required helping the parties to record settlement terms.

Attributes

These inherent personal qualities and traits include the following:

- Sensitive, empathetic understanding of issues and a respect for parties' concerns
- Sound judgment
- A creative and constructive response to problems
- Integrity and trustworthiness
- Flexibility
- Authority to manage the process and an ability to work autonomously.

Skills

These may be learned or intuitive and include the following:

- Communication skills; observing non-verbal communications; helping parties to hear and understand one another; asking questions effectively; reframing when necessary, by changing a frame of reference to give events a different yet correct perspective; and summarising
- Managing conflict and allowing parties to express their emotions without damaging the prospects of negotiating an effective outcome
- Encouraging negotiation and developing a problem-solving mode
- Managing the process in a firm, sensitive, impartial manner
- Facilitating communications, discussions and negotiations.
- Developing and narrowing settlement options
- When in an evaluative mode, expressing personal views without undue pressure and enhancing rather than damaging the prospect of agreed resolution.

Qualifications

There are no formal qualifications to act as a mediator, but special training, post-training support and continuing professional development are necessary. These are provided by various ADR organisations, most of which provide mediator accreditation, regulation and panel membership. (see Appendix 27.1) The Law Society publishes standards for mediators and is considering establishing a specialist panel of civil and commercial mediators, as in the family field.

Mediators come from a wide range of occupational backgrounds including law, medicine, accountancy, management, industry, social and community work, counselling, and other mental health fields. Two kinds of expertise can be brought into mediation. One is substance expertise, which is the specialist knowledge of the subject matter of the dispute. The other is process expertise, which is proficiency in the mediation process itself. The latter is more important, as a competent mediator can adapt to dealing with different kinds of disputes; but if a mediator has both process and substance expertise, that might be an ideal combination. Sometimes these skills can be combined, for example by having a lawyer and doctor co-mediate.

The mediation pilot scheme

It had been hoped that the mediation pilot undertaken on behalf of the NHSE would give a clear direction for the role of mediation in clinical negligence claims. Indeed, the report of the pilot was published on the Internet in January 2000, entitled *Mediating Medical Negligence Claims: an option for the future?*[48] Unfortunately the number of cases actually mediated was, for reasons explained in the report, insufficient to enable any convincing conclusions to be drawn as to the merits (or otherwise) of mediation as an improved process for resolving disputes of this kind.

It was intended that up to 40 cases would be mediated over a two-year period but, notwithstanding that the scheme was extended for an additional year, a total of only 12 cases were mediated. Settlement was reached in eleven of them. Furthermore, of the 12 cases, 6 involved one speciality, obstetrics and gynaecology, which means that even the 12 cases were not representative of all the types of clinical negligence cases that require resolution. Nevertheless, the experience of the cases mediated is instructive, and in the course of the research for the report much information was collated which gives further support for the need for developing a model for mediation in clinical negligence. For example, "a wide range of people's views were canvassed on the question of how cases which are suitable for referral to mediation can be identified." Some of the categories identified "were those involving lots of emotional overlay; cases where non-legal remedies such as apologies and explanations were being sought" as suggested above; "claims where the claimant wanted greater involvement in case management; those where speedier resolution was required; and those where the parties had a long-term relationship."

One of the problems identified with the scheme was the lack of

> *a supportive policy environment, which led to a reluctance amongst gatekeepers to refer cases. . . Concerns were expressed by many people involved in the scheme that the NHS Executive did not adopt a sufficiently strong approach to the management of the scheme and that the NHS Litigation Authority was insufficiently proactive in supporting it and directing cases towards mediation . . .*

On the other hand, concerns about low take-up of the scheme were also associated with "reticence amongst solicitors to refer cases." This suggests that in trying to devise a procedure for mediation in clinical negligence it is essential to make it effective and desirable to those who have the power to implement it. Notwithstanding the relatively small number of cases in the pilot, the researchers felt able to assert that the data suggest that there are considerable benefits to mediated settlement.

Developing the model for clinical negligence disputes

Despite the new consensual approach, it would be wrong to believe that the adversarial mode has disappeared. The protocol has undoubtedly improved procedures. However, the opportunity now exists, with a better understanding of the deep concerns of the medical profession and of patients, to use these procedures as a springboard for developing new structures for addressing clinical issues that better serve everyone's needs. This would also respond to the Committee's vision of a more integrated and clearer system and the findings of the pilot scheme.

As an initial step in the consideration of these structures, a reformed procedure for clinical negligence cases might have the following fundamental components:

- A framework structured around a staged process.
- The identification of different categories of cases and issues, for which different processes would be appropriate. This would include balancing between those cases that require extensive preparation (as covered by the protocol) and those that can be addressed more quickly and simply, for example through a modified complaints procedure that permits the award of compensation, mediation or a combination of the two.
- The appointment of a neutral assessor or "gatekeeper" whose role is to assist the parties in identifying and managing the appropriate category and process.

The following might be the sequence of stages:

Stage 1: Preliminary enquiries

Preliminary steps are taken to obtain health records. Protocol Paragraphs 3.7–3.13 provide for this. However, this should not only apply "when court proceedings are contemplated" (as now). There should be a simplified and earlier version of this enquiry so that patients can seek preliminary information and independent advice.

Stage 2: Seeking independent advice

Once the patient has initial information, he or she can seek preliminary advice from a lawyer or other agency to assess whether real cause for complaint or claim appears to exist.

531

Stage 3: Making a claim/complaint

The claimant/complainant makes a preliminary claim or complaint, providing initial relevant information. Annex C of the protocol provides a template; but there should be a simplified version of this for cases that are not as advanced in their enquiries or are not focusing on a claim.

Stage 4: The gatekeeper concept

A new concept could be introduced of an independent neutral assessor as process "gatekeeper". This assessor, who would probably have medical and/or legal expertise, would have an impartial role in considering and advising on the procedure that would most effectively apply to the case. The assessor would receive a core bundle of documents provided by the parties or their solicitors. She (feminine gender will be used for convenience) would undertake any preliminary enquiries considered helpful. For example, she might meet the lawyers separately or together, meet the parties probably separately and may perhaps have a preliminary exchange with the expert(s).

The assessor may bring in another neutral with relevant expertise if appropriate. That would lend itself to a doctor-lawyer team. (In the family field, "anchor" mediation allows a sole mediator, who might be a lawyer or counsellor, to commence the process alone, but to bring in a co-mediator from a different discipline partway through the process if that was thought helpful.) The assessor (or team), having heard both sides, forms a preliminary view about the matter. She considers into what category it should be placed. These categories should be devised and graded to indicate whether they can be dealt with speedily, with minimal expert reports (such as those now offered by medical experts at low cost to assess the merits of a claim) or documents or whether they will need a lot of preparation and expert advice.

Stage 5: The assessor's recommendations

The assessor's preliminary assessment and recommendations are not binding, but are for guidance. She would consider what process is appropriate for the case. Some may require litigation, others facilitative mediation, others an evaluative process or some permutation. Some cases may indicate an immediate process. Others might need to be deferred until further detailed information or a prognosis can be established. The assessor may anticipate whether the claimant would be satisfied with a non-pecuniary outcome, and conversely whether a respondent would not countenance a pecuniary settlement. That would influence the process recommendation and would avoid, for example, mediation being chosen where it would be unlikely to succeed.

The assessor informs the parties/lawyers of her preliminary views, discusses these and tries to agree on the procedure to be followed. Hopefully, her views will reflect those of the parties as expressed to her, but some further discussion may well be necessary to move matters forward.

Stage 6: Acting on the options

Following a non-binding recommendation, parties will decide on their course of action. It is likely that a number of options will then exist.

- Dropping further action: With the benefit of a preliminary assessment, discussion and explanation, some parties may decide not to pursue a claim or complaint.
- Seeking an explanation or apology: Where the issue is one of obtaining clarification and if appropriate an apology or other non-monetary redress, a machinery needs to be devised that will allow these issues to be addressed. There is scope for this to be a mediator, an independent panel, an official in the ombudsman's office or some other forum.
- Making a complaint: The present machinery for complaints should be reviewed and simplified. Some compensatory powers should be allowed, even if capped to provide for limited compensation.
- Mediation: Where mediation is appropriate, a lawyer–doctor co-mediation team might be helpful. That would support an evaluative element in the mediation, if that were required. The assessor, with or without another expert, could be the mediator(s).
- Evaluation: A non-binding evaluation may help the parties work towards a settlement. It could vary between a formal assessment, through to informal indications. Non binding neutral evaluative processes have been under-used and should be further explored.
- Adjudication: If adjudication is necessary, the assessor can help the parties to narrow the issues and avoid unnecessary contention. Litigation may well be used, but arbitration or expert determination might be considered.
- Case management: Where the case is adjudicated, the assessor can, where appropriate, become a neutral case manager, helping to cut through issues and continuing to search for opportunities to facilitate settlement.

Stage 7: Further investigation

Where existing information is insufficient to enable a claim or complaint to be resolved, further investigation would be necessary. The Committee urged that investigation of actual or potential adverse clinical incidents should be carried out thoroughly by well-trained, dedicated staff. The report from any such investigation should contain a detailed account of events and be robust enough to be used by other bodies.[9] The machinery for this would need to be established. The assessor would consider the outcome of any further investigation and would then be in a position to make a further recommendation.

Additional factors in developing a new process

Within this framework, there is scope for additional factors to be developed.

- The ombudsman's power (including the power to order compensation) could be increased and re-defined. For example, as in the Insurance ombudsman's scheme, the ombudsman's proposals (including compensation) could be binding on the practitioner or trust, but optional for acceptance by the complainant.
- The assessor's role and other processes, including mediation, might tie in with offers and procedures under the new Civil Procedure Rules, including in particular Part 36, which provides for settlement offers to be made at a relatively early stage of a claim.
- Although no party should ever lose the right to seek litigation, the court might impose costs sanctions for parties who do not follow these procedures.
- A further pilot scheme to develop these ideas may well be necessary.

If these neutral processes are to work effectively, they must be trusted by both claimants/complainants and the healthcare profession and their respective representatives and lawyers. It is thus essential for those who function in a neutral role to be appropriately selected, trained and regulated. Inevitably, neutrals are likely to come either from claimants' or respondents' organisations and lawyers, causing potential suspicion and concern from the other. That problem will need to be addressed, through consultation, discussion, and co-operation between the different groups. It would be more than a pity to rule out as assessors/mediators those who have the most experience in this area. The Clinical Disputes Forum has demonstrated how people with different interests can co-operate effectively. The boundaries of co-operation will have to be further extended.[10]

Summary of practicalities for risk managers

The following are the key points for risk managers.

- There is no longer an automatic assumption that litigation is appropriate for every clinical dispute. Each case can be assessed to establish the best procedure for resolving it.

- Trust's policies of the trust towards the use of ADR to resolve claims and complaints needs to be discussed, clarified and established.
- Where litigation is followed, opportunities to conclude the dispute at an early stage can be explored without involving any loss of rights or weakening of either party's position. Provision for this exists under the new Rules and in any event, non-adjudicatory ADR processes can be considered without risk.
- A dispute manager or organisation can be invited to act as an informal "gatekeeper" to assist in arriving at agreed procedures, to help simplify the issues and to facilitate settlement.
- Mediation can be considered for most disputes. There should be clarity whether the mediator offers a purely facilitative process or will provide some form of evaluation, if so required and if the mediator thinks that it would be helpful. In some cases, co-mediation by a doctor and lawyer team might be appropriate.
- Where appropriate, for example where good faith differences exist, a non-binding neutral evaluation might help to facilitate settlement negotiations. The evaluator must be skilled and authoritative.
- In some cases, a joint expert's report might be obtained. However, this would not be appropriate in many cases, because inevitably one party will feel aggrieved by it, and separate reports might be needed.
- A combination of ADR processes could be designed to meet individual situations, for example, non-binding neutral evaluation followed by mediation. Cost-effectiveness and proportionality can be built into the system.

Existing processes can produce better outcomes and save costs if managed with care and creativity. New procedures can build on these, to provide greater consistency and to make clinical negligence claims fairer and less of an ordeal for both practitioners and patients. Scope exists for all to benefit.

References

1 Brown H, Marriott A. Foreword. In: *ADR Principles and Practice*. 2nd edition. London: Sweet & Maxwell, 1999.
2 Mulcahy L. *Mediating Medical Negligence Claims: An Option for the Future?* London.
3 *Supporting doctors, protecting patients*. A consultation paper on preventing, recognizing and dealing with poor performance of doctors in the NHS in England. Dept of Helath, November 1999.
4 Brown H, Marriott A. *ADR Principles and Practice*. 2nd edition. London: Sweet & Maxwell, 1999, v.
5 House of Commons Select Committee on Health, Sixth Report, 1999 at Paragraph 20.
6 Health Service Ombudsman. Address to the UKCC on 7 June 1999.
7 Wallace H, Mulcahy L. *Cause for complaint? An evaluation of the effectiveness of the NHS Complaints Procedure*. Public Law Project, September 1999.
8 Guide to the work of the Health Service Ombudsman.

9 House of Commons Select Committee on Health, Sixth Report, 1999 at Paragraphs 58–60.
10 House of Commons Select Committee on Health, Sixth Report, 1999 at Paragraph 62 and Summary of Recommendations (h).
11 House of Commons Select Committee on Health, Sixth Report, 1999 at Paragraph 79 and Summary of Recommendations (k).
12 House of Commons Select Committee on Health, Sixth Report, 1999 Paragraphs 120 and 121.
13 National Consumer Council. *A-Z of Ombudsmen*. Published by the National Consumer Council 1997. 107–18.
14 See Lax and Sebenius, *The Manager as Negotiator*. Published by The Free Press, a division of Macmillan Inc., 1986.
15 Mackie K, Miles D, Marsh W, *Commercial Dispute Resolution*. Butterworths, 1995.
16 d'Ambrumenil P. *Mediation and Arbitration*. Cavendish Publishing, 1997.
17 *US Pound Conference report, 1976*, cited as 70 Federal Rules Decisions (FRD) 79: 113–30.

Endnotes (‡)

1‡ Complaints are dealt with in Chapter 26.
2‡ For an overview of expert determination, see John Kendall's book, *Dispute Resolution: Expert Determination* (Longman, 2nd edition, 1996).
3‡ An originator of the mini-trial, Professor Eric Green, describes the process in "Growth of the Mini-trial", (US) 9 *Litigation* 1 (Fall 1982) and in his *Mini-trial Handbook* published by the CPR Institute for Dispute Resolution, USA. The process is also described in Brown and Marriott, *ADR Principles and Practice* (Sweet & Maxwell, 2nd edition, 1999).
4‡ The City Disputes Panel created this model for financial disputes. For its use in resolving Lloyds insurance disputes, see the article by Sarah Scarlett in *Insurance Day* of 25 February 1997 "Use of ADR in Lloyd's R&R plan".
5‡ See the article "Evaluative Mediation – Oxymoron or Essential Tool" by Jonathan Marks of JAMS-Endispute: (http: //jams-endispute.com/articles/evalmed.html). Marks, with Lord Griffiths, helped resolve the largest UK mediation, the British & Commonwealth case. He says that although mostly he does not have to express a view, in a substantial minority of cases, skilful questioning and devil's advocacy are not sufficient to shift parties from their outcome predictions. In those cases he says "I think the mediator's responsibility is firmly to step over the threshold from facilitator to evaluator. If, but only if, the parties agree (and have so stated in a pre-mediation agreement), I'll tell them (with reasons) what I think a fair settlement is and what I think will happen in court if they don't settle."
6‡ US Professor Lon Fuller considers that the same person acting as mediator and then as arbitrator, may damage his efficacy as a mediator and "fatally compromise the integrity of his adjudicative role". Alternatives may allow parties the option to proceed with the arbitration if the mediation fails, to opt out of it, or to treat the mediator as an advisor whose opinion is authoritative but non-binding.
7‡ See Tony Hall's case study "Mediation: Billington v. North Staffordshire Hospital NHS Trust", *AVMA Medical and Legal Journal*, March 2000 at p. 71. Negligence proceedings followed Mrs Billington's death. In mediation, the mediator shuttled between the parties, carrying their thoughts and proposals and proactively helping them to focus their negotiations. The mediator confidentially established bands of figures, helped get issues clarified and assisted in securing an apology and reassurances. The mediator advanced the idea of an all-inclusive figure that would accommodate costs and conditional fee arrangements, which proved critical to achieving an agreed outcome.
8‡ The project was led by Linda Mulcahy and a team of researchers. Quotations and references in this section are derived from the Report and in particular its Executive Summary.
9‡ This would meet the Committee's recommendation at Paragraph 79.
10‡ The editorial by Arnold Simanowitz in *AVMA Medical and Legal Journal*, March 2000 at p. 68 suggests that "it behoves all those involved in clinical negligence litigation to

open their minds to new ways of satisfying the patient . . . .". Recent changes "provide the scope for the kind of co-operation that is necessary to achieve this, but it will need the imagination, skill and commitment of all parties. This is the challenge for the new century."

Appendix 27.1 Organisations that can advise and assist with dispute resolution

ADR Chambers (UK) Limited
1 Knightrider Court
London EC4Y 5JP
Tel: 020 7329 4909
Fax: 020 7329 4903

ADR organisation with judicial, barristers' and solicitors' panels offering arbitration, mediation, evaluation, private appeals and other ADR processes.

ADR Net/ADR Group
Grove House
Grove Road
Bristol BS6 6UN
Tel: 0117 946 7180
Fax: 0117 946 7181
E-mail: info@adrgroup. co.uk
Web site: www.adrgroup. co.uk

A national network of lawyer/mediators.

Centre for Dispute Resolution (CEDR)
Princes House
95 Gresham Street
London EC2V 7NA
Tel: 020 7600 0500
Fax: 020 7600 0501
E-mail: mediate@cedr.co.uk
Web site: www.cedr.co.uk

An independent dispute resolution organisation arranging mediation and other ADR processes for civil and commercial disputes.

Independent Mediation for Clinical Disputes Limited
Wick Villa, 63 Wick Road
Brislington, Bristol BS4 4HA
Tel: 0117 977 3415
Fax: 0117 972 0083
E-mail: imed-limited@hotmail.com
Web site: www.imcd.co.uk

An independant ADR/mediation service specializing in clinical negligence disputes.

Inter Mediation Limited
128 Cheapside
London EC2V 6BT
Tel: 020 7600 4909
Fax: 020 7600 6396
E-mail: support@intermediation.com
Web site: www.intermediation.com

CLINICAL RISK MANAGEMENT

The Academy of Experts
2 South Square, Gray's Inn
London WC1R 5HP
Tel: 020 7637 0333
Fax: 020 7637 1893
E-mail: admin@academy-experts.org
Web site: www.academy-experts.org

An organisation of experts, undertaking expert reports, mediation and other expert services.

The Chartered Institute of Arbitrators
International Arbitration Centre
24 Angel Gate, City Road
London EC1V 2RS
Tel: 020 7837 4483
Fax: 020 7837 4185
E-mail: info@arbitrators.org
Internet: http://www.arbitrators.org/ContactDet.htm

Professional body with multi-disciplinary membership promoting alternative means of dispute resolution to litigation, especially arbitration.

The Law Society of England & Wales
113 Chancery Lane
London WC2A 1PL
Tel: 020 7242 1222
Fax: 020 7831 0344
Web site: www.lawsociety.org.uk

Professional solicitors' organisation that regulates solicitors who mediate, establishes and maintains standards and is developing specialist panels of solicitor-mediators.

London Court of International Arbitration (LCIA)
Hulton House
161–166 Fleet Street
London EC4A 2DY
Tel: 020 7936 3530
Fax: 020 7936 3533
E-mail: lcia@lcia-arbitration.com
Internet:http://www.lcia-arbitration.com/town/square/xvc24/intouch/ intouch.htm

Arbitration organisation that also has provision for mediation.

28 Claims management

E JANE CHAPMAN

The cost of clinical negligence, in terms of legal costs and settlements, to the health service as a whole approached £500 million in 1998–9 and is predicted to rise steeply in the coming years. Since 1990, with the introduction of Crown Indemnity, health authorities and trusts have been both legally and financially responsible for acts of clinical negligence by their staff (this includes both agency and locum staff). The only exception to this is that an employer cannot be held responsible for any criminal acts by a member of its staff. This means that if a claim is brought by a patient (a claimant) it is the tust or health authority who is the defendant, and is financially responsible for all aspects of the claims management process. The identity of the defendant (i.e. trust or health authority) is determined by who had managerial responsibility for the care of the patient at the date of alleged negligent act. Health authorities tend only to be responsible for new cases where the allegation of negligence relates to a damaged child or person with learning difficulties who have their lifetime to sue.

Trusts are financially responsible for all cases arising since their establishment. If found to be negligent the trust has to meet its own costs as well as paying the claimant's compensation and all the claimant's costs. With individual "large cases" settling for compensation of up to £3–4 million (in for example a brain damaged baby assessed to have a normal life expectancy but to require twenty-four hour care for life), this is a is a very costly area of health service management. Good risk management practice, as described in other chapters in this book will help to reduce the exposure of the NHS to claims, both by reducing the number of negligent incidents and through the early identification and investigation of critical incidents that may lead to a claim. In practice clinical risks can never be totally eliminated and therefore robust systematic approaches to claims management are required leading to early resolution of disputes.

In recent years, claims management in the NHS has undergone radical changes. These arose first from the establishment, in 1995, of the NHS Litigation Authority (NHSLA). The NHSLA is a special health authority responsible for managing clinical (and since 1999 non-clinical) claims against the NHS. Secondly the civil law reforms that followed Lord Woolf's wide reaching investigation into all aspects of civil law in England and Wales, published in *Access to Justice* in 1997[1] have significantly changed the environment in which claims are managed. Implementing Lord Woolf's recommendations led to a major overhaul of Civil Law rules and regulations from 26 April 1999. At the time of writing both claimants and defendants are adjusting to the new ways of working, which are characterised by methods to make the systems less adversarial, less costly and faster than before.

This chapter will provide a broad overview of methods involved in claims management from the perspective of a defendant NHS trust. It will focus on how the systems operate within trusts and how trusts interact with the NHSLA, and other management arrangements for resolving disputes such as the NHS Complaints Procedure.

The chapter will outline the steps involved in the legal process, from the perspective of the defendant, starting from the identification of a claim or potential claim and ending with a full hearing of the claim before a judge. The chapter will not describe the law as applied to clinical negligence in any depth at all as readers will find a range of specific medical law textbooks available for this purpose. Rather the chapter will provide a practical overview of the claims management process from a claims manager's perspective.

The basis of clinical negligence

Recognising a claim

A clinical claim is defined as: "any demand, however made, but usually by the patient's legal adviser, for monetary compensation in respect of an adverse clinical incident leading to a personal injury."[2] A claim will usually, but not always, first be notified to a trust in the form of a letter seeking disclosure of the medical records, informing the defendant that legal action is contemplated. The letter may or may not be accompanied by a completed Law Society form[3] designed to provide basic information when requesting access in these circumstances. The letter and/or the form will usually be addressed to the claims/legal department or the medical records department. Trusts need to be certain that they have robust systems for ensuring that all such letters, where a potential claim is intimated, are directed to the claims manager as the earlier internal investigation can start the better the position for the trust.

Other indications of a claim include the following:

- a letter from a patient directly or from his next of kin or representative (for example, where the patient is a child, or has learning disabilities or has died)
- a complaint through the NHS Complaints Procedure which also includes a request for compensation
- a serious clinical incident resulting in damage to a patient can be the first indication of a potential claim
- a Summons and Particulars of Claim issued by the Court naming the trust or health authority as defendant. This means that formal legal proceedings have commenced.

Who is the defendant?

An injured patient cannot sue an individual clinician working in an NHS trust whom they consider responsible. He has to issue proceedings against the employing authority. Those involved in the alleged negligent incident act as factual witnesses in the process of preparing the defence, and through a system of vicarious liability have no individual financial liability for a civil claim.

Doctors, dentists, general practitioners and other clinicians working in private practice can be sued as individuals and are required to belong to a recognised professional indemnity organisation for example the Medical Defence Union or the Medical Protection Society.

What is clinical negligence?

In order to recover damages the claimant has to prove that the defendant was negligent. Clinical negligence is defined as "a breach of duty or care that directly results in injury or loss". For a claim to succeed the claimant needs to demonstrate both a breach of duty (liability) and loss as a direct result of the breach (causation). In simple terms this means that the clinician or team of clinical staff delivered care that was below an acceptable standard and that the patient suffered injury or loss as a direct result of the unacceptable care.

It is for the claimant to prove that negligence has occurred and for the trust or individual practitioner (defendant) to refute the claim. In determining whether negligence has occurred the legal process considers factual evidence from the records and the key staff involved, who provide witness statements, together with opinions from clinical experts instructed by each party, from the relevant field of medicine.

What can a patient recover?

Civil law is concerned with the award of financial compensation for negligent damage. The law does not directly apportion "blame". In contrast criminal law determines blame for criminal acts and issues punishment. Many clinical staff are unaware of this difference and claims managers often are called upon to assure worried clinicians that they will not get a "record" or lose their job as a result of being called as a witness in a compensation claim.

The principle underlying the calculation of damages in personal injury cases is that the sum awarded should place the claimant, as nearly as possible, in the position he would have been if the defendant had not injured him. If a patient "wins" his claim then he is awarded compensation ("*quantum*") that is calculated in two parts in the following way.

First general damages which is a sum of money awarded for the actual pain and suffering, distress, loss of opportunity, and loss of future earnings, pension rights and future costs associated with damage arising from the negligence. The sum for pain, suffering, and loss of amenity is determined by referring to previous awards made by the courts in similar circumstances. Claims managers and lawyers have a number of reference texts to consult when making this calculation.[4] Secondly an amount for special damages is also payable. Special damages are calculable damages of actual losses incurred such as actual loss of earnings, costs of travel to hospital, cost of aids or adaptations to the home that have been paid for by the claimant. The amount of special damages proposed by the claimant should be supported by receipts, pay slips, and other documentation. The Civil Procedure Rules (CPRs) require that a schedule of special damages is served with a Statement of Claim (see section on "Anatomy of a Claim", below). In addition the claimant is entitled to recover interest on the pain, suffering and loss of amenity element of the general damages, calculated at a rate of 2%, from the date of issue of the proceedings. Interest is also recoverable on the sum awarded under special damages for past losses.

In most cases when compensation is awarded lawyers acting for both parties, or for smaller claims the claims manager and the claimant's lawyer, will negotiate the level of compensation to be paid through a series of offers and counter offers. In cases where liability has been admitted but the amount of compensation cannot be agreed then the parties can go to court for a "quantum only trial".

Funding clinical negligence claims: the National Health Service Litigation Authority

Since 1990 the NHS has been responsible for the funding of clinical negligence claims against itself. Prior to that time liability was split between the doctors, funded by their defence organisations and the NHS for acts of all other staff. Form 1 January 1990 a system of Crown Indemnity was established such that all contracted staff within the NHS are covered for acts and omissions under a system of vicarious liability. Under these arrangements it is the trust hospital or health authority who is the named party in the action, and individual staff, providing they were working within the terms of their contract, are witnesses of fact but do not hold any financial risk or responsibility for the claim. Between 1990 and 1995 various regionally organised pooling arrangement operated to help off set the impact of high settlements on individual hospitals and health authorities.

In 1995 a special health authority, the NHS Litigation Authority (NHSLA), was established. Its framework document states that the overall aim of the Authority is to "promote the highest possible standards of patient care and to minimise the suffering resulting from any adverse incidents . . . ". Its objectives include minimising the costs of clinical negligence and thereby maximising the resources available for patient care, ". . . by defending unjustified actions robustly, settling justified actions efficiently, and creating incentives to reduce the number of negligent incidents."

The Clinical Negligence Scheme for Trusts (CNST)

The NHSLA has established a number of clinical and non-clinical claims schemes to help manage the NHS claims burden. Most relevant in the current context is the Clinical Negligence Scheme for Trusts (CNST) which was launched in April 1995. Trusts pay an annual contribution into a pooled fund which is used to reimburse trusts to set levels at the conclusion of cases. The scheme is not an insurance scheme but a "risk pooling scheme" offering trusts the security of obtaining reimbursements of most of the costs of their claims burden above a pre selected excess level. Currently (1999) the maximum ultimate trust liability for a settled claim is £108 000. Reimbursement of all legitimate costs over this level are made by the scheme at the conclusion of the action. With many cases settling in the hundreds of thousands or million pound range it is not surprising that virtually all trusts have opted into the scheme

In practice all claims that are valued above the trust's excess are managed by the CNST in conjunction with the trust. The claims manager is required to undertake the initial investigation and quantification of the claim and then to seek instructions for future management from the CNST. In 1997 the NHSLA established a panel of defence solicitors to provide legal advice on claims handling. Around 18 firms are on this panel, and trusts are designated one or more firms with which to work. This allows standards for claims management to be monitored and offers the NHS consistency in the quality of its legal advice.

Although the CNST is legally responsible for the management of claims above the excess chosen by each trust the scheme claims managers work closely with the trusts in a partnership approach as evidence is gathered and decisions are taken. At meetings with counsel and at trial both a scheme manager and the trust claims manager will normally attend with the appointed legal representatives.

One further important role of the CNST is the promotion of high standards in clinical risk management. All member trusts are audited against a number of standards for clinical risk management.[5] Performance in practice against these standards, which are audited by the schemes risk assessors, entitle trusts to a reduction in their membership contribution (up to 25% at Level 3 compliance with standards).

The Civil Law Reforms April 1999

Before considering the progress of a clinical claim in more detail one further part of the legal landscape requires attention. On 26 April 1999 the Civil Law in England underwent its most radical change in hundreds of years. The changes followed a review of the procedures conducted by Lord Woolf. He published his recommendations in 1997 in Access to Justice.[1] The changes, which are procedural nature, are designed to make justice fairer: in particular by putting parties on an equal footing through new rules of disclosure and evidence; by saving unnecessary legal costs through court set timetables for different legal stages; and dealing with cases in a way that reflects the estimated amount of recoverable damages (to avoid the building up of huge legal costs in low value claims).

Lord Woolf singled out clinical negligence as presenting "peculiar difficulties", and one of the most fundamental changes that has been introduced by the reforms is at the "Pre-Action" stage. This is the stage prior to the issue of proceedings through the court. Lord Woolf felt that if a greater spirit of co-operation could be established between the parties at the early stages of a potential claim, many cases would be resolved without the need for court involvement. Resolution would be either through the payment of compensation or one party (e.g. the hospital) showing the other party (the patient and his advisors) that their claim is groundless.

The pre-action protocol for clinical disputes

The task of developing the protocol was given to the Clinical Disputes Forum,[6] the multidisciplinary body formed as a result of Access to Justice. The Forum is committed to exploring and developing less adversarial and more cost-effective ways of resolving disputes about healthcare and clinical treatment. A small team of Forum members broadly representing the main "parties" in clinical disputes worked together to develop the protocol. The document was the subject of extensive consultation prior to being adopted formally by the Lord Chancellor's Department and being embedded in the justice system as part of the changed rules from April 1999.

A major feature of the protocol is the introduction of a requirement for claimants to issue a "letter of claim" at least three months prior to the issues of formal legal proceedings. This letter is quite different from the "letter before action" that previously was sent to defendants with a request to disclose records. The "letter before action" was generally a description of the alleged negligence as described to the claimant lawyer by the patient, whereas the letter of claim is to provide a reasoned argument for the basis of the claim backed up by relevant evidence and/or expert opinion. The protocol also requires the defendant to acknowledge the "letter of claim" within 14 days and provide a "letter of response" within three months. These stages are described in more detail in the following section.

This protocol is aimed at facilitating the resolution of as many cases as possible without the need to issue proceedings, and for those cases that are not resolved at the pre-proceeding stage for the issues in dispute to be narrowed down.

The requirement to be in a position to respond to a letter of claim within a limited period puts a clear pressure on the healthcare provider, who cannot afford to wait until a letter of claim is received to have its own view on liability. The key to successful defence therefore is the early investigation of cases and in cases in which there is clearly no negligence, trusts and other healthcare providers are now having to invest more resources in the early investigation of potential claims.

At the time of preparation of this chapter the protocol had been in operation for just a matter of months and therefore it is too early to comment in detail on its impact. However the writer is pleased to report early signs of a changing environment. Willingness for claimants and their representatives to share information and to discuss options for resolution are becoming more commonplace, and the writer has been able to achieve a number of creative settlements more closely reflecting what patients and their families are seeking. Settlements that include explanations of treatment, arrangements for follow up, letters of apology, and sharing evidence of changes in practice, in addition to resolving the claim itself in strictly financial terms, are now beginning to happen. This new culture will benefit the patients, future patients, staff, and the financial resources of the NHS and is to be welcomed.

Anatomy of a claim: an overview of the legal process and the role of the claims manager

Very few (probably less than 1%) clinical claims are settled in court. Many are resolved through a payment of compensation prior to the issue of proceedings, some are settled though a payment into court prior to trial, and others are dropped by the claimant for lack of evidence of negligence. However, the parties involved should conduct claims as if "trial" is to occur. The Pre-Action Protocol now governs the conduct of the parties prior to the issue of proceedings and from then the court will now set the timetable. The following section describes, in outline, the stages in the legal process with particular emphasis on the role of the claims manager at each stage.

The role of the claims manager

This section provides just an outline and should not be relied on as a full description of the claims manager's responsibilities. For those interested in further information a bibliography of useful texts is included at the conclusion of the chapter.

Each trust is required to have a named person with responsibility for the conduct of clinical claims. In some trusts, particularly those with a small number of claims, this role is frequently combined with other responsibilities. In other trusts claims management may be the sole responsibility. There is still great variation across the country as to the levels of skills, training, and delegated authority of these individuals and within this chapter only general comments as to the role can be made.

The claims manager's responsibility is to manage the conduct of all clinical claims brought against the trust. This includes internal investigation, obtaining witness statements, and internal expert opinion, instructing the trust's solicitors, and liaising with the NHSLA/CNST depending on the value of the claim and the trust's excess. The claims manager represents the trust at conferences with counsel (the barristers) at which the trust and their solicitors receive advice on the future conduct of the case. In addition the claims manager must also work closely with complaints and clinical risk colleagues so that early notification and investigation of potential claims can be achieved. Taking statements from key staff after a serious adverse event not only ensures that risk lessons are learned but also the trust can take an early view on liability and possible compensation due to the patient. Taking a proactive approach to claims management can reduce distress both to the damaged patient and his family, and to staff involved, and also helps keep legal expenses to a minimum.

Steps in the legal process

Request for records and initial internal investigation

The most usual first step in a claim comes in the form of a request for copy records. Claimants (usually the patient represented by their legal advisor) request records using the Law Society Form.[3] The claimant's solicitor should indicate in his request the period of care that he is questioning and provide some indication of the problem that his client has identified. The trust claims manager must arrange for copy records to be provided within 40 days. Copying charges can be levied.[7]

At this stage the claims manager should initiate an internal investigation into the alleged negligence. If the trust operates a robust serious incident policy it may be that the incident has previously been investigated. The objective of the initial investigation, is to obtain an early picture of the nature of the claim and its potential for being settled. The CNST has prepared a set of guidelines for this early investigation.[8] It requires that within three months of the notification of a claim the claims manager prepares a report with an initial assessment of the claim. The report should contain the following elements:

- Synopis of the case
- Breach of Duty: comments on allegations made, or if no allegations, comments from hospital staff as to whether care fell below an acceptable standard
- Causation; initial views on causation, that is whether the alleged breach of duty directly caused the injuries suffered
- Quantum: an initial estimate of the value of the claim and associated legal costs
- Future strategy: view as to what the next steps should be, for example obtaining an independent expert report, whether the claim should be robustly defended or whether there is clear evidence of liability and an early settlement should be sought.

In order to achieve this, the claims manager needs to discuss the claim with the consultant/lead clinician concerned. If the incident is recent then steps need to be taken to obtain statements from the staff involved. If staff have moved on then they should be identified from the records, and forwarding addresses should be gathered, for later use if the case proceeds. To obtain a view on quantum the claims manager can refer to previous cases or such sources as the *Judicial Studies Guide*.[4] Depending on the skill level of the claim manager and the complexity of the claim, trusts may obtain advice at this early stage from their lawyers, however the costs of such advice is not reimbursable under the CNST scheme.

This initial examination of the claim should enable the claims manager with the consultant concerned to make an assessment of whether there are grounds for a claim to succeed. It may be that the claim is obviously a legitimate one, for example a missed fracture, a missed tendon injury, a retained swab requiring a second operation, an avoidable still birth. In such clear cut cases, if there is recognition by clinical staff that acceptable standards of care were breached and the patient experienced injury or loss resulting from this, then the claims manager, in discussion with trust senior management, should consider handling this claim "in house" and making an early offer of compensation to the patient. This should be done in an effort to save unnecessary legal costs adding up on both sides. Correct legal procedures for offering the money and getting the patient to sign a letter of acceptance need to be followed, so that the trust can be assured that the compensation is accepted in full and final settlement of the claim for the particular injury/period of care.

For complex cases and for cases where potential damages and costs exceed the trust's CNST excess, the claims manager should undertake an initial investigation and seek legal and CNST advice. The claims manager should instruct the solicitor on the amount of help required. The solicitor does not have charge of the conduct of the case. He is there to ensure the correct legal conduct of the case and to advise the trust on legal tactics. Solicitors work to instructions and do not for example make admissions of liability to offers of settlement without direct instruction from their client. The trust claims manager needs to be trained and properly authorised by the trust to instruct the solicitor effectively.

Letter of claim

Any time after a request for records and no later than three months before a "statement of claim" is issued through the court, a claimant should send a "letter of claim" to the defendant. This letter should set out in detail the nature of the alleged negligence and the resultant damage, together with a valuation of the claim, "quantum", supported by medical reports. The letter of claim can include an offer to settle.

Letter of response

The defendant trust must acknowledge receipt of the "letter of claim" within 14 days and provide a fully reasoned letter of response within three months, refuting criticism with reasons and/or making admissions of liability if appropriate Any admissions made at this stage are binding. If an offer to settle has been made by the claimant then this has to be accepted or rejected with reasons. The defendant also has the opportunity at this stage of making its own offer to settle.

This short time scale is the reason for the need for attention to detail described above, during the initial claim investigation which must start soon after the claim is identified, if the trust is to be in a position to keep to this time scale. The main time pressures relate to identifying and obtaining statements from staff, particularly those who have left the trust, and obtaining sound expert advice; many experts have long waiting lists for reports. The claims manager must make every effort to track down relevant staff as soon as possible, and to obtain reports from them of their involvement. The use of "internal experts", another consultant in the same speciality as the case under review, can be helpful to the claims manager to help assess the case and better frame the questions to an external, independent expert.

The decision as to whether an offer to settle should be made involves the claims manager, often the trust lawyers, the CNST (in cases valued over the excess) and ideally the consultant/team identified in the case. The claims manager has a vital role in keeping clinical staff informed and involved at this stage. It is obviously not desirable for an admission of liability to be made without the clinical staff's knowledge. In addition the claims manager needs to play a part in ensuring that lessons are learned and risk measures are taken to reduce the chance of recurrence.

Issue of proceedings

If resolution is not achieved by this stage then the formal litigation begins. Proceedings are issued in the form of a "Statement of Claim" which must be accompanied by a medical report on condition and prognosis and a schedule of "special damages".

Defence

The "statement of claim" must be acknowledged within 14 days, and a "defence" entered (sent to the court) within a further 14 days. Limited extension of time (up to one further month) can be agreed between the parties. A barrister, who relies on factual, and expert, evidence from the defendant trust normally prepares the "defence", although this may be drafted by a solicitor. The lawyer charged with this responsibility will rely on the factual and expert evidence obtained by the claims manager.

Case management

A feature of the new procedural rules is that of "case management". In simple terms this means that for cases in litigation it is now the court, and not the parties, that set down the timetable that must be followed. There are a series of procedural steps that are followed between the serving of the "defence" and the ultimate "trial". The court will now determine the date by which these steps must be achieved. The steps include the exchange of both factual and expert evidence, and schedules/counter schedules of damages. These stages are designed to narrow down the issues in dispute. During the time before trial both parties will be making efforts to resolve the claim, either by agreeing a compensation payment or by the defendant persuading the claimant to withdraw the action. If this does not occur a "trial" will be held. At this stage of a claim the claims manager will need to monitor progress and be in a position to respond to issues around factual evidence, for example in the preparation of the list of documents. In addition they represent the trust at meetings with counsel when the trust and the CNST receive advice on whether to fight or attempt to settle the claim.

Trial

A "trial" can be held to determine both liability (whether negligence occurred) and quantum (how much compensation is to be awarded). The trial judge sits alone without a jury. The judge hears from factual witnesses, i.e. the claimant or his representative and the clinical staff involved, and from experts called by both sides. Barristers, who examine and cross-examine the factual and expert witnesses represent both parties. At this stage the claims manager supports staff called as witnesses and is available to the lawyers throughout the case. Often rapid tactical decisions need to be taken at this time and the claims manager needs to be on hand to take decisions and/or liaise with trust senior managers.

When the evidence has concluded the trial Judge will decide, "on the balance of probabilities", i.e. whether it is more likely than not that negligence occurred. This is a lower level of proof than in a criminal trial where the jury has to make a decision that is "beyond reasonable doubt".

If the judge determines the case in favour of the claimant then compensation will be awarded, and it is the judge that determines the level of damages (both "general and special damages") to be paid. In certain cases, when liability is not in dispute but the level of compensation is not agreed, then a "quantum only trial" will be held. The judge then hears evidence only relating to the level of damages and determines the amount to be paid.

In certain high value cases the parties may opt for a split trial. This decision is subject to court approval. In such cases the initial trial focuses on issues of liability and causation only, determining whether there has been negligence. If the defendant is found negligent then a second trial of "quantum only" is held, if compensation cannot be agreed.

Keys to successful claims handling

Successful claims handling is a result of early identification of claims, from a robust clinical risk management process which effectively both identifies and investigates serious adverse events, coupled with a commitment to early detailed investigation of all notified claims. In addition there needs to be a willingness to take an early view on liability (i.e. to identify when care fell below an acceptable standard and a patient was damaged) and a willingness to settle cases with minimum of delay when the evidence supports this action.

To achieve this the trust needs to be served by a competent, trained claims manager and senior clinical and managerial staff need to understand the principles of both risk management and civil litigation processes. Since the issue of the new rules many of the leading legal firms have offered client trusts support and training in this regard. Such training should be accessed not only by the claims manager but also by key members of the executive board, in particular the chief executive, medical and nursing directors and the director of finance. A joint understanding of the principles of effective investigation, the legal time restraints, and the opportunities for reducing legal costs from a proactive approach will facilitate effective claims handling, and in turn will lead to patients being able to rebuild a relationship with their local healthcare providers.

Effective claims managers work in tandem with the clinical risk department, or as in the author's case, carry dual responsibility for clinical risk and claims management. In addition they require support from the trust board, particularly the trust's medical director, and ned to work to a supportive medical director within a culture where clinical risks are faced positively, i.e. effective incident reporting and investigation is an accepted part of the culture of the organisation. In addition medico-legal awareness amongst medical staff, often fostered by staff training offered by the claims manager, can further help to avoid risks and create a spirit of co-operation by clinical staff in their roles as witnesses or internal exerts when claims arise.

Supporting claims managers

Back in the early 1990s there was little attention paid to claims management within hospitals and newly formed trusts. The general practice was for letters from claimant's solicitors to be sent to hospital solicitors with a request to act on behalf of the healthcare provider. Claims management was largely an administrative task following a solicitor's advice. As the financial extent of the claims burden became more apparent, trusts began to recognise the need to directly manage their own claims, both to minimise legal costs and to ensure that the risk lessons were learned and repeat occurrence were minimised. In response to this, specific training for claims managers was slowly developed, largely by defendant law firms.

One of the most successful training courses was established by CAPSTICKS solicitors in 1993.[9] As a direct result of support from CAPSTICKS and in response to the wishes of early students who undertook the diploma course the Association of Litigation and Risk Management (ALARM) was founded. From a small group of interested claims and risk managers, who recognised the benefit of meeting with fellow post holders the Association rapidly grew in size. It now operates from the Royal College of Medicine as a fully independent Association committed to supporting risk and claims managers in pursuit of excellence in their daily work. Its membership includes nearly 200 trusts from all geographical areas and types of trust in England. Members meet three times a year for legal updating and to have the opportunity to hear from and enter into dialogue with the policy makers of the day. In addition they network together, a most important support function in that the majority of claims managers work as single-handed practitioners within their trusts.

In its five years of existence ALARM has been able to play a very active part in the changing face of claims management. Its Chairman was a member of the Clinical Negligence Working Party during Lord Woolf's inquiry, and is a member of the Clinical Disputes Forum, and a member of the working party who drafted the Pre-Action Protocol. It has also liaised with the NHSLA, the NHSE and others as policy and practice in this expanding area is developed. Details of the Association can be obtained from the address below.[10]

In summary the role of claims management has seen unprecedented change in recent years. Trusts are responding to the ever-increasing burden of claims of negligence. Many trusts are properly integrating their claims, complaints, and risk functions to provide optimum opportunity not only for the early resolution of clinical disputes but also the learning of lessons from the adverse incident that lead to the claim. This brings many benefits, in particular to the claims managers themselves, who feel part of a team with others to discuss difficult cases and lessons to be learned. This is in contrast to the earlier days of trust claims handling which was almost invariably undertaken by one individual with little back up. The opportunities of a clinical governance approach to monitoring healthcare will only serve to strengthen the opportunity for more effective claims management in trusts.

References

1 Lord Chancellor's Department. *Access to Justice*. HMSO, 1997.
2 *Clinical negligence scheme for trusts, reporting guidelines*. NHSLA, 1995.
3 Law Society Form: *Application on Behalf of a Patient for Hospital Medical Records for use when Court Proceedings are Contemplated* included in the Pre-Action Protocol for the Resolution of Clinical Disputes, or available from The Law Society, Chancery Lane, London.
4 Judicial Studies Board. *Guidelines for the assessment of general damages in personal injury cases* (5th edition). London: Blackstone Press, 2000.
5 CNST *Risk Management Standards*, published by CNST for the NHSLA 1995 (updated 1999), copies available via CNST at Willis Corroon (fund managers CNST) Howard House, Queens Ave, Bristol BS8 1SN.
6 Clinical Disputes Forum (CDF) more details from Secretary, Sarah Leigh, Leigh Day and Co, Priory House, 25 St John's Lane, EC1M 4LB or
via web site *http: //www.clinical-disputes-forum.org.uk/*.

7 *Access to Health Records Act 1990*. London: HMSO, 1990.
8 CNST *Reporting guidelines issued to member trusts*. Copies available from the NHSLA, Napier House, 24 High Holborn, London WC1 6AZ.
9 CAPSTICKS Solicitors, 77-83 Upper Richmond Road, London SW1 6PT.
10 ALARM, Association of Litigation and Risk Management, The Royal Society of Medicine, 1 Wimpole Street, W1M 8AE. Tel 020 7290 2968.

Further reading

Montgomery J. *Health Care Law*. OUP, 1997.
Lewis C. *Medical Negligence*. Tolley, 1998.
Powers M, Harris N. *Clinical Negligence*. Butterworths, 2000.

Journals

Clinical Risk, RSM Press. Tel 020 7290 2928.
Health Care Risk Reports, The Eclipse Group. Tel 020 7354 6764.

Index

Page numbers in **bold** type refer to figures; those in *italic* refer to tables or boxed material

555